Current Topics in Behavioral Neurosciences

Volume 63

Current Topics in Behavioral Neurosciences provides critical and comprehensive discussions of the most significant areas of behavioral neuroscience research, written by leading international authorities. Each volume in the series represents the most informative and contemporary account of its subject available, making it an unrivalled reference source. Each volume will be made available in both print and electronic form.

With the development of new methodologies for brain imaging, genetic and genomic analyses, molecular engineering of mutant animals, novel routes for drug delivery, and sophisticated cross-species behavioral assessments, it is now possible to study behavior relevant to psychiatric and neurological diseases and disorders on the physiological level. The Behavioral Neurosciences series focuses on translational medicine and cutting-edge technologies. Preclinical and clinical trials for the development of new diagnostics and therapeutics as well as prevention efforts are covered whenever possible. Special attention is also drawn on epigenetical aspects, especially in psychiatric disorders.

CTBN series is indexed in PubMed and Scopus.

Deanna M. Barch • Jared W. Young
Editors

Cognitive Functioning in Schizophrenia: Leveraging the RDoC Framework

Springer

Editors
Deanna M. Barch
Departments of Psychological and Brain Sciences, Psychiatry, and Radiology
Washington University
Saint Louis, MO, USA

Jared W. Young
Department of Psychiatry
University of California San Diego
La Jolla, CA, USA

ISSN 1866-3370 ISSN 1866-3389 (electronic)
Current Topics in Behavioral Neurosciences
ISBN 978-3-031-26443-6 ISBN 978-3-031-26441-2 (eBook)
https://doi.org/10.1007/978-3-031-26441-2

This Springer imprint is published by the registered company Springer Nature Switzerland AG
The registered company address is: Gewerbestrasse 11, 6330 Cham, Switzerland

Preface

Cognition Is Vital to Living for People with Schizophrenia

Throughout the long history of conceptions of schizophrenia, dysfunctional cognition has been a hallmark feature. For example, in the late 1800s schizophrenia was first termed *dementia praecox*, meaning premature dementia. With the advent of antipsychotic therapies in the 1950s, the focus for treatment moved to the positive symptoms that characterize schizophrenia, such as hallucinations and delusions, as these were responsive to such treatments, at least in some individuals. However, antipsychotic therapies did little to address the cognitive challenge so often present for people with schizophrenia. As such, more recently (in the late 1900s), cognitive dysfunction was again identified as the pre-eminent aspect of schizophrenia that required treatment given that it most closely associated with a person's functional outcome. In other words, a patient's ability to function independently in society, their connection to their families and friends were most strongly associated with their cognitive functioning. From this evidence, researchers re-focused efforts on identifying potential treatments for the cognitive dysfunction that so frequently accompanies the disorder.

There have been many barriers faced by researchers trying to improve cognition in schizophrenia however. From the heterogeneity of cognitive dysfunction to variability in assessment tools, to rapid advancement in neuroscientific techniques, each area provides a vast array of research that requires distillation. To address potential heterogeneity and transdiagnostic qualities of cognitive dysfunction (such deficits also occur in other disorders), the National Institute of Mental Health (NIMH) began the Research Domain Criterion (RDoC) initiative. RDoC was designed as a platform by which specific domains of dysfunction could be identified irrespective of diagnosis, on the premise that the same neurobiology underlies functioning in people, thus if affected by disease it will likely be similarly affected irrespective of disease. Hence, the use of RDoC at least has the chance to reduce some of the heterogeneity limitations of research because of a greater shared language and focus on specific domains than had been used previously. The RDoC approach has only been around for ~10 years but offers great hope for tying together such a vast array of research on cognition in schizophrenia. Ultimately, our knowledge of the cognitive deficits that occur in people with schizophrenia, their potential developmental trajectory, genetic and environmental etiology, and potential neural mechanisms have greatly advanced in the past 20 years. In this book, we brought together experts on this cognitive research and where possible, they have attempted to tie such mechanistic and treatment insights to a common language utilizing RDoC. Views from across the research spectrum are incorporated and the reader will hopefully have a greater appreciation for the progress of this research in the past two decades as well as the avenues in need of further pursuit.

Cognitive deficits have been well-documented in people at high risk of developing schizophrenia and occur in people before their first psychotic episode. Dr. Karcher covers cognitive dysfunction as a risk factor for psychosis. They provide evidence that cognitive deficits may be an intermediate risk factor linking genetic and/or neural metrics to psychosis spectrum symptoms. Although specific RDoC-related domains have rarely been tested and not yet been associated with psychosis, the greatest severity of cognitive deficits has been linked to the development of psychotic symptoms. Research on potential associative mechanisms is described, which may relate to specific domains that require further research. Identification of such mechanisms and domains would enable the development of treatments that may delay/prevent the onset of psychosis.

In a more specific focus on particular domains of information processing, Dr. Giersch and Laprévote then discuss alterations in perceptual functioning in people with schizophrenia, specifically focusing on visual perception. As with cognitive deficits, abnormalities in visual perception are seen in the prodromal phase of schizophrenia, leading to difficulties adapting to surroundings. RDoC-based aspects of perception are discussed, such as contrast sensitivity, masking, visual group, and temporal perception. Identifying which domains may predict the development of psychosis, as with other cognitive domains, could enable treatment development blocking the progression to psychosis.

When first attempting to develop such treatments for cognitive dysfunction in people with schizophrenia, issues quickly arose. For one, the Federal Drug Agency (FDA) had no mechanism by which a drug could be approved that treated cognitive dysfunction associated with schizophrenia. Thus, the NIMH funded the Measurement and Treatment Research to Improve Cognition in Schizophrenia (MATRICS) initiative. The MATRICS process brought together academia, the pharmaceutical industry, and the FDA, identifying: (1) cognitive domain targets in schizophrenia; (2) promising molecular targets to enhance these domains; and importantly (3) a process of approval for potential therapeutics to treat these domains in schizophrenia. MATRICS identified seven cognitive domains most affected in people with schizophrenia including attention/vigilance, speed of processing, reasoning and problem solving, verbal learning and memory, visual learning and memory, working memory, and social cognition. From this work, they then identified the MATRICS consensus cognitive battery (MCCB), for which to quantify dysfunction in each domain and test whether treatments were efficacious in treating such cognitive difficulties. This work and an update on the research conducted to-date using their developed test battery were covered in the chapter by Dr. Neuchterlein and colleagues.

Interestingly, the evolution of MATRICS resulted in attempts to tie cognitive functioning more closely to neural mechanisms by utilizing another NIMH-funded initiative, the Cognitive Neuroscience Treatment Research to Improve Cognition in Schizophrenia (CNTRICS). This work recognized the need to move from paper-and-pen tests of cognition to more laboratory and cognitive neuroscience-based assessments. Hence, the leaders of this approach, Drs. Barch and Carter brought experts together and further narrowed the definition of cognitive deficits in people with schizophrenia so that they more likely reflect altered neural mechanisms. Importantly, this work also brought in animal researchers so that cross-species research engaging such mechanisms could be conducted. In their chapter, Dr. Barch and colleagues describe the evolution of CNTRICS and its testing platform, providing links where appropriate to domains identified by RDoC. Hence, future research will continue to be applicable when generated from this platform.

Evidence for research conducted on specific examples of RDoC-cited domains is then provided, with Dr. Luck and colleagues describing that while attention is a core area of cognitive dysfunction in people with schizophrenia, attention is complex and multifaceted, separated out by the RDoC initiative. Within this chapter, they discuss how people with schizophrenia have: (1) a reduction in global alertness, (2) deficits in visual attention only when the stimuli activate the magnocellular processing pathway, and (3) hyperfocused attention to goal-irrelevant information. By providing such detailed information on the attentional deficits in people with schizophrenia, targeted therapeutics can be generated.

The work on attention dovetails well with assessment of working memory in people with schizophrenia, as described by Drs. Gold and Luck. Using the RDoC initiative representation, they describe how working memory representations are held in a 'privileged' state that are easily retrieved and relatively immune to distracting events. Furthermore, given that working memory is fundamental to reasoning, decision-making, cognitive control, etc., detailing changes in patients with schizophrenia remains vital. Mechanisms underlying working memory deficits in patients with schizophrenia, and links to other cognitive domains, are described.

Working memory differs from other aspects of memory such as episodic memory, with research in this domain covered by Dr. Raucher-Chene and colleagues. Episodic memory refers to the associations or binding among items or elements presented together, with cognitive neuroscience relevant to RDoC domains identifying mechanisms related to such specific processes. Furthermore, fMRI biomarkers of episodic memory deficits in people with schizophrenia are identified and discussed, all distinct from those of working memory.

Importantly, these early chapters provide evidence for circuitry likely disrupted in people with schizophrenia, potentially related to specific cognitive domains. Thus, at both the neuronal and local levels, treatments can be targeted at these regions. Drs. I-

Wei Shu and Eric Granholm provide an overview on how targeting frontal gamma – affected in people with schizophrenia measurable during cognitive testing – with neurofeedback offers opportunities to selectively target structures affected by the disease process. This top-down process of identifying cognitive deficits and directly targeting circuits affected has provided compelling data for efficacy, but the work requires further exploration. Regarding pharmacological treatments, Dr. Horan and colleagues then provide an update on such studies for cognitive dysfunction in people with schizophrenia. Although no treatments have passed Phase III trials to-date, there is a glutamatergic-based drug that is currently undergoing testing that shows some promise. Importantly, positive findings have been reported and the authors highlight this work and how transdiagnostic approaches may aid in more targeted therapeutics via the identification of homogeneous subgroups. Hence, future opportunities continue to arise for the targeted therapeutic development of cognitive impairment associated with schizophrenia.

A great deal of additional research has been conducted from a bottom-up perspective also, trying to discover mechanisms affected by the disease process and how they affect cognitive dysfunction that occurs in people with schizophrenia. For example, Dr. Tiffany Greenwood describes the evidence for the multiple genetic abnormalities that occur in people with schizophrenia, describing genetic networks that largely underpin synaptic pruning and neural development at a very young age. Dr. Lipner et al describe how environmental factors can play a role in driving neural changes that are associated with cognitive deficits in people with schizophrenia. Each of these mechanisms may work alone and/or synergistically to result in the cognitive deficits in people with schizophrenia, but understanding their mechanisms offers targeting opportunities for therapeutic development.

The information on potential causes underlying schizophrenia, alterations in neural mechanisms, and information on positive and negative therapeutic effects are all vital for preclinical researchers, such as the work of Dr. Kentner and colleagues. This group describes early-life developmental manipulations that can be conducted in rodents and tools to assess cognitive outcomes based on RDoC-relevant tasks. The validity of these disease-relevant manipulations, the impact of potential treatments, and their utility for treatment-development research are all discussed. Furthermore, Dr. Chaffee provides a similar overview, but utilizing primate models to explore the theory of the failure cascade leading to prefrontal circuit collapse in people with schizophrenia. The importance of using non-human primates is that prefrontal networks are similarly anatomically organized between monkeys and humans, with similar imaging tools used across species in a consistent developmental timeline. Tying these changes to behavioral outcome is vital and the authors highlight the opportunity for RDoC to more closely tie such neural developmental changes to outcome consistent across species.

From the approach of these research chapters, the authors cover a great deal of research and standard areas of assessment toward developing therapies for cognitive dysfunction in people with schizophrenia. Other avenues of research exist however, including focusing on the impact of substance use in people with schizophrenia from a developmental to treatment perspective. Dr. Khokar and colleagues describe this research, noting that healthy people who initiated cannabis use at earlier ages exhibited poorer cognition, while cannabis use in people with schizophrenia has been associated with the exacerbation of symptoms, but better overall cognitive performance, including in earlier age of use. Animal studies are then described to attempt to provide directionality of these effects, including specific cannabinoid agents.

Another important research area for cognitive disruption in people with schizophrenia is that of neuroinflammation and immunity, led by Dr. Deakin and colleagues. They describe that despite hypotheses, increased levels of cytokines detectable in the prodromal period were unlikely to be the driver of cognitive dysfunction in people with schizophrenia. Specifically, multiple meta-analyses did not however reveal any link between cytokine levels with cognitive impairment in people with high risk. Thus, the authors conclude that neuroinflammation is unlikely to be a core feature of schizophrenia or a driver in cognitive dysfunction, instead proposing that such deficits arise as a convergence of genetic and immune-neurodevelopmental dysregulation.

Another key area of research that is of great importance is that of potential sex/gender differences that occur in schizophrenia and cognition in general, led by Drs. Freeman and Lee. Initial studies demonstrate comparable sex effects in people with schizophrenia to healthy populations across multiple domains and phases of the illness. Further questions remain unresolved however, which may provide clues between cognitive impairment and pathophysiological processes.

Often overlooked is the potential deleterious impact that current therapeutics may exert on cognitive functioning. Acetylcholine plays a major role in cognitive functioning and several antipsychotics exert anticholinergic effects. This potential anticholinergic burden effect is described by Dr. Joshi, as is future directions that can detail potential detrimental effects and future directions for research.

Finally, almost all of the cognitive research described above utilize visual stimuli, and in some cases auditory stimuli. Oft-overlooked, however, are the olfactory cognitive deficits that arise as a result of the disease. Given that olfactory functioning develops early and dysfunction is seen across psychiatric conditions, Dr. MacQueen describes domains affected and paradigms that can be used to assess such functioning. Furthermore, this research offers opportunities for cross-species translational testing given faster cognitive training for rodents using olfactory cues.

In aggregate, this book provides an overview of research into the cognitive deficits associated with schizophrenia, where possible tying this research together utilizing language from the RDoC initiative. Although focused on schizophrenia, this transdiagnostic approach also provides insight into platforms of research approaches that can be used to determine mechanisms and treatments for other disorders that also involve cognitive challenges, such as bipolar disorder with psychotic features and individuals with chronic depression.

La Jolla, CA, USA — Jared W. Young
Saint Louis, MO, USA — Deanna M. Barch

Contents

The MATRICS Consensus Cognitive Battery: An Update

Keith H. Nuechterlein, Michael F. Green, and Robert S. Kern

Contents

Abstract Through a series of NIMH-supported consensus-building meetings of experts and empirical comparisons of candidate tests, the Measurement and Treatment Research to Improve Cognition in Schizophrenia (MATRICS) initiative

K. H. Nuechterlein (✉)
Department of Psychiatry and Biobehavioral Sciences, Semel Institute for Neuroscience and Human Behavior, University of California, Los Angeles, Los Angeles, CA, USA

Department of Psychology, University of California, Los Angeles, Los Angeles, CA, USA
e-mail: keithn@ucla.edu

M. F. Green and R. S. Kern
Department of Psychiatry and Biobehavioral Sciences, Semel Institute for Neuroscience and Human Behavior, University of California, Los Angeles, Los Angeles, CA, USA

VISN 22 Mental Illness Research, Education, and Clinical Center, VA Greater Los Angeles Healthcare System, Los Angeles, CA, USA

Curr Topics Behav Neurosci (2023) 63: 1–18
https://doi.org/10.1007/7854_2022_395
Published Online: 29 October 2022

developed a battery of standardized cognitive measures to allow reliable evaluation of results from clinical trials of promising interventions for core cognitive deficits in this disorder. Ten tests in seven cognitive domains were selected for the MATRICS Consensus Cognitive Battery (MCCB). The MCCB has now been translated into 39 languages/dialects and has been employed in more than 145 clinical trials. It has become the standard cognitive change measure for studies of both pharmacological and training-based interventions seeking to improve cognitive deficits in schizophrenia. We summarize its applications and its relationship to the subsequent development of the NIMH RDoC Matrix.

Keywords Cognition · Clinical trials · International · MATRICS · Schizophrenia

1 Background of the MATRICS Initiative and Its Consensus Cognitive Battery

The Food and Drug Administration (FDA) and the National Institute of Mental Health (NIMH) in the USA came to recognize in the initial years after 2000 that development of interventions to improve cognitive deficits in schizophrenia was a critical unmet need. Standardized procedures for evaluating potential new agents for this purpose were not available and were limiting development in this area. Cognitive deficits in schizophrenia were known to be prominent predictors of functional outcome, more than the severity of positive symptoms (Green 1996; Green and Nuechterlein 1999; Green et al. 2000), but effective interventions to improve these cognitive deficits were not available. Although a few early clinical trials of potential cognitive enhancers were beginning, the FDA was unwilling to approve any drug for improving cognition in schizophrenia without consensus on cognitive domains, measurement of cognition, and study design (Hyman and Fenton 2003; Marder and Fenton 2004). Thus, the NIMH invited applications for a contract to develop a consensus among experts from academia, NIMH, the pharmaceutical industry, and consumer advocacy on recommended research design and cognitive measurement procedures.

After a competitive application process, the NIMH awarded a contract to UCLA to launch the Measurement and Treatment Research to Improve Cognition in Schizophrenia (MATRICS) Initiative with Stephen R. Marder, M.D., as PI. As part of the broader MATRICS process, study design recommendations were developed (Buchanan et al. 2005, 2011) and promising neuropharmacological targets were identified (Geyer and Tamminga 2004). Another key aspect of the MATRICS Initiative was to identify the separable dimensions of cognition in schizophrenia and to develop a consensus measurement instrument to detect cognitive improvement in these domains in clinical trials (Green et al. 2004). While the MATRICS process preceded the development of the RDoC framework for clinical research, identification of separable cognitive domains within the MATRICS initiative served as one influence on the later content of the NIMH RDoC Matrix.

A Neurocognition Committee was formed with experts from academia, NIMH, and consumer advocacy, led by Co-Chairs Keith Nuechterlein and Michael Green. It included representatives from academia (Drs. Deanna Barch, Jonathan Cohen, Susan Essock, James Gold, Robert Heaton, Richard Keefe, and Helena Kraemer), NIMH (Drs. Wayne Fenton, Terry Goldberg, Ellen Stover, Daniel Weinberger, and Steven Zalcman), and consumer advocacy (Dr. Frederick Frese). The key separable domains of cognition relevant to clinical trials in schizophrenia were identified by integrating data from factor analytic studies (Nuechterlein et al. 2004) and a survey of experts (Kern et al. 2004). A consensus was reached on seven domains to be included in a cognitive battery (Green et al. 2004). The cognitive domains were speed of processing, attention/vigilance, working memory, verbal learning, visual learning, reasoning and problem-solving, and social cognition.

The criteria for selecting tests for the battery were also determined at an initial MATRICS consensus meeting of experts in multiple relevant fields (Green et al. 2004). They were high test-retest reliability, utility as a repeated measure, demonstrated relationship to functional outcome, potential changeability in response to pharmacological agents, and practicality and tolerability. In addition, given that the maximum length of a cognitive battery for clinical trials was believed to be 2 h, individual tests needed to require less than 15 min of administration time.

A series of consensus meetings among experts were held, typically involving more than 100 experts from academia, NIMH, industry, and consumer advocacy. Initially, over 90 tests were nominated as possible indices of the seven cognitive domains. Then, a series of steps were completed to reach a final battery of 10 tests representing the seven cognitive domains. Initial discussion of the suitability of each test for a clinical trials battery narrowed to the nominations to six or fewer tests per cognitive domain, often based on the administration time required or the practicality of training time or scoring. This initial review produced 36 candidate tests across the seven cognitive domains. Then, a database of existing test information relevant to the selection criteria was created for each test. A structured consensus process, the RAND/UCLA Appropriateness Method (Young et al. 2000; Fitch et al. 2001), was used by an expert panel to systematically evaluate the 36 tests. Based on a review of all relevant scientific evidence regarding the selection criteria, the RAND/UCLA method applied, iteratively, procedures to help increase agreement among members of the expert panel representing key stakeholder groups. This step led to the selection of the 20 most promising tests.

The final step in the selection process involved administering the 20 tests to 176 individuals with schizophrenia at five sites across the USA to directly compare the properties of these tests. A four-week follow-up assessment was completed with 167 of these participants to assess test-retest reliability, practicality of administration and scoring, and tolerability of the test with the participants. The final group of 10 tests was selected by the MATRICS Neurocognition Committee based on these data (Nuechterlein et al. 2008). A normative community sample of 300 individuals drawn from the same five sites, stratified by age, gender, and education, was also

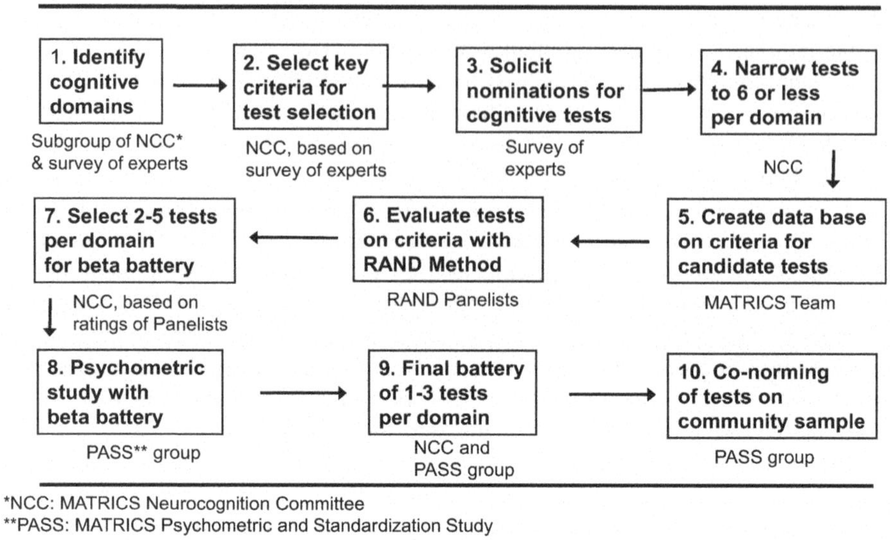

Fig. 1 Steps to create the MATRICS consensus cognitive battery

administered the 20 tests to allow co-norming, which places each test on the same measurement scale and allows correction for demographic effects in the general population (Kern et al. 2008). Because the FDA indicated that a co-primary measure of everyday functioning or functional capacity would also be needed in clinical trials, candidate measures for this co-primary role were also administered to the schizophrenia participants and evaluated for their promise (Green et al. 2008). The steps to create the MCCB™ are summarized in Fig. 1.

A non-profit company, MATRICS Assessment, Inc., was formed to allow compilation of the 10 tests into a published battery, with licensing agreements with the individual copyright holders (Nuechterlein and Green 2006). A MATRICS Computer Scoring Program was developed to convert the test raw scores into T scores, cognitive domain T scores, and an Overall Composite T score, with options to correct for age and gender (recommended for schizophrenia) or age, gender, and education (for application to disorders that typically occur after educational periods are completed). Distribution of the battery was arranged with three psychological test corporations (Multi-Health Systems, Inc., Pearson, Inc., and Psychological Assessment Resources, Inc.).

2 Translation and Normative Data with the MCCB™ in Additional Languages

2.1 Translations

It quickly became apparent that the application of the MCCB™ in large clinical trials of new agents for improving cognition in schizophrenia would require that it be available in multiple languages, as many of these trials involve international data collection. Thus, a government-industry collaboration, MATRICS-CT (Co-primary and Translation), was formed soon after the completion of the MATRICS Initiative to fund the professional translation of the MCCB™ and the collection of normative data in six languages/dialects: Chinese, German, Hindi, Russian, Spanish for Spain, and Spanish for Central/South America.

MATRICS Assessment, Inc., supervised the translations using the following steps for each language (Hambleton et al. 2005). First, a professional translation company was selected and the English version of the tests and the MCCB™ Manual was provided to them. Second, two professional translators completed a forward translation of the test materials and the MCCB™ Manual chapters on administration and scoring. The two translators then reconciled their translations. A third professional translator then back translated the materials into English and checked for discrepancies from the original English version. After these translators reached consensus on a forward translation, the translation was provided to a psychologist or psychiatrist experienced with neuropsychological testing who was a native language speaker in the target language. That local professional expert reviewed the translation for tone and phrasing appropriate to a psychological testing situation. This feedback was provided to the professional translators, who adapted the translation accordingly.

The resulting refined version was then set into a PDF format and printed for pilot work. It was provided to a trained psychological testing professional in the target country to pilot test 3–5 schizophrenia patients or individuals with similar disorders. Feedback from this pilot work was used to determine whether any phrasing of instructions to patients was unclear. In addition, the results were scored and examined by the authors of this chapter to detect any unusual patterns that needed to be queried further. Once a final translated version was reached, a print-ready version of all materials was sent to a professional printer company and an initial batch of MCCB™ kits in the language were printed and assembled. The steps in translating and culturally adapting the MCCB™ are summarized in Fig. 2.

In addition to the professional translations that are appropriate for clinical trials and all other applications, MATRICS Assessment, Inc. also established a process by which individual academic researchers could obtain permission to translate the MCCB™ for their non-commercial research. This translation process also includes forward and back translation and review of the back translation by MATRICS Assessment, Inc., and test copyright holders, but does not involve the other steps. These translations are not commercially available and are not appropriate for commercial clinical trials. Academic research translations have been completed for some languages for which a professional translation has not been done, including Brazilian Portuguese. Other academic research translations have subsequently been replaced by professional translations.

The demand for translation of the MCCB™ into multiple languages has remained strong over the years since the initial publication of the English version in 2006 (see www.matricsinc.org). The MCCB™ is currently available in 39 languages (see Table 1).

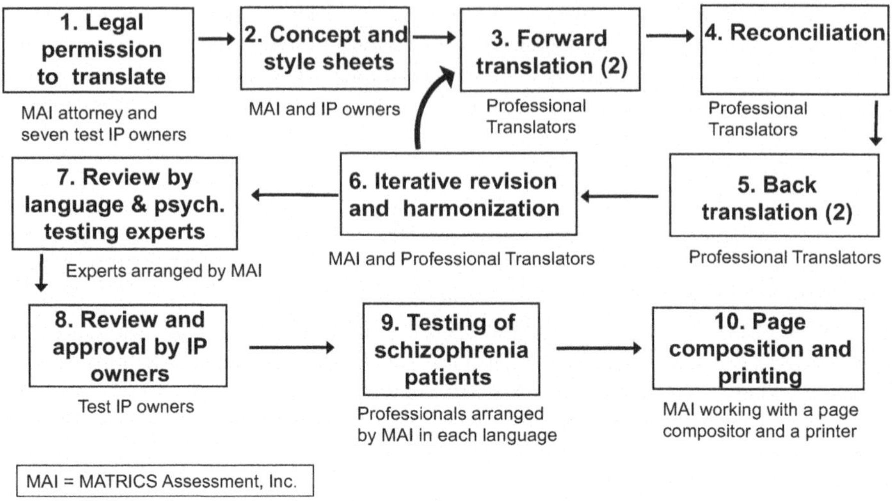

Fig. 2 Steps in translation and cultural adaptation of the MATRICS consensus cognitive battery

Table 1 Languages in which the MCCB™ is currently available

Armenian (academic research only)	Greek	Portuguese – Brazil (academic research only)
Bulgarian	Hebrew	Portuguese – Portugal
Chinese – simplified	Hindi	Romanian
Chinese – traditional	Hungarian	Russian
Croatian	Italian	Serbian
Czech	Japanese	Slovak
Danish	Kannada	Spanish for Central and South America
Dutch	Korean	Spanish for Spain
English	Lithuanian	Swedish
English – Malaysia	Malay	Tamil
French	Marathi	Telugu
Finnish	Norwegian	Turkish
German	Polish	Ukrainian

2.2 *Community Norming in Other Languages*

For several of the MCCB™ translations that are most typically used in international clinical trials, community normative data have been collected through a process paralleling the norming of the English MCCB™ in North America. For each language, 200 to 300 community members stratified by age, gender, and education were administered the translated MCCB™, mainly with funding from the MATRICS-CT collaboration between NIMH and industry. The results were analyzed by the MATRICS Assessment, Inc., team and T scores were created that parallel those for the English MCCB™. The MCCB™ Computer Scoring Program was updated to provide these T scores for Simplified Chinese, German, Hindi, Italian, Japanese, Russian, Spanish for Spain, and Spanish for Central/South America (Nuechterlein and Green 2016).

2.3 *International Scoring System for the MSCEIT Managing Emotions Branch*

Because the items in the social cognition test in the MCCB™, the MSCEIT Managing Emotions Branch, appeared to be less universal in cultural context than the other tests in the MCCB™, research was completed to evaluate the extent to which the frequency of alternative answers and their correlation with the total test score differed from the English version (Hellemann et al. 2017).

The MSCEIT Managing Emotions Branch uses a "consensus based" scoring method in which the score assigned to a response is the proportion of a population that selected that response in the normative sample. Thus, rather than a "correct" response, the scores reflect the extent to which a response agrees with the responses by community members. Multi-Health Systems, Inc., developed the original norms of the MSCEIT Managing Emotions Branch using a large sample ($N = 2{,}112$) of participants drawn from seven English-speaking countries.

To examine the degree to which responses of community members from other cultures differed from those in the English-speaking countries, we examined the individual item data from the community normative samples from China, India (Hindi), Japan, Russia, Spain, and Central and South America. Each sample was stratified by age, sex, and education according to its region's population. We used a measure known as L1 (Manhattan norm) to measure the discrepancies across cultures/countries. It is defined as the sum of the absolute differences between the percentages of choices for each of the response options (Hellemann et al. 2017). We also examined whether items were reverse scored across cultures/countries. That is, whether a response considered to be an effective handling of certain emotions in one culture was usually considered to be an ineffective method in another culture.

Three items were found to be reverse scored across cultures, while three additional items had high discrepancy scores. Thus, 6 of 29 items were excluded from the International MSCEIT Branch 4 Scoring Program. Correlations between the original scores and those generated by the international scoring system were high (generally $r > 0.80$) for each country, but the international scoring produced less discrepancy from country to country (Hellemann et al. 2017). The International MSCEIT Branch 4 Scoring Program is therefore recommended for non-English-speaking applications of the MCCB™.

3 Development of the Neurocognitive Composite Score

The growing awareness that neurocognition (non-social cognition) and social cognition are separable dimensions (Fett et al. 2011; Lee et al. 2013; Green et al. 2019) led us to develop a composite score that summarizes performance across the six neurocognitive domains. Some interventions might impact social cognition and non-social cognition differently, or might target one or the other, such as the effect of oxytocin on social cognition (Davis et al. 2014). To allow investigators to examine non-social cognition only, we developed the Neurocognitive Composite score, which is distributed as a T score in the normative samples based on the six non-social cognitive domains. We incorporated an option to generate the Neurocognitive Composite score into the 2016 version of the MCCB™ Computer Scoring Program. This additional composite score was reviewed and approved by the MATRICS™ Neurocognition Committee.

4 Website for Downloading the MCCB™ Computer Programs

Three computer programs were supplied on CDs with the original MCCB™ kit (Nuechterlein and Green 2006): the CPT-IP administration and scoring program, the MSCEIT Branch 4 Scoring Program, and the MCCB Computer Scoring Program. With the multiple translations of the MCCB™, the translated directions to subjects were added to the CPT-IP.

MATRICS International Version 2 program. In 2016, the International MSCEIT Branch 4 Scoring Program was added to the CDs. As PC laptops increasingly were designed without built-in CD/DVD drives and were often the most convenient way to administer the CPT-IP and score the MCCB, particularly in multisite clinical trials, the demand for downloadable MCCB programs grew.

As a result, we worked with a website developer to make it possible for those who purchased an MCCB™ kit to download the four MCCB computer programs as an alternative to loading them from CDs. Starting in 2021, this became a standard feature of the MCCB™.

5 Applications of the MCCB™ in Clinical Trials

The primary goal for the development of the MCCB™ was to provide a standardized cognitive battery for use in clinical trials that would allow cognitive gains to be compared across trials (Green et al. 2004; Kern et al. 2008; Nuechterlein et al. 2008). The MCCB™ has been very successful in this regard. The FDA has called the MCCB™ the gold standard for measuring cognitive change in clinical trials for schizophrenia. A search of ClinicalTrials.gov for the term MATRICS yields 245 studies, which documents the overall impact of the MATRICS Initiative on clinical trials of potential interventions to improve cognition in severe mental disorders. Although not all studies used the abbreviation MCCB in their study descriptions, a ClinicalTrials.gov search for MCCB indicates that at least 145 clinical trials did include this consensus cognitive battery. The fact that these studies have been conducted in many different countries is evidence that the MCCB™ is widely accepted as the standard battery for clinical trials internationally. Some studies of bipolar disorder and other severe mental illnesses are also among the applications listed in ClinicalTrials.gov.

5.1 Pharmacological Clinical Trials with the MCCB

In the years since the MCCB™ was published in 2006, many clinical trials have been completed to evaluate the safety and efficacy of potential pharmacological cognitive enhancers for schizophrenia. A 2018 meta-analysis examined results from 93 randomized clinical trials that evaluated cognitive improvement with neuropsychological tests, 76 of which were reported from 2007 through 2017 (Sinkeviciute et al. 2018). Although not all 76 clinical trials reported since the publication of the MCCB™ used this battery to measure cognitive change, the MCCB™ has become the most common choice as the primary cognitive outcome measure, either focusing on the Overall Composite T Score or, less frequently, on one of the cognitive domain T scores from the MCCB™. Even when the MCCB™ is not used in the earliest phases of clinical trials, it is usually adopted in later phases due to its acceptance as the gold standard by the FDA.

After initial enthusiasm for examining new agents that targeted a wide range of neurotransmitter systems (Geyer and Tamminga 2004; Geyer and Heinssen 2005), most randomized clinical trials have unfortunately yielded negative results. The Sinkeviciute et al. (2018) meta-analysis found that the effect size across all cognitive enhancers in the 93 studies, with 5,630 participating patients, was positive and significant, but quite small (Hedge's $g = 0.10$, $p = 0.023$). The most promising pharmacological targets were the glutamatergic system (overall cognition Hedge's $g = 0.19$, $p = 0.01$; working memory $g = 0.13$, $p = 0.04$) and cholinesterase inhibitors (working memory $g = 0.26$, $p = 0.03$). A common pattern was positive results in early Phase II trials followed by failure to replicate the positive findings in larger late Phase II trials or Phase III trials. This pattern led to a search for factors in research design, sample selection, and cognitive measurement that might be limiting detection of a cognitive signal (Green et al. 2019; Keefe 2019).

The clinical trials with new pharmacological agents targeting cognition in schizophrenia since 2018 have recently been reviewed by Horan et al. (in press). Of the 9 trials that they list, 8 use either the MCCB Overall Composite or Neurocognitive Composite Score or the MCCB Working Memory domain score as their primary cognitive endpoint. While it remains the case that no drug for enhancing cognition associated with schizophrenia has been approved by the FDA, and 2 of the 9 trials are completed with negative results, one completed trial was positive for MCCB™ composite gains and 6 remain active at this point (Horan et al. in press). The most promising compound at this time is Boehringer Ingelheim's glycine transporter-1 (glyT1) inhibitor, BI 425809, which is currently in large Phase III trials after positive MCCB Overall Composite results in a multisite Phase II trial. The FDA granted BI 425809 Breakthrough Therapy Designation for cognitive impairment associated with schizophrenia in May 2021 (Horan et al. in press). Another glutamatergic drug, BIIB-104, a positive allosteric modulator (PAM) of the AMPA receptor (AMPAR), is currently being examined in a phase IIb study by Biogen. The cognitive target in that case is the MCCB Working Memory domain score.

5.2 Psychometric Properties of the MCCB™

As the earlier negative results of clinical trials of potential pharmacological cognitive enhancers multiplied, one concern was whether the psychometric properties of the MCCB™ were leading to too much measurement noise, practice effects, and ceiling effects, thereby reducing sensitivity to the drug effects. These concerns have been allayed by careful examination of the psychometric properties of the battery. First, the selection criteria for tests in the MCCB™ emphasized the need for high test-retest reliability, utility as a repeated measure, and potential changeability in response to pharmacological agents (Nuechterlein et al. 2008). In the 5-site psychometric study with 167 schizophrenia patients assessed twice 4 weeks apart, the selected individual tests had high test-retest reliability (ICC of 0.68–0.85) and the Overall Composite Score had an ICC of 0.90. In addition, the effect sizes for practice effects for the individual tests ranged from Cohen's $d = 0.00$ to 0.22 (Nuechterlein et al. 2008). Those data also showed that the obtained scores were rarely or never at the floor or ceiling of the tests. Thus, the initial data supporting test selection indicated high test-retest reliability, small practice effects, and absence of floor or ceiling effects.

A question remained, however, about the psychometric properties of the MCCB™ in actual clinical trials. This issue was well addressed by Keefe and colleagues through the examination of data from a 29-site clinical trial with 323 outpatients with schizophrenia (Keefe et al. 2011). Patients were assessed at screening and a median of 15 days later at baseline. The test-retest reliability of the Overall Composite Score was very high (ICC = 0.88). Furthermore, the practice effect for the composite score was quite small (Cohen's $d = 0.18$) and not statistically significant. Individual cognitive domain T scores were also generally above ICC of 0.70, except for Verbal Learning (0.58) and Visual Learning (0.65) and only Reasoning and Problem-Solving showed a significant practice effect (Cohen's $d = 0.14$). When one considers that the mean Overall Composite T score for these schizophrenia patients was about 25 (general population mean = 50 with SD = 10) and that the practice effect is about 2T scores from first to second administration, it becomes clear that practice effects are very small and that ceiling effects are not suppressing drug effects. Furthermore, any practice effects would be maximum from first to second administration, so further repeated administrations would be even less impacted by practice.

5.3 Clinical Trials with Training-Based Interventions

The sensitivity of the MCCB™ to cognitive change becomes clear when the results of clinical trials with cognitive remediation and other training-based interventions are considered. The popularity of the MCCB™ to evaluate cognitive effects for training-based interventions is evident based on a search of ClinicalTrials.gov. Forty-three trials of cognitive training use either the MCCB Overall Composite score or one of its cognitive domain scores to evaluate the efficacy of the intervention. Recently physical exercise has become another training-based intervention that is being actively evaluated for improving cognition in psychosis. ClinicalTrials.gov lists nine studies of physical exercise effects on the MCCB, four of which examine physical exercise combined with cognitive training. One additional study is examining the impact of mindfulness training on cognition using the MCCB.

Of the 43 cognitive training studies, only nine have yet posted results and most are ongoing. A series of studies completed by Vinogradov, Fisher, and colleagues at UC San Francisco using a slightly modified MCCB have demonstrated significant differential cognitive improvement in schizophrenia with Posit Science auditory processing modules (now part of BrainHQ) compared with a computer games control group. The effect sizes have been medium to large for the global cognition score with patients with multi-episode schizophrenia ($d = 0.86$) (Fisher et al. 2009), relatively recent-onset schizophrenia ($d = 0.73$) (Fisher et al. 2015), and clinical high risk for psychosis (Loewy et al. 2016). When these modules were administered remotely with relatively recent-onset patients, the improvement was present 6 months after training (Loewy et al. 2022). A similar large differential effect of Posit Science Brain Works modules versus nonspecific computer games was demonstrated in bipolar patients ($d = 0.80$) for the MCCB Overall Composite Score (Lewandowski et al. 2017). Using a different set of cognitive training modules drawn from NET (Bell et al. 2001) and NEAR (Medalia et al. 2000, 2001), Nuechterlein and colleagues at UCLA showed that first-episode schizophrenia outpatients had substantial differential MCCB Overall Composite gains (equivalent to $d = 0.72$) with cognitive training compared to a healthy behavior training comparison group (Nuechterlein et al. 2020) when medication adherence was covaried. This study also demonstrated generalization of effects to everyday work/school functioning (equivalent to $d = 0.78$).

One limitation of the cognitive training literature thus far has been to show similar substantial MCCB™ improvements in large multisite studies. Thus, a multisite Posit Science study (Mahncke et al. 2019) of 150 schizophrenia patients failed to find a differential cognitive effect of cognitive training versus computer games using the

MCCB Overall Composite Score. Limitations in patient treatment engagement were a possible contributor. Similarly, a multisite study in which all schizophrenia patients were first stabilized on lurasidone before randomization did not find significant differential MCCB gains from randomization to the study endpoint (Kantrowitz et al. 2016), although substantial cognitive improvements during the lurasidone stabilization period complicated the analyses. Thus, the sensitivity of the MCCB™ to cognitive gains produced by cognitive training is well demonstrated by well-controlled studies at single academic sites. Why multisite studies do not reveal the same strong effects needs further examination, as these factors may be impacting both pharmacological and cognitive training multisite clinical trials.

Clinical trials of physical exercise have also demonstrated that the MCCB™ can sensitively detect cognitive gains. Kimhy and colleagues (2015) showed that an X-Box aerobic exercise program produced large cognitive improvements ($d = 0.93$) on the MCCB Overall Composite Score. Furthermore, Nuechterlein and collaborators (2022) demonstrated that adding an aerobic exercise program to cognitive training could produce a large boost in the magnitude of cognitive gain (equivalent to $d = 0.86$) in 3 months and generalization to larger work/school functioning gains (equivalent to $d = 1.06$) by 6 months compared to cognitive training alone.

6 Applications of the MCCB™ within Psychopathology Research

6.1 Factor Analytic Studies of the MCCB™

Several studies have reported results of factor analyses of the MCCB™. While the number of factors derived from the 10 tests of the final MCCB™ has varied somewhat, the most common result has been three factors (Burton et al. 2013; Lo et al. 2016; Mohn et al. 2017; Kuo et al. 2020). Usually these factors represent processing speed, attention/working memory, and learning (Burton et al. 2013; Lo et al. 2016; Kuo et al. 2020), but sometimes a slightly different structure (Holmen et al. 2019). The major limitation of these factor analytic studies is that they include only the 10 scores from the final MCCB™. Most of the seven cognitive domains in the MCCB™ are represented by only one test to keep the battery as brief as possible for clinical trials. However, at least two measures of a hypothesized dimension are generally considered necessary to identify a factor through factor analysis. Thus, the confirmatory factor analysis by McCleery and colleagues (2015) is distinctive in that it used the beta battery from the MCCB development process (Nuechterlein et al. 2008), which includes at least two measures of each hypothesized cognitive domain. McCleery et al. (2014) confirm that a seven-factor solution is the best fit, significantly better than a single factor, three correlated factors, or a hierarchical model. These results support the seven cognitive domains that were the basis for the development of the MCCB™.

6.2 Profile of Cognitive Deficits in Schizophrenia

Using the original five-site sample of schizophrenia patients and healthy adults which led to the selection of the final 10 tests in the MCCB™, Kern and colleagues demonstrated that each of the seven domain T scores was very sensitive to cognitive impairment in schizophrenia, with T scores ranging from 33 to 39 (community mean of 50 with SD of 10) (Kern et al. 2011). Speed of processing and working memory was most impaired, while reasoning and problem-solving was least impaired. As Kern et al. (2011) discuss, the lower scores for speed of processing and working memory might be due to the fact that these domains are measured by more than one test in the MCCB, which would tend to increase their sensitivity to deficits. McCleery and collaborators compared this sample of multi-episode schizophrenia patients (mean age of 44 years) with a first-episode schizophrenia sample (mean age of 22 years) to examine whether evidence of progression of cognitive deficit was present (McCleery et al. 2014). They found that the level of impairment was comparable for most cognitive domains, but working memory and social cognition deficits were significantly less severe in the first-episode patients.

Subsequent examinations of the profile of cognitive deficits in schizophrenia across domains using translations of the MCCB have confirmed that the deficits are present in all seven cognitive domains in countries outside the USA, usually between one and two standard deviations below the healthy community mean (Rodriguez-Jimenez et al. 2015; Fonseca et al. 2017; Mucci et al. 2018; Bezdicek et al. 2020). When Spanish samples of multi-episode and first-episode schizophrenia patients were compared, the deficits of first-episode patients were again generally comparable, but in this case verbal and visual memory and attention/vigilance were somewhat less severely impaired than in multi-episode patients (Rodriguez-Jimenez et al. 2019). Thus, the sensitivity of the MCCB™ to cognitive deficits in schizophrenia is clear across multiple languages and cultures. The specific cognitive domains that may show progression in the severity of deficits from the first episode to later stages of schizophrenia need further investigation.

6.3 Sensitivity of MCCB™ to Cognitive Deficits in Biological Relatives and Familial Aggregation

The Italian Network for Research on Psychosis administered the Italian translation of the MCCB to 852 outpatients with schizophrenia, 342 unaffected relatives, and a normative Italian sample of 774 healthy subjects (Mucci et al. 2018). They found that the schizophrenia patients were one to two standard deviations below the normative mean in each cognitive domain and the biological relatives were about 0.5 standard deviations below the normative mean. Relatives were significantly below the normative mean in each domain except social cognition, but they had significantly less severe deficits than the patients in each domain. Proband scores significantly predicted their relatives scores for every domain except visual learning (Mucci et al. 2018). Thus, the MCCB™ detects subtle cognitive deficits in biological relatives of schizophrenia probands which show significant familiality.

The MATRICS initiative also was one influence on the later development of the RDoC approach to NIMH clinical research. The emphasis on consensus processes was also a prominent feature of the construction of the NIMH RDoC Matrix. The focus on establishing cognitive domains of importance in major psychopathology was further elaborated in the NIMH RDoC Matrix. Some domains in the NIMH RDoC Matrix are similar to those selected by the MATRICS initiative (Green et al. 2004; Nuechterlein et al. 2004), designated as either Cognitive Systems (i.e., attention, working memory, declarative memory) or Social Processes (social communication, perception and understanding of self, perception and understanding of others).

7 Summary

The MCCB™, developed through multiple steps by a wide range of experts participating in the NIMH MATRICS Initiative, has had a major impact on the measurement of cognitive deficits in schizophrenia and particularly on the evaluation of cognitive change in clinical trials.

The MCCB™ has been applied in psychopathology research to examine the separable cognitive dimensions in individuals with schizophrenia, the profile of deficits across those cognitive domains in patients with schizophrenia and their biological relatives, and the familiality of these cognitive deficits. When multiple tests of each hypothesized domain are included, the seven separable domains underlying MCCB™ development are confirmed. The mean scores of samples of patients with schizophrenia are one to two standard deviations below community norms, their biological relatives are only about a half standard deviation below community norms, and there is a significant familiality of cognitive performance.

The development of the MCCB™ has allowed comparisons of the degree of cognitive improvement achieved in many different clinical trials, as desired by the FDA. The translation of the MCCB™ into more than 30 languages has greatly facilitated international clinical trials of interventions to improve cognition in schizophrenia. The co-norming of the MCCB™ tests in multiple languages and cultures has further aided international use of the battery. While most trials of possible pharmacological cognitive enhancers have thus far been negative, some promising new compounds are currently being tested. Clinical trials of cognitive training and physical exercise programs have shown that it is possible to achieve medium to large cognitive gains in schizophrenia and these can be sensitively detected by the MCCB™. The applications of the MCCB™ in clinical trials can be expected to continue expanding as it has become the primary tool through which the promise of interventions to improve the core cognitive deficits in schizophrenia is judged.

While the MATRICS initiative and development of the MCCB preceded the development of the RDoC approach to clinical research, its emphasis on multiple cognitive domains and consensus among experts was an influence on the later construction of the NIMH RDoC Matrix. Some dimensions identified for the MCCB (i.e., attention, working memory, learning, social cognition) are represented in the NIMH RDoC Matrix, sometimes using different terms. Additional influences on the NIMH RDoC Matrix came from the later Cognitive Neuroscience Treatment Research to Improve Cognition in Schizophrenia (CNTRICS) meetings (Barch et al. 2009; Carter et al. 2008). The CNTRICS meetings led to additional distinctions among different cognitive control processes and working memory components that were derived from the neuroscience literature rather than from factor analytic studies of cognitive dimensions in schizophrenia. The processes identified by the CNTRICS meetings and incorporated into the NIMH RDoC Matrix emphasize cognitive components that can be disassociated from each other rather than combined into broader composite scores. Thus far the broad composite scores have been adopted as the primary outcome by most clinical trials of cognitive enhancers to maximize sensitivity to cognitive gains that are correlated. Targeted interventions might address only certain cognitive processes that are dysfunctional in schizophrenia, as both the individual MCCB cognitive domains and the tasks developed from the CNTRICS initiative allow for this possibility. Until this point less effort has been devoted to trials of such more targeted cognitive interventions.

References

Barch DM, Carter CS, Arnsten A, Buchanan RW, Cohen JD, Geyer M, Green MF, Krystal JH, Nuechterlein K, Robbins T, Silverstein S, Smith EE, Strauss M, Wykes T, Heinssen R (2009) Selecting paradigms from cognitive neuroscience for translation into use in clinical trials: proceedings of the third CNTRICS meeting. Schizophr Bull 35(1):109–114

Bell M, Bryson G, Greig T, Corcoran C, Wexler BE (2001) Neurocognitive enhancement therapy with work therapy: effects on neuropsychological test performance. Arch Gen Psychiatry 58: 763–768

Bezdicek O, Michalec J, Kalisova L, Kufa T, Dechterenko F, Chlebovcova M, Havlik F, Green MF, Nuechterlein KH (2020) Profile of cognitive deficits in schizophrenia and factor structure of the Czech MATRICS consensus cognitive battery. Schizophr Res 218:85–92

Buchanan RW, Davis M, Goff D, Green MF, Keefe RS, Leon AC, Nuechterlein KH, Laughren T, Levin R, Stover E, Fenton W, Marder SR (2005) A summary of the FDA-NIMH-MATRICS workshop on clinical trial design for neurocognitive drugs for schizophrenia. Schizophr Bull 31: 5–19

Buchanan RW, Keefe RS, Umbricht D, Green MF, Laughren T, Marder SR (2011) The FDA-NIMH-MATRICS guidelines for clinical trial design of cognitive-enhancing drugs: what do we know 5 years later? Schizophr Bull 37:1209–1217

Burton CZ, Vella L, Harvey PD, Patterson TL, Heaton RK, Twamley EW (2013) Factor structure of the MATRICS consensus cognitive battery (MCCB) in schizophrenia. Schizophr Res 146:244–248

Carter CS, Barch DM, Buchanan RW, Bullmore E, Krystal JH, Cohen J, Geyer M, Green M, Nuechterlein KH, Robbins T, Silverstein S, Smith EE, Strauss M, Wykes T, Heinssen R (2008)

Identifying cognitive mechanisms targeted for treatment development in schizophrenia: an overview of the first meeting of the cognitive neuroscience treatment research to improve cognition in schizophrenia initiative. Biol Psychiatry 64(1):4–10
Davis MC, Green MF, Lee J, Horan WP, Senturk D, Clarke AD, Marder SR (2014) Oxytocin-augmented social cognitive skills training in schizophrenia. Neuropsychopharmacology 39: 2070–2077
Fett AKJ, Viechtbauer W, Dominguez MG, Penn DL, Van Os J, Krabbendam L (2011) The relationship between neurocognition and social cognition with functional outcomes in schizophrenia: a meta-analysis. Neurosci Biobehav Rev 35:573–588
Fisher M, Holland C, Merzenich MM, Vinogradov S (2009) Using neuroplasticity-based auditory training to improve verbal memory in schizophrenia. Am J Psychiatr 166:805–811
Fisher M, Loewy R, Carter C, Lee A, Ragland JD, Niendam T, Schlosser D, Pham L, Miskovich T, Vinogradov S (2015) Neuroplasticity-based auditory training via laptop computer improves cognition in young individuals with recent onset schizophrenia. Schizophr Bull 41:250–258
Fitch K, Bernstein SJ, Aguilar MD, Burnand B, Lacalle JR, Lazaro P, Van Het Loo M, McDonnell J, Vader JP, Kahan JP (2001) The RAND/UCLA appropriateness method user's manual. RAND, Santa Monica
Fonseca AO, Berberian AA, De Meneses-Gaya C, Gadelha A, Vicente MO, Nuechterlein KH, Bressan RA, Lacerda ALT (2017) The Brazilian standardization of the MATRICS consensus cognitive battery (MCCB): psychometric study. Schizophr Res 185:148–153
Geyer MA, Heinssen R (2005) New approaches to measurement and treatment research to improve cognition in schizophrenia (MATRICS). Schizophr Bull 4:806–809
Geyer MA, Tamminga CA (2004) Measurement and treatment research to improve cognition in schizophrenia: Neuropharmacological aspects. Psychopharmacology 174:1–2
Green MF (1996) What are the functional consequences of neurocognitive deficits in schizophrenia? Am J Psychiatry 153:321–330
Green MF, Nuechterlein KH (1999) Should schizophrenia be treated as a neurocognitive disorder? Schizophr Bull 25:309–319
Green MF, Kern RS, Braff DL, Mintz J (2000) Neurocognitive deficits and functional outcome in schizophrenia: are we measuring the "right stuff"? Schizophr Bull 26:119–136
Green MF, Nuechterlein KH, Gold JM, Barch DM, Cohen J, Essock S, Fenton WS, Frese F, Goldberg TE, Heaton RK, Keefe RS, Kern RS, Kraemer H, Stover E, Weinberger DR, Zalcman S, Marder SR (2004) Approaching a consensus cognitive battery for clinical trials in schizophrenia: the NIMH-MATRICS conference to select cognitive domains and test criteria. Biol Psychiatry 56:301–307
Green MF, Nuechterlein KH, Kern RS, Baade LE, Fenton WS, Gold JM, Keefe RS, Mesholam-Gately R, Seidman LJ, Stover E, Marder SR (2008) Functional co-primary measures for clinical trials in schizophrenia: results from the MATRICS psychometric and standardization study. Am J Psychiatr 165:221–228
Green MF, Horan WP, Lee J (2019) Nonsocial and social cognition in schizophrenia: current evidence and future directions. World Psychiatry 18:146–161
Hambleton RK, Merenda PF, Spielberger CD (2005) Adapting educational and psychological tests for cross-cultural assessment. Lawrence Erlbaum
Hellemann GS, Green MF, Kern RS, Sitarenios G, Nuechterlein KH (2017) Developing an international scoring system for a consensus-based social cognition measure: MSCEIT-managing emotions. Psychol Med 47:2494–2501
Holmen TL, Engh JA, Andersen E, Andreassen OA, Martinsen EW, Bigseth TT, Bang-Kittilsen G, Egeland J (2019) Cardio-respiratory fitness is associated with a verbal factor across cognitive domains in schizophrenia. Schizophr Res 206:157–162
Horan WP, Catalano L, Green MF (in press) An update on treatment of cognitive impairment associated with schizophrenia. In: Barch D, Young JW (eds) Current topics in behavioral neurosciences, cognitive functioning in schizophrenia: leveraging the RDoC framework
Hyman SE, Fenton WS (2003) What are the right targets for psychopharmacology? Science 299: 350–351

Kantrowitz JT, Sharif Z, Medalia A, Keefe RS, Harvey P, Bruder G, Barch DM, Choo T, Lee S, Lieberman JA (2016) A multicenter, rater-blinded, randomized controlled study of auditory processing-focused cognitive remediation combined with open-label lurasidone in patients with schizophrenia and schizoaffective disorder. J Clin Psychiatry 77:799–806

Keefe RSE (2019) Why are there no approved treatments for cognitive impairment in schizophrenia? World Psychiatry 18:167–168

Keefe RSE, Fox KH, Harvey PD, Cucchiaro J, Siu C, Loebel A (2011) Characteristics of the MATRICS consensus cognitive battery in a 29-site antipsychotic schizophrenia clinical trial. Schizophr Res 125:161–168

Kern RS, Green MF, Nuechterlein KH, Deng BH (2004) NIMH-MATRICS survey on assessment of neurocognition in schizophrenia. Schizophr Res 72:11–19

Kern RS, Nuechterlein KH, Green MF, Baade LE, Fenton WS, Gold JM, Keefe RS, Mesholam-Gately R, Mintz J, Seidman LJ, Stover E, Marder SR (2008) The MATRICS consensus cognitive battery, part 2: co-norming and standardization. Am J Psychiatr 165:214–220

Kern RS, Gold JM, Dickinson D, Green MF, Nuechterlein KH, Baade LE, Keefe RS, Mesholam-Gately RI, Seidman LJ, Lee C, Sugar CA, Marder SR (2011) The MCCB impairment profile for schizophrenia outpatients: results from the MATRICS psychometric and standardization study. Schizophr Res 126:124–131

Kimhy D, Vakhrusheva J, Bartels MN, Armstrong HF, Ballon JS, Khan S, Chang RW, Hansen MC, Ayanruoh L, Lister A, Castren E, Smith EE, Sloan RP (2015) The impact of aerobic exercise on brain-derived neurotrophic factor and neurocognition in individuals with schizophrenia: a single-blind, randomized clinical trial. Schizophr Bull 41:859–868

Kuo SS, Wojtalik JA, Mesholam-Gately RI, Keshavan MS, Eack SM (2020) Transdiagnostic validity of the MATRICS consensus cognitive battery across the autism-schizophrenia spectrum. Psychol Med 50:1623–1632

Lee J, Altshuler L, Glahn DC, Miklowitz DJ, Ochsner K, Green MF (2013) Social and nonsocial cognition in bipolar disorder and schizophrenia: relative levels of impairment. Am J Psychiatry 170:334–341

Lewandowski KE, Sperry SH, Cohen BM, Norris LA, Fitzmaurice GM, Ongur D, Keshavan MS (2017) Treatment to enhance cognition in bipolar disorder (TREC-BD): efficacy of a randomized controlled trial of cognitive remediation versus active control. J Clin Psychiatry 78:e1242–e1249

Lo SB, Szuhany KL, Kredlow MA, Wolfe R, Mueser KT, McGurk SR (2016) A confirmatory factor analysis of the MATRICS consensus cognitive battery in severe mental illness. Schizophr Res 175:79–84

Loewy R, Fisher M, Schlosser DA, Biagianti B, Stuart B, Mathalon DH, Vinogradov S (2016) Intensive auditory cognitive training improves verbal memory in adolescents and young adults at clinical high risk for psychosis. Schizophr Bull 42(Suppl 1):S118–S126

Loewy R, Fisher M, Ma S, Carter C, Ragland JD, Niendam TA, Stuart B, Schlosser D, Amirfathi F, Yohannes S, Vinogradov S (2022) Durable cognitive gains and symptom improvement are observed in individuals with recent-onset schizophrenia 6 months after a randomized trial of auditory training completed remotely. Schizophr Bull 48:262–272

Mahncke HW, Kim SJ, Rose A, Stasio C, Buckley P, Caroff S, Duncan E, Yasmin S, Jarskog LF, Lamberti JS, Nuechterlein K, Strassnig M, Velligan D, Ventura J, Walker T, Stroup TS, Keefe RSE (2019) Evaluation of a plasticity-based cognitive training program in schizophrenia: results from the eCaesar trial. Schizophr Res 208:182–189

Marder SR, Fenton WS (2004) Measurement and treatment research to improve cognition in schizophrenia: NIMH MATRICS initiative to support the development of agents for improving cognition in schizophrenia. Schizophr Res 72:5–10

McCleery A, Ventura J, Kern RS, Subotnik KL, Gretchen-Doorly D, Green MF, Hellemann GS, Nuechterlein KH (2014) Cognitive functioning in first-episode schizophrenia: MATRICS consensus cognitive battery (MCCB) profile of impairment. Schizophr Res 157:33–39

McCleery A, Green MF, Hellemann GS, Baade LE, Gold JM, Keefe RS, Kern RS, Mesholam-Gately RI, Seidman LJ, Subotnik KL, Ventura J, Nuechterlein KH (2015) Latent structure of cognition in schizophrenia: a confirmatory factor analysis of the MATRICS consensus cognitive battery (MCCB). Psychol Med 45:2657–2666

Medalia A, Revheim N, Casey M (2000) Remediation of memory disorders in schizophrenia. Psychol Med 30:1451–1459

Medalia A, Revheim N, Casey M (2001) The remediation of problem-solving skills in schizophrenia. Schizophr Bull 27:259–267

Mohn C, Lystad JU, Ueland T, Falkum E, Rund BR (2017) Factor analyzing the Norwegian MATRICS consensus cognitive battery. Psychiatry Clin Neurosci 71:336–345

Mucci A, Galderisi S, Green MF, Nuechterlein K, Rucci P, Gibertoni D, Rossi A, Rocca P, Bertolino A, Bucci P, Hellemann G, Spisto M, Palumbo D, Aguglia E, Amodeo G, Amore M, Bellomo A, Brugnoli R, Carpiniello B, Dell'osso L, Di Fabio F, Di Giannantonio M, Di Lorenzo G, Marchesi C, Monteleone P, Montemagni C, Oldani L, Romano R, Roncone R, Stratta P, Tenconi E, Vita A, Zeppegno P, Maj M, Italian Network for Research On Psychosis (2018) Familial aggregation of MATRICS consensus cognitive battery scores in a large sample of outpatients with schizophrenia and their unaffected relatives. Psychol Med 48:1359–1366

Nuechterlein KH, Green MF (2006) MATRICS consensus cognitive battery. MATRICS Assessment, Inc.

Nuechterlein KH, Green MF (2016) MATRICS consensus cognitive battery manual, 3rd edn. MATRICS Assessment, Inc.

Nuechterlein KH, Barch DM, Gold JM, Goldberg TE, Green MF, Heaton RK (2004) Identification of separable cognitive factors in schizophrenia. Schizophr Res 72:29–39

Nuechterlein KH, Green MF, Kern RS, Baade LE, Barch DM, Cohen JD, Essock S, Fenton WS, Frese FJ 3rd, Gold JM, Goldberg T, Heaton RK, Keefe RS, Kraemer H, Mesholam-Gately R, Seidman LJ, Stover E, Weinberger DR, Young AS, Zalcman S, Marder SR (2008) The MATRICS consensus cognitive battery, part 1: test selection, reliability, and validity. Am J Psychiatr 165:203–213

Nuechterlein KH, Ventura J, Subotnik KL, Gretchen-Doorly D, Turner LR, Casaus LR, Luo J, Boucher ML, Hayata JN, Bell MD, Medalia A (2020) A randomized controlled trial of cognitive remediation and long-acting injectable risperidone after a first episode of schizophrenia: improving cognition and work/school functioning. Psychol Med:1–10

Nuechterlein KH, McEwen SC, Ventura J, Subotnik KL, Turner LR, Boucher M, Casaus LR, Distler MD, Hayata JN (2022) Aerobic exercise enhances cognitive training effects in first episode schizophrenia: randomized clinical trial demonstrates cognitive and functional gains. Psychol Med:1–11

Rodriguez-Jimenez R, Dompablo M, Bagney A, Santabarbara J, Aparicio AI, Torio I, Moreno-Ortega M, Lopez-Anton R, Lobo A, Kern RS, Green MF, Jimenez-Arriero MA, Santos JL, Nuechterlein KH, Palomo T (2015) The MCCB impairment profile in a Spanish sample of patients with schizophrenia: effects of diagnosis, age, and gender on cognitive functioning. Schizophr Res 169:116–120

Rodriguez-Jimenez R, Santos JL, Dompablo M, Santabarbara J, Aparicio AI, Olmos R, Jimenez-Lopez E, Sanchez-Morla E, Lobo A, Palomo T, Kern RS, Green MF, Nuechterlein KH, Garcia-Fernandez L (2019) MCCB cognitive profile in Spanish first episode schizophrenia patients. Schizophr Res 211:88–92

Sinkeviciute I, Begemann M, Prikken M, Oranje B, Johnsen E, Lei WU, Hugdahl K, Kroken RA, Rau C, Jacobs JD, Mattaroccia S, Sommer IE (2018) Efficacy of different types of cognitive enhancers for patients with schizophrenia: a meta-analysis. NPJ Schizophr 4:22

Young AS, Forquer SL, Tran A, Starzynski M, Shatkin J (2000) Identifying clinical competencies that support rehabilitation and empowerment in individuals with severe mental illness. J Behav Health Serv Res 27:321–333

Cognitive [Computational] Neuroscience Test Reliability and Clinical Applications for Serious Mental Illness (CNTRaCS) Consortium: Progress and Future Directions

Deanna M. Barch, Megan Ann Boudewyn, Cameron C. Carter, Molly Erickson, Michael J. Frank, James M. Gold, Steven J. Luck, Angus W. MacDonald III, J. Daniel Ragland, Charan Ranganath, Steven M. Silverstein, and Andy Yonelinas

Contents

D. M. Barch (✉)
Department of Psychological & Brain Sciences, Washington University in St. Louis, St. Louis, MO, USA
e-mail: dbarch@wustl.edu

M. A. Boudewyn
University of California, Santa Cruz, CA, USA

C. C. Carter, S. J. Luck, J. D. Ragland, C. Ranganath, and A. Yonelinas
University of California, Davis, CA, USA

M. Erickson
University of Chicago, Chicago, IL, USA

M. J. Frank
Brown University, Providence, RI, USA

J. M. Gold
Maryland Psychiatric Research Center, Baltimore, MD, USA

A. W. MacDonald III
University of Minnesota, Minneapolis, MN, USA

S. M. Silverstein
University of Rochester, Rochester, NY, USA

Curr Topics Behav Neurosci (2023) 63: 19–60
https://doi.org/10.1007/7854_2022_391
Published Online: 30 September 2022

Abstract The development of treatments for impaired cognition in schizophrenia has been characterized as the most important challenge facing psychiatry at the beginning of the twenty-first century. The Cognitive Neuroscience Treatment Research to Improve Cognition in Schizophrenia (CNTRICS) project was designed to build on the potential benefits of using tasks and tools from cognitive neuroscience to better understanding and treat cognitive impairments in psychosis. These benefits include: (1) the use of fine-grained tasks that measure discrete cognitive processes; (2) the ability to design tasks that distinguish between specific cognitive domain deficits and poor performance due to generalized deficits resulting from sedation, low motivation, poor test taking skills, etc.; and (3) the ability to link cognitive deficits to specific neural systems, using animal models, neuropsychology, and functional imaging. CNTRICS convened a series of meetings to identify paradigms from cognitive neuroscience that maximize these benefits and identified the steps need for translation into use in clinical populations. The *Cognitive Neuroscience Test Reliability and Clinical Applications for Schizophrenia (CNTRaCS) Consortium* was developed to help carry out these steps. CNTRaCS consists of investigators at five different sites across the country with diverse expertise relevant to a wide range of the cognitive systems identified as critical as part of CNTRICs. This work reports on the progress and current directions in the evaluation and optimization carried out by CNTRaCS of the tasks identified as part of the original CNTRICs process, as well as subsequent extensions into the Positive Valence systems domain of Research Domain Criteria (RDoC). We also describe the current focus of CNTRaCS, which involves taking a computational psychiatry approach to measuring cognitive and motivational function across the spectrum of psychosis. Specifically, the current iteration of CNTRaCS is using computational modeling to isolate parameters reflecting potentially more specific cognitive and visual processes that may provide greater interpretability in understanding shared and distinct impairments across psychiatric disorders.

Keywords CNTRaCS · CNTRICS · Cognitive neuroscience · Positive valence systems · Schizophrenia

Cognitive impairments in schizophrenia are present prior to illness onset (see Karcher et al.'s chapter in this volume), persist throughout the lifespan, are associated with poor outcome and functional disability, and are largely treatment refractory. Hence, development of treatments for impaired cognition in schizophrenia has been characterized as the most important challenge facing psychiatry at the beginning of the twenty-first century (Carter and Barch 2007). The past several decades have seen a rapidly growing understanding of the neurobiology and neuropharmacology of cognition, and research has identified many molecular targets for enhancing cognitive processing in schizophrenia and other psychiatric disorders (Arnsten 2004; Friedman 2004; Lewis et al. 2004; Martin et al. 2004; Moghaddam 2004; Roth et al. 2004; Tamminga 2006). However, despite this growing knowledge, there was no established mechanism for developing cognitive enhancing drugs for schizophrenia until the National Institute of Mental Health (NIMH)-funded Measurement and Treatment Research to Improve Cognition in Schizophrenia (MATRICS, see Nuechterlein et al.'s chapter in this volume) initiative was created. The MATRICS (Green et al. 2004; Marder and Fenton 2004) process brought together academia, the pharmaceutical industry, and the Food and Drug Administration to: (1) identify cognitive domain targets in schizophrenia; (2) identify promising molecular targets to enhance those cognitive domains; and (3) develop a process by which new therapeutic agents could be approved for the treatment of cognition in schizophrenia.

One of the challenges MATRICS faced was the need to produce a consensus based set of cognitive measures quickly. Thus, MATRICS selected standardized tests with well-known and strong measurement properties (test-retest reliability, low practice effects, etc.). As such, the measurement approach in the MATRICS battery primarily reflects the experience of the field with clinical neuropsychological tests used in the clinical trials of atypical antipsychotics during the 1980s and 1990s. Measures derived from cognitive neuroscience were considered, but were not included primarily because they did not have already established measurement properties. The Cognitive Neuroscience Treatment Research to Improve Cognition in Schizophrenia (CNTRICS) project grew out of the final MATRICS meeting, where the potential benefits of using tasks and tools from cognitive neuroscience were broadly acknowledged. These benefits include: (1) the use of fine-grained tasks that measure discrete cognitive processes; (2) the ability to design tasks that distinguish between specific cognitive domain deficits and poor performance due to generalized deficits resulting from sedation, low motivation, poor test taking skills, etc.; and (3) the ability to link cognitive deficits to specific neural systems, using animal models, neuropsychology, and functional imaging. Measuring the function of specific cognitive systems linked to specific neural systems using a cognitive neuroscience approach offers unique advantages, especially for translational research. One of the key advantages is the ability to use the results of animal as well as human studies to *identify* molecular targets that modulate specific cognitive systems. Many such targetable systems, such as working memory and episodic memory (WM and EM, respectively), attention, perceptual processing, and cognitive control are conserved across many mammalian species and measurable using parallel versions of experimental cognitive tasks. CNTRICS was developed collaboratively with the leadership of the NIMH including Drs. Robert Heinssen, Director Tom Insel, and the late Wayne Fenton and supported by two R13 conference grants.

At the first meeting, CNTRICS identified a set of constructs across six cognitive systems to be targeted (Carter and Barch 2007; Carter et al. 2008), including executive control, WM, EM, attention, and perception. At the second meeting measurement issues were laid out together with strategies for addressing them in future research (Barch and Carter 2008). At the third meeting tasks were identified that were promising measures of these cognitive systems (Barch et al. 2009a, b). Task selection was guided by the following principles: (1) tasks have strong construct validity from cognitive neuroscience as measures of the cognitive processes to be targeted; (2) there are strong data from cognitive neuroscience linking the processes engaged by the task to specific neural systems; (3) the tasks have designs that will allow us to distinguish between a specific cognitive deficit and a generalized deficit; (4) tasks are readily incorporated into functional imaging (EEG and fMRI) studies that can measure medication effects on cognition related brain activity; (5) tasks assay distinct neural systems, and provide coverage of deficits in both early "bottom-up" and later "top-down" processes in order to enhance the utility of these tools for different pharmacological agents; and (6) where possible tasks have the possibility for use across-species. These tasks are known to be sensitive to deficits in schizophrenia, though in some cases the tasks needed to be studied using new parameters designed to meet the six properties outlined above.

After initial CNTRICS meetings, the NIMH issued a Request for Proposals to fund research that would optimize and psychometrically evaluate these tasks identified through the CNTRICs process. In response to this call, the *Cognitive Neuroscience Test Reliability and Clinical Applications for Schizophrenia (CNTRaCS) Consortium* was developed consisting of investigators at five different sites across the country with diverse expertise relevant to a wide range of the cognitive systems identified as critical as part of CNTRICs. These five sites were Washington University in St. Louis (led by Deanna Barch), Maryland Psychiatric Research Center (led by Jim Gold), Rutgers University (led by Steve Silverstein), the University of California at Davis (led by Cameron Carter and Daniel Ragland), and the University of Minnesota (led by Angus MacDonald). Here, we report on the progress and current directions in the evaluation and optimization carried out by CNTRaCS of the tasks identified as part of the original CNTRICs process, as well as subsequent extensions into the Positive Valence systems domain of Research Domain Criteria (RDoC). All tasks and a description of the validation process are available for download at https://cntracs.ucdavis.edu/. We end by discussing the current focus of CNTRaCS, which involves taking a computational psychiatry approach to measuring cognitive and motivational function across the spectrum of psychosis. Specifically, the current iteration of CNTRaCS is using computational modeling to isolate parameters reflecting potentially more specific cognitive and visual processes that may provide greater interpretability in understanding shared and distinct impairments across psychiatric disorders.

1 Goal Maintenance

We define goal maintenance as processes involved in activating task related goals or rules based on endogenous or exogenous cues, actively representing them in a highly accessible form, and maintaining this information over an interval during which that information is needed to bias and constrain attention and response selection (Cohen and Servan-Schreiber 1992; Kane and Engle 2000, 2002, 2003; Kane et al. 2001a, b; Miller and Cohen 2001; Engle and Kane 2004; Barch et al. 2009a, b). Goals also include task set representations that help determine what information is relevant for the current contents of WM, also referred to as "context" information (Cohen and

Servan-Schreiber 1992). Active goal maintenance has been linked to the function of dorsolateral prefrontal cortex (DLPFC), with additional work implicating dopaminergic inputs to DLPFC are critical as well (though recent work has also specified an important role for both glutamate (Durstewitz and Gabriel 2007) and norepinephrine (Arnsten 2004)). Such mechanisms by which goals could be actively maintained and bias ongoing information processing have been explicitly implemented in biologically plausible computational models designed to formalize the interactions between prefrontal and basal ganglia systems in goal maintenance (Braver et al. 1995; Anderson et al. 1996; Just et al. 1996; Braver and Cohen 2000; Miller and Cohen 2001; Hazy et al. 2007; Collins and Frank 2013). Further, a number of functional imaging studies revealed activation of DLPFC when individuals are required to maintain goals in WM (Barch et al. 1997; MacDonald et al. 2000; Passingham and Sakai 2004; Fassbender et al. 2006). Thus, this construct has confirmed validity at both the psychological and neural levels of analysis.

As previously reviewed (Barch et al. 2009a, b), numerous studies provide evidence that both medicated and unmedicated individuals with schizophrenia have difficulties with goal maintenance, at both acute and chronic stages of the illness (Servan-Schreiber et al. 1996a, b; Schooler et al. 1997; Stratta et al. 1998; Cohen et al. 1999; Javitt et al. 2000; Stratta et al. 2000; Barch et al. 2001; Chen et al. 2001; Henik et al. 2002; Bagner et al. 2003; MacDonald and Carter 2003; Barch et al. 2004a, b; Henik and Salo 2004; Holmes et al. 2005; Ettinger et al. 2006; Lee and Park 2006; Radant et al. 2007; Wilde et al. 2007). In addition, goal maintenance deficits are found in first-degree relatives of individuals with schizophrenia (MacDonald et al. 2003; Calkins et al. 2004; Delawalla et al. 2007), and in individuals with schizotypal personality disorder (Barch et al. 2004a, b; Calkins et al. 2004), indicative of a potential genetic and broad-based underlying mechanisms. This construct was identified for measurement development for three of the six domains addressed by CNTRICS ((attention, WM, and executive functions (Carter et al. 2008)). That is, deficits in goal maintenance were thought to be responsible for many of the impairments observed across attention, WM, and executive control in schizophrenia, suggesting that this may be a critical core deficit in the illness (Carter et al. 2008).

One task used to understand the psychological and neural mechanisms underlying goal maintenance is the expectancy manipulation of the traditional AX-CPT (Servan-Schreiber et al. 1996a, b), which has been used in both its original form (AX-CPT) and in a form (called the dot pattern expectancy task, or DPX, see below) that uses non-verbal stimuli (reducing confounds associated with native language and literacy, and decrease administration time (MacDonald et al. 2005a, b)). In the expectancy AX-CPT, participants view a series of letters one at a time. They respond with the non-target button to every letter except X when it follows an A, which requires a target response. The vast majority of trials are A-then-X trials, creating a prepotent pattern of responding. Whether the cue was an A or any other letter (hereafter called B) provided the context for preparing a response. In BX trials, which occurred ~10% of the time, the B provided the context that the subsequent X was not a target, although generally X's are valid targets. Individuals with schizophrenia had difficulty representing and maintaining this context and were more likely to be lured into mistaking this invalid X for a target (BX maintenance error). Thus, this condition tested the ability to maintain crucial goal information. In AY trials, which also occurred ~10% of the time, the A provided the context that the subsequent stimulus was likely to be a valid target. When any invalid probe occurred (hereafter Y), individuals who have prepared for a target response have to overcome that prepared response. Thus, the expectancy AX task can produce a double-dissociation in performance whereby individuals with a goal maintenance deficit show impaired performance on BX trials, whereas those with intact goal maintenance but poor cognitive control perform poorly on AY trials.

CPT paradigms are domain general, and any number of stimuli can be defined as valid cues or probes. A limitation of using letter stimuli is that a very strong prepotency, many trials, and a longer cue-probe delay are required to identify a specific deficit associated with schizophrenia. Such tasks can take up to 45 min (Cohen et al. 1999; MacDonald et al. 2003). This limitation may be related to the ease with which over-learned letter stimuli are stored. Thus, we developed the DPX, which uses under-learned dot pattern stimuli (originally based on Braille letter patterns). The DPX had the added advantage of making AY trials harder for controls, thereby increasing the likelihood that differences the BX condition would be interpretable as a specific deficit in goal maintenance (MacDonald et al. 2005a, b). Confirmatory factor analysis supported the convergent validity of the letter version of the expectancy AX and the formally equivalent DPX (MacDonald et al. 2005a, b).

CNTRaCS chose this DPX paradigm because it fulfills the criteria the field (in CNTRICS Meeting two), identified as important for task selection (Barch et al. 2009a, b). The AX-CPT was discussed during MATRICS as a candidate task but due to its long duration of administration and unknown psychometric properties further consideration was deferred. CNTRaCS compared five DPX versions that manipulated the strength of prepotency and the length of the interstimulus interval (ISI) between cues and probes. As shown in Fig. 1, results indicated that the best compromise between task duration and interpretability occurred on a version with a short ISI (2,000 ms vs. 4,000 ms) and a strong prepotency (69% "AX" trials, which elicited clear deficits in both schizophrenia and schizoaffective disorder (Henderson et al. 2012). This version of the task correlated with negative symptoms, daily living skills, and functional status (Gold et al. 2012a, b). In addition, a subsequent CNTRaCS test-retest study indicated that the optimized DPX shows acceptable internal consistency (Henderson et al. 2012) and good to excellent test-retest reliability (Strauss et al. 2014), as well as modest practice effects. In addition, there is a version of the DPX for use in primates (Blackman et al. 2016).

In subsequent work, CNTRaCS was funded to develop the DPX (and AX-CPT) into imaging biomarkers that could be used to assess the neural systems supporting goal maintenance and identify the neural correlations of impairments in goal maintenance. The signature of goal maintenance is activation of DLPFC (BA 9/46) in conditions where active representation is necessary for task appropriate behavior, as seen in numerous AC-CPT studies (Barch et al. 1997; Braver and Bongiolatti 2002). Individuals with schizophrenia also show consistent evidence of impaired prefrontal

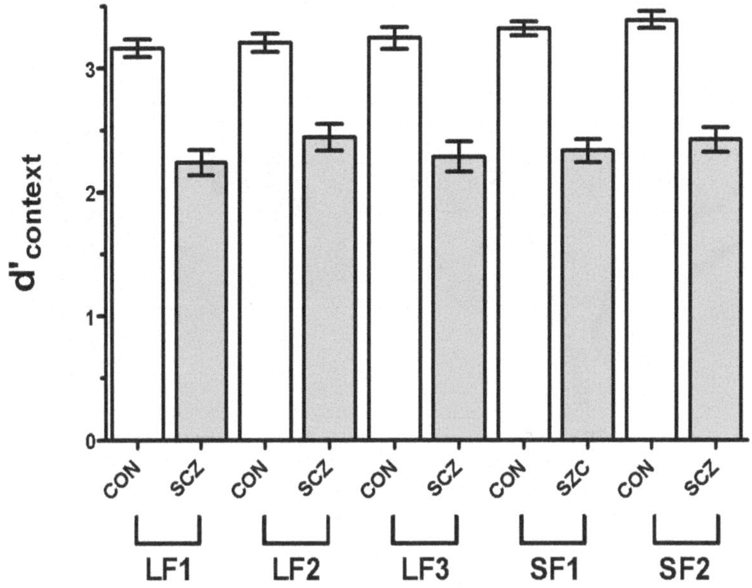

Fig. 1 Mean and standard error of d'$_{context}$ for patient and control groups for each of five DPX tasks. LF1 (long form 1) and SF1 (short form 1) had 69%, LF2 and SF2 62%, and LF3 58% AX trials. Reprinted with permission from Henderson et al. (2012)

activity, particularly in DLFPC regions, during tasks requiring goal maintenance (Barch et al. 2001; Holmes et al. 2005; MacDonald et al. 2005a, b; Harrison et al. 2006; Tu et al. 2006; Van Snellenberg et al. 2006). Again, first-degree relatives of individuals with schizophrenia also showed impaired DLPFC activation during goal maintenance (MacDonald et al. 2006; Delawalla et al. 2007). Evidence from the CNTRaCS Imaging Biomarker study indicated that both of the CNTRaCS AX-CPT and DPX tasks robustly engage the frontal-parietal network in conditions that require the use of goal information to guide behavior (Lopez-Garcia et al. 2016). Consistent with early work using the AX-CPT (Barch et al. 1999, 2001; Holmes et al. 2005; MacDonald et al. 2005a, b), as shown in Fig. 2, the CNTRaCS imaging DPX robustly identified reduced activation in dorsal frontal and parietal regions among individuals with schizophrenia (Poppe et al. 2016). Thus, the DPX provides a novel symbol-agnostic method to measure DLPFC activity during goal maintenance in individuals and is sensitive to deficits in individuals with schizophrenia.

2 Relational Encoding and Retrieval in Episodic Memory

Another cognitive domain identified by CNTRICS is that of EM, specifically relational encoding and retrieval. EM depends on representations that link together information about items and the context that they were encountered in, as well as

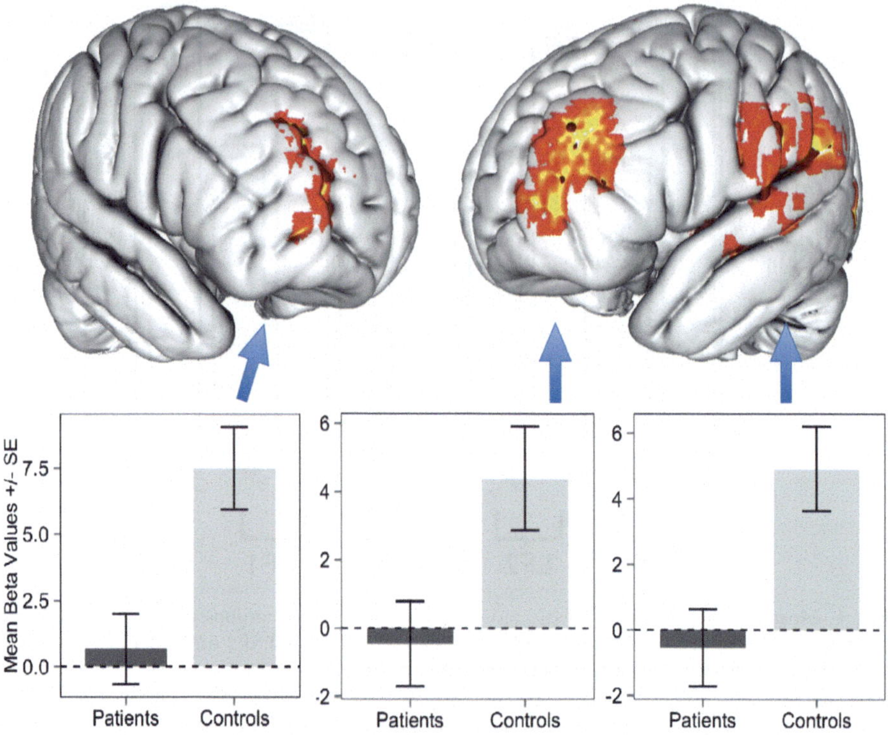

Fig. 2 Whole brain functional magnetic resonance imaging (fMRI) GLM results. Beta values represent B Cues – A Cues contrast. Regions with greater activation in healthy controls (HC) than schizophrenia (SCHIZOPHRENIA; 3 clusters). Reprinted with permission Poppe et al. (2016)

strategies that help us form these representations. For instance, one can use "item-specific" encoding strategies that focus attention on distinctive aspects of particular items (e.g., pleasantness or animacy judgments), or "relational" encoding strategies that focus attention on relationships between items encountered at a particular moment (e.g., imagine two items interacting, or link two or more words in the context of a sentence or story (Bower 1970a, b; Hunt and Einsten 1981; Hunt and McDaniel 1993)). Relative to item-specific processing, relational processing disproportionately depends on DLPFC (Postle et al. 1999), and engagement of the DLPFC during relational WM processing predicts successful EM for inter-item associations (Blumenfeld and Ranganath 2006, 2007; Murray and Ranganath 2007). There is near consensus that the hippocampus is essential for EM, supporting recollection of contextual information associated with specific items, particularly relationships between items (Ranganath 2010). Available evidence, therefore, indicates that the construct of relational encoding and retrieval has validity at both cognitive and neural levels of analysis and is supported by both hippocampal- and DLPFC mediated mechanisms.

Individuals with schizophrenia have pronounced EM impairment (Heinrichs and Zakzanis 1998; Aleman et al. 1999; Ranganath 2010), with evidence of hippocampal abnormalities (Heckers and Konradi 2010; Benes 2015; Roeske et al. 2021), but the pattern is task-dependent (Pelletier et al. 2005). Like frontal lobe lesion individual, individuals with schizophrenia become more impaired as retrieval tasks become less structured. Meta-analytic reviews demonstrate moderate-to-large effect sizes of schizophrenia on free recall tasks, medium effects on cued recall tasks, and lesser impairments during recognition testing (Paulsen et al. 1995; Aleman et al. 1999). Individuals with schizophrenia also fail to spontaneously use item-specific semantic information to categorize related word lists during initial encoding (Gold et al. 1992; Paulsen et al. 1995; Iddon et al. 1998). This failure appears due to difficulty self-generating item-specific organizational strategies rather than lack of semantic knowledge (Brebion et al. 1997; Iddon et al. 1998; Stone et al. 1998), since recognition can be remediated by instructing individuals to make semantic decisions about individual words on a learning list (McClain 1983; Brebion et al. 1997; Stone et al. 1998; Ragland et al. 2003; Bonner-Jackson et al. 2005). However, individuals with schizophrenia continue to show impairment on tasks that require relational encoding (Titone et al. 2004; Ongur et al. 2006) and may not benefit from being provided with a relational encoding strategy, either because of specific difficulties implementing DLPFC relational control functions (Ragland et al. 2007) or because of impaired hippocampally-mediated binding functions (Heckers et al. 1998; Weiss et al. 2003; Heckers 2004; Weiss et al. 2004).

Many cognitive neuroscience paradigms designed to assess relational encoding and retrieval suffer from a problem that limits their application to clinical populations – they leave the nature of the encoding strategy up to the individual, opening the possibility that poor task performance simply reflects a failure to apply relational processing, rather than a fundamental deficit in the ability to engage in such processing. Ranganath and colleagues developed a task to investigate cognitive and neural mechanisms underlying relational encoding and retrieval (Blumenfeld and Ranganath 2006) that explicitly controls the type of relational processing in which participants engage. This paradigm did a good job meeting the CNTRICS selection criteria of strong construct validity, a specific neural mechanism, and appropriateness for functional imaging.

As shown in Fig. 3, CNTRaCS created a variation of the Ranganath paradigm named the relational and item-specific encoding and retrieval task (RiSE). This task manipulated encoding by requiring participants to decide whether stimuli are "living/nonliving" (item-specific) or whether one stimulus fits inside the other (relational). This task also allows one to estimate familiarity (F) and recollection (R) by examining receiver operator characteristics (ROC) and assessing item (old or new judgment) and associative (were these items presented together or not) recognition. CNTRaCS compared word and object versions of the RiSE, with objects more effective in identifying impairments in relational encoding and retrieval in schizophrenia. Specifically, CNTRACS studies (Ragland et al. 2012) confirmed that individuals with schizophrenia had a disproportionate recognition deficit following relational-versus item-specific encoding, most striking for familiarity-based

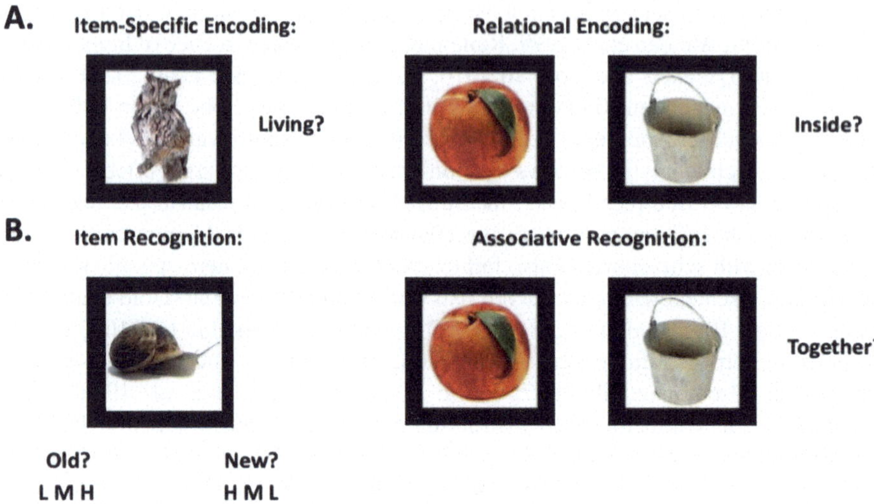

Fig. 3 Illustration of item-specific and relational test procedures and task stimuli. (**a**) Memory encoding, (**b**) Memory retrieval. Reprinted with permission from Ragland et al. (2012)

retrieval. Moreover, RiSE performance was positively correlated with functional abilities and had good internal consistency, retest reliability (more so for item than associative recognition), and good alternate-form reliability (Ragland et al. 2012). Further, CNTRaCS created three parallel versions of the RiSE with good psychometric properties to enable repeated testing. Thus, this task is useful for both group studies, individual differences, and treatment studies.

Like goal maintenance, CNTRaCS was supported to create a version of the RiSE task for use as an imaging biomarker measure. Murray and Ranganath (Murray and Ranganath 2007) found that activity in the DLPFC was higher during relational than item-specific encoding and specifically predicted successful memory for associations amongst items. Activity in the VLPFC also increased for relational encoding, but was nonspecific and predicted success in item-specific and associative recognition conditions. This work suggests that DLPFC may contribute to EM through its role in active processing of relationships during encoding and that DLPFC will show greater activation in relational than item encoding. In contrast, the VLPFC may have a more general role in encoding processes for both relational and item encoding (Blumenfeld and Ranganath 2007). The RiSE was also designed to reveal anatomical dissociations within the medial temporal lobe by examining separate components of episodic retrieval. The hippocampus and parahippocampal cortex (PHC) play central roles in creating memories of the relationships between specific items and the context in which they were encountered (Eichenbaum et al. 2007; Ranganath 2010) and then retrieving these contextual details to support associative recognition or recollection of the event (Davachi 2006). As shown in Fig. 4 and described above, consistent with these hypotheses, we found that relational versus item-specific encoding activated both DLPFC and VLPFC prefrontal cortex, but activity was

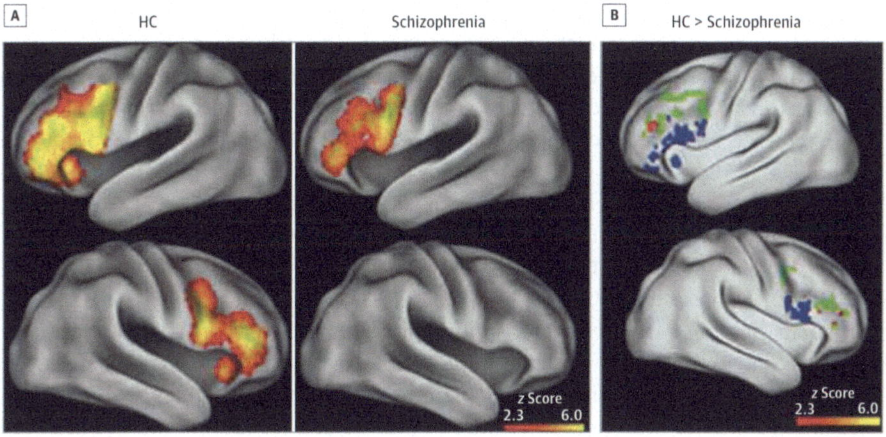

Fig. 4 Brain activation in RiSE task in schizophrenia. (**a**) Surface rendering of left (top) and right (bottom) hemisphere PFC activation shown separately for healthy controls (HC) and individuals with schizophrenia. Hotter colors reflect greater activation (range, $z = 2.3$-6.0). (**b**) Significant group differences (HC-schizophrenia) in dorsolateral PFC activation during relational versus item-specific encoding in left (top) and right (bottom) hemispheres. Group differences are indicated in red, with hotter colors reflecting greater activation (range, z 2.3-6.0) and are overlaid on dorsolateral PFC (green) and ventrolateral PFC (blue) regions of interest to illustrate the regional specificity of prefrontal dysfunction in schizophrenia. Reprinted with permission from Ragland et al. (2012)

reduced in schizophrenia relative to healthy controls only in the DLPFC (Ragland et al. 2015). Retrieval success (hits > misses) was associated with activation of the hippocampus in controls during associative recognition and item recognition following relational encoding and was reduced in individuals with schizophrenia for item recognition following relational encoding. Thus, these data support the construct validity of the RiSE in revealing expected DLPFC and medial temporal lobe memory effects during specific encoding and retrieval conditions. Group differences support the presence of a disproportionate memory deficit in schizophrenia for relational versus item-specific information, accompanied by regionally and functionally specific deficits in DLPFC and hippocampus activation.

3 Gain Control

A critical component of perception highlighted at the first CNTRICS meeting was gain control, which refers to processes that amplify or attenuate overall levels of neural activity to optimize operation of systems with limited, dynamic signaling range. Sensory gain control operates via intracellular mechanisms, direct excitatory and inhibitory connections between neurons, and feedback. Gain control mechanisms have been demonstrated using various behavioral tasks, including those involving pop-out phenomena (where neurons coding similar features inhibit each other, leading to increased salience of a single different element) (Derrington 1996), effects of surrounding contrast on contrast thresholds (Chubb et al. 1989), texture segregation (where texture elements near texture borders are increased in salience) (Nothdurft et al. 2000), and figure-ground segregation (Lamme 1995). Moreover, there is convergence between theoretical work (e.g., Heeger 1992), psychophysical studies (e.g., Foley 1994), electrophysiology (Bonds 1989, 1991), and functional MRI (Zenger-Landolt and Heeger 2003), in supporting the existence of gain control mechanisms and their effects on neurons in the visual cortex.

Gain control impairments in individuals with schizophrenia are found for both vision (e.g., Yeap et al. 2006) and audition (e.g., Javitt et al. 1997). For example, individuals demonstrate less visual suppression (as assessed by contrast sensitivity functions) due to the effects of surrounding contrast (Dakin et al. 2005; Linares et al. 2020). In addition, individuals with schizophrenia show clear, magnocellular (M)-pathway dysfunction, typically as assessed by either contrast sensitivity or backward masking functions (Cadenhead et al. 1998; Slaghuis and Thompson 2003; Keri et al. 2004; Butler et al. 2005, 2007; Kim et al. 2005, 2006a, b). The M-pathway has several properties (speed of processing, low spatial resolution) that suggest it is a physiological substrate for gain control (Lennie 1980) so that deficits in M-processing may be the physiological basis for gain control abnormalities in schizophrenia. Mechanisms of gain control dysfunction also include NMDA and GABA-ergic dysfunction. Indeed, NMDA dysfunction appears to be linked to gain control in the M-pathway, and it is linked to schizophrenia (Javitt and Zukin 1991). There is also evidence that gain control deficits are important in outcome. For instance, impaired contrast detection in steady-state and transient visual evoked potential studies is related to poorer functional outcome in schizophrenia as assessed with the Problem Solving Factor of the Independent Living Scales (ILS) (Schechter et al. 2005). Finally, abnormal contrast sensitivity and backward masking functions are linked to negative symptoms and poor treatment outcome in individuals with schizophrenia (Slaghuis 1998). Thus, aspects of gain control may be an important target for overall treatment in individuals with schizophrenia.

There are a number of different approaches to measuring gain control. One such approach – referred to as the Contrast-Contrast Effect task is to study the perception of contrast utilizing an illusion in which the contrast of the elements in a small target circle appears reduced when presented within a high contrast surround compared to when the same target is presented in isolation (Chubb et al. 1989). When asked to match a variable contrast patch to the central patch, controls indicated that the central patch had a substantially lower contrast than it actually did, reflecting affected gain control. Individuals with schizophrenia were less susceptible to the illusion and in fact 12 of 15 individuals were more accurate than the most-accurate control (Dakin et al. 2005). These results are consistent with decreased center-surround antagonism and hence decreased gain control in schizophrenia individuals.

Given that this approach affords the ability to rule out a generalized deficit interpretation, CNTRaCS used the Contrast-Contrast Effect task (Saccuzzo and Schubert 1981; Green and Walker 1984) in the first set of studies. More specifically, we compared versions of the Contrast-Contrast Effect task that manipulated duration and included catch trials to measure off-task performance (attention lapsing) (Barch et al. 2012). In the first CNTRaCS study using this task, we were able to replicate previous findings of reduced surround effects in schizophrenia (a putative indication of reduced gain control), but found that such effects were almost entirely accounted for by off-task performance as measured by lapses on easy catch trials. In a subsequent test-retest reliability study, the gain control task once again failed to provide evidence of impairments in schizophrenia that were independent of attention lapsing. Thus, the CNTRaCS consortium ultimately did not recommend the version of this task to assess impaired gain control in schizophrenia.

4 Visual Integration

Visual integration includes processes beyond the registration of color, orientation, motion, and depth cues that can bind these features to create higher-level, emergent, holistic, representations (i.e., shapes, and eventually objects) that are suitable to guide behavior. Integration occurs both via long-range lateral connections between feature detectors within early visual cortex areas and via recurrent innervation of visual cortex by temporal visual regions involved in object recognition, and frontal and parietal regions supporting visual attention. Integration is relevant to phenomena such as gestalt perception, object recognition, and coherent motion perception. The existence of integrative mechanisms in vision is supported by data from a variety of sources. First, animal studies (e.g., cats) using microelectrode recording demonstrate effects of information from outside of classical receptive fields on target processing (e.g., Kapadia et al. 1995). Second, psychophysical studies of perceptual organization in healthy humans (e.g., Pomerantz and Pristach 1989; Kovacs 1996) demonstrate integrative processing. Third, electrophysiological recording of healthy humans during visual integration tasks (e.g., Han et al. 2001, 2002) and fMRI studies of integration in healthy human subjects and in monkeys (e.g., Altmann et al. 2003; Kourtzi et al. 2003) all provide evidence of integrative mechanisms. Converging data from these lines of research indicate that, along the ventral visual stream from V1 to inferior and lateral temporal areas, receptive fields of cells become increasingly larger, more responsive to global stimulus features, and invariant with respect to retinotopic position of the stimulus. Data also indicate that the firing rates of these cells are increasingly more dependent on the extent to which sets of individual features possess statistical regularities indicative of a contour or shape (e.g., correlations between element orientations) (Kanwisher 2004).

Numerous studies demonstrate a reduction in visual feature integration abilities in individuals with schizophrenia (Silverstein et al. 2015a, b, 2020; Keane et al. 2016). Moreover, in several of these studies, the reduced ability to integrate information resulted in superior overall performance of the task compared to controls, in making decisions about individual features (see gain control section above). This superiority includes a reduced susceptibility to visual illusions in which the grouping of information interferes with accurate perception (Uhlhaas et al. 2006). Therefore, evidence for impairments in visual integration is convincingly demonstrated independent of a generalized deficit (Knight and Silverstein 2001). Integration impairments in individuals with schizophrenia are demonstrated with both static (Silverstein et al. 2000) and moving cues (Chen et al. 2005). Furthermore, integration impairments in schizophrenia are disease-specific/medication independent as deficits are seen in unmedicated individuals (Uhlhaas et al. 2005; Uhlhaas and Silverstein 2005), with performance not correlated with medication dose in medicated individuals (Spencer et al. 2003, 2004).

Researchers typically measure visual integration by manipulating a single stimulus parameter and determine the effect of this manipulation on the ability to perceive stimulus configurations. The most common manipulations include those of contour element orientation and contour element spacing. CNTRaCS examined a version of the task that manipulated the orientation of the elements. Specifically, participants are asked to determine which direction an egg-shaped contour, made up of Gabor elements, is pointing. Gabor elements are Gaussian-modulated sinusoidal luminance distributions that closely model the known spatial frequency processing properties of cells in area V1. Therefore, use of Gabor elements provides superior measurement of orientation sensitivity, and grouping of orientation cues, compared to stimuli with unknown effects on V1 neurons (e.g., arbitrarily constructed lines and dots). The embedded contours in stimuli utilizing Gabor elements cannot be detected by purely local filters or by known types of orientation tuned neurons with large receptive fields (e.g., Dakin and Hess 1998). The long-range orientation correlations along the path of the contour can only be found by integration of local orientation measurements into an emergent shape representation. Numerous studies using such tasks have explored the conditions under which human observers perceive or do not perceive contours. CNTRaCS refers to this task as the Jittered Orientation Visual Integration (JOVI) task. Participants press one of two keys to indicate whether the shape was leftward or rightward pointing. Trials are blocked according to the amount of orientational jitter that was added to the contour elements: ±0°, 7–8°, 11–12°, 15–16°, 19–20°, or 23–24° (see Fig. 5). An advantage of having a broad range of jitter values is that one can plot each subject's complete psychometric function – from floor to ceiling. In the first CNTRaCS study with this task, we found prominent ceiling and floor effects and there were no between-group differences in threshold or slope (Silverstein et al. 2012). In a follow-up study, we utilized a narrower range of difficulty levels (eliminating 19–20°, or 23–24°) and found that patient thresholds were worse than those of controls (Silverstein et al. 2012). This difference in performance remained even when only the first half of the trials were analyzed and when we controlled for catch trials (Silverstein et al. 2012; Strauss et al. 2013). Thus, the JOVI provides a brief (six-minute), sensitive measure of visual integration deficits in individuals with schizophrenia. Accuracy on this task shows good test-retest reliability, though threshold estimates are less optimal in terms of test-retest reliability (Strauss et al. 2013).

CNTRaCS also aided in the creation of an imaging biomarker version of the JOVI. The contour integration task has demonstrated sensitivity to visual integration deficits in both anisometropic and strabismic amblyopia, disorders where integration

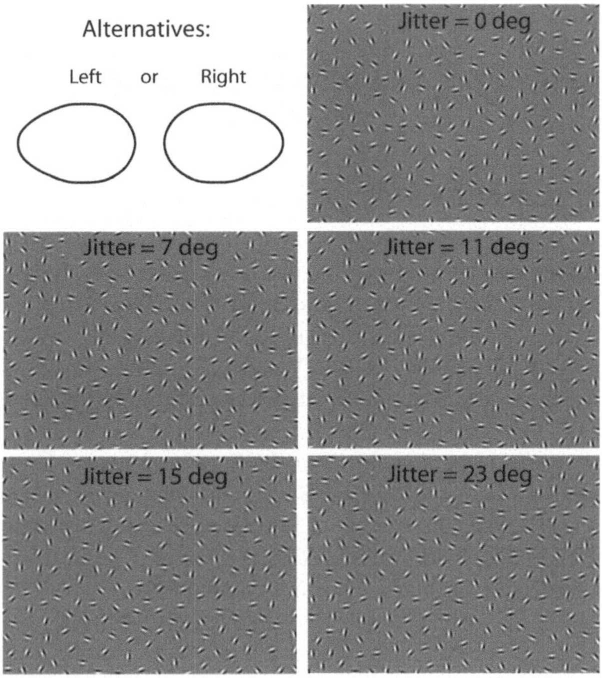

Fig. 5 Task and stimuli for JOVI experiments. Top left panel depicts the two basic shapes that subjects discriminated. Other panels show examples of stimuli from several of the conditions across the two versions of the task. The stimuli on the left are rightward pointing and those on the right are leftward pointing. Reprinted with permission from Silverstein et al. (2012)

deficits are limited to early visual cortex regions subserving the disordered eye, showing clear differences between amblyopic and fellow eyes (Kovacs et al. 2000; Chandna et al. 2001). FMRI data in humans (Altmann et al. 2003) and monkeys (Kourtzi et al. 2003) indicate a visual cortex basis for contour integration. We used a version of the JOVI for imaging with +/– 0°, 7–8°, 9–10°, 11–12°, and 13–14° trials. We also administered two types of catch trials (i.e., where no errors were expected) to ensure that all subjects were properly attending to and understanding the task. *Outline* catch trials consisted of 0° jitter stimuli with a black line tracing out the entire contour, obviating the need for integration; *no-background* catch trials also had 0°jitter, but these contained no-background noise elements (obviating the need for suppression of background noise). After covarying for number of catch trial errors, there were significant main effects of group, with overall worse performance in schizophrenia that did not vary as a function of jitter (Silverstein et al. 2015a, b). These results replicate prior studies (Kozma-Wiebe et al. 2006; Silverstein et al. 2009, 2012), in indicating that performance deficits in individuals with schizophrenia were relatively consistent across difficulty levels, with no differences between groups in early visual cortex (V1-V4). However, individuals with schizophrenia demonstrated increased (and presumably compensatory) activation across all jitter levels in the lateral occipital complex, an area critical for shape and object processing (Silverstein et al. 2015a, b; Keane et al. 2021). Individuals also demonstrated increased activation across all jitter levels in the superior parietal lobules, a region involved in binding of visual features and in distribution of visual-spatial attention.

Thus, the JOVI captures visual integration deficits in individuals with schizophrenia and reveals potential new regions of interest as biomarkers of deficits, including the lateral occipital complex and superior parietal lobules.

5 CNTRaCS Phase Two

After completing work on the tasks described above, the CNTRaCS consortium moved toward conducting similar work with new paradigms measuring additional features of the RdoCs Cognitive Systems, namely WM, plus constructs included as part of the RdoCs Positive Valence Systems. While task selection for the Positive Valence system domain had not gone through the same selection process as originally conducted for CNTRICS, CNTRaCS used the same principles in selecting measures to be examined for the Positive Valence Systems domain. Further, in the second phase of CNTRaCS, patient populations expanded to include individuals with Bipolar Disorder with Psychotic features to better understand transdiagnostic impairments within the psychosis spectrum, so at this time we changed the "S" in CNTRaCS to stand for Serious Mental Illness.

6 Working Memory

WM continues to be one of the most well-studied cognitive domains in schizophrenia (Lee and Park 2005; Forbes et al. 2009; Grot et al. 2014; Zhang et al. 2016; Liu et al. 2021) and is highlighted as part of the RdoCs Cognitive Systems domain. Importantly, there is a rich body of work examining both the psychological and neurobiological mechanisms that underlie WM (Goldman-Rakic 1995), with a general consensus that there are a number of different subcomponents of WM that may have dissociable neural mechanisms (Cowan 1988; Baddeley 2000). A common definition of WM is that it refers to the maintenance and manipulation of information over a short period of time (up to ~30 s), serving as a temporary workspace (e.g., a "mental blackboard") supporting complex cognitive operations. This maintained information can be either specific stimuli or task goals used to guide the current action plan, and the contents of WM can be protected from interference due to either distracting information or decay over time.

Many studies demonstrate that individuals with schizophrenia exhibit deficits on a wide range of WM tasks and that these deficits are associated with functional impairments in neural circuits that support WM (Lee and Park 2005; Forbes et al. 2009; Grot et al. 2014; Zhang et al. 2016; Liu et al. 2021). Given the body of work on WM in schizophrenia, CNTRICS initially identified measures of two aspects of WM as ready for immediate translation for development and use in clinical trials in schizophrenia: (1) Goal Maintenance (see above); and (2) Interference Control. *Goal Maintenance* was defined as: "The processes involved in activating task related goals or rules based on endogenous or exogenous cues, actively representing them in a highly accessible form, and maintaining this information over an interval during which that information is needed to bias and constrain attention and response selection." *Interference Control* was defined as: "The processes involved in protecting the contents of WM from interference from either other competing internal representations or external stimuli." As described above, the first set of CNTRaCS projects focused on goal maintenance, and work by other investigators, see chapter "Working Memory in People with Schizophrenia" Luck and Gold, focused on interference control in relationship to attention, another RdoCs cognitive systems domain. However, as new data continued to emerge, CNTRaCS Phase Two turned to the critical issue of WM capacity, a construct highlighted at the first RdoC cognitive systems meeting and CNTRICs. WM capacity is sharply limited (typically 3–5 simple objects (Cowan 2010)). Individual differences in WM capacity are robustly correlated with a range of higher order cognitive abilities including IQ, fluid reasoning, language comprehension, and cognitive control (Brewin and Beaton 2002; Unsworth et al. 2009; Fukuda et al. 2010; Gold et al. 2010). Thus, pathological reductions in WM capacity should be expected to have widespread negative consequences. In the domain of WM capacity, Gold and Luck used change detection tasks in several experiments to show that individuals with schizophrenia demonstrate sizeable and replicable WM capacity impairments (Gold et al. 2002, 2006, 2010), typically manifest as a downward shift in a computed measure of capacity ("K"). Such K scores are substantially correlated with neuropsychological performance as indexed by the MATRICS total score ($N = 76$, $r = 0.52$). Although perceptual deficits might artifactually lead to the appearance of reduced capacity in many WM tasks (Haenschel et al. 2007; Dias et al. 2011), robust patient deficits can be observed in variants of this task when perceptual ability is factored out (Gold et al. 2010).

Visual change detection tasks provide a purer estimate of storage capacity than many traditional WM tests (Cowan 2010). Participants are shown a brief "sample array" (100–200 ms) containing N items (e.g., 5 color patches; see Fig. 6). After a short delay (~1,000 ms), subjects are shown a "test array" that is either identical to the sample or includes an item that has changed. Participants must indicate whether a change is detected. An ideal subject with a storage capacity of "K" items will be 100% correct when $N <= K$. As N increases above K, there is increasing probability that the changed item is not in memory, so accuracy declines. Capacity (K) can be robustly measured from task performance.

In the second set of CNTRaCS projects, we also used the *multiple change detection task, which was* developed to address two problems that are acute in animal paradigms (Gibson et al. 2011). First, subjects may have occasional lapses of attention, leading to random responding. Our previous CNTRaCS studies indicated that such lapses can dramatically impair the construct validity of a measure (Barch et al. 2012). Second, larger set sizes are more difficult and subjects may exert less effort as "N" increases. Both factors would artificially decrease the estimated capacity for a subject. To address these issues, the multiple change detection task keeps *N* constant at one value (e.g., 5 items), while varying unpredictably the number of items that change. Again, subjects simply report whether a change was

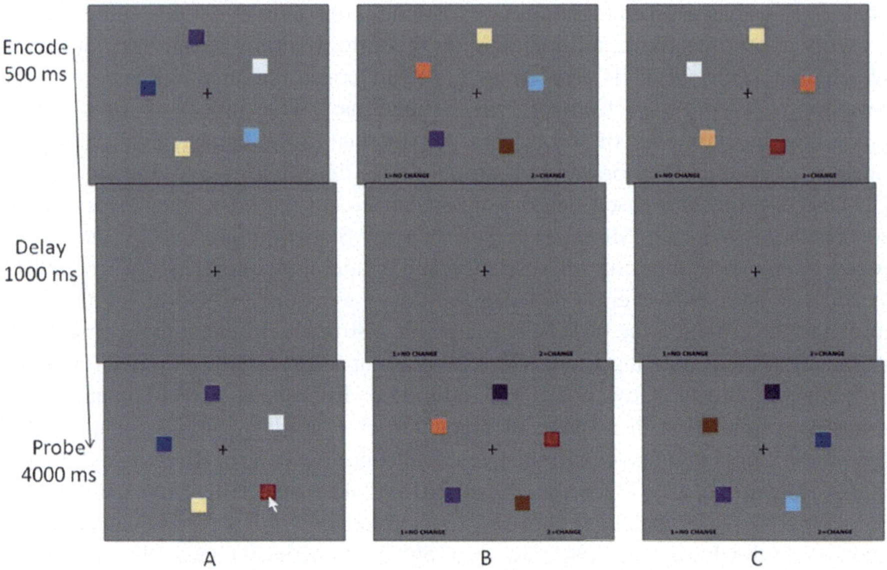

Fig. 6 Illustration (not to scale) of the Change Localization (**a**) and Multiple Change Detection tasks (**b**, **c**). In Change Localization a single item (circled) always differed between the encoding array and the test array. Panel (**b**) illustrates a trial where two items change from the encoding array to the test array. Panel (**c**) illustrates a "catch trial" from the Multiple Change Detection task where all five items changed on the test array. Reprinted with permission from Gold et al. (2018)

detected or not. Many of the trials are very easy (e.g., when all items change), keeping motivation high, and all trials seem equally easy to the subject. In addition, the subject should always be able to detect changes when all N items change, making it possible to measure lapse rates and factor them out from the WM capacity (K) measure. To minimize contributions of sensory imprecision, the changed color is always 180° (in color space) from the original color (see Fig. 6). Psychophysical studies show that color representations are sufficiently precise in both individuals and controls (Zhang and Luck 2008; Gold et al. 2010), and that there is a vanishingly small probability that an 180° color change would fail to be detected due to encoding imprecision. Thus, sensory precision reductions in individuals with schizophrenia cannot meaningfully distort capacity estimates. One consideration is that 7-10% of males have red-green color blindness, hence we also included a version using multidimensional objects where all dimensions change (and color changes are between wavelengths that can be discriminated by color-blind individuals). Multidimensional objects are stored just as easily as single-dimension objects in both controls (Luck and Vogel 1997) and individuals with schizophrenia (Gold et al. 2003) and multidimensional changes produce optimal performance levels (Awh et al. 2007). This design eliminates any effects of sensory imprecision on performance for anyone whose vision is good enough to qualify for participation. CNTRaCS compared this multiple change detection task to a change localization task (two versions, one with just colored squares and one with color objects to parallel the multiple change detection task where one stimulus always changed each trial and the person had to use the cursor to identify which item changed (see Fig. 6 for example). For change localization we examined accuracy while for multiple change detection, we applied a mathematical modeling procedure to the accuracy scores for each trial type providing an estimate of WM capacity (K), the probability that the participant was paying attention on a given trial (A), and a guessing bias parameter (G).

Overall, healthy participants had higher capacity in both versions of the multiple change detection and change localization tasks compared to a combined patient group of schizophrenia, schizoaffective disorder, and bipolar disorder (Gold et al. 2018). However, capacity reduction was actually strongest in bipolar disorder and not significantly different in individuals with schizophrenia in the multiple change detection task. However all patient groups showed reductions in the "a" parameter as a measure of lapses of attention and higher guessing rates. The color square and color objects versions of each task yielded similar results, but anecdotally participants reported finding the color object versions of the task distracting and complicated. Thus, we moved the color square versions into a test-retest reliability study. We found excellent internal consistency for both the multiple change detection and change localization tasks, and moderate test-retest reliability for accuracy in individual conditions. However, test-retest reliability for the mathematically estimated capacity parameter was moderate and low for attention and guessing. Thus, accuracy measures on this task will be good for both group and individual difference/treatment studies, but the computationally derived parameters are currently better suited for group difference studies and will need enhancement for robust use in individual different and treatment studies.

7 Positive Valence Systems

The original CNTRICS process focused on constructs in the Cognitive Systems domain. However, both RDoCs and subsequent CNTRICS work focused on human/animal translational paradigms included a focus on the Positive Valence domain due, in part, to: a) a burgeoning affective neuroscience literature in human and animal systems revealing core neural systems that process and integrate reward and penalty signals, and translate these signals into value and/or utility estimates that can be used to drive action selection and planning and b) a growing literature suggesting that disruptions in components of the Positive Valence domain are associated with motivation and life function impairments in schizophrenia. Positive Valence domain includes a number of constructs, including hedonics (initial responsiveness to reward attainment), reinforcement learning (RL), and preference-based decision making. Within RL, distinctions were made between negative and positive RL, and RL with and without conscious perception. In subsequent meetings, reversal learning, or the ability to update stimulus response contingencies, was identified as another key aspect of positive valence systems.

RL is thought to be mediated by the midbrain dopamine (DA) system projections to ventral and dorsal striatal regions of the basal ganglia (Berridge 2004; Schultz 2007). The degree to which these neurons respond to rewards depends on predictability. Unpredicted rewards induce DA neurons to fire strongly (positive prediction error). If a predicted reward does not occur, transient depression in DA neuron firing occurs (negative prediction error) (Schultz 1992, 2004, 2007; Schultz et al. 1993, 1997). Over time, DA neurons learn to fire in response to cues that predict reward, rather than to rewards themselves. In humans there is evidence from fMRI for activation of ventral and dorsal striatum to cues that predict reward (Knutson et al. 2000, 2001) as well as both positive and negative prediction error responses (McClure et al. 2003; Abler et al. 2006). These DA/striatal responses are captured by temporal difference models that learn about stimuli in the environment that predict rewards (Montague and Sejnowski 1994; Montague et al. 1996). These mechanisms are thought to underlie aspects of RL that may occur *without* conscious awareness (Dayan and Balleine 2002; Frank et al. 2004). While there are common mechanisms that may contribute to RL with and without conscious awareness for both positive (reward) and negative (loss or punishment) feedback, there are also dissociable mechanisms. For example, there is evidence for striatal cells that mediate "go" or reward based learning versus cells that mediate "no-go" or punishment based learning, with a hypothesized role for D1 receptors in go learning and D2 receptors in no-go learning (Frank et al. 2004; Frank and O'Reilly 2006; Hazy et al. 2007; Frank and Hutchison 2009). There is also growing evidence of a role for serotonin in negative RL (Evers et al. 2005; Crockett et al. 2009; Bari et al. 2010). Theories of RL postulate that *RL with conscious awareness* involves interactions between striatal learning systems and orbitofrontal cortex (OFC) (Schoenbaum and Roesch 2005; Frank and O'Reilly 2006). A number of theories suggest that the OFC supports the ability to represent value information, taking into account both the hedonic properties of a stimulus and the motivational state of the organism (e.g., value of juice when thirsty versus not) (Rolls et al. 1989), during the delay before the reward occurs (Roesch and Olson 2005; Rudebeck et al. 2006), different reward options available (e.g., juice vs wine after a hard day) (Padoa-Schioppa and Assad 2006; Padoa-Schioppa 2007), and changing contingencies associated with stimuli (a previously rewarded response is now punished) (Dias et al. 1996). Some researchers described the OFC as being involved in "working memory" for value, the ability to explicitly maintain, update, and integrate different sources of information about value (Frank and O'Reilly 2006; Wallis 2007). Human fMRI shows activation of OFC in conditions requiring value representations (O'Doherty et al. 2003; O'Doherty J 2007), including those in which response contingencies need to be updated, such as reversal learning (Cools et al. 2002, 2007; O'Doherty et al. 2003). Humans with OFC lesions also show reversal learning impairments (Fellows and Farah 2003, 2005; Hornak et al. 2004), consistent with numerous targeted animal OFC lesion studies (McAlonan and Brown 2003; Clarke et al. 2008; Man et al. 2009).

The literature on RL in schizophrenia is mixed, though distinctions between with and without conscious awareness and between positive and negative RL help shed light on these data. If one focuses on studies using paradigms engaging RL without conscious awareness, many studies suggest intact learning in schizophrenia. For example, intact learning of initial discriminations in reversal learning (Waltz et al. 2007) and ID-ED tasks (Elliott et al. 1995; Hutton et al. 1998; Joyce et al. 2002; Turner et al. 2004; Tyson et al. 2004; Jazbec et al. 2007; Ceaser et al. 2008), and intact learning *rates* on probabilistic learning tasks (Keri et al. 2000; Weickert et al. 2002, 2009; Beninger et al. 2003; Keri et al. 2005; Weiler et al. 2009) are repeatedly observed, with a few exceptions (Oades 1997; Pantelis et al. 1999; Foerde et al. 2008; Horan et al. 2008). Further, both Gold's (Heerey et al. 2008) and Barch's groups found evidence for intact positive RL in schizophrenia using the Pizzagalli bias learning task (Pizzagalli et al. 2005). In contrast, one finds more robust evidence for deficits in SCHIZOPHRENIA on explicit RL tasks that may engage OFC (Gold et al. 2008) as well as striatal mechanisms (Waltz et al. 2007, 2011; Morris et al. 2008; Koch et al. 2009; Strauss et al. 2011). This literature also suggests distinctions between learning from positive and negative feedback in individuals with schizophrenia, with a series of studies showing impaired positive RL ("Go" learning), but intact negative RL ("No-Go") (Waltz et al. 2007, 2011; Polgar et al. 2008; Strauss et al. 2011), though see Somlai et al. (2011) for exception. The literature also provides evidence for impaired reversal learning in schizophrenia (Pantelis et al. 1999; Jazbec et al. 2007; Waltz et al. 2007; Murray et al. 2008; Leeson et al. 2009; McKirdy et al. 2009; Weiler et al. 2009). Importantly, there is robust evidence that the magnitude of RL and reversal learning impairments in schizophrenia is correlated with severity of anhedonia/amotivation symptoms (Farkas et al. 2008; Murray et al. 2008; Polgar et al. 2008; Somlai et al. 2011; Strauss et al. 2011; Waltz et al. 2011), with some evidence that negative symptoms are specifically related to positive compared to negative RL (Polgar et al. 2008; Somlai et al. 2011). Hence, RL paradigms provide insight into potential neural mechanisms underlying deficient cognition in individuals with schizophrenia, with largely consistent findings highlight the importance of conscious vs. unconscious awareness, and the impact of positive vs. negative RL.

Reinforcement Learning Without Conscious Awareness. Relatively few tasks isolate RL without conscious awareness, as they frequently conflate both with and without awareness constructs (e.g., the Weather Prediction Task (Gluck et al. 2002)). Thus, CNTRaCS used a bias learning task to specifically isolate RL without conscious awareness, as participants are consistently unaware of reinforcement contingencies (Pizzagalli et al. 2005, 2007; Bogdan and Pizzagalli 2006, 2009; Bogdan et al. 2010). This task has an animal analogue that was recommended for further development in CNTRICs (Moore et al. 2013). Participants decide whether a briefly presented mouth on a face is either short or long. One type of correct response is reinforced at a higher rate than another. Signal detection indices assess accuracy (d-prime) and bias to respond with the more highly rewarded or more highly punished response type (beta). The original Pizzagalli task focused on *positive* feedback. CNTRaCS also developed a version that focuses on *negative* feedback.

The logic of this version is identical to the positive version, as one type of incorrect response is provided with feedback at a higher rate than the other type. Individuals also develop a bias about the response type that receives more feedback, which increases across blocks. CNTRaCS also developed multiple stimulus sets for these tasks, to allow for repeated testing. In both CNTRaCS studies of these tasks we found robust evidence that participants developed the expected bias about the more rewarded versus more punished stimulus. Like prior research, we found that RL without conscious awareness was intact in schizophrenia (as well as in bipolar disorder) (Barch et al. 2017; Pratt et al. 2021), though we found some evidence of increased reward bias associated with greater mania symptoms. A CNTRaCS test-retest reliability study found that performance on these RL tasks showed good internal consistency, but poor test-retest reliability, particularly for patient groups (Pratt et al. 2021). Thus, this task may be good for characterizing group differences in RL without conscious awareness, but is likely not as useful for individual difference or treatment studies.

Reinforcement Learning with Conscious Awareness. For RL with conscious awareness, CNTRaCS optimized a task paradigm developed by Pessiglione (Pessiglione et al. 2006) and Kim (Kim et al. 2006a, b). Participants are asked to learn which image in a pair of images is either more associated with winning (e.g., potential gains) or more associated with not losing (potential loses). Gold and colleagues (2012a, b) demonstrated that schizophrenia participants with high versus low negative symptoms are impaired learning from positive feedback, but do not differ in learning from negative feedback. As shown in Fig. 7a, on potential gain trials, if the correct item is selected, participants see an image of a nickel and the word "Win," whereas if the incorrect item is selected, they see "Not a winner, try again." On correct potential loss trials (Fig. 7b, participants see "Keep your money," whereas if the incorrect item is selected, they see a nickel with a red cross through it and the word "Lose." The correct response is reinforced on either 90% of trials (one condition) or 80% (another condition). Thus, there were a total of four types of trials: (1) Win/Not Win at 90/10 probability distribution; (2) Win/Not Win at 80/20 probability distribution; (3) Not Lose/Lose at 90/10 probability distribution; and (4) Not Lose/Lose at 80/10 probability distribution. To generate multiple parallel versions that could be used in longitudinal or treatment studies, we developed four different sets of stimuli. As dependent measures we compute both model based learning rates for achieving gains and avoiding losses (Gold et al. 2012a, b) and accuracy in the last block. Following training, a transfer test phase is presented. In these 72 trials, the original four training pairs are each presented four times, with novel pairings presented on 58 trials. For novel pairings, each trained item is presented with every other trained item. Of most interest were pairings that pitted stimuli that had experienced different types of reinforcement histories against each other (referred to as pairings). Participants were instructed to pick the item in the pair that they thought was "best" based on their earlier learning. No feedback was administered during this phase. Thus, this straightforward task provides a rich set of RL measures.

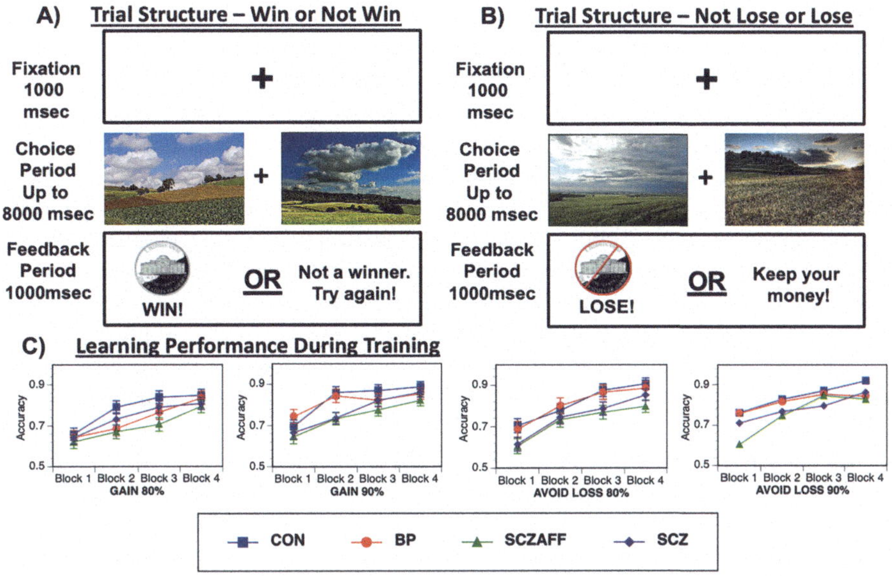

Fig. 7 Schematic and stimulus examples for the Explicit Probabilistic Incentive Learning Task (EPILT) for (**a**) obtaining reward; and (**b**) avoiding punishment, as well as Training Performance in the EPILT as a function of Diagnostic Group. Reprinted with permission from Barch et al. (2017)

As shown in Fig. 7c, and consistent with other work (Gold et al. 2012a, b; Abohamza et al. 2020), in two CNTRaCS studies, both individuals with schizophrenia and schizoaffective disorder performed significantly worse than controls in the learning phase (Barch et al. 2017; Pratt et al. 2021), and in one study individuals with bipolar also performed poorly (Pratt et al. 2021). In the transfer phase, all patient groups showed intact sensitivity to which stimuli were more associated with losing versus winning, but individuals with schizophrenia and schizoaffective disorder showed less sensitivity to the frequency of winning. Taken together, these data indicate some evidence of reduced sensitivity to frequent reward amongst patient groups. This finding is generally consistent with prior work (Gold et al. 2012a, b), who also found impaired sensitivity to the frequency of winning among individuals, but only among those with impairments in motivation. Importantly, worse performance on the explicit RL task was related to worse motivation and pleasure symptoms across all individuals and was also related to WM. Relationships between explicit RL learning and WM accounted for some of the diagnostic group differences, but did not explain relationships between explicit RL and motivation and pleasure symptoms. These findings suggest transdiagnostic relationships across the spectrum of psychotic disorders between motivation and pleasure impairments and RL with conscious awareness. Like the RL without conscious awareness tasks, internal consistency was strong for the training phase of explicit RL, though less so for the transfer phase (Pratt et al. 2021). Test-retest reliability was modest for the training phase and poor for the transfer phase (Pratt et al. 2021). Thus, the training/

learning measures of RL with conscious awareness will be useful for both group discrimination and individual difference/treatment studies, but not the transfer phase measures are likely most useful for group difference studies only.

Reversal Learning. CNTRaCS optimized Cools' paradigm previously used in human and animal studies (Clark et al. 2004), including fMRI (Cools et al. 2002, 2007; Funkiewiez et al. 2006; Robinson et al. 2010) and PET studies of dopaminergic and serotonergic influences on reversal learning (Evers et al. 2005; Cools et al. 2007; Clatworthy et al. 2009). It was recommended for further development during CNTRICs. Participants are presented with pairs of items and told that one stimulus from each pair is "correct," and that they have to figure out which one. They are told that no stimulus is correct all the time, and that the "correct" stimulus changes occasionally. The choice of one of the stimuli is positively reinforced 80% of the time (the other stimulus is reinforced 20%). Once participants reach an initial criterion, the contingencies are reversed. This type of task can also be conducted in rodents (Bari et al. 2010; Amitai et al. 2014; Milienne-Petiot et al. 2018), and results in consistent EEG biomarkers of performance (Cavanagh et al. 2021). Participants are required to detect the shift in reinforcement contingencies and learn to choose the stimulus now reinforced 80% of the time. If participants succeed in reaching criterion in this phase, they are considered to have successfully achieved a *reversal*. Gold has shown that individuals with schizophrenia learn the initial discrimination, but make fewer reversals and more errors before successful reversals (Waltz and Gold 2007). This task has excellent construct validity and elegant animal literature to support the involvement of striatal and OFC systems. However, the ability to interpret selective deficits in reversal is hampered by the fact that the initial discrimination stage is easier and has lower discriminating power. Thus, CNTRaCS developed a version in which the initial discrimination and reversal are better-matched psychometrically in controls, by reducing the difficulty of the reversal learning trials (90% rather than 80%), making the initial discrimination and reversal conditions better psychometrically matched in controls. Individuals with schizophrenia, schizoaffective disorder, and bipolar disorder were all impaired on both initial discrimination and reversal. Bayesian hidden Markov modeling (Rouder et al. 2009; Wagenmakers et al. 2017a, b) within a series of hierarchically nested models (Daw et al. 2011) revealed that all three groups made more errors due to a greater tendency to shift away from rewarded categories. Formal modeling showed a reduction in $\beta_{temperature}$, implicating a reduction in exploitation of known rewards, and allowed us to rule out two other hypotheses, namely that this behavior reflects deficits in belief states ($\delta_{transition}$) or attention lapses ($\lambda_{lapse\ rate}$). Thus, reversal learning tasks offer an opportunity to reveal positive RL deficits in patient populations, as seen in individuals with schizophrenia.

8 Future Directions of CNTRACS: Phase Three

As the field advances toward precision psychiatry, we need clinically informative measures with good psychometric properties that: (1) optimally differentiate individuals and controls, (2) capture variance in important symptom dimensions and functional outcomes, and (3) are sensitive to treatment effects. The CNTRaCS initiative has helped move the field from traditional neuropsychological measurement to cognitive-neuroscience-based approaches, including the development of imaging biomarkers, made freely available to the field and industry (http://cntracs.ucdavis.edu). Psychiatric research is now undergoing significant advances in a new subspecialty of computational psychiatry, complementing cognitive neuroscience constructs with an expanding paradigm of neurocomputational modeling. The scientific premise of this work is that the computations (i.e., algorithm-based transformations of information) performed by neural circuits can be estimated, and that these parameter estimates bridge the gap between neural circuit function, cognition, and behavior. Consequently, the ways in which pathophysiology generates psychopathology can be specified and tested using mathematical formalisms (Redish and Gordon 2016). Within this context, the CNTRaCS consortium modified its acronym again, such that the "C" now referred to Computational Neuroscience, allowed us to maintain continuity while growing our goal. Thus, the third phase of CNTRaCS aims to provide the field with a set of "vetted" tasks and associated computational models that meet the measurement standards needed for clinical research. We selected task + model combinations on the basis of four criteria: (1) a rich clinical literature suggesting relevance for a broad range of psychopathology; (2) the ability to quantify underlying processes that contribute to a broad range of tasks; (3) the ability to distinguish between specific deficits and non-specific or generalized deficits; and (4) when possible, paradigms for which neural measures can be used to provide biological validation of the model parameters. The first study of this third phase is ongoing, recruiting healthy controls, as well as individuals with schizophrenia, schizoaffective disorder, bipolar disorder with psychotic features, and major depression.

These criteria led us to focus on the domains of visual perception, WM, EM, reinforcement learning (RL), and effort-based decision making – functions that span much of the behavioral geography of the brain and which are part of the RDoC matrix (Insel et al. 2010; Morris and Cuthbert 2012; Cuthbert and Kozak 2013). Each of these domains has clear relevance to psychotic disorders and is also increasingly relevant to affective, substance use, and personality disorders. Whereas existing measures often treat each of these domains as monolithic constructs, the computational models we propose can disentangle multiple processes that underlie each domain, illuminating the neural basis of comorbidity and heterogeneity. For example, we expect that a significant proportion of impairments in visual perception, WM and EM in individuals with psychotic disorders will be accounted for by a single computational parameter reflecting the *precision* with which information is represented. Conversely, we predict that both psychotic and depressed individuals will exhibit deficits in RL but will differ in the model parameters that are impaired, reflecting different pathways by which performance is disrupted.

To be concrete, consider the domain of visual perception and the computational parameter of *precision*, defined as the degree to which a neural representation consistently matches the properties of a particular stimulus. A more narrowly tuned neuron provides a more precise representation of orientation, making it easier to discriminate between similar line orientations. Behaviorally, schizophrenia individuals exhibit impaired precision in the form of broadened orientation tuning (Yoon et al. 2010; Rokem et al. 2011; Schallmo et al. 2013), hypothesized to reflect altered excitation/inhibition (E/I) balance (Krystal et al. 2017) and/or coarsening of representations to compensate for excessive neural noise (Silverstein et al. 2017). Because these alterations may impact neural function in schizophrenia at multiple levels of analysis (Krystal et al. 2017), reduced precision is hypothesized to contribute to aberrant representations across domains of cognition, including perception, memory, and belief formation (Javitt et al. 1997; Rokem et al. 2011; Schallmo et al. 2013; Krystal et al. 2017). Moreover, reduced precision contributes to both orientation discrimination deficits and impaired WM in schizophrenia (Rokem et al. 2011; Starc et al. 2017). These data are consistent with animal and human data showing that precision is a critical variable in orientation tuning (Edden et al. 2009; Katzner et al. 2011), in WM performance (van den Berg et al. 2012), and in hippocampally-mediated EM (Koen et al. 2017; Kolarik et al. 2018). Whereas these domains have historically been conceptualized as independent constructs, we are using tasks and models that isolate a precision parameter (a construct with significant links with functional outcome measures) (Green et al. 2012; Sheffield et al. 2014; Zaragoza Domingo et al. 2015; MacQueen and Memedovich 2017; Soni et al. 2017) across domains to determine the extent to which reduced precision may account for multiple aspects of cognitive pathology in psychotic (Park and Gooding 2014; Berna et al. 2016; Silverstein 2016) and affective disorders (Bubl et al. 2015; Bora 2018; Dillon and Pizzagalli 2018).

In many behavioral tasks, incorrect responses can arise either from imprecise neural coding or from lapses of attention. Indeed, a previous CNTRaCS study demonstrated that a putative perceptual deficit in schizophrenia individuals could be explained by attentional lapses (Barch et al. 2012). This premise underscores the need for the task-model combinations that provide independent estimates of precision and lapse rate for each participant. Lapses of attention often reflect failures of goal maintenance (Smeekens and Kane 2016; Kane et al. 2017), an aspect of cognitive control that has been shown to be specifically impaired in psychotic disorders and is associated with atypical activation and connectivity in the frontal-parietal attention network (Phillips et al. 2015). Importantly, we are also including EEG recordings in our ongoing CNTRaCS study to identify potential neural correlates of the computationally derived metrics, using cost-effective EEG/ERP methods that are feasible to use in larger-scale studies. For example, we are measuring pre-trial alpha-band oscillations, which are shown to predict lapses in attention (Erickson et al. 2016; Boudewyn and Carter 2018).

In addition to precision and lapsing, *capacity* (the number of items that can be simultaneously represented) is a key factor in the efficient performance of complex tasks. Like precision, WM capacity depends critically on E/I balance (Wei et al. 2012), and it also appears to depend on the balance of D1 and D2 receptor activity (Durstewitz and Seamans 2008). However, impaired performance on WM tasks may be due to poor precision, high lapse rate, or a true capacity deficit, and the computational modeling in CNTRaCS will separate each of these parameters for each subject. Using both behavioral and EEG (Erickson et al. 2016) methodology, we have shown that individuals across a spectrum of psychotic disorders – including bipolar disorder – exhibit separable deficits attributable to capacity limits and lapsing.

In addition to measures of "cold" cognition, CNTRaCS III includes task + model combinations examining abnormalities in motivation and goal-directed behavior relevant for affective and psychotic disorders. Specifically, we are studying reinforcement learning (RL) and effort valuation, two key constructs from the Positive Valence Systems in the RDoC matrix. We and others consistently found these constructs to relate to motivational symptoms in schizophrenia, bipolar disorder, and depression (Gold et al. 2012a, b, 2013; Barch et al. 2016, 2017). However, the unique contributions of multiple neural and cognitive systems that give rise to RL and effort valuation deficits differ across disorders in ways that cannot be detected without specialized tasks and models. For example, in RL, abnormalities may occur in the ability to signal *reward prediction errors* (RPEs). RPEs are events that are better or worse than expected and are linked to dopaminergic function (Schultz 2016). Altered RPEs can have marked motivational consequences across mental illnesses (Maia and Frank 2011, 2017). Alternatively, changes in RL could arise due to alterations in downstream targets of the RPEs (e.g., in striatum) and in updating of *value representations*. In effort-based decision making, changes in the willingness to invest effort can arise not only from an amplification of the cost of effort, but also from impairments in maintaining prospective reward *value representations* in WM. Reduced WM capacity can therefore lead to impaired performance in these tasks. As shown in Preliminary Data, our computational models demonstrate that the RL deficits widely observed in schizophrenia are secondary to reduced WM capacity rather than reflecting impairments in reward signaling and prediction errors (Collins et al. 2014, 2017), whereas the latter appears may be a more primary deficit in affective disorders (Zhang et al. 2013; Barch et al. 2016). Such a distinction has important implications for the development and assessments of new treatments. This type of insight is only achieved with optimized experimental designs accompanied by quantitative modeling. This approach also maps behavioral task parameters to EEG markers of RL, such as the well-validated Reward Positivity (Fromer et al. 2016; Heydari and Holroyd 2016) also seen in mice (Cavanagh et al. 2021), and newer decoding-based EEG indices of RL (Frank et al. 2015; Collins and Frank 2016).

Acknowledgments and Disclosures Funding for this work was provided by NIMH ROI1s MH084840 (DMB), MH084826 (CSC), MH084821 (JMG), MH084861 (AWM), and MH084828 (SMS).

DMB has received grants from the National Institutes of Health (NIH) and the Brain & Behavior Research Foundation.

MAB has received research grants from the National Institutes of Health (NIH) and the Brain & Behavior Research Foundation.

CSC has received research grants from the National Institutes of Health (NIH), the Brain & Behavior Foundation, the Burroughs Wellcome foundation, GlaxoSmithKline, and the Robert Wood Johnson Foundation and has been an external consultant for Lilly, Merck, Pfizer, Roche, and Servier.

JMG has received grants from National Institutes of Health (NIH), receives royalty payments from Brief Assessment of Cognition in Schizophrenia, and has acted as a consultant to Amgen, AstraZeneca, GlaxoSmithKline, Hoffmann-La Roche, Merck, Pfizer, and Solvay.

SJL has received research grants from the National Institutes of Health (NIH), the National Science Foundation (NSF), McDonnell-Pew Program in Cognitive Neuroscience, and the Human Frontier Science Program.

AWM has received research grants from the National Institutes of Health (NIH) and the Brain & Behavior Research Foundation.

JDR has received research grants from the National Institutes of Health (NIH), the Brain & Behavior Research Foundation, the EJLB Foundation, and the Robert Wood Johnson Foundation.

SMS has received research grants from the National Institutes of Mental Health (NIMH), the Brain & Behavior Research Foundation, the van Ameringen Foundation, the Jacob and Valeria Langeloth Foundation, the New England Research Institutes, the New York State Office of Mental Health, the New Jersey Division of Mental Health and Addiction Services, Janssen Pharmaceutica, AstraZeneca, and Pfizer.

MJF has received grants from the National Institutes of Health (NIH), the National Science Foundation (NSF), and has been an external consultant for Roche, Pfizer, and Boehringer.

References

Abler B, Walter H et al (2006) Prediction error as a linear function of reward probability is coded in human nucleus accumbens. Neuroimage 31(2):790–795

Abohamza E, Weickert T et al (2020) Reward and punishment learning in schizophrenia and bipolar disorder. Behav Brain Res 381:112298

Aleman A, Hij R et al (1999) Memory impairment in schizophrenia: a meta-analysis. Am J Psychiatry 156(9):1358–1366

Altmann CF, Bulthoff HH et al (2003) Perceptual organization of local elements into global shapes in the human visual cortex. Curr Biol 13(4):342–349

Amitai N, Young JW, Higa K, Sharp RF, Geyer MA, Powell SB (2014) Isolation rearing effects on probabilistic learning and cognitive flexibility in rats. Cogn Affect Behav Neurosci 14(1):388–406

Anderson JR, Reder LM et al (1996) Working memory: activation limiations on retrieval. Cogn Psychol 30(3):221–256

Arnsten AF (2004) Adrenergic targets for the treatment of cognitive deficits in schizophrenia. Psychopharmacology (Berl) 174(1):25–31

Awh E, Barton B et al (2007) Visual working memory represents a fixed number of items regardless of complexity. Psychol Sci 18(7):622–628

Baddeley AD (2000) The episodic buffer: a new component of working memory? Trends Cogn Sci 4:417–423

Bagner DM, Melinder MR et al (2003) Language comprehension and working memory language comprehension and working memory deficits in patients with schizophrenia. Schizophr Res 60(2-3):299–309

Barch DM, Carter CS (2008) Measurement issues in the use of cognitive neuroscience tasks in drug development for impaired cognition in schizophrenia: a report of the second consensus building conference of the CNTRICS initiative. Schizophr Bull 34(4):613–618

Barch DM, Braver TS et al (1997) Dissociating working memory from task difficulty in human prefrontal cortex. Neuropsychologia 35(10):1373–1380

Barch DM, Carter CS et al (1999) Prefrontal cortex and context processing in medication-naive first-episode patients with schizophrenia. Schizophr Res 36(1-3):217–218

Barch DM, Carter CS et al (2001) Selective deficits in prefrontal cortex regions in medication naive schizophrenia patients. Arch Gen Psychiatry 50:280–288

Barch DM, Carter CS et al (2004a) Factors influencing Stroop performance in schizophrenia. Neuropsychology 18(3):477–484

Barch DM, Mitropoulou V et al (2004b) Context-processing deficits in schizotypal personality disorder. J Abnorm Psychol 113(4):556–568

Barch DM, Braver TS et al (2009a) CNTRICS final task selection: executive control. Schizophr Bull 35(1):115–135

Barch DM, Carter CS et al (2009b) Selecting paradigms from cognitive neuroscience for translation into use in clinical trials: proceedings of the third CNTRICS meeting. Schizophr Bull 35(1): 109–114

Barch DM, Carter CS et al (2012) The clinical translation of a measure of gain control: the contrast-contrast effect task. Schizophr Bull 38(1):135–143

Barch DM, Pagliaccio D et al (2016) Mechanisms underlying motivational deficits in psychopathology: similarities and differences in depression and schizophrenia. Curr Top Behav Neurosci 27:411–449

Barch DM, Carter CS et al (2017) Explicit and implicit reinforcement learning across the psychosis spectrum. J Abnorm Psychol 126(5):694–711

Bari A, Theobald DE et al (2010) Serotonin modulates sensitivity to reward and negative feedback in a probabilistic reversal learning task in rats. Neuropsychopharmacology 35(6):1290–1301

Benes FM (2015) Building models for postmortem abnormalities in hippocampus of schizophrenics. Schizophr Res 167(1-3):73–83

Beninger RJ, Wasserman J et al (2003) Typical and atypical antipsychotic medications differentially affect two nondeclarative memory tasks in schizophrenic patients: a double dissociation. Schizophr Res 61(2-3):281–292

Berna F, Potheegadoo J et al (2016) A meta-analysis of autobiographical memory studies in schizophrenia spectrum disorder. Schizophr Bull 42(1):56–66

Berridge KC (2004) Motivation concepts in behavioral neuroscience. Physiol Behav 81(2): 179–209

Blackman RK, Crowe DA et al (2016) Monkey prefrontal neurons reflect logical operations for cognitive control in a variant of the AX continuous performance task (AX-CPT). J Neurosci 36(14):4067–4079

Blumenfeld RS, Ranganath C (2006) Dorsolateral prefrontal cortex promotes long-term memory formation through its role in working memory organization. J Neurosci 26(3):916–925
Blumenfeld RS, Ranganath C (2007) Prefrontal cortex and long-term memory encoding: an integrative review of findings from neuropsychology and neuroimaging. Neuroscientist 13(3): 280–291
Bogdan R, Pizzagalli DA (2006) Acute stress reduces reward responsiveness: implications for depression. Biol Psychiatry 60(10):1147–1154
Bogdan R, Pizzagalli DA (2009) The heritability of hedonic capacity and perceived stress: a twin study evaluation of candidate depressive phenotypes. Psychol Med 39(2):211–218
Bogdan R, Perlis RH et al (2010) The impact of mineralocorticoid receptor ISO/VAL genotype (rs5522) and stress on reward learning. Genes Brain Behav 9(6):658–667
Bonds AB (1989) Role of inhibition in the specification of orientation selectivity of cells in the cat striate cortex. Vis Neurosci 2(1):41–55
Bonds AB (1991) Temporal dynamics of contrast gain in single cells of the cat striate cortex. Vis Neurosci 6(3):239–255
Bonner-Jackson A, Haut K et al (2005) The influence of encoding strategy on episodic memory and cortical activity in schizophrenia. Biol Psychiatry 58:47–55
Bora E (2018) Neurocognitive features in clinical subgroups of bipolar disorder: a meta-analysis. J Affect Disord 229:125–134
Boudewyn MA, Carter CS (2018) Electrophysiological correlates of adaptive control and attentional engagement in patients with first episode schizophrenia and healthy young adults. Psychophysiology 55(3)
Bower BH (1970a) Imagery as a relational organizer in associative learing. J Verb Learning Verb Behav 9:529–533
Bower GH (1970b) Organizational factors in memory. Cogn Psychol 1:18–46
Braver TS, Bongiolatti SR (2002) The role of the frontopolar prefrontal cortex in subgoal processing during working memory. Neuroimage 15:523–536
Braver TS, Cohen JD (2000) On the control of control: the role of dopamine in regulating prefrontal function and working memory. In: Monsell S, Driver J (eds) Attention and performance XVIII. MIT Press, Cambridge, pp 713–738
Braver TS, Cohen JD et al (1995) A computational model of prefrontal cortex function. Advances in neural information processing systems. In: Touretzky DS, Tesauro G, Leen TK (eds) , vol 7. MIT Press, Cambridge, pp 141–148
Brebion G, Amador X et al (1997) Mechanisms underlying memory impairment in schizophrenia. Psychol Med 27:383–393
Brewin CR, Beaton A (2002) Thought suppression, intelligence, and working memory capacity. Behav Res Ther 40(8):923–930
Bubl E, Kern E et al (2015) Retinal dysfunction of contrast processing in major depression also apparent in cortical activity. Eur Arch Psychiatry Clin Neurosci 265(4):343–350
Butler PD, Zemon V et al (2005) Early-stage visual processing and cortical amplification deficits in schizophrenia. Arch Gen Psychiatry 62(5):495–504
Butler PD, Martinez A et al (2007) Subcortical visual dysfunction in schizophrenia drives secondary cortical impairments. Brain 130(Pt 2):417–430
Cadenhead KS, Serper Y et al (1998) Transient versus sustained visual channels in the visual backward masking deficits of schizophrenia patients. Biol Psychiatry 43(2):132–138
Calkins ME, Curtis CE et al (2004) Antisaccade performance is impaired in medically and psychiatrically healthy biological relatives of schizophrenia patients. Schizophr Res 71(1): 167–178
Carter CS, Barch DM (2007) Cognitive neuroscience-based approaches to measuring and improving treatment effects on cognition in schizophrenia: the CNTRICS initiative. Schizophr Bull 33(5):1131–1137

Carter CS, Barch DM et al (2008) Identifying cognitive mechanisms targeted for treatment development in schizophrenia: an overview of the first meeting of the cognitive neuroscience treatment research to improve cognition in schizophrenia initiative. Biol Psychiatry 64(1):4–10
Cavanagh JF, Gregg D, Light GA, Olguin SL, Sharp RF, Bismark AW, Bhakta SG, Swerdlow NR, Brigman JL, Young JW (2021) Electrophysiological biomarkers of behavioral dimensions from cross-species paradigms. Transl Psychiatry 11(1):482
Ceaser AE, Goldberg TE et al (2008) Set-shifting ability and schizophrenia: a marker of clinical illness or an intermediate phenotype? Biol Psychiatry 64(9):782–788
Chandna A, Pennefather PM et al (2001) Contour integration deficits in anisometropic amblyopia. Invest Ophthalmol Vis Sci 42(3):875–878
Chen EYH, Wong AWS et al (2001) Stroop interference and facilitation effects in first-episode schizophrenia patients. Schizophr Res 48:29–44
Chen Y, Bidwell LC et al (2005) Visual motion integration in schizophrenia patients, their first-degree relatives, and patients with bipolar disorder. Schizophr Res 74(2-3):271–281
Chubb C, Sperling G et al (1989) Texture interactions determine perceived contrast. Proc Natl Acad Sci U S A 86(23):9631–9635
Clark L, Cools R et al (2004) The neuropsychology of ventral prefrontal cortex: decision-making and reversal learning. Brain Cogn 55(1):41–53
Clarke HF, Robbins TW et al (2008) Lesions of the medial striatum in monkeys produce perseverative impairments during reversal learning similar to those produced by lesions of the orbitofrontal cortex. J Neurosci 28(43):10972–10982
Clatworthy PL, Lewis SJ et al (2009) Dopamine release in dissociable striatal subregions predicts the different effects of oral methylphenidate on reversal learning and spatial working memory. J Neurosci 29(15):4690–4696
Cohen JD, Servan-Schreiber D (1992) Context, cortex and dopamine: a connectionist approach to behavior and biology in schizophrenia. Psychol Rev 99(1):45–77
Cohen JD, Barch DM et al (1999) Context-processing deficits in schizophrenia: converging evidence from three theoretically motivated cognitive tasks. J Abnorm Psychol 108:120–133
Collins AG, Frank MJ (2013) Cognitive control over learning: creating, clustering, and generalizing task-set structure. Psychol Rev 120(1):190–229
Collins AGE, Frank MJ (2016) Neural signature of hierarchically structured expectations predicts clustering and transfer of rule sets in reinforcement learning. Cognition 152:160–169
Collins AG, Brown JK et al (2014) Working memory contributions to reinforcement learning impairments in schizophrenia. J Neurosci 34(41):13747–13756
Collins AGE, Albrecht MA et al (2017) Interactions among working memory, reinforcement learning, and effort in value-based choice: a new paradigm and selective deficits in schizophrenia. Biol Psychiatry 82(6):431–439
Cools R, Clark L et al (2002) Defining the neural mechanisms of probabilistic reversal learning using event-related functional magnetic resonance imaging. J Neurosci 22(11):4563–4567
Cools R, Lewis SJ et al (2007) L-DOPA disrupts activity in the nucleus accumbens during reversal learning in Parkinson's disease. Neuropsychopharmacology 32(1):180–189
Cowan N (1988) Evolving conceptions of memory storage, selective attention, and their mutual constraints within the human information-processing system. Psychol Bull 104:163–191
Cowan N (2010) The magical mystery four: how is working memory capacity limited, and why? Curr Dir Psychol Sci 19(1):51–57
Crockett MJ, Clark L et al (2009) Reconciling the role of serotonin in behavioral inhibition and aversion: acute tryptophan depletion abolishes punishment-induced inhibition in humans. J Neurosci Off J Soc Neurosci 29(38):11993–11999
Cuthbert BN, Kozak MJ (2013) Constructing constructs for psychopathology: the NIMH research domain criteria. J Abnorm Psychol 122(3):928–937
Dakin SC, Hess RF (1998) Spatial-frequency tuning of visual contour integration. J Opt Soc Am A Opt Image Sci Vis 15(6):1486–1499

Dakin S, Carlin P et al (2005) Weak suppression of visual context in chronic schizophrenia. Curr Biol 15(20):R822–R824

Davachi L (2006) Item, context and relational episodic encoding in humans. Curr Opin Neurobiol 16(6):693–700

Daw ND, Gershman SJ et al (2011) Model-based influences on humans' choices and striatal prediction errors. Neuron 69(6):1204–1215

Dayan P, Balleine BW (2002) Reward, motivation, and reinforcement learning. Neuron 36:285–298

Delawalla Z, Csernansky JG et al (2007) Prefrontal cortex function in nonpsychotic siblings of individuals with schizophrenia. Biol Psychiatry

Derrington A (1996) Vision: filling in and pop out. Curr Biol 6(2):141–143

Dias R, Robbins TW et al (1996) Dissociation in prefrontal cortex of affective and attentional shifts. Nature 380:69–72

Dias EC, Butler PD et al (2011) Early sensory contributions to contextual encoding deficits in schizophrenia. Arch Gen Psychiatry 68(7):654–664

Dillon DG, Pizzagalli DA (2018) Mechanisms of memory disruption in depression. Trends Neurosci

Durstewitz D, Gabriel T (2007) Dynamical basis of irregular spiking in NMDA-driven prefrontal cortex neurons. Cereb Cortex 17(4):894–908

Durstewitz D, Seamans JK (2008) The dual-state theory of prefrontal cortex dopamine function with relevance to catechol-o-methyltransferase genotypes and schizophrenia. Biol Psychiatry 64(9):739–749

Edden RA, Muthukumaraswamy SD et al (2009) Orientation discrimination performance is predicted by GABA concentration and gamma oscillation frequency in human primary visual cortex. J Neurosci 29(50):15721–15726

Eichenbaum H, Yonelinas AP et al (2007) The medial temporal lobe and recognition memory. Annu Rev Neurosci 30:123–152

Elliott R, McKenna PJ et al (1995) Neuropsychological evidence for frontostriatal dysfunction in schizophrenia. Psychol Med 25(3):619–630

Engle RW, Kane MJ (2004) Executive attention, working memory capacity and a two-factor theory of cognitive control. In: Ross B (ed) The psychology of learning and motivation. Elsevier, New York, p 44

Erickson MA, Albrecht MA et al (2016) Impaired suppression of delay-period alpha and beta is associated with impaired working memory in schizophrenia. Biol Psychiatry Cogn Neurosci Neuroimaging 2(3):272–279

Ettinger U, Picchioni M et al (2006) Antisaccade performance in monozygotic twins discordant for schizophrenia: the Maudsley twin study. Am J Psychiatry 163(3):543–545

Evers EA, Cools R et al (2005) Serotonergic modulation of prefrontal cortex during negative feedback in probabilistic reversal learning. Neuropsychopharmacology 30(6):1138–1147

Farkas M, Polgar P et al (2008) Associative learning in deficit and nondeficit schizophrenia. Neuroreport 19(1):55–58

Fassbender C, Foxe JJ et al (2006) Mapping the functional anatomy of task preparation: priming task-appropriate brain networks. Hum Brain Mapp 27(10):819–827

Fellows LK, Farah MJ (2003) Ventromedial frontal cortex mediates affective shifting in humans: evidence from a reversal learning paradigm. Brain 126(Pt 8):1830–1837

Fellows LK, Farah MJ (2005) Different underlying impairments in decision-making following ventromedial and dorsolateral frontal lobe damage in humans. Cereb Cortex 15(1):58–63

Foerde K, Poldrack RA et al (2008) Selective corticostriatal dysfunction in schizophrenia: examination of motor and cognitive skill learning. Neuropsychology 22(1):100–109

Foley JM (1994) Human luminance pattern-vision mechanisms: masking experiments require a new model. J Opt Soc Am A Opt Image Sci Vis 11(6):1710–1719

Forbes NF, Carrick LA et al (2009) Working memory in schizophrenia: a meta-analysis. Psychol Med 39(6):889–905

Frank MJ, Hutchison K (2009) Genetic contributions to avoidance-based decisions: striatal D2 receptor polymorphisms. Neuroscience 164(1):131–140

Frank MJ, O'Reilly RC (2006) A mechanistic account of striatal dopamine function in human cognition: psychopharmacological studies with cabergoline and haloperidol. Behav Neurosci 120(3):497–517

Frank MJ, Seeberger LC et al (2004) By carrot or by stick: cognitive reinforcement learning in parkinsonism. Science 306(5703):1940–1943

Frank MJ, Gagne C et al (2015) fMRI and EEG predictors of dynamic decision parameters during human reinforcement learning. J Neurosci 35(2):485–494

Friedman JI (2004) Cholinergic targets for cognitive enhancement in schizophrenia: focus on cholinesterase inhibitors and muscarinic agonists. Psychopharmacology (Berl) 174(1):45–53

Fromer R, Sturmer B et al (2016) The better, the bigger: the effect of graded positive performance feedback on the reward positivity. Biol Psychol 114:61–68

Fukuda K, Awh E et al (2010) Discrete capacity limits in visual working memory. Curr Opin Neurobiol 20(2):177–182

Funkiewiez A, Ardouin C et al (2006) Effects of levodopa and subthalamic nucleus stimulation on cognitive and affective functioning in Parkinson's disease. Mov Disord 21(10):1656–1662

Gibson B, Wasserman E et al (2011) Qualitative similarities in the visual short-term memory of pigeons and people. Psychon Bull Rev 18:979–984

Gluck MA, Shohamy D et al (2002) How do people solve the "weather prediction" task?: individual variability in strategies for probabilistic category learning. Learn Mem 9(6):408–418

Gold JM, Randolph C et al (1992) Forms of memory failure in schizophrenia. J Abnorm Psychol 101(3):487–494

Gold JM, Goldberg RW et al (2002) Cognitive correlates of job tenure among patients with severe mental illness. Am J Psychiatry 159(8):1395–1402

Gold JM, Wilk CM et al (2003) Working memory for visual features and conjunctions in schizophrenia. J Abnorm Psychol 112(1):61–71

Gold JM, Fuller RL et al (2006) Intact attentional control of working memory encoding in schizophrenia. J Abnorm Psychol 115(4):658–673

Gold JM, Waltz JA et al (2008) Reward processing in schizophrenia: a deficit in the representation of value. Schizophr Bull 34(5):835–847

Gold JM, Hahn B et al (2010) Reduced capacity but spared precision and maintenance of working memory representations in schizophrenia. Arch Gen Psychiatry 67(6):570–577

Gold JM, Barch DM et al (2012a) Clinical, functional, and intertask correlations of measures developed by the cognitive neuroscience test reliability and clinical applications for schizophrenia consortium. Schizophr Bull 38(1):144–152

Gold JM, Waltz JA et al (2012b) Negative symptoms and the failure to represent the expected reward value of actions: behavioral and computational modeling evidence. Arch Gen Psychiatry 69(2):129–138

Gold JM, Strauss GP et al (2013) Negative symptoms of schizophrenia are associated with abnormal effort-cost computations. Biol Psychiatry

Gold JM, Barch DM et al (2018) Working memory impairment across psychotic disorders. Schizophr Bull

Gold JM, Barch DM et al (in submission) Modelling of working memory across the spectrum of psychotic disorders: dissociation capacity from attention lapsing

Goldman-Rakic (1995) Cellular basis of working memory. Neuron 14:477–485

Green M, Walker E (1984) Susceptibility to backward masking in schizophrenic patients with positive or negative symptoms. Am J Psychiatry 141(10):1273–1275

Green MF, Nuechterlein KH et al (2004) Approaching a consensus cognitive battery for clinical trials in schizophrenia: the NIMH-MATRICS conference to select cognitive domains and test criteria. Biol Psychiatry 56(5):301–307

Green MF, Hellemann G et al (2012) From perception to functional outcome in schizophrenia: modeling the role of ability and motivation. Arch Gen Psychiatry 69(12):1216–1224

Grot S, Potvin S et al (2014) Is there a binding deficit in working memory in patients with schizophrenia? A meta-analysis. Schizophr Res 158(1-3):142–145
Haenschel C, Bittner RA et al (2007) Contribution of impaired early-stage visual processing to working memory dysfunction in adolescents with schizophrenia: a study with event-related potentials and functional magnetic resonance imaging. Arch Gen Psychiatry 64(11):1229–1240
Han S, Song Y et al (2001) Neural substrates for visual perceptual grouping in humans. Psychophysiology 38(6):926–935
Han S, Ding Y et al (2002) Neural mechanisms of perceptual grouping in humans as revealed by high density event related potentials. Neurosci Lett 319(1):29–32
Harrison BJ, Yucel M et al (2006) Dysfunction of dorsolateral prefrontal cortex in antipsychotic-naive schizophreniform psychosis. Psychiatry Res 148(1):23–31
Hazy TE, Frank MJ et al (2007) Towards an executive without a homunculus: computational models of the prefrontal cortex/basal ganglia system. Philo Trans R Soc Lond B Biol Sci 362(1485):1601–1613
Heckers S (2004) The hippocampus in schizophrenia. Am J Psychiatry 161(11):2138–2139
Heckers S, Konradi C (2010) Hippocampal pathology in schizophrenia. Curr Top Behav Neurosci 4:529–553
Heckers S, Rauch SL et al (1998) Impaired recruitment of the hippocampus during conscious recollection in schizophrenia. Nat Neurosci 1(4):318–323
Heeger DJ (1992) Normalization of cell responses in cat striate cortex. Vis Neurosci 9(2):181–197
Heerey EA, Bell-Warren KR et al (2008) Decision-making impairments in the context of intact reward sensitivity in schizophrenia. Biol Psychiatry 64(1):62–69
Heinrichs RW, Zakzanis KK (1998) Neurocognitive deficit in schizophrenia: a quantitative review of the evidence. Neuropsychology 12(3):426–445
Henderson D, Poppe AB et al (2012) Optimization of a goal maintenance task for use in clinical applications. Schizophr Bull 38(1):104–113
Henik A, Salo R (2004) Schizophrenia and the stroop effect. Behav Cogn Neurosci Rev 3(1):42–59
Henik A, Carter CS et al (2002) Attentional control and word inhibition in schizophrenia. Psychiatry Res 110(2):137–149
Heydari S, Holroyd CB (2016) Reward positivity: reward prediction error or salience prediction error? Psychophysiology 53(8):1185–1192
Holmes AJ, MacDonald A 3rd et al (2005) Prefrontal functioning during context processing in schizophrenia and major depression: an event-related fMRI study. Schizophr Res 76(2-3): 199–206
Horan WP, Green MF et al (2008) Impaired implicit learning in schizophrenia. Neuropsychology 22(5):606–617
Hornak J, O'Doherty J et al (2004) Reward-related reversal learning after surgical excisions in orbito-frontal or dorsolateral prefrontal cortex in humans. J Cogn Neurosci 16(3):463–478
Hunt RR, Einsten GO (1981) Relational and item-specific information in memory. J Verbal Learn Verbal Behav 920:497–514
Hunt RR, McDaniel MA (1993) The enigma of organization and distinctiveness. J Mem Lang 32: 421–445
Hutton SB, Puri BK et al (1998) Executive function in first-epsiode schizophrenia. Psychol Med 28(2):463–473
Iddon JL, McKenna PJ et al (1998) Impaired generation and use of strategy in schizophrenia: evidence from visuospatial and verbal tasks. Psychol Med 28(5):1049–1062
Insel T, Cuthbert B et al (2010) Research domain criteria (RDoC): toward a new classification framework for research on mental disorders. Am J Psychiatry 167(7):748–751
Javitt DC, Zukin SR (1991) Recent advances in the phencyclidine model of schizophrenia. Am J Psychiatry 148(10):1301–1308
Javitt DC, Strous RD et al (1997) Impaired precision, but normal retention, of auditory sensory ("echoic") memory information in schizophrenia. J Abnorm Psychol 106:315–324

Javitt DC, Shelley A et al (2000) Deficits in auditory and visual context-dependent processing in schizophrenia. Arch Gen Psychiatry 57:1131–1137

Jazbec S, Pantelis C et al (2007) Intra-dimensional/extra-dimensional set-shifting performance in schizophrenia: impact of distractors. Schizophr Res 89(1-3):339–349

Joyce E, Hutton S et al (2002) Executive dysfunction in first-episode schizophrenia and relationship to duration of untreated psychosis: the West London study. Br J Psychiatry Suppl 43:s38–s44

Just MA, Carpenter PA et al (1996) The capacity theory of comprehension: new frontiers of evidence and arguments. Psychol Rev 103:773–780

Kane MJ, Engle RW (2000) Working-memory capacity, proactive interference, and divided attention: limits on long-term memory retrieval. J Exp Psychol Learn Mem Cogn 26(2):336–358

Kane MJ, Engle RW (2002) The role of prefrontal cortex in working-memory capacity, executive attention, and general fluid intelligence: an individual-differences perspective. Psychon Bull Rev 9(4):637–671

Kane MJ, Engle RW (2003) Working-memory capacity and the control of attention: the contributions of goal neglect, response competition, and task set to Stroop interference. J Exp Psychol Gen 132(1):47–70

Kane MJ, Bleckley MK et al (2001a) A controlled-attention view of working-memory capacity. J Exp Psychol Gen 130(2):169–183

Kane MJ, Bleckley MK et al (2001b) A controlled-attention view of working memory capacity. J Exp Psychol Gen 130:169–183

Kane MJ, Gross GM et al (2017) For whom the mind wanders, and when, varies across laboratory and daily-life settings. Psychol Sci 28(9):1271–1289

Kanwisher N (2004) The ventral visual object pathway in humans: evidence from fMRI. In: Chalupa LM, Werner JS (eds) The visual neurosciences. MIT Pres, Cambridge, pp 1179–1189

Kapadia MK, Ito M et al (1995) Improvement in visual sensitivity by changes in local context: parallel studies in human observers and in V1 of alert monkeys. Neuron 15(4):843–856

Katzner S, Busse L et al (2011) GABAA inhibition controls response gain in visual cortex. J Neurosci 31(16):5931–5941

Keane BP, Paterno D et al (2016) Visual integration dysfunction in schizophrenia arises by the first psychotic episode and worsens with illness duration. J Abnorm Psychol 125(4):543–549

Keane BP, Barch DM et al (2021) Brain network mechanisms of visual shape completion. Neuroimage 236:118069

Keri S, Kelemen O et al (2000) Schizophrenics know more than they can tell: probabilistic classification learning in schizophrenia. Psychol Med 30(1):149–155

Keri S, Kelemen O et al (2004) Vernier threshold in patients with schizophrenia and in their unaffected siblings. Neuropsychology 18(3):537–542

Keri S, Juhasz A et al (2005) Habit learning and the genetics of the dopamine D3 receptor: evidence from patients with schizophrenia and healthy controls. Behav Neurosci 119(3):687–693

Kim D, Zemon V et al (2005) Dysfunction of early-stage visual processing in schizophrenia: harmonic analysis. Schizophr Res 76(1):55–65

Kim D, Wylie G et al (2006a) Magnocellular contributions to impaired motion processing in schizophrenia. Schizophr Res 82(1):1–8

Kim H, Shimojo S et al (2006b) Is avoiding an aversive outcome rewarding? Neural substrates of avoidance learning in the human brain. PLoS Biol 4(8):e233

Knight RA, Silverstein SM (2001) A process-oriented approach for averting confounds resulting from general performance deficiencies in schizophrenia. J Abnorm Psychol 110(1):15–30

Knutson B, Westdorp A et al (2000) FMRI visualization of brain activity during a monetary incentive delay task. Neuroimage 12:20–27

Knutson B, Adams CM et al (2001) Anticipation of increasing monetary reward selectively recruits nucleus accumbens. J Neurosci 21

Koch K, Schachtzabel C et al (2009) Altered activation in association with reward-related trial-and-error learning in patients with schizophrenia. Neuroimage 50(1):223–232

Koen JD, Borders AA et al (2017) Visual short-term memory for high resolution associations is impaired in patients with medial temporal lobe damage. Hippocampus 27(2):184–193
Kolarik BS, Baer T et al (2018) Close but no cigar: spatial precision deficits following medial temporal lobe lesions provide novel insight into theoretical models of navigation and memory. Hippocampus 28(1):31–41
Kourtzi Z, Tolias AS et al (2003) Integration of local features into global shapes: monkey and human FMRI studies. Neuron 37(2):333–346
Kovacs I (1996) Gestalten of today: early processing of visual contours and surfaces. Behav Brain Res 82(1):1–11
Kovacs I, Polat U et al (2000) A new test of contour integration deficits in patients with a history of disrupted binocular experience during visual development. Vision Res 40(13):1775–1783
Kozma-Wiebe P, Silverstein S et al (2006) Development of a word-wide web based contour integration test: reliablity and validity. Comput Hum Behav 22:971–980
Krystal JH, Anticevic A et al (2017) Impaired tuning of neural ensembles and the pathophysiology of schizophrenia: a translational and computational neuroscience perspective. Biol Psychiatry 81(10):874–885
Lamme VA (1995) The neurophysiology of figure-ground segregation in primary visual cortex. J Neurosci 15(2):1605–1615
Lee J, Park S (2005) Working memory impairments in schizophrenia: a meta-analysis. J Abnorm Psychol 114(4):599–611
Lee J, Park S (2006) The role of stimulus salience in CPT-AX performance of schizophrenia patients. Schizophr Res 81(2-3):191–197
Leeson VC, Robbins TW et al (2009) Discrimination learning, reversal, and set-shifting in first-episode schizophrenia: stability over six years and specific associations with medication type and disorganization syndrome. Biol Psychiatry 66(6):586–593
Lennie P (1980) Parallel visual pathways: a review. Vision Res 20(7):561–594
Lewis DA, Volk DW et al (2004) Selective alterations in prefrontal cortical GABA neurotransmission in schizophrenia: a novel target for the treatment of working memory dysfunction. Psychopharmacology (Berl) 174(1):143–150
Linares D, Amoretti S et al (2020) Spatial suppression and sensitivity for motion in schizophrenia. Schizophrenia Bull Open 1(1):sgaa045
Liu Y, Gu N et al (2021) Effects of transcranial electrical stimulation on working memory in patients with schizophrenia: a systematic review and meta-analysis. Psychiatry Res 296:113656
Lopez-Garcia P, Lesh TA et al (2016) The neural circuitry supporting goal maintenance during cognitive control: a comparison of expectancy AX-CPT and dot probe expectancy paradigms. Cogn Affect Behav Neurosci 16(1):164–175
Luck SJ, Vogel EK (1997) The capacity of visual working memory for features and conjunctions. Nature 390(6657):279–281
MacDonald AW 3rd, Carter CS (2003) Event-related FMRI study of context processing in dorsolateral prefrontal cortex of patients with schizophrenia. J Abnorm Psychol 112(4):689–697
MacDonald AW 3rd, Cohen JD et al (2000) Dissociating the role of the dorsolateral prefrontal and anterior cingulate cortex in cognitive control. Science 288(5472):1835–1838
MacDonald AW 3rd, Becker TM et al (2006) Functional magnetic resonance imaging study of cognitive control in the healthy relatives of schizophrenia patients. Biol Psychiatry 60(11): 1241–1249
MacDonald AW III, Patzelt E et al (in submission) Shared reversal learning impairments in schizophrenia and bipolar disorder reflect a failure to exploit rewards in computational model
MacDonald AW, Pogue-Geile MF et al (2003) A specific deficit in context processing in the unaffected siblings of patients with schizophrenia. Arch Gen Psychiatry 60:57–65
MacDonald A, Carter CS et al (2005a) Specificity of prefrontal dysfunction and context processing defícts to schizophrenia in a never medicated first-episode psychotic sample. Am J Psychiatry 162:475–484

MacDonald AW, 3rd, Goghari VM et al (2005b) A convergent-divergent approach to context processing, general intellectual functioning, and the genetic liability to schizophrenia. Neuropsychology 19(6):814–821
MacQueen GM, Memedovich KA (2017) Cognitive dysfunction in major depression and bipolar disorder: assessment and treatment options. Psychiatry Clin Neurosci 71(1):18–27
Maia TV, Frank MJ (2011) From reinforcement learning models to psychiatric and neurological disorders. Nat Neurosci 14(2):154–162
Maia TV, Frank MJ (2017) An integrative perspective on the role of dopamine in schizophrenia. Biol Psychiatry 81(1):52–66
Man MS, Clarke HF et al (2009) The role of the orbitofrontal cortex and medial striatum in the regulation of prepotent responses to food rewards. Cereb Cortex 19(4):899–906
Marder SR, Fenton W (2004) Measurement and treatment research to improve cognition in schizophrenia: NIMH MATRICS initiative to support the development of agents for improving cognition in schizophrenia. Schizophr Res 72(1):5–9
Martin LF, Kem WR et al (2004) Alpha-7 nicotinic receptor agonists: potential new candidates for the treatment of schizophrenia. Psychopharmacology (Berl) 174(1):54–64
McAlonan K, Brown VJ (2003) Orbital prefrontal cortex mediates reversal learning and not attentional set shifting in the rat. Behav Brain Res 146(1-2):97–103
McClain L (1983) Encoding and retrieval in schizophrenic's free recall. J Nerv Ment Dis 171:471–479
McClure SM, Berns GS et al (2003) Temporal prediction errors in a passive learning task activate human striatum. Neuron 38(2):339–346
McKirdy J, Sussmann JE et al (2009) Set shifting and reversal learning in patients with bipolar disorder or schizophrenia. Psychol Med 39(8):1289–1293
Milienne-Petiot M, Higa KK, Grim A, Deben D, Groenink L, Twamley EW, Geyer MA, Young JW (2018) Nicotine improves probabilistic reward learning in wildtype but not alpha7 nAChR null mutants, yet alpha7 nAChR agonists do not improve probabilistic learning. Eur Neuropsychopharmacol 28(11):1217–1231
Miller EK, Cohen JD (2001) An integrative theory of prefrontal cortex function. Annu Rev Neurosci 21:167–202
Moghaddam B (2004) Targeting metabotropic glutamate receptors for treatment of the cognitive symptoms of schizophrenia. Psychopharmacology (Berl) 174(1):39–44
Montague PR, Sejnowski TJ (1994) The predictive brain: temporal coincidence and temporal order in synaptic learning mechanisms. Learn Mem 1:1–33
Montague PR, Dayan P et al (1996) A framework for mesencephalic dopamine systems based on predictive Hebbian learning. J Neurosci 16:1936–1947
Moore H, Geyer MA et al (2013) Harnessing cognitive neuroscience to develop new treatments for improving cognition in schizophrenia: CNTRICS selected cognitive paradigms for animal models. Neurosci Biobehav Rev 37(9 Pt B):2087–2091
Morris SE, Cuthbert BN (2012) Research domain criteria: cognitive systems, neural circuits, and dimensions of behavior. Dialogues Clin Neurosci 14(1):29–37
Morris SE, Heerey EA et al (2008) Learning-related changes in brain activity following errors and performance feedback in schizophrenia. Schizophr Res 99(1-3):274–285
Murray LJ, Ranganath C (2007) The dorsolateral prefrontal cortex contributes to successful relational memory encoding. J Neurosci 27(20):5515–5522
Murray GK, Cheng F et al (2008) Reinforcement and reversal learning in first-episode psychosis. Schizophr Bull 34(5):848–855
Nothdurft HC, Gallant JL et al (2000) Response profiles to texture border patterns in area V1. Vis Neurosci 17(3):421–436
Oades RD (1997) Stimulus dimension shifts in patients with schizophrenia, with and without paranoid hallucinatory symptoms, or obsessive compulsive disorder: strategies, blocking and monoamine status. Behav Brain Res 88(1):115–131

O'Doherty JP (2007) Lights, camembert, action! The role of human orbitofrontal cortex in encoding stimuli, rewards and choices. Ann N Y Acad Sci 1121:254–272
O'Doherty J, Critchley H et al (2003) Dissociating valence of outcome from behavioral control in human orbital and ventral prefrontal cortices. J Neurosci 23(21):7931–7939
Ongur D, Cullen TJ et al (2006) The neural basis of relational memory deficits in schizophrenia. Arch Gen Psychiatry 63(4):356–365
Padoa-Schioppa C (2007) Orbitofrontal cortex and the computation of economic value. Ann N Y Acad Sci 441(7090):223–226
Padoa-Schioppa C, Assad JA (2006) Neurons in the orbitofrontal cortex encode economic value. Nature 441(7090):223–226
Pantelis C, Barber FZ et al (1999) Comparison of set-shifting ability in patients with chronic schizophrenia and frontal lobe damage. Schizophr Res 37(3):251–270
Park S, Gooding DC (2014) Working memory impairment as an endophenotypic marker of a schizophrenia diathesis. Schizophr Res Cogn 1(3):127–136
Passingham D, Sakai K (2004) The prefrontal cortex and working memory: physiology and brain imaging. Curr Opin Neurobiol 14(2):163–168
Paulsen JS, Heaton RK et al (1995) The nature of learning and memory impairments in schizophrenia. J Int Neuropsychol Soc 1(1):88–99
Pelletier M, Achim AM et al (2005) Cognitive and clinical moderators of recognition memory in schizophrenia: a meta-analysis. Schizophr Res 74(2–3, 233):–252
Pessiglione M, Seymour B et al (2006) Dopamine-dependent prediction errors underpin reward-seeking behaviour in humans. Nature 442(7106):1042–1045
Phillips RC, Salo T et al (2015) Distinct neural correlates for attention lapses in patients with schizophrenia and healthy participants. Front Hum Neurosci 9:502
Pizzagalli DA, Jahn AL et al (2005) Toward an objective characterization of an anhedonic phenotype: a signal-detection approach. Biol Psychiatry 57(4):319–327
Pizzagalli DA, Bogdan R et al (2007) Increased perceived stress is associated with blunted hedonic capacity: potential implications for depression research. Behav Res Ther 45(11):2742–2753
Polgar P, Farkas M et al (2008) How to find the way out from four rooms? The learning of "chaining" associations may shed light on the neuropsychology of the deficit syndrome of schizophrenia. Schizophr Res 99(1-3):200–207
Pomerantz JR, Pristach EA (1989) Emergent features, attention, and perceptual glue in visual form perception. J Exp Psychol Hum Percept Perform 15(4):635–649
Poppe AB, Barch DM et al (2016) Reduced frontoparietal activity in schizophrenia is linked to a specific deficit in goal maintenance: a multisite functional imaging study. Schizophr Bull 42(5): 1149–1157
Postle BR, Berger JS et al (1999) Functional neuroanatomical double dissociation of mnemonic and executive control processes contributing to working memory performance. Proc Natl Acad Sci 96:12959–12964
Pratt DN, Barch DM et al (2021) Reliability and replicability of implicit and explicit reinforcement learning paradigms in people with psychotic disorders. Schizophr Bull 47(3):731–739
Radant AD, Dobie DJ et al (2007) Successful multi-site measurement of antisaccade performance deficits in schizophrenia. Schizophr Res 89(1–3):320–329
Ragland JD, Moelter ST et al (2003) Levels-of-processing effect on word recognition in schizophrenia. Biol Psychiatry 54:1154–1161
Ragland JD, Yoon J et al (2007) Neuroimaging of cognitive disability in schizophrenia: search for a pathophysiological mechanism. Int Rev Psychiatry 19(4):417–427
Ragland JD, Ranganath C et al (2012) Relational and item-specific encoding (RISE): task development and psychometric characteristics. Schizophr Bull 38(1):114–124
Ragland JD, Ranganath C et al (2015) Functional and neuroanatomic specificity of episodic memory dysfunction in schizophrenia: a functional magnetic resonance imaging study of the relational and item-specific encoding task. JAMA Psychiat 72(9):909–916

Ranganath C (2010) A unified framework for the functional organization of the medial temporal lobes and the phenomenology of episodic memory. Hippocampus 20(11):1263–1290

Redish AD, Gordon JA (2016) Breakdowns and failure modes: an engineer's view. In: Redish AD, Gordon JA (eds) Computational psychiatry: new perspectives on mental illness. MIT Press, Cambridge, pp 15–29

Robinson OJ, Frank MJ et al (2010) Dissociable responses to punishment in distinct striatal regions during reversal learning. Neuroimage 51(4):1459–1467

Roesch MR, Olson CR (2005) Neuronal activity in primate orbitofrontal cortex reflects the value of time. J Neurophysiol 94(4):2457–2471

Roeske MJ, Konradi C et al (2021) Hippocampal volume and hippocampal neuron density, number and size in schizophrenia: a systematic review and meta-analysis of postmortem studies. Mol Psychiatry 26(7):3524–3535

Rokem A, Yoon JH et al (2011) Broader visual orientation tuning in patients with schizophrenia. Front Hum Neurosci 5:127

Rolls ET, Sienkiewicz ZJ et al (1989) Hunger modulates the responses to gustatory stimuli of single neurons in the caudolateral orbitofrontal cortex of the macaque monkey. Eur J Neurosci 1(1): 53–60

Roth BL, Hanizavareh SM et al (2004) Serotonin receptors represent highly favorable molecular targets for cognitive enhancement in schizophrenia and other disorders. Psychopharmacology (Berl) 174(1):17–24

Rouder JN, Speckman PL et al (2009) Bayesian t tests for accepting and rejecting the null hypothesis. Psychon Bull Rev 16(2):225–237

Rudebeck PH, Walton ME et al (2006) Separate neural pathways process different decision costs. Nat Neurosci 9(9):1161–1168

Saccuzzo DP, Schubert DL (1981) Backward masking as a measure of slow processing in schizophrenia spectrum disorders. J Abnorm Psychol 90(4):305–312

Schallmo MP, Sponheim SR et al (2013) Abnormal contextual modulation of visual contour detection in patients with schizophrenia. PLoS One 8(6):e68090

Schechter I, Butler PD et al (2005) Impairments in generation of early-stage transient visual evoked potentials to magno- and parvocellular-selective stimuli in schizophrenia. Clin Neurophysiol 116(9):2204–2215

Schoenbaum G, Roesch M (2005) Orbitofrontal cortex, associative learning, and expectancies. Neuron 47(5):633–636

Schooler C, Neumann E et al (1997) A time course analysis of Stroop interference and facilitation: comparing normal and schizophrenic individuals. J Exp Psychol Gen 126:19–36

Schultz W (1992) Activity of dopamine neurons in the behaving primate. Semin Neurosci 4:129–138

Schultz W (2004) Neural coding of basic reward terms of animal learning theory, game theory, microeconomics, and behavioral ecology. Curr Opin Neurobiol 14:139–147

Schultz W (2007) Multiple dopamine functions at different time courses. Annu Rev Neurosci 30: 259–288

Schultz W (2016) Dopamine reward prediction-error signalling: a two-component response. Nat Rev Neurosci 17(3):183–195

Schultz W, Apicella P et al (1993) Responses of monkey dopamine neurons to reward and conditioned stimuli during successive steps of learning a delayed response task. J Neurosci 13(3):900–913

Schultz W, Dayan P et al (1997) A neural substrate of prediction and reward. Science 275:1593–1599

Servan-Schreiber D, Cohen J et al (1996a) Schizophrenic deficits in the processing of context: a test of a theoretical model. Arch Gen Psychiatry 53:1105–1112

Servan-Schreiber D, Cohen JD et al (1996b) Schizophrenic deficits in the processing of context: a test of a theoretical model. Arch Gen Psychiatry 53(Dec):1105–1113

Sheffield JM, Gold JM et al (2014) Common and specific cognitive deficits in schizophrenia: relationships to function. Cogn Affect Behav Neurosci 14(1):161–174
Silverstein SM (2016) Visual perception disturbances in schizophrenia: a unified model. Nebr Symp Motiv 63:77–132
Silverstein SM, Kovacs I et al (2000) Perceptual organization, the disorganization syndrome, and context processing in chronic schizophrenia. Schizophr Res 43(1):11–20
Silverstein SM, Berten S et al (2009) An fMRI examination of visual integration in schizophrenia. J Integr Neurosci 8(2):175–202
Silverstein SM, Keane BP et al (2012) Optimization and validation of a visual integration test for schizophrenia research. Schizophr Bull 38(1):125–134
Silverstein S, Keane BP et al (2015a) Vision in schizophrenia: why it matters. Front Psychol 6:41
Silverstein SM, Harms MP et al (2015b) Cortical contributions to impaired contour integration in schizophrenia. Neuropsychologia 75:469–480
Silverstein SM, Demmin DL et al (2017) Computational Modeling of contrast sensitivity and orientation tuning in first-episode and chronic schizophrenia. Comput Psychiatr 1:102–131
Silverstein SM, Keane BP et al (2020) Visual impairments in schizophrenia: their significance and unrealized clinical potential. Psychiatr Danub 32(1):72–73
Slaghuis WL (1998) Contrast sensitivity for stationary and drifting spatial frequency gratings in positive- and negative-symptom schizophrenia. J Abnorm Psychol 107(1):49–62
Slaghuis WL, Thompson AK (2003) The effect of peripheral visual motion on focal contrast sensitivity in positive- and negative-symptom schizophrenia. Neuropsychologia 41(8):968–980
Smeekens BA, Kane MJ (2016) Working memory capacity, mind wandering, and creative cognition: an individual-differences investigation into the benefits of controlled versus spontaneous thought. Psychol Aesthet Creat Arts 10(4):389–415
Somlai Z, Moustafa AA et al (2011) General functioning predicts reward and punishment learning in schizophrenia. Schizophr Res 127(1-3):131–136
Soni A, Singh P et al (2017) Impact of cognition and clinical factors on functional outcome in patients with bipolar disorder. East Asian Arch Psychiatry 27(1):26–34
Spencer KM, Nestor PG et al (2003) Abnormal neural synchrony in schizophrenia. J Neurosci 23(19):7407–7411
Spencer KM, Nestor PG et al (2004) Neural synchrony indexes disordered perception and cognition in schizophrenia. Proc Natl Acad Sci U S A 101(49):17288–17293
Starc M, Murray JD et al (2017) Schizophrenia is associated with a pattern of spatial working memory deficits consistent with cortical disinhibition. Schizophr Res 181:107–116
Stone M, Gabrieli JD et al (1998) Working and strategic memory deficits in schizophrenia. Neuropsychology 12:278–288
Stratta P, Daneluzzo E et al (1998) Schizophrenic deficits in the processing of context. Arch Gen Psychiatry 55:186–187
Stratta P, Daneluzzo E et al (2000) Processing of context information in schizophrenia: relation to clinical symptoms and WCST performance. Schizophr Res 44:57–67
Strauss GP, Frank MJ et al (2011) Deficits in positive reinforcement learning and uncertainty-driven exploration are associated with distinct aspects of negative symptoms in schizophrenia. Biol Psychiatry 69(5):424–431
Strauss ME, McLouth CJ et al (2013) Temporal stability and moderating effects of age and sex on CNTRaCS task performance. Schizophr Bull
Strauss ME, McLouth CJ et al (2014) Temporal stability and moderating effects of age and sex on CNTRaCS task performance. Schizophr Bull 40(4):835–844
Tamminga CA (2006) The neurobiology of cognition in schizophrenia. J Clin Psychiatry 67(9):e11
Titone D, Ditman T et al (2004) Transitive inference in schizophrenia: impairments in relational memory organization. Schizophr Res 68(2-3):235–247
Tu PC, Yang TH et al (2006) Neural correlates of antisaccade deficits in schizophrenia, an fMRI study. J Psychiatr Res 40(7):606–612

Turner DC, Aitken MR et al (2004) The role of the lateral frontal cortex in causal associative learning: exploring preventative and super-learning. Cereb Cortex 14(8):872–880

Tyson PJ, Laws KR et al (2004) Stability of set-shifting and planning abilities in patients with schizophrenia. Psychiatry Res 129(3):229–239

Uhlhaas PJ, Silverstein SM (2005) Perceptual organization in schizophrenia spectrum disorders: empirical research and theoretical implications. Psychol Bull 131(4):618–632

Uhlhaas PJ, Phillips WA et al (2005) The course and clinical correlates of dysfunctions in visual perceptual organization in schizophrenia during the remission of psychotic symptoms. Schizophr Res 75(2-3):183–192

Uhlhaas PJ, Phillips WA et al (2006) Perceptual grouping in disorganized schizophrenia. Psychiatry Res 145(2-3):105–117

Unsworth N, Redick TS et al (2009) Complex working memory span tasks and higher-order cognition: a latent-variable analysis of the relationship between processing and storage. Memory 17(6):635–654

van den Berg R, Shin H et al (2012) Variability in encoding precision accounts for visual short-term memory limitations. Proc Natl Acad Sci U S A 109(22):8780–8785

Van Snellenberg JX, Torres IJ et al (2006) Functional neuroimaging of working memory in schizophrenia: task performance as a moderating variable. Neuropsychology 20(5):497–510

Wagenmakers EJ, Love J et al (2017a) Bayesian inference for psychology. Part II: example applications with JASP. Psychon Bull Rev

Wagenmakers EJ, Marsman M et al (2017b) Bayesian inference for psychology. Part I: theoretical advantages and practical ramifications. Psychon Bull Rev

Wallis JD (2007) Orbitofrontal cortex and its contribution to decision-making. Annu Rev Neurosci 30:31–56

Waltz JA, Gold JM (2007) Probabilistic reversal learning impairments in schizophrenia: further evidence of orbitofrontal dysfunction. Schizophr Res 93(1-3):296–303

Waltz JA, Frank MJ et al (2007) Selective reinforcement learning deficits in schizophrenia support predictions from computational models of striatal-cortical dysfunction. Biol Psychiatry

Waltz JA, Frank MJ et al (2011) Altered probabilistic learning and response biases in schizophrenia: behavioral evidence and neurocomputational modeling. Neuropsychology 25(1):86–97

Wei Z, Wang XJ et al (2012) From distributed resources to limited slots in multiple-item working memory: a spiking network model with normalization. J Neurosci 32(33):11228–11240

Weickert TW, Terrazas A et al (2002) Habit and skill learning in schizophrenia: evidence of normal striatal processing with abnormal cortical input. Learn Mem 9(6):430–442

Weickert TW, Goldberg TE et al (2009) Neural correlates of probabilistic category learning in patients with schizophrenia. J Neurosci 29(4):1244–1254

Weiler JA, Bellebaum C et al (2009) Impairment of probabilistic reward-based learning in schizophrenia. Neuropsychology 23(5):571–580

Weiss AP, Schacter DL et al (2003) Impaired hippocampal recruitment during normal modulation of memory performance in schizophrenia. Biol Psychiatry 53:48–55

Weiss EM, Hofer A et al (2004) Brain activation patterns during a verbal fluency test-a functional MRI study in healthy volunteers and patients with schizophrenia. Schizophr Res 70(2-3): 287–291

Wilde OM, Bour L et al (2007) Antisaccade deficit is present in young first-episode patients with schizophrenia but not in their healthy young siblings. Psychol Med:1–5

Yeap S, Kelly SP et al (2006) Early visual sensory deficits as endophenotypes for schizophrenia: high-density electrical mapping in clinically unaffected first-degree relatives. Arch Gen Psychiatry 63(11):1180–1188

Yoon JH, Maddock RJ et al (2010) GABA concentration is reduced in visual cortex in schizophrenia and correlates with orientation-specific surround suppression. J Neurosci 30(10):3777–3781

Zaragoza Domingo S, Bobes J et al (2015) Cognitive performance associated to functional outcomes in stable outpatients with schizophrenia. Schizophr Res Cogn 2(3):146–158

Zenger-Landolt B, Heeger DJ (2003) Response suppression in v1 agrees with psychophysics of surround masking. J Neurosci 23(17):6884–6893

Zhang W, Luck SJ (2008) Discrete fixed-resolution representations in visual working memory. Nature 453(7192):233–235

Zhang WN, Chang SH et al (2013) The neural correlates of reward-related processing in major depressive disorder: a meta-analysis of functional magnetic resonance imaging studies. J Affect Disord 151(2):531–539

Zhang R, Picchioni M et al (2016) Working memory in unaffected relatives of patients with schizophrenia: a meta-analysis of functional magnetic resonance imaging studies. Schizophr Bull 42(4):1068–1077

Attention in Schizophrenia

Steven J. Luck and James M. Gold

Contents

Abstract Attention is clearly a core area of cognitive dysfunction in schizophrenia, but the concept of "attention" is complex and multifaceted. This chapter focuses on three different aspects of attentional function that are of particular interest in schizophrenia. First, we discuss the evidence that schizophrenia involves a reduction in global alertness, leading to an inward focusing of attention and a neglect of external stimuli and tasks. Second, we discuss the control of attention, the set of processes that allow general goals to be translated into shifts of attention toward task-relevant information. When a goal is adequately represented, people with schizophrenia often show no deficit in using the goal to direct attention in the visual modality unless challenged by stimuli that strongly activate the magnocellular processing pathway. Finally, we discuss the implementation of selection, the

S. J. Luck (✉)
Department of Psychology, Center for Mind and Brain, University of California, Davis, CA, USA
e-mail: sjluck@ucdavis.edu

J. M. Gold
Department of Psychiatry, Maryland Psychiatric Research Center, University of Maryland School of Medicine, Baltimore, MD, USA

Curr Topics Behav Neurosci (2023) 63: 61–78
https://doi.org/10.1007/7854_2022_380
Published Online: 29 July 2022

processes that boost relevant information and suppress distractors once attention has been directed to a given source of information. Although early evidence indicated an impairment in selection, more recent evidence indicating that people with schizophrenia actually focus their attention more narrowly and more intensely that healthy individuals (hyperfocusing). However, this hyperfocused attention may be directed toward goal-irrelevant information, creating the appearance of impaired attentional filtering.

Keywords Alertness · Attentional control · Attentional selection · Hyperfocusing

1 Defining Attention

Attentional dysfunction has been a part of the clinical description of schizophrenia since the days of Bleuler (1911) and Kraepelin (1919). Consider, for example, this self-report (Djinn (pseudonym) 2014): "I remember one day when I got caught in the rain. Each drop felt like an electric shock and I found it hard to move because of how intense and painful the feeling was." This sort of sensory flooding was classically attributed to an inability to focus attention on relevant information and filter out irrelevant information (McGhie and Chapman 1961; Venables 1963).

Much more is now known about the nature of attention in the healthy brain and the dysfunction of attention in people with schizophrenia (PSZ), and the story is now richer and more complex than the simple idea of a "broken filter." This richness and complexity requires that we subdivide attention into three key components: (1) the global state of alertness; (2) the control of attention; and (3) the implementation of selection. In the Research Domain Criteria (RDoC) framework (RDoC Matrix 2022), global alertness is related to the *arousal* construct, whereas control and implementation are distinguished within the *attention* construct.

All three of these components combine to influence behavior, but they must be carefully distinguished to understand the nature of attentional dysfunction in schizophrenia. To preview the conclusions of this chapter: current research indicates that schizophrenia involves a reduction in global attentiveness, an impairment in the ability to direct attention toward relevant sources of information under some but not all conditions, and a tendency to hyperfocus on the currently selected object of attention.

2 Global Alertness

Global alertness is a general state of the organism that ranges from unfocused on one end of the continuum to vigilant on the other (Posner 2008). In a low state of alertness, the mind wanders (Braboszcz and Delorme 2011) and is occupied by internal thoughts rather than external tasks. Low alertness is often accompanied by an increase in alpha-band EEG activity (8–12 Hz) and increased activity in the default mode network (Compton et al. 2019; Arnau et al. 2020; Boudewyn and Carter 2018; Christoff et al. 2009), which are potential biomarkers for alertness.

Decreased alertness can potentially lead to impaired behavioral performance across a broad range of tasks, and impaired performance in a given task may reflect decreased alertness rather than an impairment in the processes the task is designed to tap. In neurotypical young adults, for example, individual differences in the performance of working memory tasks and intelligence tests appear to be at least partially a result of individual differences in mind wandering (which is associated with decreased alertness (Braboszcz and Delorme 2011; Mrazek et al. 2012)). Similarly, in psychophysical procedures designed to assess sensory thresholds, lapses in attention can make it appear (incorrectly) that sensory processing is impaired (Clark and Merfeld 2021; Wichmann and Hill 2001). That is, if participants have lapses of attention on a significant proportion of trials, this will lead to increased sensory thresholds even if there is nothing wrong with the sensory systems per se. Thus, it is important to factor out differences in global alertness when attempting to quantify deficits in sensory or cognitive function in PSZ. However, it is nontrivial to isolate deficits in specific sensory or cognitive abilities from deficits in global alertness.

One approach to solving this problem is to use paradigms that include occasional "catch trials" that are so easy that errors on these trials likely reflect lapses of attention. The error rate on these trials can be used to estimate the lapse rate. For example, an initial study of visuospatial integration found that PSZ are less impacted by a task-irrelevant stimulus surrounding the target than are HCS (Dakin et al. 2005), but a subsequent study that included catch trials found that the apparent difference in surround processing was eliminated when the lapse rate was included as a covariate (Barch et al. 2012).

Similarly, a recent study examined whether reduced working memory performance in PSZ relative to HCS could be explained by differences in the lapse rate (Gold et al. 2020). Figure 1a shows the experimental design, which used a modified change detection task. In a standard change detection task (Luck and Vogel 2013), subjects view a sample array consisting of multiple colored squares, followed by a delay interval and then a test array that is either identical to the sample array or differs in the color of one item. Subjects report "change" or "no change" on each trial. Performance on this task can be used to estimate working memory capacity (K), but storage capacity will be underestimated if lapses of attention occur. To factor out lapses of attention, the paradigm was modified so that more than one item might change on each trial, but the task was still to report "change" (if one or more changes were detected) or "no change" (if no changes were detected) (Gibson et al. 2011). When all of the items change, it should be trivially easy for the subject to detect the change as long as the subject is paying attention. The error rate on these trials can therefore be used to determine how often attention lapsed. As shown in Fig. 1b, a model can be fit to the data to separately estimate the storage capacity and the lapse rate (see (Feuerstahler et al. 2019) for limitations).

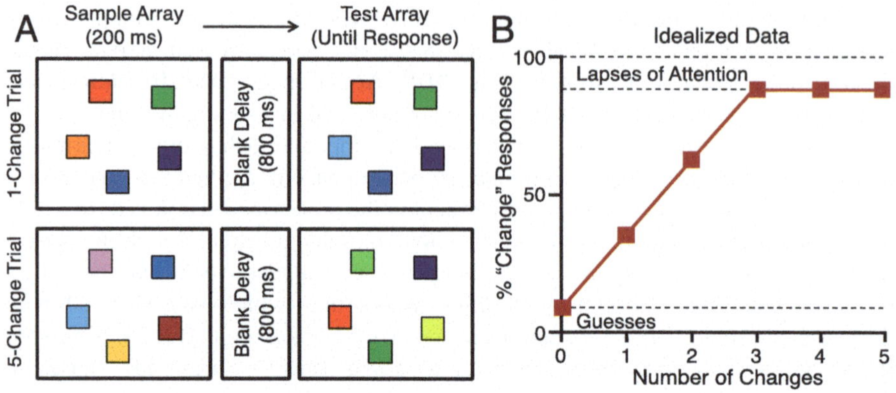

Fig. 1 Modified change detection task (**a**) and idealized data (**b**). The task is report whether or not any colors changed between the sample and test array (regardless of the number of changes). When most or all of the items change, the changes should always be detected unless attention has lapsed

The study that used this task (Gold et al. 2020) examined several different diagnostic groups (schizophrenia, schizoaffective disorder, bipolar disorder, and matched control subjects). Storage capacity was found to be only modestly reduced in the patient groups compared to the healthy control group, but the lapse rate was substantially higher in each of the patient groups than in the control group. In addition, when performance on multiple working memory tasks was combined into a factor analysis, the lapse rate formed a distinct factor, indicating that it represents a separate source of variance that can be dissociated from working memory capacity (see also chapter "Working Memory in People with Schizophrenia" this volume).

Unfortunately, lapses of attention have been carefully isolated in only a few studies of schizophrenia. However, it is plausible that PSZ exhibit greater lapse rates as a result of decreased global alertness across multiple laboratory tasks. In everyday life, decreased global alertness may have a variety of practical consequences, such as increased accidents, decreased learning, and impaired social interactions. Indeed, the lapse rate in the study shown in Fig. 1 was correlated with the UPSA-B measure of functional capacity (Gold et al. 2020).

Relatively little is known at this point about the neural systems that underlie decreased global alertness in schizophrenia. In a task similar to that shown in Fig. 1, greater alpha-band EEG activity during the pretrial interval (indicated decreased global alertness) was significantly correlated with a measure of the lapse rate in PSZ (Erickson et al. 2017). However, this is really just further evidence that the lapses were caused by decreased alertness rather than being an explanation of the decreased alertness.

One possible explanation is that PSZ have difficulty inhibiting the default mode network (DMN), which is activated during states of decreased alertness and increased mind wandering (Fernández-Espejo et al. 2012; Sämann et al. 2011; Fox et al. 2015). Indeed, differences in DMN activation are associated with differences in sustained attention among healthy individuals (Compton et al. 2019; Arnau et al.

2020; Boudewyn and Carter 2018; Christoff et al. 2009). Psychotic symptoms such as hallucinations might also lead PSZ to focus more on their internal thoughts and less on external stimuli and goals. However, although some studies have found evidence of reduced task-elicited DMN inhibition in PSZ, others have found the opposite pattern (Hahn et al. 2017). Another possibility is that the reduction in global alertness is a consequence of a general reduction in cognitive control. Consistent with this possibility, one study found that lapses of attention were associated with greater DMN activation in HCS whereas lapses were associated with reduced activity in the frontoparietal attention network in PSZ (Phillips et al. 2015).

To conclude this section on global alertness, we would like to note that no clinician would be surprised to hear that PSZ exhibit greater mind wandering and tend to focus on internal thoughts rather than the external environment. However, this aspect of attention has received relatively little study over the past two decades even though it is likely of significant importance for the daily life of PSZ. Earlier research examined this issue but often focused on the question of whether performance falls more rapidly over time in PSZ than in HCS (a vigilance decrement). These studies typically found that PSZ exhibited impaired performance relative to HCS from the very beginning of the session, without much evidence of a faster decline in PSZ ((Nuechterlein et al. 1994), but see (Hahn et al. 2012a)). The reduced performance observed throughout the session could potentially be attributed to impairments in a wide range of sensory or cognitive processes, so this research could not isolate global alertness from other factors. Methods are now available to distinguish between these processes (such as the task shown in Fig. 1), so this important aspect of cognitive impairment in schizophrenia is now ripe for more detailed research.

3 Control of Attention in Schizophrenia

Attention is often conceptualized as a mental spotlight (Norman 1968; Posner et al. 1980). The control of attention in this analogy would be the set of mechanisms that determine where the spotlight is pointing, whereas the implementation of selection would be the set of mechanisms that control the brightness of the beam (Luck and Gold 2008). Attentional control is largely determined by the frontoparietal attention network, whereas the implementation of selection largely occurs within specific processing systems (e.g., within visual cortex for visual perception tasks) (Posner and Petersen 1990). Attentional control is also impacted by the ability to maintain the correct task set in memory. In many experiments, reduced task performance in a patient group can be explained by reduced maintenance of the task set, by impaired control per se, or by impaired selection, so special care is needed to determine the cause of reduced performance in attentional paradigms.

A simple way to minimize the impact of impaired task maintenance is to provide a constant reminder of the task. For example, in experiments that involve selecting targets of one color and ignoring distractors of another color, the color of the to-be-selected target can be indicated by the fixation point ("R" for attend-red and "B" for attend-blue, as in Sawaki et al. (2017)).

3.1 Control of Attention: Evidence from Salient Distractors

To distinguish between impaired control and impaired selection, one can vary the difficulty of control by using distractor stimuli that vary in physical salience. If schizophrenia involves impaired attentional control, then PSZ should be particularly impaired when asked to focus on a low-salience target object in the presence of a highly salient distractor object.

Several studies have confirmed this hypothesis. For example, Fig. 2a illustrates a spatial working memory experiment (Hahn et al. 2012b) in which six checkerboards were presented on each trial, three of which were flickering (high salience) and three of which were static (low salience). When subjects were asked to prioritize the high-salience checkerboards, both HCS and PSZ remembered the high-salience checkerboards better than the low-salience checkerboards. When asked to prioritize the low-salience checkerboards, however, PSZ failed to filter out the high-salience checkerboards (see also (Erickson et al. 2015)).

Figure 2b shows an analogous visual search task, in which subjects were asked to find a target (a circle with a gap on the top or bottom) among a large set of distractors (Bansal et al. 2019). Each object was either low-contrast (light gray) or high-contrast (black). Subjects were instructed that the target would always be high-contrast in some trial blocks and that it would always be low-contrast in others. Eye tracking data indicated that both HCS and PSZ could avoid directing gaze toward the low-contrast items when searching for a high-contrast target, but PSZ were impaired at avoiding the high-contrast items when searching for a low-contrast target.

Although these results appear to support the hypothesis of impaired attentional control in schizophrenia, there is another possible explanation: The salient items in

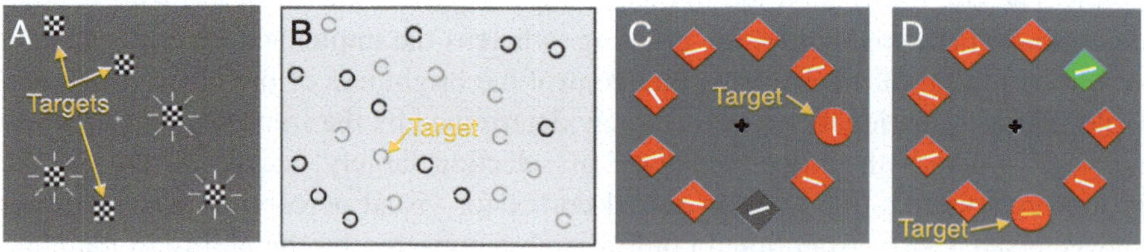

Fig. 2 (**a**) Example stimulus from the working memory task used in Hahn et al. (2012b), with three flickering checkerboards and two static checkerboards. The key task was to remember the less salient static checkerboards and ignore the flickering checkerboards. (**b**) Example stimulus from the visual search task used in Bansal et al. (2019). The key task was to find a low-contrast circle with a gap on the bottom or top, ignoring the high-contrast distractors. (**c**, **d**) Example stimulus from the visual search task used in Leonard et al. (2014). The task was to report the orientation of the line inside the target (the circle). The displays could contain a luminance singleton distractor (**c**) or a color singleton distractor (**d**), which were equally salient in healthy individuals

these experiments also presumably activated the magnocellular visual pathway, which appears to be dysregulated in schizophrenia (Butler et al. 2003; Cadenhead et al. 1998; Green et al. 1994a). Support for this alternative was provided by a study using the paradigm shown in Fig. 2c, d (Leonard et al. 2014). The target in this study was a shape singleton (a circle among diamonds or a diamond among circles), and some trials also contained a salient distractor singleton. The distractor singleton was either a luminance singleton (black among either red or green) or a color singleton that was isoluminant with the other objects (red among green or green among red). The luminance singleton was designed to be easily detectable by the magnocellular pathway, whereas the color singleton was designed to be invisible to this pathway. Importantly, pretesting showed that luminance and color singletons were equally salient to healthy individuals (Leonard and Luck 2011). However, PSZ showed more capture by the luminance singleton than by the color singleton, and they showed no more capture by the color singleton than did HCS. A follow-up study using eye tracking to measure attention found that PSZ could suppress a potentially distracting color singleton just as well as HCS (Bansal et al. 2021). Together, these results suggest that schizophrenia does not involve a general impairment in attentional control but instead show an exaggerated allocation of attention to stimuli that strongly activate the magnocellular pathway.

3.2 Control of Attention: Evidence from Implicit Priming

Another approach to examining the control of attention is to pit explicit task goals against implicit priming from previous trials. Research from the basic cognitive science literature has shown that what happens on one trial can strongly influence the allocation of attention on the next trial. For example, studies of healthy young adults using variations on the paradigm shown in Fig. 2d have shown that gaze is often directed to the location that had contained the target on the previous trial, even though this location is no more likely than any other location to contain the current-trial target (Talcott and Gaspelin 2020). This priming effect is stronger in PSZ than in HCS (Bansal et al. 2019). Similarly, when the color of a target is incidental but varies from trial to trial, healthy young adults detect the current-trial target more rapidly when its color matches the previous-trial targets (Kristjansson 2008), and this effect is significantly enhanced in PSZ (Leonard et al. 2020).

These implicit priming effects suggest that schizophrenia reduces the voluntary control of attention, allowing irrelevant information from previous trials to have a larger effect on the direction of attention on the current trial. However, an alternative possibility is that the irrelevant information from the previous trials is simply stronger in PSZ than in HCS. In either case, task goals are more likely to be overridden by persisting information from the past in PSZ, which may lead to increased perseverative behavior (Crider 1997; Bilder and Goldberg 1987).

4 Selection in Schizophrenia: Impaired Focusing or Hyperfocusing?

Classic research supported the idea that schizophrenia involves a "broken filter" and that PSZ are unable to filter out irrelevant information (reviewed by Luck et al. (2019a)). However, more recent research has led to the opposite conclusion, namely that schizophrenia involves a tendency to "hyperfocus" attention (reviewed by Luck et al. (2019b)). Here we will review the evidence for both of these conclusions and then propose a potential reconciliation.

4.1 Early Studies of Impaired Focusing

Many early studies of attention in schizophrenia used a dichotic listening paradigm in which subjects were instructed to "shadow" (listen to and repeat) speech delivered to one ear and ignore the other ear. In HCS, this research found that shadowing was more difficult when irrelevant speech was simultaneously delivered to the other ear compared to when no speech was delivered to the other ear. This effect was even larger in PSZ. That is, PSZ were much more impaired by the irrelevant speech than were HCS (Payne et al. 1970; Wahl 1976; Wishner and Wahl 1974; Schneider 1976; Wielgus and Harvey 1988). Moreover, PSZ tended to remember more information from the irrelevant speech signal than HCS (Payne et al. 1970; Wishner and Wahl 1974), providing positive evidence that they failed to filter speech inputs from the to-be-ignored ear.

Other classic research used a short-term memory distraction paradigm, in which subjects had to remember a sequence of letters and digits spoken in a female voice. PSZ became highly impaired in this task when the task-relevant information was interspersed with to-be-ignored letters and digits spoken in a male voice (Lawson et al. 1967; McGhie et al. 1965).

Several important caveats must be raised with regard to these classic findings. First, the dichotic listening effects could reflect a psychometric artifact: Patient deficits in dichotic listening were primarily found under the conditions that were also most difficult for HCS (Oltmanns 1978; Oltmanns and Neale 1975; Oltmanns et al. 1978) (although this was not an issue with the short-term memory distraction studies). Second, these findings could reflect an impairment in attentional control rather than an impairment in the filtering process itself (Hugdahl et al. 2003). Third, they could be a consequence of active psychosis rather than reflecting the relatively stable cognitive deficits that characterize schizophrenia. Specifically, most of these studies used inpatients, and many of the effects were correlated with positive symptoms, were reduced by antipsychotic medications, or were present only during periods of relatively severe psychosis (Oltmanns et al. 1978; Green et al. 1994b; Hugdahl et al. 2012). Finally, these effects were largely limited to the auditory modality. For example, no patient impairment was found in visual versions of the short-term memory distraction paradigm (Lawson et al. 1967; McGhie et al. 1965).

4.2 Hyperfocusing: Narrow But Intense Focusing of Attention

More recent studies – mainly using visual stimuli and testing medicated outpatients – have often found evidence that PSZ exhibit hyperfocusing, focusing their attention more narrowly and intensely than HCS, especially when the task was designed to require a broad distribution of processing resources (Luck et al. 2019b; Ashinoff and Abu-Akel 2021). In other words, HCS can focus their attention narrowly and intensely when necessitated by the task, but PSZ tend to focus narrowly and intensely even when this is unnecessary or counterproductive.

Figure 3a shows an example case of hyperfocusing in a spatial cueing paradigm (Hahn et al. 2012c). On each trial, a central cue indicated either a single location that should be attended or that attention should be divided equally among all four locations. A peripheral target stimulus was then presented. HCS performed the task equally well when a single location was cued and when all four locations were cued, with similar error rates for both trial types. However, PSZ were impaired when four locations were cued compared to when one location was cued. That is, PSZ were unimpaired when asked to focus on a single location but had difficulty distributing their attention broadly. These results have been replicated twice (Hahn et al. 2013, 2016), and similar results were obtained by another lab using a similar paradigm (Spencer et al. 2011).

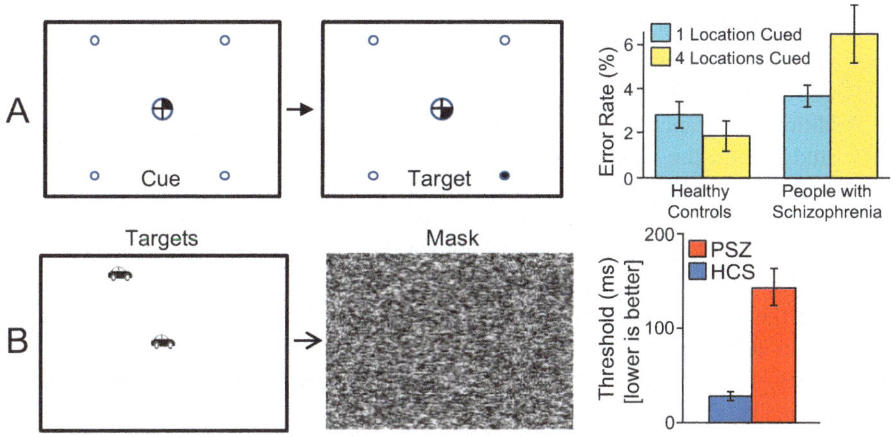

Fig. 3 (**a**) Stimuli and results from Hahn et al. (2012c). (**b**) Stimuli and results from Gray et al. (2014)

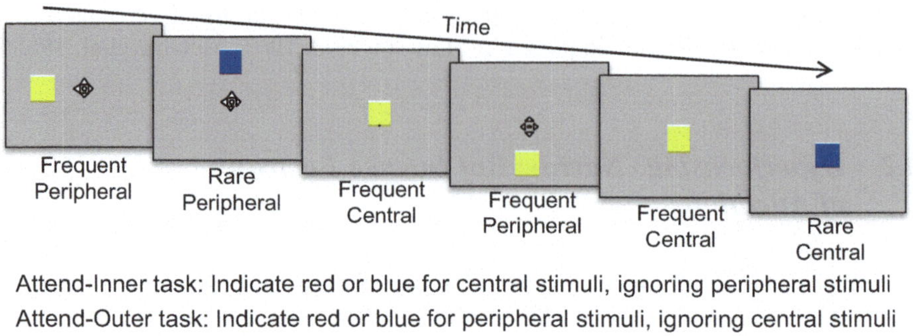

Fig. 4 Experimental task from Kreither et al. (2017)

A similar impairment in attending broadly was observed in a study using the useful field of view task (Gray et al. 2014), which predicts real-world outcomes such as automobile driving performance (Clay et al. 2005). In the key condition (see Fig. 3b), subjects must discriminate whether a central stimulus is a car or a truck and also report the location of a simultaneously presented peripheral stimulus. The stimulus display is masked, and the stimulus exposure duration prior to the mask is varied using a staircase procedure to determine the time needed for subjects to reach 75% correct on both the central and peripheral tasks (the threshold). A greater threshold indicates that a longer exposure duration is needed to reach a given accuracy level, so larger values indicate a poorer ability to divide attention between the central target and the peripheral target. The mean threshold was more than five times as great in PSZ than in HCS, with an effect size (Cohen's d) of 1.33. Thus, PSZ exhibit a massive impairment in the ability to distribute attention broadly in this task.

Visuospatial attention is ordinarily biased toward the center of gaze, and multiple pieces of evidence indicate that PSZ tend to hyperfocus on the center of gaze. For example, when required to make an eye movement toward a peripheral location, PSZ are more likely than HCS to make short (hypometric) saccades, as if they cannot shift their gaze as easily away from the current point of fixation (Leonard et al. 2013; Luck et al. 2014; Everling et al. 1996; Hutton et al. 2001).

Additional evidence for hyperfocusing on the center of gaze was obtained in an ERP study using the task shown in Fig. 4 (Kreither et al. 2017). A sequence of stimuli was presented, with some stimuli at fixation (inner location) and others in the periphery (outer locations). There were two colors, one of which was rare (shown as blue in Fig. 4) and one of which was frequent (shown as yellow in Fig. 4). In some trial blocks, subjects were asked to perform an Attend-Inner task in which they indicated the color of the inner stimuli with a buttonpress response, making no response to the outer stimuli. In other blocks, they performed an Attend-Outer task in which they indicated the color of the outer stimuli and ignored the inner stimuli. Thus, subjects were required either to attend narrowly at fixation or broadly in the periphery.

In general, the hyperfocusing hypothesis would predict that PSZ would tend to focus narrowly on fixation, allowing them to filter out the peripheral stimuli more effectively than HCS in the Attend-Inner condition. However, hyperfocusing would also lead to increased processing of the central stimuli in PSZ relative to HCS in the Attend-Outer condition. These predictions were verified with both a measure of sensory processing (the P1 ERP component) and cognitive processing (the P3b ERP component).

Specifically, PSZ were impaired relative to HCS at suppressing the P1 component for the central stimulus in the Attend-Outer condition, but PSZ were actually significantly better than HCS at suppressing the peripheral stimulus in the Attend-Inner condition. Similar results were observed for cognitive processing, quantified as the difference in P3b amplitude between the rare and frequent stimuli. That is, PSZ had a smaller P3b effect than HCS for peripheral stimuli in the Attend-Inner condition, but PSZ actually had a larger P3b effect than HCS for central stimuli in the Attend-Outer condition. In other words, PSZ were impaired relative to HCS at suppressing central stimuli when asked to attend broadly, but PSZ were actually superior to HCS at suppressing peripheral stimuli when asked to attend narrowly at fixation.

4.3 *Hyperfocusing: Exaggerated Focusing on Partial Matches*

Another important aspect of the greater intensity of attention proposed by the hyperfocusing hypothesis is that PSZ will "go all in" when focusing attention onto a given source of information. This has been observed in several paradigms in which a given nontarget item partially matches the desired target item (Sawaki et al. 2017; Mayer et al. 2012; Leonard et al. 2017). These items will typically attract some attention in healthy individuals (Folk et al. 1992, 2002), but this allocation of attention is exaggerated in PSZ.

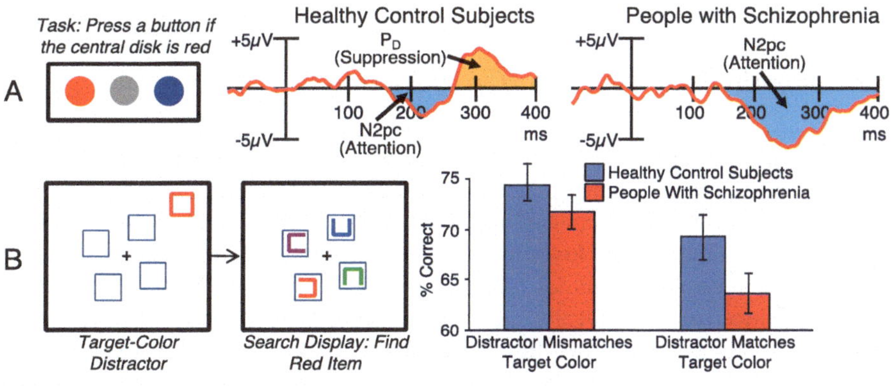

Fig. 5 (**a**) Stimuli and data from Sawaki et al. (2017). (**b**) Stimuli and data from Mayer et al. (2012)

An example using ERPs is illustrated in Fig. 5a (Sawaki et al. 2017). On each trial, three colored disks appeared, and the task was to press a button if the central disk was a particular target color (e.g., red) and ignore the flanking disks. Occasionally a flanking disk is drawn in the target color, in which case it partially matches the target description (i.e., it is the correct color but an incorrect location). Two different ERP components are of interest in this task: the *N2pc* component, which reflects the focusing of attention; and the P_D component, which reflects a suppressive process (Luck 2012). A study of a neurotypical college population found that target-colored flankers elicit a brief N2pc followed by a large P_D, indicating that attention is briefly captured by the flanker, followed by suppression (Sawaki et al. 2012). When this paradigm was used in PSZ and matched HCS, the HCS showed the same pattern as the college population, namely a brief N2pc followed by a P_D (attention followed by suppression; see Fig. 5a, middle). However, PSZ exhibited a large and sustained N2pc component (Fig. 5a, right), indicating that they focused their attention more intensely on the target-colored flanker. Note that this exaggerated focusing of attention in PSZ cannot be explained by extraneous factors such as reduced motivation or a failure to remember which color was task-relevant.

An analogous pattern of results was obtained in the behavioral experiment shown in Fig. 5b (Mayer et al. 2012). In this study, the task was to find an item of a target color (e.g., red) and press a button to indicate the shape of this item. A peripheral distractor appeared immediately prior to the target display. Target discrimination performance was reduced in both HCS and PSZ when the distractor was the same color as the target compared to when the distractor was drawn in a task-irrelevant color. However, this distraction effect was substantially larger in PSZ than in HCS (Fig. 5b, right). In other words, a distractor that partially matches the to-be-discriminated target attracted attention in both HCS and PSZ, reducing target discrimination performance, but the target-colored distractor created a stronger shift of attention in PSZ than in HCS. Again, this stronger shift cannot be explained by factors such as reduced motivation or impaired memory for which color was relevant. A similar pattern was observed in a study using a completely different behavioral task (Leonard et al. 2017).

4.4 Impaired Focusing or Hyperfocusing?

We have now discussed early studies indicating that the selective focusing of attention is impaired in schizophrenia and more recent studies that have reached the opposite conclusion, concluding that schizophrenia involves an aberrant hyperfocusing of attention. How can we resolve this apparent discrepancy?

There are several possibilities (see (Luck et al. 2019a) for further discussion). First, the older studies typically examined inpatients with fairly high levels of positive symptoms, so impaired filtering in PSZ may be associated with periods of acute psychosis. In contrast, the more recent evidence for hyperfocusing comes primarily from studies of medicated outpatients. Thus, hyperfocusing may be part of the pattern of cognitive dysfunction that is observed during periods of clinical stability.

A second possibility is that the discrepancy reflects differences between the auditory and visual modalities. The early studies showing impaired filtering primarily used auditory stimuli, whereas the more recent studies showing hyperfocusing have used visual stimuli. Consistent with this possibility, two early studies using the short-term memory distraction paradigm found increased distraction in PSZ relative to HCS with auditory stimuli but not with visual stimuli (Lawson et al. 1967; McGhie et al. 1965). It would be useful for researchers to examine the issue of modality differences using contemporary methods for defining diagnostic groups and for measuring attentional function.

A third possibility is that PSZ are able to focus their attention quite strongly – and may even focus more narrowly and intensely than HCS – but they may focus on the wrong sources of information. Indeed, the studies shown in Fig. 5 show that PSZ may focus more intensely than HCS on objects that are not targets but contain one or more task-relevant properties. Similarly, impairments in cognitive control or context maintenance could lead PSZ to focus on irrelevant sources of information. Such factors would lead to the appearance of an inability to focus attention when in fact attention is being focused very strongly, but on inappropriate information. Thus, we suggest that apparent failures to focus are often not a result of random lapses of attention, distraction by internal states, or a consequence of reduced alertness. Instead, these errors may arise when attention is being focused strongly, but overly narrowly, on information that a typical person would consider to be irrelevant or unimportant.

This third possibility suggests a reframing of the self-report described at the beginning of the chapter (Djinn (pseudonym) 2014): "I remember one day when I got caught in the rain. Each drop felt like an electric shock and I found it hard to move because of how intense and painful the feeling was." This does not sound like someone who failed to focus attention. Instead, it sounds like someone who focused intensely and narrowly on a sensory signal that might receive only cursory attention from a neurotypical individual. In this way, hyperfocusing may be a more refined way of accounting for greater distractibility in people with schizophrenia.

5 Open Questions and Future Directions

As we have reviewed, perspectives on the nature of attentional dysfunction in schizophrenia have evolved substantially over time. The ability to focus attention onto one source of information and filter out others is not impaired in schizophrenia (at least in the visual modality). Instead, schizophrenia appears to involve a hyperfocusing of attention, but PSZ may focus on task-irrelevant sources of information and therefore appear to be distracted. In addition, schizophrenia involves a reduction in global alertness, which may impact many tasks in the laboratory and in daily life.

Several open questions remain. First, new research is needed to fully resolve the apparent incompatibility between the older research showing impaired filtering and the newer research showing hyperfocusing. Second, additional work is needed to determine whether and how the attentional control deficits in schizophrenia are related to broader deficits in cognitive control (see chapter "Working Memory in People with Schizophrenia" this volume). Third, relatively little is known about the circuitry and pharmacology of the attentional abnormalities described in this chapter. Posterior parietal cortex is a key hub for attention, and some evidence implicates this region in hyperfocusing (Hahn et al. 2018). In addition, computational modeling suggests that a change in the balance of D1 and D2 dopamine receptor activation could lead to hyperfocusing-like changes in cortical processing (Luck et al. 2019b). Much more research would be needed to nail down the neural mechanisms underlying impaired attention in schizophrenia.

Finally, it will be important for future research to develop and test new treatments that target global alertness and/or hyperfocusing. New treatments could take the form of biological interventions, such as compounds that impact D1/D2 balance or neurostimulation. Cognitive training interventions may also be effective. For example, video games have been shown to be effective in helping older adults distribute their attention broadly rather than narrowly (Anguera et al. 2013; Rolle et al. 2017), and this approach could potentially reduce hyperfocusing in schizophrenia.

Acknowledgements Preparation of this chapter was made possible by NIH grant R01MH065034 to J.M.G. and S.J.L.

References

Anguera JA, Boccanfuso J, Rintoul JL, Al-Hashimi O, Faraji F, Janowich J et al (2013) Video game training enhances cognitive control in older adults. Nature 501(7465):97–101. https://doi.org/10.1038/nature12486

Arnau S, Löffler C, Rummel J, Hagemann D, Wascher E, Schubert A-L (2020) Inter-trial alpha power indicates mind wandering. Psychophysiology 57(6):e13581. https://doi.org/10.1111/psyp.13581

Ashinoff BK, Abu-Akel A (2021) Hyperfocus: the forgotten frontier of attention. Psychol Res 85(1):1–19. https://doi.org/10.1007/s00426-019-01245-8

Bansal S, Robinson BM, Leonard CJ, Hahn B, Luck SJ, Gold JM (2019) Failures in top-down control in schizophrenia revealed by patterns of saccadic eye movements. J Abnorm Psychol 128:415–422

Bansal S, Gaspelin N, Robinson BM, Hahn B, Luck SJ, Gold JM (2021) Oculomotor inhibition and location priming in schizophrenia. J Abnorm Psychol 130:651–664. https://doi.org/10.1037/abn0000683

Barch DM, Carter CS, Dakin SC, Gold JM, Luck SJ, MacDonald A III et al (2012) The clinical translation of a measure of gain control: the contrast-contrast effect task. Schizophr Bull 38: 135–143

Bilder RM, Goldberg E (1987) Motor perseverations in schizophrenia. Arch Clin Neuropsychol 2(3):195–214

Bleuler E (1911) Dementia praecox or the group of schizophrenias. In: Zinkin L (Trans.). International Universities Press, New York
Boudewyn MA, Carter CS (2018) I must have missed that: alpha-band oscillations track attention to spoken language. Neuropsychologia 117:148–155. https://doi.org/10.1016/j.neuropsychologia.2018.05.024
Braboszcz C, Delorme A (2011) Lost in thoughts: neural markers of low alertness during mind wandering. Neuroimage 54(4):3040–3047. https://doi.org/10.1016/j.neuroimage.2010.10.008
Butler PD, DeSanti LA, Maddox J, Harkavy-Friedman JM, Amador XF, Goetz RR et al (2003) Visual backward-masking deficits in schizophrenia: relationship to visual pathway function and symptomatology. Schizophr Res 59(2):199–209. https://doi.org/10.1016/S0920-9964(01)00341-3
Cadenhead KS, Serper Y, Braff DL (1998) Transient versus sustained visual channels in the visual backward masking deficits of schizophrenia patients. Biol Psychiatry 43(2):132–138. https://doi.org/10.1016/S0006-3223(97)00316-8
Christoff K, Gordon AM, Smallwood J, Smith R, Schooler JW (2009) Experience sampling during fMRI reveals default network and executive system contributions to mind wandering. Proc Natl Acad Sci 106(21):8719–8724. https://doi.org/10.1073/pnas.0900234106
Clark TK, Merfeld DM (2021) Statistical approaches to identifying lapses in psychometric response data. Psychon Bull Rev 28(5):1433–1457. https://doi.org/10.3758/s13423-021-01876-2
Clay OJ, Wadley VG, Edwards JD, Roth DL, Roenker DL, Ball KK (2005) Cumulative meta-analysis of the relationship between useful field of view and driving performance in older adults: current and future implications. Optom Vis Sci 82(8):724–731
Compton RJ, Gearinger D, Wild H (2019) The wandering mind oscillates: EEG alpha power is enhanced during moments of mind-wandering. Cogn Affect Behav Neurosci 19(5):1184–1191. https://doi.org/10.3758/s13415-019-00745-9
Crider A (1997) Perseveration in schizophrenia. Schizophr Bull 23(1):63–74
Dakin S, Carlin P, Hemsley D (2005) Weak suppression of visual context in chronic schizophrenia. Curr Biol 15:R822–R824
Djinn (pseudonym) (2014) Sensory overload. Schizophrenia.com. Retrieved January 4, 2019, from https://forum.schizophrenia.com/t/sensory-overload/4910
Erickson MA, Hahn B, Leonard CJ, Robinson BM, Gray B, Luck SJ, Gold JM (2015) Impaired working memory capacity is not caused by failures of selective attention in schizophrenia. Schizophr Bull 41:366–373
Erickson MA, Albrecht MA, Robinson BM, Luck SJ, Gold JM (2017) Impaired suppression of delay-period alpha and beta is associated with impaired working memory in schizophrenia. Biol Psychiatry Cogn Neurosci Neuroimaging 2:272–279
Everling S, Krappmann P, Preuss S, Brand A, Flohr H (1996) Hypometric primary saccades of schizophrenics in a delayed-response task. Exp Brain Res 111(2):289–295
Fernández-Espejo D, Soddu A, Cruse D, Palacios EM, Junque C, Vanhaudenhuyse A et al (2012) A role for the default mode network in the bases of disorders of consciousness. Ann Neurol 72(3):335–343. https://doi.org/10.1002/ana.23635
Feuerstahler LM, Luck SJ, MacDonald A III, Waller NG (2019) A note on the identification of change detection task models to measure storage capacity and attention in visual working memory. Behav Res Methods 51:1360–1370
Folk CL, Remington RW, Johnston JC (1992) Involuntary covert orienting is contingent on attentional control settings. J Exp Psychol Hum Percept Perform 18:1030–1044
Folk CL, Leber AB, Egeth HE (2002) Made you blink! Contingent attentional capture produces a spatial blink. Percept Psychophys 64(5):741–753
Fox KCR, Spreng RN, Ellamil M, Andrews-Hanna JR, Christoff K (2015) The wandering brain: meta-analysis of functional neuroimaging studies of mind-wandering and related spontaneous thought processes. Neuroimage 111:611–621. https://doi.org/10.1016/j.neuroimage.2015.02.039

Gibson B, Wasserman E, Luck SJ (2011) Qualitative similarities in the visual short-term memory of pigeons and people. Psychon Bull Rev 18:979–984

Gold JM, Barch DM, Feuerstahler LM, Carter CS, MacDonald AW III, Ragland JD et al (2020) Working memory impairment across psychotic disorders. Schizophr Bull 45:804–812

Gray BE, Hahn B, Robinson BM, Harvey A, Leonard CJ, Luck SJ, Gold JM (2014) Relationships between divided attention and working memory impairment in people with schizophrenia. Schizophr Bull 40:1462–1471

Green MF, Nuechterlein KH, Mintz J (1994a) Backward masking in schizophrenia and mania: II. Specifying the visual channels. Arch Gen Psychiatry 51(12):945–951. https://doi.org/10.1001/archpsyc.1994.03950120017004

Green MF, Hugdahl K, Mitchell S (1994b) Dichotic listening during auditory hallucinations in patients with schizophrenia. Am J Psychiatry 151(3):357

Hahn B, Robinson BM, Kaiser ST, Matveeva TM, Harvey AN, Luck SJ, Gold JM (2012a) Kraepelin and Bleuler had it right: people with schizophrenia have deficits sustaining attention over time. J Abnorm Psychol 121:641–648

Hahn B, Hollingworth A, Robinson BM, Kaiser ST, Leonard CJ, Beck VM et al (2012b) Control of working memory content in schizophrenia. Schizophr Res 12:70–75

Hahn B, Robinson BM, Harvey AN, Kaiser ST, Leonard CJ, Luck SJ, Gold JM (2012c) Visuospatial attention in schizophrenia: deficits in broad monitoring. J Abnorm Psychol 121:119–128

Hahn B, Harvey AN, Concheiro-Guisan M, Huestis MA, Holcomb HH, Gold JM (2013) A test of the cognitive self-medication hypothesis of tobacco smoking in schizophrenia. Biol Psychiatry 74(6):436–443

Hahn B, Harvey AN, Gold JM, Fischer BA, Keller WR, Ross TJ, Stein EA (2016) Hyperdeactivation of the default mode network in people with schizophrenia when focusing attention in space. Schizophr Bull 42:1158–1166

Hahn B, Harvey AN, Gold JM, Ross TJ, Stein EA (2017) Load-dependent hyperdeactivation of the default mode network in people with schizophrenia. Schizophr Res

Hahn B, Robinson BM, Leonard CJ, Luck SJ, Gold JM (2018) Posterior parietal cortex dysfunction is central to working memory storage and broad cognitive deficits in schizophrenia. J Neurosci 37:8378–8387. https://doi.org/10.1523/JNEUROSCI.0913-18.2018

Hugdahl K, Lund A, Asbjørnsen A, Egeland J, Landrø NI, Roness A et al (2003) Attentional and executive dysfunctions in schizophrenia and depression: evidence from dichotic listening performance. Biol Psychiatry 53(7):609–616

Hugdahl K, Løberg E-M, Falkenberg LE, Johnsen E, Kompus K, Kroken RA et al (2012) Auditory verbal hallucinations in schizophrenia as aberrant lateralized speech perception: evidence from dichotic listening. Schizophr Res 140(1):59–64

Hutton SB, Cuthbert I, Crawford TJ, Kennard C, Barnes TR, Joyce EM (2001) Saccadic hypometria in drug-naive and drug-treated schizophrenic patients: a working memory deficit? Psychophysiology 38(1):125–132

Kraepelin E (1919) In: Mary Barclay R (Trans.) Dementia praecox and paraphrenia, vol 3. 8th edn., Livingstone, Edinburgh

Kreither J, Lopez-Calderon J, Leonard CJ, Robinson BM, Ruffle A, Hahn B et al (2017) Electrophysiological evidence for spatial hyperfocusing in schizophrenia. J Neurosci 37:3813–3823

Kristjansson A (2008) "I know what you did on the last trial" – a selective review of research on priming in visual search. Front Biosci 13:1171–1181. https://doi.org/10.2741/2753

Lawson JS, McGhie A, Chapman J (1967) Distractibility in schizophrenia and organic cerebral disease. Br J Psychiatry 113(498):527–535

Leonard CJ, Luck SJ (2011) The role of magnocellular signals in oculomotor attentional capture. J Vis 11:1–12. https://doi.org/10.1167/11.13.11

Leonard CJ, Robinson BM, Kaiser ST, Hahn B, McClenon C, Harvey AN et al (2013) Testing sensory and cognitive explanations of the antisaccade deficit in schizophrenia. J Abnorm Psychol 122:1111–1120

Leonard CJ, Robinson BM, Hahn B, Gold JM, Luck SJ (2014) Enhanced distraction by magnocellular salience signals in schizophrenia. Neuropsychologia 56:359–366
Leonard CJ, Robinson BM, Hahn B, Luck SJ, Gold JM (2017) Altered spatial profile of distraction in people with schizophrenia. J Abnorm Psychol 126:1077–1086
Leonard CJ, Robinson BM, Hahn B, Gold JM, Luck SJ (2020) Increased influence of a previously attended feature in people with schizophrenia. J Abnorm Psychol 129:305–311
Luck SJ (2012) Electrophysiological correlates of the focusing of attention within complex visual scenes: N2pc and related ERP components. In: Luck SJ, Kappenman ES (eds) The oxford handbook of ERP components. Oxford University Press, New York, pp 329–360
Luck SJ, Gold JM (2008) The construct of attention in schizophrenia. Biol Psychiatry 64:34–39
Luck SJ, Vogel EK (2013) Visual working memory capacity: from psychophysics and neurobiology to individual differences. Trends Cogn Sci 17:391–400
Luck SJ, McClenon C, Beck VM, Hollingworth A, Leonard CJ, Hahn B et al (2014) Hyperfocusing in schizophrenia: evidence from interactions between working memory and eye movements. J Abnorm Psychol 123:783–795
Luck SJ, Leonard CJ, Hahn B, Gold JM (2019a) Is selective attention impaired in schizophrenia? Schizophr Bull 45:1001–1011. https://doi.org/10.1093/schbul/sbz045
Luck SJ, Hahn B, Leonard CJ, Gold JM (2019b) The hyperfocusing hypothesis: a new account of cognitive dysfunction in schizophrenia. Schizophr Bull 45:991–1000. https://doi.org/10.1093/schbul/sbz063
Mayer JS, Fukuda K, Vogel EK, Park S (2012) Impaired contingent attentional capture predicts reduced working memory capacity in schizophrenia. PLoS One 7(11):e48586. https://doi.org/10.1371/journal.pone.0048586
McGhie A, Chapman J (1961) Disorders of attention and perception in early schizophrenia. Br J Med Psychol 34:103–116
McGhie A, Chapman J, Lawson JS (1965) The effect of distraction on schizophrenic performance (1) perception and immediate memory. Br J Psychiatry 111(474):383–390
Mrazek MD, Smallwood J, Franklin MS, Chin JM, Baird B, Schooler JW (2012) The role of mind-wandering in measurements of general aptitude. J Exp Psychol Gen 141(4):788–798. https://doi.org/10.1037/a0027968
Norman DA (1968) Toward a theory of memory and attention. Psychol Rev 75(6):522–536. https://doi.org/10.1037/h0026699
Nuechterlein KH, Dawson ME, Green MF (1994) Information-processing abnormalities as neuropsychological vulnerability indicators for schizophrenia. Acta Psychiatr Scand 90(s384):71–79
Oltmanns TF (1978) Selective attention in schizophrenic and manic psychoses: the effect of distraction on information processing. J Abnorm Psychol 87(2):212–225
Oltmanns TF, Neale JM (1975) Schizophrenic performance when distractors are present: attentional deficit or differential task difficulty? J Abnorm Psychol 84(3):205
Oltmanns TF, Ohayon J, Neale JM (1978) The effect of anti-psychotic medication and diagnostic criteria on distractibility in schizophrenia. J Psychiatr Res 14:81–91
Payne RW, Hockberg AC, Hawks DV (1970) Dichotic stimulation as a method of assessing disorder of attention in overinclusive schizophrenic patients. J Abnorm Psychol 76:185–193
Phillips RC, Salo T, Carter CS (2015) Distinct neural correlates for attention lapses in patients with schizophrenia and healthy participants. Front Hum Neurosci 9:502. https://doi.org/10.3389/fnhum.2015.00502
Posner MI (2008) Measuring alertness. Ann N Y Acad Sci 1129(1):193–199. https://doi.org/10.1196/annals.1417.011
Posner MI, Petersen SE (1990) The attention system of the human brain. Annu Rev Neurosci 13:25–42
Posner MI, Snyder CRR, Davidson BJ (1980) Attention and the detection of signals. J Exp Psychol Gen 109:160–174
RDoC Matrix (2022). National Institute of Mental Health (NIMH). Retrieved February 15, 2022, from https://www.nimh.nih.gov/research/research-funded-by-nimh/rdoc/constructs/rdoc-matrix

Rolle CE, Anguera JA, Skinner SN, Voytek B, Gazzaley A (2017) Enhancing spatial attention and working memory in younger and older adults. J Cogn Neurosci 29(9):1483–1497. https://doi.org/10.1162/jocn_a_01159

Sämann PG, Wehrle R, Hoehn D, Spoormaker VI, Peters H, Tully C et al (2011) Development of the brain's default mode network from wakefulness to slow wave sleep. Cereb Cortex 21(9): 2082–2093. https://doi.org/10.1093/cercor/bhq295

Sawaki R, Geng JJ, Luck SJ (2012) A common neural mechanism for preventing and terminating the allocation of attention. J Neurosci 32:10725–10736

Sawaki R, Kreither J, Leonard CJ, Kaiser ST, Hahn B, Gold JM, Luck SJ (2017) Hyperfocusing on goal-related information in schizophrenia: evidence from electrophysiology. J Abnorm Psychol 126:106–116

Schneider SJ (1976) Selective attention in schizophrenia. J Abnorm Psychol 85:167–173

Spencer KM, Nestor PG, Valdman O, Niznikiewicz MA, Shenton ME, McCarley RW (2011) Enhanced facilitation of spatial attention in schizophrenia. Neuropsychology 25(1):76–85. https://doi.org/10.1037/a0020779

Talcott TN, Gaspelin N (2020) Prior target locations attract overt attention during search. Cognition 201:104282. https://doi.org/10.1016/j.cognition.2020.104282

Venables PH (1963) Input dysfunction in schizophrenia. Prog Exp Pers Res 72:1–47

Wahl O (1976) Schizophrenic patterns of dichotic shadowing performance. J Nerv Ment Dis 163: 401–407

Wichmann FA, Hill NJ (2001) The psychometric function: I. Fitting, sampling, and goodness of fit. Percept Psychophys 63:1293–1313

Wielgus MS, Harvey PD (1988) Dichotic listening and recall in schizophrenia and mania. Schizophr Bull 14(4):689–700. https://doi.org/10.1093/schbul/14.4.689

Wishner J, Wahl O (1974) Dichotic listening in schizophrenia. J Consult Clin Psychol 42:538–546

Perceptual Functioning

Anne Giersch and Vincent Laprévote

Contents

Abstract Perceptual disorders are not part of the diagnosis criteria for schizophrenia. Yet, a considerable amount of work has been conducted, especially on visual perception abnormalities, and there is little doubt that visual perception is altered in patients. There are several reasons why such perturbations are of interest in this

---

A. Giersch (✉)
University of Strasbourg, INSERM U1114, Centre Hospitalier Régional Universitaire de Strasbourg, Strasbourg, France
e-mail: giersch@unistra.fr

V. Laprévote
University of Strasbourg, INSERM U1114, Centre Hospitalier Régional Universitaire de Strasbourg, Strasbourg, France

CLIP Centre de Liaison et d'Intervention Précoce, Centre Psychothérapique de Nancy, Laxou, France

Faculté de Médecine, Université de Lorraine, Vandoeuvre-lès-Nancy, France

Curr Topics Behav Neurosci (2023) 63: 79–114
https://doi.org/10.1007/7854_2022_393
Published Online: 29 October 2022

pathology. They are observed during the prodromal phase of psychosis, they are related to the pathophysiology (clinical disorganization, disorders of the sense of self), and they are associated with neuronal connectivity disorders. Perturbations occur at different levels of processing and likely affect how patients interact and adapt to their surroundings. The literature has become very large, and here we try to summarize different models that have guided the exploration of perception in patients. We also illustrate several lines of research by showing how perception has been investigated and by discussing the interpretation of the results. In addition to discussing domains such as contrast sensitivity, masking, and visual grouping, we develop more recent fields like processing at the level of the retina, and the timing of perception.

Keywords Masking · Perception · Retina · Schizophrenia · Timing · Visual integration

Perceptual disorders are not at the forefront of the symptoms typically looked for in individuals with schizophrenia. Yet a number of self-descriptions of patients suggest that they suffer from unusual perceptual experiences, especially at the beginning of the pathology, and a large number of studies have explored various aspects of perception impairments. The link between perception impairments and the pathophysiology of psychosis is now supported by a number of results. For example, several studies describe a link between early anomalous experiences and the risk of developing psychosis. Perception is one of the domains identified in the Research Domain Criteria (RDoC), and the link with schizophrenia is documented. However, anomalous perceptual experiences and in general perceptual difficulties are not included in the definition of schizophrenia. There is a need to develop tools to explore perception to understand how the anomalous experiences emerge, and how they participate to the pathophysiology of schizophrenia. We will start by describing clinical observations and self-reports, which are especially rich before the onset of psychosis and in early stages of psychosis. We will then describe existing tools which can help in assessing perception in individuals at risk of developing schizophrenia as well as in individuals with chronic schizophrenia. This field of research is highly dynamic, with theoretical contexts changing with time. Instead of making an exhaustive review of the exploration tools, we will give contextual information that will allow the reader to orientate him or herself in a dense literature, with experiments realized in different theoretical contexts and with distinct tools. Many reviews have been written and we will cite them as much as possible to allow the interested reader to find complementary information, should they wish to do so.

1 Anomalous Perceptual Experiences in Psychosis: Clinical Observations

Chapman (1966) listed a number of citations that illustrate the difficulties reported by patients with schizophrenia: 'Things go too quick for my mind. Everything is too fast and too big for me, too quick to study. Things get blurred and it's like being blind. I can't make them out clearly. It's as if you were seeing one picture one minute and another picture the next. I just stop and watch my feet. If I move, everything alters every minute and I have no control over my legs'. Another patient says: 'I've to put things together in my head. If I look at my watch I see the watch, watchstrap, face, hands and so on, then I have got to put them together to get it into one piece'. Self-reports can be difficult to interpret. It is difficult to know if they reveal an attention or a perception anomaly, and the patients might have a difficulty to describe their perceptual experience (Giersch et al. 2021). Nonetheless, it is remarkable that perceptual complaints predate the conversion to psychosis and the treatment.

Patients with psychosis may experience subtle clinical changes up to several years before the onset of frank psychosis, with important functional consequences (Riecher-Rössler et al. 2006). On this basis, the construct of Clinical High-Risk (CHR) state for psychosis has emerged (Fusar-Poli et al. 2013), combining late-onset attenuated psychotic symptoms known as Ultra High-Risk (UHR) criteria (Yung et al. 2005) with earlier-onset alterations known as basic symptoms (Schultze-Lutter 2009). UHR criteria are based on the presence of identifiable psychotic symptoms whose intensity, duration, or frequency are below the threshold for a diagnosis of psychotic disorder. Besides, the concept of basic symptoms combines subjective symptoms, experienced by the patients themselves as deviations from their usual functioning, which may affect different cognitive domains. They are the earliest phase of clinical high-risk states for psychosis and may persist after remission of psychotic symptoms. Based on the pioneering work of Gerd Huber (Gross and Huber 1985), 142 basic symptoms were grouped in the Bonn Scale for the Assessment of Basic Symptoms (BSABS; Gross et al. 2008). Derived from this scale, the most widely used instruments for the clinical characterization of basic symptoms are the Schizophrenia Proneness Instrument, Adult Version (SPI-A) and Schizophrenia Proneness Instrument, Child and Youth Version (SPI-CY;) (Schultze-Lutter et al. 2012). Perceptual symptoms play an important role in these assessments. Importantly, the criterion 'disturbances of visual perception' is included in the Cognitive-Perceptive basic symptoms (COPER) (Cognitive-Perceptive Basic Symptoms) criteria of the SPI-A (Klosterkötter et al. 2001; Häfner et al. 2004; Ruhrmann et al. 2003) and the criterion 'attention focused on details of the visual field' in the COGDIS (High-Risk Criterion Cognitive Disturbances) criteria (Klosterkötter et al. 2001), both of which define the initial prodromal state of psychosis (Schultze-Lutter et al. 2007).

A significant number of other visual symptoms are also present in the basic symptoms. Thus, among at-risk patients who later make a transition to psychosis, 12% display hypersensitivity to light or visual stimuli, 9% photopsia, 7% perceptual changes in face and/or shape of others, and 11% report a sensory hypervigilance

(Schultze-Lutter 2001). These results are in line with those of Gourzis et al. (2002) who investigated prodromal symptoms on the basis of the DSM III and found unusual perceptual experiences in 35% of patients before the initial phase of schizophrenia. It has been suggested that among basic symptoms, perceptual abnormalities are those symptoms best predicting the conversion from a high-risk state to psychosis (Klosterkötter et al. 2001). As a matter of fact, basic perceptual symptoms are not isolated and are related to other psychiatric symptoms. For instance, Granö et al. (2015) found an independent association between visual distortions and the occurrence of suicidal ideation, which is a major outcome in clinical states at high risk of psychosis. At later stages, Keane et al. (2018) found visual perceptual symptoms of BSABS (Bonn Scale for the Assessment of Basic Symptoms) at a comparable level in patients with First-Episode Psychosis (FEP) and patients with schizophrenia, and demonstrated a link between these symptoms and crucial clinical markers such as earlier age of onset, delusions, or hallucinations. In their pioneering work, Cutting and Dunne (1986) explored qualitatively the perception of remitted patients with schizophrenia. They found that 60% of their sample of 66 patients with schizophrenia reported experiencing perceptual distortions, which were mainly visual distortions of basic properties of the environment.

Such results highlight the importance of assessing these disorders both in individuals at risk of developing psychosis and in those with chronic schizophrenia. With this in mind, instruments for measuring visual distortions have been developed to quantify anomalous perceptions. Bunney et al. (1999) developed a structured interview for assessing perceptual anomalies (SIAPA) specifically for schizophrenia. This 15-item instrument explores perceptual increases or flooding in the five senses. They found that 32.8% of patients in their sample reported subjective visual abnormalities, regardless of the presence of hallucinations. Nikitova et al. (2019) recently proposed the Audio-Visual Abnormalities Questionnaire (AVAQ). It is a self-administered questionnaire based on both phenomenological reviews of sensory experiences and the results of experimental studies exploring perceptual processes in schizophrenia. It is a very promising questionnaire, but to the authors' knowledge, there are no published results on clinical populations with schizophrenia.

A limit of the questionnaires is the difficulty for the patients to verbalize and describe what they perceive. Besides, exploring the mechanisms of the reported perceptual abnormalities requires an experimental approach, because most of the mechanisms leading to conscious perceptual experiences are inaccessible to consciousness. Approaching anomalous perceptual experiences with an experimental approach is all the more justified that some studies have shown that they are correlated with impairments in visual perception tasks. Kéri et al. (2005) explored anomalous perceptual experiences with the Bonn Scale for the Assessment of Basic Symptoms (BSABS) in parallel with various psychophysical tests of visual information processing and found that BSABS scores and various visual dysfunctions were correlated. Kiss et al. (2010) measured the visual contrast sensitivity in unmedicated patients with a first episode of schizophrenia and found decreased sensitivity was associated with the anomalous visual experiences measured by the SIAPA (Bunney et al. 1999).

In the following, we focus on different tools that can be used to explore visual perception in schizophrenia, associated electrophysiological and fMRI markers, and highlight how various perceptual impairments link with various clinical symptoms. It is to be noted that changes in perception also affect tactile and auditory information. We will refer to some results that extend those obtained in visual perception to other modalities, but we will mainly focus on visual perception, given it has been explored more extensively than any other sense. It should be kept in mind that auditory or tactile anomalous perceptions may be especially pertinent when exploring, e.g. language or bodily self-impairments (Liu et al. 2020; Zopf et al. 2021; Dondé et al. 2020; Meyer et al. 2021; Richards et al. 2021; Senkowski and Moran 2022), and that such explorations can be expected to be developed further in the future. Similarly, we will only allude to the role of eye movements, even though saccades, fixations, or smooth pursuit would merit a whole chapter. We refer to reviews for interested readers (Holzman 2000; Trillenberg et al. 2004; Keshavan et al. 2005; Reilly et al. 2008; Myles et al. 2017; Thakkar and Rolfs 2019).

The exploration of perception in psychosis has been influenced by different theoretical backgrounds that changed over the years. They modified the experimental approaches and sometimes the interpretation of results. For this reason, we start with a quick reminder of the basic mechanisms of perception, and then develop the theoretical backgrounds that guided the exploration of visual perception in psychosis.

2 Basic Mechanisms of Visual Perception and Methodological Issues

Even though we have the subjective impression of perceiving the outer world in a direct and immediate way, what we know about visual processing is in stark contrast with our everyday impression. Information is conveyed from a multi-layered retina to the occipital cortex via the geniculate nuclei. In the primary visual cortex, information is processed by specialized neurons with small receptive fields, effectively decomposing visual information into small bits of partial information, e.g. orientation, luminance, colour (Hubel and Wiesel 1959; Campbell and Robson 1968; Grossberg 1991; Boucart et al. 1994). Spatial and 3D information, or action, is processed in the dorsal pathway, going from the primary visual cortex to the parietal cortex (Humphreys et al. 1994, 2010; de Haan et al. 2012; Freud et al. 2016; Xu et al. 2017). On the other hand, contour and surface information are processed in separate pathways, both of them going from the primary visual cortex to the temporal cortex (Livingstone and Hubel 1987; Humphreys 2003). The distinction between the ventral and dorsal pathway overlaps partially with the distinction between the parvo- and magnocellular pathways (Breitmeyer 2014). The former conveys high spatial frequencies, i.e. detail information corresponding to the contour details, whereas the latter conveys low spatial frequencies, i.e. the global form of the objects.

The magnocellular pathway also processes information faster and in a more phasic way than the parvocellular pathway. This pathway allows us to categorize information in a 'fast and dirty' way, before identifying the details of the visual information (Thorpe et al. 1996; Bar 2004). Identifying an object in our environment requires to bring the different contour parts together (the 'binding' problem), to associate the surface of the object with its contour, and to match the re-built form with representations in memory (Boucart et al. 1994; Humphreys 2003). To localize the object it is further required to associate the form information processed in the ventral pathway with the spatial information processed in the dorsal pathway (Humphreys 2003). In all, the processing of visual information is much more complex than our subjective feeling suggests. This complexity explains why a number of experimental approaches have been developed to assess the different steps of visual processing.

Experimental approaches to explore visual perception can be used with different objectives when applied to schizophrenia, with distinct methodological issues. This point has some impact on the literature. When trying to find biomarkers of anomalous perceptual experiences, the main issue is to relate the marker with its associated clinical consequences, whatever the mechanisms involved in the perceptual experience. On the other hand, when trying to understand the origin of the perceptual disorders, the difficulty is to dissociate the different mechanisms possibly involved in the anomalous perception. Here we would like to attract the attention of the reader to three main difficulties, i.e. the generalized deficit, the impact of attention, and the access of information to consciousness. These difficulties are mainly encountered when trying to understand the origin of the perceptual experiences of the patients. They should also be taken into account in experimental settings that are often far from everyday experiences. As a matter of fact, the results in such experimental settings may not necessarily generalize to everyday perception if they are due to something else than perception itself.

The generalized deficit refers to the possibility that deficient performance in a given task is related to the difficulty of the task rather than to the selective processes involved in the task. Instead of evaluating those selective mechanisms, performance would rather reflect the ability of the patients to engage in the difficult task. A very thorough development on this question can be found in Knight and Silverstein (2001). A second issue is the impact of attention on visual perception. Attention can affect any task through a decrease of vigilance or attentional lapses (Phillips et al. 2015a; Chidharom et al. 2021). However, attention can also impact perception in a more selective way. There are massive feedback connections on the visual cortex (Bullier et al. 2001), which allow for feedback influences on visual processing by 100 ms after the onset of a stimulus (Lamme and Roelfsema 2000). The influences can be varied (Gilbert and Li 2013) and include an impact of attention on response gain, i.e. an enhancement of responses within the focus of attention and a suppression outside this focus (Moran and Desimone 1985). Influences can also be task-dependent: which information is required and which not clearly varies across tasks. In monkeys, it has been shown that neurons can respond differently to the same stimulus depending on the task at hand (Li et al. 2004). More recent studies have confirmed that in humans, attention mechanisms help to select appropriate modality-specific signals (Limanowski and Friston 2020), or select multiple objects (Wutz et al. 2020), depending on the task. How attention affects visual perception has been and still is a matter of intense debate (Schneider 1993; Walther and Koch 2007; Theeuwes 2018; Gaspelin and Luck 2018), and detailing all the existing models is beyond the aim of this chapter. Yet, it is clear that our conscious perception is both the result of unconscious perceptual processes and attention, and most likely an interaction between the two. This should be kept in mind when interpreting the data in individuals with schizophrenia. When perception is explored experimentally, participants are given instructions that may affect how they process information. An alteration might be the result of perception disruptions per se, but it may also be the result of a maladaptation of the processes required for the task, or a difficulty to increase the gain of the to-be-detected signal.

An additional potential confound is the access to consciousness. In visual tasks, participants are usually asked to emit a conscious judgement about the stimuli. We have seen that most perceptual mechanisms are non-conscious. Several models of conscious perception propose that attention is involved when visual information becomes conscious (Mashour et al. 2020). This question is again a matter of intense debate (Koch and Tsuchiya 2007), but some results have shown that in individuals with chronic schizophrenia, conscious access to information is disrupted per se (Del Cul et al. 2006), in relation with altered brain connectivity (Berkovitch et al. 2021). These results are not specific to schizophrenia and are also observed in multiple sclerosis (Reuter et al. 2007). Nonetheless, they should be kept in mind when interpreting the literature on perception in individuals with schizophrenia.

Beside methodological difficulties, explorations on visual perception in individuals with schizophrenia have been conducted within different theoretical frameworks. Inasmuch theoretical backgrounds may influence the interpretation of the data, it seems important to describe those backgrounds in order to facilitate the understanding of the literature. Hereafter, we describe the main theoretical frameworks, or models, at the background of studies on visual perception in individuals with schizophrenia. They are not necessarily incompatible with each other, and we only shortly summarize some of them.

3 Different Models

3.1 Signal-to-Noise Ratio

The idea that there is a decreased signal-to-noise ratio in schizophrenia was not originally been developed for sensory disorders and has been rather proposed as a general consequence of abnormalities in dopamine transmission (Winterer and Weinberger 2004; Rolls et al. 2008). However, perceiving is about detecting signals, and perceptual detection has been conceptualized as the ability to discriminate signal from noise (Green and Swets 1966). Some authors have proposed that, e.g., face processing is altered due to a decreased signal-to-noise ratio (Christensen et al.

2013). Place and Gilmore (1980) and Wells and Leventhal (1984) showed that when visual information was spatially disorganized rather than organized, this affected controls more so than patients with schizophrenia. This result might be interpreted as a higher level of noise in patients when information is organized. However, not all results are compatible with a decreased signal-to-noise ratio. A lack of sensitivity to illusions (Notredame et al. 2014; King et al. 2017) or an abnormal sensitivity to small delays in sensory signals (Marques-Carneiro et al. 2021; Foerster et al. 2021) is difficult to explain by noisy information.

3.2 A Disruption of the Magnocellular Pathway

There has been much work on the hypothesis of a deficit of the magnocellular pathway, which is reputedly more fragile than the parvocellular pathway and more susceptible to neurodevelopmental disorders (Bosworth et al. 2013). It has been argued that a disruption of the magnocellular pathway may impair visual processing in a bottom-up manner (Javitt 2009), ultimately affecting occupational and social functions. Bottom-up processing is strongly emphasized in this model. The magnocellular specificity as well as the exact level of the alteration (subcortical or cortical) has been discussed (Skottun and Skoyles 2007, 2013). Yet any visual discrimination difficulty may have a functional impact, and recent results on retinal transmission have renewed this field of investigation. Hypotheses on the magnocellular pathway are at the background of investigations on masking and spatial vision and are further developed in the methodological descriptions.

3.3 Context-Modulation Model

As emphasized in the description of visual processing mechanisms, in the primary visual cortex neurons are highly specialized and have small receptive fields, requiring information to be secondarily bound together. Although we experience no difficulty in identifying objects in a cluttered environment, such a performance requires to determine which contour belongs to which object, what is in the background and what is in the foreground, and more generally to disambiguate visual signals (Rensink and Enns 1998; Giersch et al. 2000; Berzhanskaya et al. 2007). We may not be aware that our environment includes ambiguities, but those are numerous. They happen when a contour can be attributed to one or another object, when the information is blurred or poorly contrasted, at night (Joos et al. 2020). These ambiguities are efficiently processed thanks to the adaptation mechanisms taking place at the cortical level. A number of signal modulations help to adjust processing by increasing the tuning of signal processing, by suppressing redundant signal, and ultimately grouping the signal into neuronal assemblies. These modulation mechanisms have been proposed to be altered in patients and they all have been grouped into the generic term of context-modulation (Phillips et al. 2015b; Silverstein 2016). They are meant to be a general mechanism and can include top-down attention modulations, as well as gain through lateral interactions between neurons, i.e. local or global connections. Inasmuch as contextual modulation is a way of adapting the processing of signal to a complex environment, it could include adaptations to the task at hand. When considering that adaptation may evolve with time this model may not be that far from predictive coding.

3.4 Predictive Coding Model

The predictive coding model has been proposed as a general model of brain functioning (Friston 2005), inspired from motor control (Tschacher et al. 2017). In motor control action is programmed, the sensory consequences are predicted, and the outcome of the action is verified online. This closed-loop regulation allows the motor programme to be adjusted in case of unexpected sensory signal (Wolpert et al. 1995). Predictive coding can be easily applied to perception. Perception can be seen as a dynamic process in which perception is predicted and adjusted in order to follow information in a changing environment (Rao and Ballard 1999; Kok and de Lange 2015). When everything occurs as planned information can be ignored, whereas any unexpected signal is processed to adjust perceptual predictions. These close-loop mechanisms would occur at different levels of processing and would help to maximize the difference between expected and unexpected events, i.e. the ability to adapt and adjust. The mechanisms used to adjust perception may be similar to those described in the context-modulation model and may help in contour processing (Rao and Ballard 1999). The main difficulty when applying this model to pathology is to understand which mechanisms exactly are impaired: the ability to predict, the ability to detect a prediction error, the adjustment to the error, or all of those. Yet, the literature inspired by this approach is blooming and already helps to relate visual impairments with clinical symptoms in schizophrenia (Sterzer et al. 2018).

In the following, we detail some of the tests currently in use with individuals with schizophrenia, their relationships with clinical symptoms, and the associated impairments in fMRI or EEG. We discuss also, whenever possible, if the disorders are rather trait or state markers.

4 Methodological Descriptions

4.1 Masking

Masking has been used since the early 80s and has often been believed to reflect early visual mechanisms. This is probably true, but it may also reveal attentional gain mechanisms. The literature on this task has been abundant and still is. We will only provide some guidelines for the interested readers. We selected masking in this review because it illustrates how the interpretation of the results in this task has evolved in time and has been adapted to changing theoretical backgrounds.

In masking tasks, a visual target is presented briefly in close temporal and spatial proximity with a mask. The relative delays and spatial characteristics of the target and mask define different types of masking tasks (Breitmeyer and Öğmen 2006), but the general principle is that the mask reduces the visibility of the target. The participant identifies or localizes the target. Individuals with schizophrenia typically need larger asynchronies between target and mask onset to detect the target (Saccuzzo and Braff 1981; Green and Walker 1986; Rund 1993; Cadenhead et al. 1998). The results are robust and have been replicated throughout the literature, but the mechanisms proposed as an explanation for the impairment in patients have evolved with time.

Masking has been attributed to interactions between the magno- and parvocellular pathways (Keesey 1972; Kulikowski and Tolhurst 1973; Tolhurst 1973; Breitmeyer and Ganz 1976; Green and Walker 1984). When the mask follows the target (backward masking, which is among the most frequently used task in patients) both integration and interruption mechanisms are involved. Integration refers to a fusion between the target and the mask, i.e. an integration of the sustained activities associated with the two successive stimuli. Integration occurs when the onset of target and mask is separated by 0–30 ms. Interruption occurs when the mask is displayed after a longer delay after the target. Since the onset of the mask is transient, it activates the magnocellular pathway that 'interrupts' the processing of the target, i.e. the processing of visual details in the parvocellular pathway. It is this interruption that would then reduce the visibility of the target (Breitmeyer and Ganz 1976; Breitmeyer and Öğmen 2006). Several hypotheses have been derived from this general framework and proposed to explain the patients' difficulties at detecting a masked target. Although the simplest explanation would have been excessive interruption through the magnocellular pathway, several studies suggested an impairment at the level of the magnocellular pathway (Butler et al. 2001; Schechter et al. 2003). A lack of interruption by the mask was proposed to have a detrimental effect, by leading to a fusion between the target and the mask (Slaghuis 2004). This explanation is coherent with the results suggesting a deficit on the magnocellular pathway, but unlikely explains the deficits in all types of masking tasks. In metacontrast and paracontrast masking, the mask is displayed in close spatial proximity to the target, but its localization does not overlap with the target (metacontrast and paracontrast refer to the cases where the mask respectively follows or precedes the target in time). The target and the mask cannot be fused in space, but individuals with schizophrenia are impaired in a similar way in all types of masking (Rassovsky et al. 2004).

These findings yielded the introduction of a theoretical framework used to explain metacontrast and paracontrast, i.e. 'object substitution' (Enns and di Lollo 1997). This theory relies on the assumption that the target and the mask both elicit feedforward and feedback processing. Since the stimuli succeed each other in time, the feedback processing elicited by the first stimulus would coincide in time with the feedforward processing elicited by the second stimulus. This would lead the first stimulus to be substituted by the second one before the first stimulus has been identified.

As for the first theory, these hypotheses are consistent with existing masking models, but do not explain the whole pattern of results with masking tasks in individuals with schizophrenia. In all the tasks described until now, patients are asked to explicitly detect the target, and the difficulty of patients has been replicated again and again. Several authors have also used implicit tasks, though. Implicit means that even though visual information is masked the task of the participants is not to explicitly identify this information. Depending on the task, participants may not even know that there is information in addition to the mask. The aim of such tasks is to examine whether the masked information incidentally influences the processing of information that follows. Several studies showed that masked stimuli influenced the performance of patients and controls in the same way, despite the fact that patients had difficulties at explicitly detecting the masked signals (Herzog et al. 2004; Del Cul et al. 2009). These results suggest that at least the subconscious processing of the masked signal is processed efficiently in patients with schizophrenia. It also means that feedback mechanisms, conscious access or other mechanisms may play a role, and not only the initial processing of sensory information. Several authors have suggested a reduced gain control (Butler et al. 2008; Herzog et al. 2013; Skottun and Skoyles 2013), i.e. a deficit in the amplification of signals elicited by stimuli with a poor visibility. A few studies more directly support the possibility of an involvement of attention. Granholm et al. (2009) measured pupil dilation as a proxy for the allocation of attentional resources during backward masking tasks and showed impairments in patients. Another study used monetary rewards and showed this helped to improve patients' performance, although the improvement was weak (Rassovsky et al. 2005). Finally, it was shown that when the participants were unable to focus attention selectively on the masked target because the target was duplicated, then performance was equalized in patients and controls (Lalanne et al. 2012a).

4.2 Electroencephalographic Correlates of Masking Impairments

A number of studies have compared electroencephalographic signals elicited by masked stimuli in patients and controls. They regularly found decreased amplitudes of signals, already 100 ms after the stimulus onset (Neuhaus et al. 2011; Plomp et al. 2013; Wynn et al. 2013). Yet, some results point towards the involvement of top-down gain amplification. The use of distracters during the task showed that the amplitude of electroencephalographic signals was mainly reduced when attention could be mobilized (Berkovitch et al. 2018). In another study the analysis of the brain source of electroencephalographic signals showed reduced signals at around 200 ms and in the ventral stream. This latency corresponds to re-entry processing, which allows for an enhancement of detailed information processing (Plomp et al. 2013). Those results fit with an explanation in terms of reduced attentional gain and impaired conscious access to masked information. In a complementary way, one study explored neuronal oscillations and showed that oscillations in the gamma range were decreased in patients during a backward masking task (Green et al. 2003). Since such analyses are pertinent for a range of visual perception tasks, they are further developed in the Sect. 4.5.2.

In all, there is no doubt that patients with schizophrenia have difficulty to consciously identify masked visual stimuli. It is to be noted that the deficit may not be specific to schizophrenia, although the literature on this topic is somewhat contradictory. Some studies have shown similar deficits in patients with schizophrenia and with bipolar disorders (Garobbio et al. 2021; Reavis et al. 2017), whereas others showed differences (Goghari and Sponheim 2008). It has also been suggested that backward masking may help to make a difference between siblings of patients with schizophrenia and with bipolar disorders (McClure 1999; Kéri et al. 2001; MacQueen et al. 2004), but whether or not masking deficits are related to a specific vulnerability remains to be ascertained.

The most recent studies point towards a top-down gain deficit in patients with schizophrenia, which may originate a deficit shared across visual tasks, beyond masking tasks. However, this explanation does not necessarily exclude the possibility of impairments at more basic level. For example, Reavis et al. (2017) linked backward masking impairments in schizophrenia with the volume of optic radiations. Besides, recent results have highlighted transmission impairments at the retina level that may also impact the ability of the patients to detect short and barely visible stimuli, and or low spatial frequencies. These possibilities are developed in Sects. 4.3 and 4.4.

4.3 Spatial Vision

The spatial vision model postulates that the visual system behaves as a sum of psychophysical channels specific of different spatial frequencies and orientations. This model finds a neural substrate in the anatomical and physiological segregations from retina to the magnocellular and parvocellular pathways that has been already alluded to in Sects. 2 and 4.1. As a reminder, the magnocellular pathway is considered to be more sensitive to low contrast and low spatial frequency information, whereas the parvocellular pathway is more sensitive to high spatial frequency information and less sensitive to low contrast. The contrast sensitivity function is a reference method assessing spatial vision. It consists in presenting gratings at different spatial frequencies and determining the minimum contrast threshold for them to be perceived. Dynamic stimuli can be used in order to stimulate preferentially the magnocellular pathway. This behavioural method and several of its variants have been used to measure spatial vision in psychosis. As already emphasized several studies (Butler et al. 2007; Kantrowitz et al. 2009; Revheim et al. 2006; Schwartz et al. 1987) found a decrease in behavioural performance specifically for the lowest spatial frequencies, i.e. spatial frequencies below 1.5 c.p.d. These results have been interpreted as evidence of impaired magnocellular function. However, it should be noted that a number of studies found an alteration in performance for all spatial frequencies (Slaghuis 1998, 2004; Kéri and Benedek 2007; Martínez et al. 2008, 2012; Shoshina et al. 2021). For example, Slaghuis and Thompson (2003) found a drop in performance for low frequencies (below 1.5 CPD) as well as for intermediate frequencies (between 1.5 and 7 cpd) and high frequencies (over 7 cpd).

It is interesting to note that alterations in contrast sensitivity function may vary with the stage or progression of the disease. Using the contrast sensitivity paradigm of Pokorny and Smith (1997), Kéri and Benedek (2007) showed a hypersensitivity to magnocellular biased stimuli in UHR. Interestingly this magnocellular hypersensitivity was correlated to the clinical measure of perceptual anomalies by the structured interview for assessing perceptual anomalies (SIAPA, Bunney et al. 1999). In a comparable setting, Kiss et al. (2010) evidenced an increase in performance at low spatial frequencies in first-episode schizophrenia patients. Meanwhile, Almeida et al. (2020) found greater contrast sensitivity deficits in patients with longer duration of illness, as well as a combined effect of duration of illness and use of atypical antipsychotics. These results could be interpreted as the presence of two different processes, with visual hyperexcitability in the early phases and an alteration in performance as the disorder progresses.

In all the impairments described until now can be expected to dim vision. However, it is likely that dim vision (Kantrowitz et al. 2009) interacts with other difficulties to produce the whole pattern of strange experiences encountered in the pathology. This point is further developed in Sect. 4.5.2.

Several studies have found neurobiological correlates of the perceptual deficit by 100 ms after the onset of low spatial frequency stimuli, and especially a decrease in the amplitude of EEG P1 and N1 waves (Butler et al. 2007), or a decrease in V1 activation measured by fMRI (Martínez et al. 2008; Calderone et al. 2013). However, inasmuch attention is believed to modulate the transmission of sensory information by 100 ms (Lamme and Roelfsema 2000), such results are not decisive regarding an interpretation in terms of bottom-up or top-down mechanisms. One way to resolve this conundrum is to look at even earlier stages of visual processing. Samani et al. (2018) recently measured the presence of retinal structural abnormalities in patients with schizophrenia using spectral domain optical coherence tomography (SD-OCT) and showed that these structural abnormalities correlated with decreased performance in contrast sensitivity at low spatial frequencies. At the functional level, our team recently measured that a decrease in the amplitude of the P1 wave in EEG during the presentation of high or low spatial frequencies was associated with an alteration in the functioning of ganglion cells measured by electroretinogram (Remy et al. 2022). The latter result was not yet observed in schizophrenia, but it still suggests a link between retinal transmission and contrast sensitivity. Those results suggest that the alteration of contrast sensitivity function in schizophrenia could be explained by the presence of retinal abnormalities that would result in an alteration of subsequent cortical processing of spatial frequencies. Such alterations might be more pronounced at low spatial frequencies either because deficits are easier to evidence at low than at high spatial frequencies or because the magnocellular pathway is more sensitive to an alteration of visual input processing. In the following sections, we summarize the recent results observed at the retina level.

4.4 Retinal Function

The retina is the first stage of visual processing, and it has recently been the subject of increasing interest in research on psychosis. Besides studies showing structural abnormalities of the retina (for a review, see Silverstein et al. 2020), the use of the electroretinogram (ERG) is a non-invasive procedure allowing for a detailed analysis of the functioning of the different cell layers of the retina. The standards for the execution of Electroretinogram (ERGs) are set out in the guidelines of the International Society for Clinical Electrophysiology of Vision (Robson et al. 2018). Briefly, the flash ERG (fERG) technique uses a flash of variable intensity, in scotopic or photopic conditions. The fERG helps to isolate an a-wave that reflects the functioning of the photoreceptors, and a b-wave that reflects the depolarization of the ON-bipolar and Müller cells complex. The photopic negative response (PhNR) calculation allows an indirect measurement of ganglion cell activity. The pattern ERG (pERG) measures the response to reversal black and white checkerboards and reflects ganglion cell function. Other measures are also possible, including oscillatory potentials, which are thought to reflect the activity of amacrine cells in the inner retina (Wachtmeister 1981).

Since the pioneering work of Warner et al. (1999), who found a decrease in the amplitude of the photopic and scotopic a-waves, a dozen studies have confirmed the presence of retinal processing disorders in schizophrenia. These include decreases in the amplitude of the photopic a-wave indicating cone dysfunctions (Balogh et al. 2008; Hébert et al. 2015, 2020; Demmin et al. 2018, 2020a, b; Bernardin et al. 2020), decreases in the amplitudes of the scotopic a-wave indicating rod dysfunctions (Hébert et al. 2015, 2020; Demmin et al. 2018, 2020b; Bernardin et al. 2020), and decreases in the amplitudes of the b-wave indicating bipolar cell dysfunctions (Hébert et al. 2015, 2020; Demmin et al. 2018, 2020b; Bernardin et al. 2020). Some studies also found alterations in the pattern ERG (Bernardin et al. 2020) or alterations in the photopic negative response (PhNR) (Demmin et al. 2018) indicating dysfunctions in the ganglion cells. These latter dysfunctions are of particular interest because ganglion cells are the closest to brain neurons.

Several variations should be noted depending on the clinical presentation. For example, Balogh et al. (2008) showed that fERG abnormalities were particularly marked in the acute phase. Several studies have also found a correlation of fERG abnormalities with the intensity of symptomatology (Balogh et al. 2008; Demmin et al. 2018) and Bernardin et al. (2021) have shown an association between ganglion cell dysfunction and the presence of visual hallucinations. It is interesting to note that the latter association is mediated by disturbed visual cognition, as explored with the Visual and Object Space Perception battery (VOSP) (James and Warrington 1991). Bernardin et al. (2022) also noted that central retinal abnormalities in fERG and the presence of oscillatory potentials abnormalities could serve as a marker of hypodopaminergia in patients with treated schizophrenia. Finally, it should be noted that Hébert et al. (2010) found rod response abnormalities on the fERG in first-degree relatives of people with schizophrenia or bipolar disorder, indicating that certain retinal parameters could be a marker of risk for psychosis. Furthermore, they described different abnormalities in chronic patients with schizophrenia vs. bipolar disorders, suggesting a possibility for selective markers (Hébert et al. 2020).

All in all, it seems that the functioning of the main cell layers of the retina is altered in schizophrenia. New research should now focus on determining the impact of these retinal abnormalities on subsequent visual processing, including simultaneous measurements of retinal and cortical processing. The relationship with cortical processing may not be enough to uncover all perceptual disorders in individuals with schizophrenia, though. Till this point, we described impairments in the extraction of elementary visual features, with or without top-down influences. However, it has also been suggested that individuals with schizophrenia have difficulties at grouping the different features composing visual objects. These difficulties concern a later step of visual processing and have been related to disruptions in the neuronal connectivity disorders. In the following, we summarize this line of research.

4.5 Relationship Between Visual Impairments and Disruptions in the Neuronal Connectivity

The exploration of visual binding deficits has been conducted in parallel with the investigation of disruptions of the neuronal connectivity, since neuronal connectivity has been proposed as a neurobiological mean to group visual features and identify objects (Gray et al. 1989). We describe them together thereafter, but first describe what is known about contour integration deficits in individuals with schizophrenia.

4.5.1 Contour Integration Deficits

A large number of studies have suggested that patients with schizophrenia experience difficulties to integrate information when processing visual form (reviewed in Silverstein and Keane 2011, and Silverstein 2016). As a reminder contour information is processed by specialized neurons with small receptive fields in V1, and this information requires to be bound together to recover the objects form, and to distinguish objects from one another (Boucart et al. 1994). Contour information is integrated based on collinearity (alignment) of contour information, but also other types of grouping, like, e.g., proximity or similarity. Many studies have suggested deficient performance in individuals with schizophrenia when the task requires grouping (Uhlhaas et al. 2006a, b; Kurylo et al. 2007; Kéri et al. 2009; Keane et al. 2012). Those studies are based on the use of various types of fragmented figures, where different parts have to be bound together correctly in order to recover the object form. Interestingly, the deficit is less in bipolar disorders (Keane et al. 2016a, 2022) and absent in Body Dysmorphic Disorder (Silverstein et al. 2015a). It is already found in first-episode patients (Rivolta et al. 2014; Feigenson et al. 2014) and appears to aggravate with the occurrence of acute episodes (Feigenson et al. 2014; Keane et al. 2016b).

It should be noted that grouping is not systematically altered in patients with schizophrenia. As a rule, impairments are more easily found in patients in acute phases, or when grouping requires to bind fragments of information that are far from each other or are intermingled with distracters, i.e. when grouping is not straightforward. Else individuals with schizophrenia are often sensitive to grouping effect or contextual influences (van Assche and Giersch 2011; Yang et al. 2013; Tibber et al. 2013; Roinishvili et al. 2015). This observation might raise the question of a generalized deficit, i.e. impaired performance due to the difficulty of the task (e.g. when information becomes ambiguous, or unclear) rather than an impairment in the precise mechanisms involved in the task. However, a number of studies suggest otherwise. Several studies show both preserved and impaired contextual modulations in the same population (Tibber et al. 2013, 2015; Yang et al. 2013) suggesting that the impairments are selective (albeit which mechanisms are impaired and why requires further explorations). Besides, grouping difficulties are often related to clinical disorganization specifically (review in Silverstein and Keane 2011) and have been proposed to be related to a general mechanism of loose associations. Finally, grouping impairments appear to be specific to schizophrenia (Silverstein 2016), which should not be the case if they were related to a generalized deficit.

Another debate regards the impact of top-down attention effects on the integration of visual information. There is no question that information can be bound together through bottom-up processes (Giersch et al. 2000; Driver et al. 2001). However, it is also possible to group items mentally, through top-down processes (Beck and Palmer 2002), like, e.g., when we compare two identical fruits from different baskets. In that case the two items belong to different groups but can still be mentally re-grouped. Van Assche and Giersch (2011) have suggested this ability to be impaired in patients with schizophrenia. Furthermore, top-down processes may also affect bottom-up grouping. It has been suggested, in both animal and humans, that top-down attention modulates the strength of grouping, e.g., by modulating lateral connectivity between neurons coding for orientation (Freeman et al. 2003; Li et al. 2004; Gilbert and Li 2013). It is thus possible that the modulation of contour integration is affected in individuals with schizophrenia, rather than the feedforward integration of contour. As a matter of fact, the deficit in contour integration observed in individuals with schizophrenia is not improved when the task incites participants to focus on contours (Kéri et al. 2009). There are only few fMRI studies related to visual perception, but a Diffusion Tensor Imaging (DTI) study recently evidenced disorders in the anatomical connectivity of the visuospatial attentional network in schizophrenia (Leroux et al. 2020). fMRI studies confirm the involvement of widespread activation reductions during grouping by collinearity (alignment) of contour elements, that do not fit with an impairment restricted to early visual processing. Silverstein et al. (2015b) showed reduced activations in patients with schizophrenia relative to controls, in the visual cortex, but not in V1. Similarly Wynn et al. (2008) showed abnormal spatial organization of the lateral occipital cortex. Moreover, Silverstein et al. (2015b), as well as Sehatpour et al. (2010) showed these reductions to be accompanied by a lack of activation in regions outside the occipital cortex, and especially in the attentional network (see also Dima et al. 2010). It is to be noted that a recent approach by Hettwer et al. (2022) capitalizes on known polygenic resilience factors to evidence that this resilience is associated with an increased volume of the left fusiform gyrus. Although it is premature to interpret this finding, this original approach is promising and may help to complement existing studies.

Visual perception has been widely explored in relation with the disruptions of neuronal connectivity, partly for historical reasons. Those studies are summarized in the following section.

4.5.2 Visual Perception and Disruptions of Neuronal Connectivity

Since the initial description of neuronal synchronization in the late 80s (Gray et al. 1989), we have moved from a model of brain functioning whereby information was believed to converge on specialized brain areas to a model in which information processing relies on large-range connectivity between brain areas. This understanding of normal brain functioning has opened up new avenues for the understanding of brain diseases in general, and especially for schizophrenia. Disruptions of neuronal connectivity have been described and are included in the models of the pathophysiology of, e.g., schizophrenia (Uhlhaas and Singer 2010). Their relation with perception initially came from evidence about the functional role of neural synchrony in visual binding, i.e. the ability to connect information coded by specialized neurons with small receptive fields and to derive a global form (Gray et al. 1989; Bertrand and Tallon-Baudry 2000). This observation led to several studies linking visual integration difficulties in schizophrenia with disruptions of neuronal connectivity (Uhlhaas and Singer 2010).

It is known today that neural synchrony plays a more general role in large-scale integration of distributed neural activity than only on the binding mechanisms. It occurs between distant cortical areas and is involved in visual attention, memory, and consciousness (Tallon-Baudry 2003; Sergent and Dehaene 2004). Impairments in neuronal networks may thus be related to many abnormal cognitive and conscious activities. There is abundant evidence about disruptions of neuronal connectivity in patients with schizophrenia (Spencer 2008; Uhlhaas and Singer 2010, 2012), which may play an important role in the pathophysiology of schizophrenia.

A first series of studies relies on the observation that a rhythmic auditory or visual stimulation elicits, or 'entrains' a rhythmic activity in the brain. When applied to schizophrenia, this technique has consistently shown reduced amplitude- and phase-modulation of neuronal responses to stimulation at various frequencies in patients relative to controls (Kwon et al. 1999; Krishnan et al. 2005; Spencer et al. 2008a; Hamm et al. 2011). However, similar impairments are observed in Bipolar Disorder and in Autism Spectrum Disorders and are thus not specific of schizophrenia (O'Donnell et al. 2004; Wilson et al. 2007).

Several studies have shown disruptions of neuronal connectivity during perceptual tasks, though. Neural responses can be evoked, i.e. at a constant delay after the stimulus. In contrast, they are called 'induced' when they are not time-locked to the stimulus (Bertrand and Tallon-Baudry 2000). Results in patients have shown reduced amplitude of both types of signals for beta/gamma frequencies (Spencer et al. 2003, 2008b; Grützner et al. 2013; Sun et al. 2013). Abnormalities have additionally been evidenced regarding phase-synchronization between electrode pairs (Spencer et al. 2003; Uhlhaas et al. 2006a, b). Phase-synchronization is especially important for the phase-locking of the different areas involved in perception, attention, and executive processes (Varela et al. 2001). Importantly disruptions of neuronal connectivity have also been observed in the prodromal stage of psychosis, which is encouraging for the discovery of biomarkers of psychosis vulnerability (Mikanmaa et al. 2019).

In summary disruptions of neuronal connectivity may impact visual perception directly, and indirectly through top-down mechanisms. Such disruptions may also underlie the impact of eye movements on perception, especially by affecting the ability to predict the sensory consequences of saccades. Disruptions of neuronal connectivity are important for both attentional gain, context-modulation and predictive coding. The latter entails a dialogue between motor and sensory areas and thus can be affected by disruptions of neuronal connectivity. Predictive coding entails the prediction of the sensory consequences of action, whether a motor action or an ocular saccade (Sperry 1950). Sensory cortices thus require to receive information from motor or oculomotor areas, i.e. the 'efference' copy of the motor programme, or the 'corollary discharge'. This information transmission has been repeatedly proposed to be impaired in schizophrenia (Feinberg 1978; Franck et al. 2001; Frith 2005; Ford and Mathalon 2005). It may again impact cognition in several ways (Ford et al. 2002, 2008; Ford and Mathalon 2005). It may especially impact the ability to predict and adjust perception when making saccades (Thakkar and Rolfs 2019, but see Lencer et al. 2021). In can be noted that ocular movements are beyond the objectives of the present paper, but several reviews are helpful to discover smooth pursuit, saccadic control or free ocular exploration abnormalities (Holzman 2000; Trillenberg et al. 2004; Beedie et al. 2011).

We still need a more in-depth understanding of the relationships between clinical symptoms and impairments at the level of neuronal networks, but the accumulated knowledge already guides the development of both drug and stimulation methods. Stimulation techniques aim a normalization of the connectivity between brain areas (Lefaucheur et al. 2014; Moseley et al. 2015). Similarly, drug development is guided by the observation that the balance between excitatory/inhibitory transmission is important for efficient connectivity (Uhlhaas 2013). Drugs are developed to restore the excitatory/inhibitory balance and thus synchronized activity in neuronal networks (Sears and Hewett 2021). In the longer term, the analyses of connectivity impairments (e.g. connectomics, Crossley et al. 2016) may provide biomarkers for distinct states or symptoms of the pathology (Northoff and Duncan 2016). A promising avenue is the distinction between those disruptions of neuronal connectivity that are already present in patients' siblings, and represent trait markers, and those that are associated with the illness expression (Yao et al. 2020).

The consequences of the impairments reviewed until now have been nicely summarized in a chapter by Silverstein (2016). It may account for complaints like 'Things get blurred and it's like being blind' or 'I've to put things together in my head'. However, it might be asked whether this is the whole story, especially as visual grouping/integration difficulties in patients appear to develop more clearly as the pathology evolves in a chronic state. A striking and somewhat overlooked aspect of the patients' descriptions reviewed by e.g. Chapman (1966) is that they often include a mention about self-motion. Citations include the precision 'if I move', or 'if your run', 'I can't move properly', which appears to accompany perceptual disorders. This observation is also supported by studies exploring different aspects of the dynamics of perception, i.e. motion perception and saccades, predictive coding and the time structure of perception, which are summarized in the next sections.

4.6 Dynamic Aspects of Perception

Perception is inherently dynamic, as any mental activity. Our environment is itself highly dynamic, and sensory information unfolds in time. A first straightforward example is the perception of motion. The dorsal pathway that processes spatial information includes specialized areas of motion processing and allows for several stages of information processing. First-order motion processing allows localized motion to be encoded, whereas second-order motion results from the integration of several first-order signals. For example, if several dots are moving in different directions (which is one of the approaches most often used in individuals with schizophrenia), it is still possible to derive a global motion if there is enough coherence between the different local motions. Patients appear to be mainly impaired for second-order motion (see the review by Chen 2011). Whether this difficulty is related with impaired binding mechanisms, like when a contour must be derived from local oriented elements, is a matter of debate, though. First Tibber et al. (2015), have shown that individuals with schizophrenia are more impaired when static rather than dynamic elements have to be integrated. Second, some studies have suggested that motion processing may be difficult for individuals with schizophrenia due to eye movements' impairments. Those studies have shown that no impairment is found when motion is too short to allow for an impact of eye movements (Hong et al. 2009) or when motion intervenes incidentally in the task (Kaliuzhna et al. 2020; but in that case motion is first-order motion). Whether motion impairments are solely due to eye-tracking difficulties for long durations remains a matter of debate (Chen 2011). Whatever the mechanisms of these difficulties, the results, nonetheless, suggest a difficulty to process at least second-order motion, and this difficulty is attested to by reduced activation of the V5 complex in fMRI in patients relative to control in a smooth pursuit task (Lencer et al. 2005).

Other results also suggest a difficulty in the dynamic aspects of perception, even in the absence of motion information. A major theoretical development has been the application of predictive coding to the understanding of the pathophysiology of schizophrenia (Friston 2005; Sterzer et al. 2018). As already described above, the main principle of predictive coding is the coding of predictions at several levels of information processing, and the detection of mismatches (prediction errors) between the predictions and real sensory information (Friston 2005; Kok and de Lange 2015; Rao and Ballard 1999). This strategy is believed to minimize energy inasmuch only error signals are propagated, but not predictable and stable information (Alink et al. 2010; Schellekens et al. 2016). Importantly, higher level expectations may modulate activity in early sensory areas (Kok et al. 2014; Muckli et al. 2005; Todorovic and de Lange 2012; van Kemenade et al. 2022), by activating primary sensory cortex in the absence of expected information (Kok et al. 2014; Muckli et al. 2005) or attenuating processing of the expected sensory information (Todorovic and de Lange 2012). People with schizophrenia are globally less susceptible to visual illusions (Notredame et al. 2014), which may suggest that they rely less on their structural biases and more on sensory evidence (see also Weilnhammer et al. 2020). In other tasks, however, patients with schizophrenia sometimes show stronger adaptation-based biases compared to healthy controls (Stuke et al. 2021; Ueda et al. 2022). Different alternative models have been proposed to explain these empirical findings (Frith 2005; Fletcher and Frith 2009; Jardri and Denève 2013). In a nutshell what is unclear is when and whether priors are too weak and lead to excessive confidence in sensory information, and when and whether priors are too strong and inflexible. One possibility to resolve this conundrum might be to consider how prediction errors are processed over time. A recent study by Bansal et al. (2022) used moving dots that changed, or not, direction after 500 ms. Participants were asked to report the last direction, but patients with schizophrenia tended to report the first one. These results were interpreted as a failure in perceptual updating and too strong weight attributed to the initial perception. These results fit also with a difficulty to process information in time.

Timing impairments have since long been described, and related to disorders of the sense of self, that are observed in subjects at risk of developing psychosis (Parnas et al. 2011). Patients themselves report a link between those disorders, as illustrated by the following patient's citation: 'Time splits up and doesn't run forward anymore. There arise uncountable disparate now, now, now, all crazy and without rule or order. It is the same with myself. From moment to moment, various 'selves' arise and disappear entirely at random. There is no connection between my present ego and the one before' (Kimura, cited in Fuchs 2007). Such reports have led phenomenologists to hypothesize a link between the sense of self and timing (Fuchs 2007; Vogeley and Kupke 2007; Stanghellini et al. 2016; Fuchs and van Duppen 2017). The observation of a time fragmentation can hardly be accounted for by duration perception (Thoenes and Oberfeld 2017; Coull and Giersch 2022). Rather, the roots of a time fragmentation are to be found in what allows time to have a structure, i.e. succession, order, and simultaneity (Martin et al. 2014; Vogel et al. 2019). From this point of view, it is interesting to note that the ability to predict the occurrence of a visual stimulus in time is impaired in those patients displaying a disturbed sense of self (Martin et al. 2017) and that the abnormal reaction to short temporal asynchronies in individuals with schizophrenia leads to a loss of feeling of control, i.e. agency disorders, when asynchronies occur during manual movement (Foerster et al. 2021). Such results are consistent with the idea of a link between time and self-disorders and justify the focus on this topic.

A number of studies have evidenced difficulties in patients with schizophrenia when they have to process information in time. When two signals are displayed in close temporal proximity (but in different locations) patients have a hard time detecting the asynchrony, whether the signals are visual, auditory, tactile, or audio-visual (Foucher et al. 2007; Giersch et al. 2009; Lalanne et al. 2012b; Schmidt et al. 2011; Martin et al. 2013; Stevenson et al. 2017; Di Cosmo et al. 2021). Patients have even more difficulties to order signals in time (Capa et al. 2014). This difficulty may already account for a difficulty to follow information fluently (Martin et al. 2014). However, in addition to the conscious ability to distinguish information in time, automatic mechanisms allow us to predict the moment of occurrence of the incoming signal, on the basis of previous experience. This has been observed at the level of seconds (Vallesi et al. 2013) and at the level of milliseconds (Marques-Carneiro et al. 2020). These mechanisms are critical to follow information in time, and to avoid lagging behind information (Herzog et al. 2020). Predicting information is critical for timely interactions with the environment. Lalanne et al. (2012b, c) suggested that patients with schizophrenia have a difficulty to predict sequences of events at the level of milliseconds. Instead of orienting their attention towards the end of the sequence like controls, it is as if they are stuck with the first stimulus of the sequence. The difficulty to follow information in time may explain the patients' feeling of being disconnected from their environment: 'Things go too quick for my mind. Everything is too fast and too big for me, too quick to study' (citation excerpt from Chapman 1966). Such observations are encouraging results and may represent a useful addition to other known perceptual disorders, in that they may help to relate perceptual disorders to the complaints of the individuals during the prodromal phase preceding the conversion to psychosis.

Imaging results on timing are still too scarce to be reviewed (but see Ciullo et al. 2018a; Marques-Carneiro et al. 2021). However, MMN (Mismatch Negativity) may be related to predictive coding impairments in schizophrenia, and especially to time prediction impairments. MMN is a wave recorded with electroencephalography, and whose amplitude increases in response to a rare event, i.e. an oddball. Predictive coding has been proposed to be involved in the detection of the oddball, because it represents an irregularity in the series of information displayed during the task, i.e. a prediction error (Lieder et al. 2013; Wacongne 2016). The amplitude of the MMN is typically reduced in individuals with schizophrenia (Neuhaus et al. 2013; Farkas et al. 2015; Corcoran et al. 2018). It is interesting to note that duration deviants attenuate patients' MMN response more so than pitch deviants (Umbricht and Krljes 2005; Erickson et al. 2016; see Coull and Giersch 2022 for a more lengthy development on this point). Such results point to the potential importance of time relative to space in the impairments of patients (see also Ciullo et al. 2018b).

5 Conclusion

We have reviewed a broad range of perceptual disorders observed in individuals with schizophrenia. The approaches are diverse and concern different levels of visual processing, from the retina to top-down attention mechanisms. Much remains to be done to understand the link between the observed disorders and the subjective reports of the patients, as well as their link to prodromal symptoms. However, the number of possible causes for abnormal perceptual experiences is in stark contrast with the fact that these disorders are absent from typical diagnostic criteria. They might be used in the future to help detecting the risk of developing psychosis during prodromes.

References

Alink A, Schwiedrzik CM, Kohler A et al (2010) Stimulus predictability reduces responses in primary visual cortex. J Neurosci 30:2960–2966. https://doi.org/10.1523/JNEUROSCI.3730-10.2010

Almeida NL, Fernandes TP, Lima EH et al (2020) Combined influence of illness duration and medication type on visual sensitivity in schizophrenia. Braz J Psychiatry 42:27–32. https://doi.org/10.1590/1516-4446-2018-0331

Balogh Z, Benedek G, Kéri S (2008) Retinal dysfunctions in schizophrenia. Prog Neuropsychopharmacol Biol Psychiatry 32:297–300. https://doi.org/10.1016/j.pnpbp.2007.08.024

Bansal S, Bae G-Y, Robinson BM et al (2022) Association between failures in perceptual updating and the severity of psychosis in schizophrenia. JAMA Psychiat 79:169–177. https://doi.org/10.1001/jamapsychiatry.2021.3482

Bar M (2004) Visual objects in context. Nat Rev Neurosci 5:617–629. https://doi.org/10.1038/nrn1476

Beedie SA, Benson PJ, St Clair DM (2011) Atypical scanpaths in schizophrenia: evidence of a trait- or state-dependent phenomenon? J Psychiatry Neurosci 36:150–164. https://doi.org/10.1503/jpn.090169

Beck DM, Palmer SE (2002) Top-down influences on perceptual grouping. J Exp Psychol Hum Percept Perform 28:1071–1084

Berkovitch L, Del Cul A, Maheu M, Dehaene S (2018) Impaired conscious access and abnormal attentional amplification in schizophrenia. Neuroimage Clin 18:835–848. https://doi.org/10.1016/j.nicl.2018.03.010

Berkovitch L, Charles L, Del Cul A et al (2021) Disruption of conscious access in psychosis is associated with altered structural brain connectivity. J Neurosci 41:513–523. https://doi.org/10.1523/JNEUROSCI.0945-20.2020
Bernardin F, Schwitzer T, Angioi-Duprez K et al (2020) Retinal ganglion cells dysfunctions in schizophrenia patients with or without visual hallucinations. Schizophr Res 219:47–55. https://doi.org/10.1016/j.schres.2019.07.007
Bernardin F, Schwitzer T, Angioi-Duprez K et al (2021) Retinal ganglion cell dysfunction is correlated with disturbed visual cognition in schizophrenia patients with visual hallucinations. Psychiatry Res 298:113780. https://doi.org/10.1016/j.psychres.2021.113780
Bernardin F, Schwitzer T, Schwan R et al (2022) Altered central vision and amacrine cells dysfunction as marker of hypodopaminergic activity in treated patients with schizophrenia. Schizophr Res 239:134–141. https://doi.org/10.1016/j.schres.2021.11.049
Bertrand O, Tallon-Baudry C (2000) Oscillatory gamma activity in humans: a possible role for object representation. Int J Psychophysiol 38:211–223. https://doi.org/10.1016/s0167-8760(00)00166-5
Berzhanskaya J, Grossberg S, Mingolla E (2007) Laminar cortical dynamics of visual form and motion interactions during coherent object motion perception. Spat Vis 20:337–395. https://doi.org/10.1163/156856807780919000
Bosworth RG, Robbins SL, Granet DB, Dobkins KR (2013) Delayed luminance and chromatic contrast sensitivity in infants with spontaneously regressed retinopathy of prematurity. Doc Ophthalmol 127:57–68. https://doi.org/10.1007/s10633-013-9395-9
Boucart M, Delord S, Giersch A (1994) The computation of contour information in complex objects. Perception 23:399–409. https://doi.org/10.1068/p230399
Breitmeyer BG (2014) Contributions of magno- and parvocellular channels to conscious and non-conscious vision. Philos Trans R Soc Lond B Biol Sci 369:20130213. https://doi.org/10.1098/rstb.2013.0213
Breitmeyer BG, Ganz L (1976) Implications of sustained and transient channels for theories of visual pattern masking, saccadic suppression, and information processing. Psychol Rev 83:1–36
Breitmeyer BG, Öğmen H (2006) Visual masking: time slices through conscious and unconscious vision, 2nd edn. Oxford University Press, New York
Bullier J, Hupé JM, James AC, Girard P (2001) The role of feedback connections in shaping the responses of visual cortical neurons. Prog Brain Res 134:193–204. https://doi.org/10.1016/s0079-6123(01)34014-1
Bunney WE Jr, Hetrick WP, Bunney BG et al (1999) Structured interview for assessing perceptual anomalies (SIAPA). Schizophr Bull 25:577–592. https://doi.org/10.1093/oxfordjournals.schbul.a033402
Butler PD, Schechter I, Zemon V et al (2001) Dysfunction of early-stage visual processing in schizophrenia. Am J Psychiatry 158:1126–1133. https://doi.org/10.1176/appi.ajp.158.7.1126
Butler PD, Martinez A, Foxe JJ et al (2007) Subcortical visual dysfunction in schizophrenia drives secondary cortical impairments. Brain 130:417–430. https://doi.org/10.1093/brain/awl233
Butler PD, Silverstein SM, Dakin SC (2008) Visual perception and its impairment in schizophrenia. Biol Psychiatry 64:40–47. https://doi.org/10.1016/j.biopsych.2008.03.023
Cadenhead KS, Serper Y, Braff DL (1998) Transient versus sustained visual channels in the visual backward masking deficits of schizophrenia patients. Biol Psychiatry 43:132–138. https://doi.org/10.1016/S0006-3223(97)00316-8
Calderone DJ, Martinez A, Zemon V et al (2013) Comparison of psychophysical, electrophysiological, and fMRI assessment of visual contrast responses in patients with schizophrenia. Neuroimage 67:153–162. https://doi.org/10.1016/j.neuroimage.2012.11.019
Campbell FW, Robson JG (1968) Application of Fourier analysis to the visibility of gratings. J Physiol 197:551–566. https://doi.org/10.1113/jphysiol.1968.sp008574
Capa RL, Duval CZ, Blaison D, Giersch A (2014) Patients with schizophrenia selectively impaired in temporal order judgments. Schizophr Res 156:51–55. https://doi.org/10.1016/j.schres.2014.04.001

Chapman J (1966) The early symptoms of schizophrenia. Br J Psychiatry 112:225–251
Chen Y (2011) Abnormal visual motion processing in schizophrenia: a review of research progress. Schizophr Bull 37:709–715. https://doi.org/10.1093/schbul/sbr020
Chidharom M, Krieg J, Marques-Carneiro E et al (2021) Investigation of electrophysiological precursors of attentional errors in schizophrenia: toward a better understanding of abnormal proactive control engagement. J Psychiatr Res 140:235–242. https://doi.org/10.1016/j.jpsychires.2021.05.079
Christensen BK, Spencer JMY, King JP et al (2013) Noise as a mechanism of anomalous face processing among persons with schizophrenia. Front Psychol 4:401. https://doi.org/10.3389/fpsyg.2013.00401
Ciullo V, Vecchio D, Gili T et al (2018a) Segregation of brain structural networks supports Spatio-temporal predictive processing. Front Hum Neurosci 12:212. https://doi.org/10.3389/fnhum.2018.00212
Ciullo V, Piras F, Vecchio D et al (2018b) Predictive timing disturbance is a precise marker of schizophrenia. Schizophr Res Cogn 12:42–49. https://doi.org/10.1016/j.scog.2018.04.001
Corcoran CM, Stoops A, Lee M et al (2018) Developmental trajectory of mismatch negativity and visual event-related potentials in healthy controls: implications for neurodevelopmental vs. neurodegenerative models of schizophrenia. Schizophr Res 191:101–108. https://doi.org/10.1016/j.schres.2017.09.047
Coull JT, Giersch A (2022) The distinction between temporal order and duration processing, and implications for schizophrenia. Nat Rev Psychol:1–15. https://doi.org/10.1038/s44159-022-00038-y
Crossley NA, Fox PT, Bullmore ET (2016) Meta-connectomics: human brain network and connectivity meta- analyses. Psychol Med 46:897–907. https://doi.org/10.1017/S0033291715002895
Cutting J, Dunne F (1986) The nature of the abnormal perceptual experiences at the onset of schizophrenia. Psychopathology 19:347–352. https://doi.org/10.1159/000284459
de Haan B, Karnath H-O, Driver J (2012) Mechanisms and anatomy of unilateral extinction after brain injury. Neuropsychologia 50:1045–1053. https://doi.org/10.1016/j.neuropsychologia.2012.02.015
Del Cul A, Dehaene S, Leboyer M (2006) Preserved subliminal processing and impaired conscious access in schizophrenia. Arch Gen Psychiatry 63:1313–1323. https://doi.org/10.1001/archpsyc.63.12.1313
Del Cul A, Dehaene S, Reyes P et al (2009) Causal role of prefrontal cortex in the threshold for access to consciousness. Brain 132:2531–2540. https://doi.org/10.1093/brain/awp111
Demmin DL, Davis Q, Roché M, Silverstein SM (2018) Electroretinographic anomalies in schizophrenia. J Abnorm Psychol 127:417–428. https://doi.org/10.1037/abn0000347
Demmin DL, Mote J, Beaudette DM et al (2020a) Retinal functioning and reward processing in schizophrenia. Schizophr Res 219:25–33. https://doi.org/10.1016/j.schres.2019.06.019
Demmin DL, Netser R, Roché MW et al (2020b) People with current major depression resemble healthy controls on flash electroretinogram indices associated with impairment in people with stabilized schizophrenia. Schizophr Res 219:69–76. https://doi.org/10.1016/j.schres.2019.07.024
Di Cosmo G, Costantini M, Ambrosini E et al (2021) Body-environment integration: temporal processing of tactile and auditory inputs along the schizophrenia continuum. J Psychiatr Res 134:208–214. https://doi.org/10.1016/j.jpsychires.2020.12.034
Dima D, Dietrich DE, Dillo W, Emrich HM (2010) Impaired top-down processes in schizophrenia: a DCM study of ERPs. Neuroimage 52:824–832. https://doi.org/10.1016/j.neuroimage.2009.12.086
Dondé C, Brunelin J, Haesebaert F (2020) Duration, pitch and intensity features reveal different magnitudes of tone-matching deficit in schizophrenia. Schizophr Res 215:460–462. https://doi.org/10.1016/j.schres.2019.10.003

Driver J, Davis G, Russell C et al (2001) Segmentation, attention and phenomenal visual objects. Cognition 80:61–95. https://doi.org/10.1016/s0010-0277(00)00151-7
Enns JT, Di Lollo V (1997) Object substitution: a new form of masking in unattended visual locations. Psychol Sci 8:135–139. https://doi.org/10.1111/j.1467-9280.1997.tb00696.x
Erickson MA, Ruffle A, Gold JM (2016) A meta-analysis of mismatch negativity in schizophrenia: from clinical risk to disease specificity and progression. Biol Psychiatry 79:980–987. https://doi.org/10.1016/j.biopsych.2015.08.025
Farkas K, Stefanics G, Marosi C, Csukly G (2015) Elementary sensory deficits in schizophrenia indexed by impaired visual mismatch negativity. Schizophr Res 166:164–170. https://doi.org/10.1016/j.schres.2015.05.011
Feigenson KA, Keane BP, Roché MW, Silverstein SM (2014) Contour integration impairment in schizophrenia and first episode psychosis: state or trait? Schizophr Res 159:515–520. https://doi.org/10.1016/j.schres.2014.09.028
Feinberg I (1978) Efference copy and corollary discharge: implications for thinking and its disorders. Schizophr Bull 4:636–640. https://doi.org/10.1093/schbul/4.4.636
Fletcher PC, Frith CD (2009) Perceiving is believing: a Bayesian approach to explaining the positive symptoms of schizophrenia. Nat Rev Neurosci 10:48–58. https://doi.org/10.1038/nrn2536
Foerster FR, Weibel S, Poncelet P et al (2021) Volatility of subliminal haptic feedback alters the feeling of control in schizophrenia. J Abnorm Psychol 130:775–784. https://doi.org/10.1037/abn0000703
Ford JM, Mathalon DH (2005) Corollary discharge dysfunction in schizophrenia: can it explain auditory hallucinations? Int J Psychophysiol 58:179–189. https://doi.org/10.1016/j.ijpsycho.2005.01.014
Ford JM, Mathalon DH, Whitfield S et al (2002) Reduced communication between frontal and temporal lobes during talking in schizophrenia. Biol Psychiatry 51:485–492. https://doi.org/10.1016/s0006-3223(01)01335-x
Ford JM, Roach BJ, Faustman WO, Mathalon DH (2008) Out-of-synch and out-of-sorts: dysfunction of motor-sensory communication in schizophrenia. Biol Psychiatry 63:736–743. https://doi.org/10.1016/j.biopsych.2007.09.013
Foucher JR, Lacambre M, Pham B-T et al (2007) Low time resolution in schizophrenia lengthened windows of simultaneity for visual, auditory and bimodal stimuli. Schizophr Res 97:118–127. https://doi.org/10.1016/j.schres.2007.08.013
Franck N, Farrer C, Georgieff N et al (2001) Defective recognition of one's own actions in patients with schizophrenia. Am J Psychiatry 158:454–459. https://doi.org/10.1176/appi.ajp.158.3.454
Freeman E, Driver J, Sagi D, Zhaoping L (2003) Top-down modulation of lateral interactions in early vision: does attention affect integration of the whole or just perception of the parts? Curr Biol 13:985–989. https://doi.org/10.1016/s0960-9822(03)00333-6
Freud E, Plaut DC, Behrmann M (2016) "What" is happening in the dorsal visual pathway. Trends Cogn Sci 20:773–784. https://doi.org/10.1016/j.tics.2016.08.003
Friston K (2005) A theory of cortical responses. Philos Trans R Soc Lond B Biol Sci 360:815–836. https://doi.org/10.1098/rstb.2005.1622
Frith C (2005) The neural basis of hallucinations and delusions. C R Biol 328:169–175. https://doi.org/10.1016/j.crvi.2004.10.012
Fuchs T (2007) The temporal structure of intentionality and its disturbance in schizophrenia. Psychopathology 40:229–235. https://doi.org/10.1159/000101365
Fuchs T, Van Duppen Z (2017) Time and events: on the phenomenology of temporal experience in schizophrenia (ancillary article to EAWE domain 2). Psychopathology 50:68–74. https://doi.org/10.1159/000452768
Fusar-Poli P, Borgwardt S, Bechdolf A et al (2013) The psychosis high-risk state: a comprehensive state-of- the-art review. JAMA Psychiat 70:107–120. https://doi.org/10.1001/jamapsychiatry.2013.269

Garobbio S, Roinishvili M, Favrod O et al (2021) Electrophysiological correlates of visual backward masking in patients with bipolar disorder. Psychiatry Res Neuroimaging 307: 111206. https://doi.org/10.1016/j.pscychresns.2020.111206
Gaspelin N, Luck SJ (2018) "Top-down" does not mean "Voluntary". J Cogn 1:25. https://doi.org/10.5334/joc.28
Giersch A, Humphreys GW, Boucart M, Kovacs I (2000) The computation of occluded contours in visual agnosia: evidence for early computation prior to shape binding and figure-ground coding. Cogn Neuropsychol 17:731–759. https://doi.org/10.1080/026432900750038317
Giersch A, Lalanne L, Corves C et al (2009) Extended visual simultaneity thresholds in patients with schizophrenia. Schizophr Bull 35:816–825. https://doi.org/10.1093/schbul/sbn016
Giersch A, Huard T, Park S, Rosen C (2021) The Strasbourg visual scale: a novel method to assess visual hallucinations. Front Psych 12:685018. https://doi.org/10.3389/fpsyt.2021.685018
Gilbert CD, Li W (2013) Top-down influences on visual processing. Nat Rev Neurosci 14:350–363. https://doi.org/10.1038/nrn3476
Goghari VM, Sponheim SR (2008) Divergent backward masking performance in schizophrenia and bipolar disorder: association with COMT. Am J Med Genet B Neuropsychiatr Genet 147B:223–227. https://doi.org/10.1002/ajmg.b.30583
Gourzis P, Katrivanou A, Beratis S (2002) Symptomatology of the initial prodromal phase in schizophrenia. Schizophr Bull 28:415–429. https://doi.org/10.1093/oxfordjournals.schbul.a006950
Granholm E, Fish SC, Verney SP (2009) Pupillometric measures of attentional allocation to target and mask processing on the backward masking task in schizophrenia. Psychophysiology 46: 510–520. https://doi.org/10.1111/j.1469-8986.2009.00805.x
Granö N, Salmijärvi L, Karjalainen M et al (2015) Early signs of worry: psychosis risk symptom visual distortions are independently associated with suicidal ideation. Psychiatry Res 225:263–267. https://doi.org/10.1016/j.psychres.2014.12.031
Gray CM, König P, Engel AK, Singer W (1989) Oscillatory responses in cat visual cortex exhibit inter- columnar synchronization which reflects global stimulus properties. Nature 338:334–337. https://doi.org/10.1038/338334a0
Green DM, Swets JA (1966) Signal detection theory and psychophysics, vol 1. Wiley, New York, p 1969
Green M, Walker E (1984) Susceptibility to backward masking in schizophrenic patients with positive or negative symptoms. Am J Psychiatry 141:1273–1275. https://doi.org/10.1176/ajp.141.10.1273
Green M, Walker E (1986) Symptom correlates of vulnerability to backward masking in schizophrenia. Am J Psychiatry 143:181–186. https://doi.org/10.1176/ajp.143.2.181
Green MF, Mintz J, Salveson D et al (2003) Visual masking as a probe for abnormal gamma range activity in schizophrenia. Biol Psychiatry 53:1113–1119. https://doi.org/10.1016/s0006-3223(02)01813-9
Gross G, Huber G (1985) Psychopathology of basic stages of schizophrenia in view of formal thought disturbances. Psychopathology 18:115–125. https://doi.org/10.1159/000284224
Gross G, Huber G, Klosterkötter J, Linz M (2008) Bonn scale for the assessment of basic symptoms. Shaker Verlag, Aachen
Grossberg S (1991) Why do parallel cortical systems exist for the perception of static form and moving form? Percept Psychophys 49:117–141. https://doi.org/10.3758/bf03205033
Grützner C, Wibral M, Sun L et al (2013) Deficits in high- (>60 Hz) gamma-band oscillations during visual processing in schizophrenia. Front Hum Neurosci 7:88. https://doi.org/10.3389/fnhum.2013.00088
Häfner H, Maurer K, Ruhrmann S et al (2004) Early detection and secondary prevention of psychosis: facts and visions. Eur Arch Psychiatry Clin Neurosci 254:117–128. https://doi.org/10.1007/s00406-004-0508-z

Hamm JP, Gilmore CS, Picchetti NAM et al (2011) Abnormalities of neuronal oscillations and temporal integration to low- and high-frequency auditory stimulation in schizophrenia. Biol Psychiatry 69:989–996. https://doi.org/10.1016/j.biopsych.2010.11.021
Hébert M, Gagné A-M, Paradis M-E et al (2010) Retinal response to light in young nonaffected offspring at high genetic risk of neuropsychiatric brain disorders. Biol Psychiatry 67:270–274. https://doi.org/10.1016/j.biopsych.2009.08.016
Hébert M, Mérette C, Paccalet T et al (2015) Light evoked potentials measured by electroretinogram may tap into the neurodevelopmental roots of schizophrenia. Schizophr Res 162:294–295. https://doi.org/10.1016/j.schres.2014.12.030
Hébert M, Mérette C, Gagné A-M et al (2020) The electroretinogram may differentiate schizophrenia from bipolar disorder. Biol Psychiatry 87:263–270. https://doi.org/10.1016/j.biopsych.2019.06.014
Herzog MH, Kopmann S, Brand A (2004) Intact figure-ground segmentation in schizophrenia. Psychiatry Res 129:55–63. https://doi.org/10.1016/j.psychres.2004.06.008
Herzog MH, Roinishvili M, Chkonia E, Brand A (2013) Schizophrenia and visual backward masking: a general deficit of target enhancement. Front Psychol 4:254. https://doi.org/10.3389/fpsyg.2013.00254
Herzog MH, Drissi-Daoudi L, Doerig A (2020) All in good time: long-lasting postdictive effects reveal discrete perception. Trends Cogn Sci 24:826–837. https://doi.org/10.1016/j.tics.2020.07.001
Hettwer MD, Lancaster TM, Raspor E et al (2022) Evidence from imaging resilience genetics for a protective mechanism against schizophrenia in the ventral visual pathway. Schizophr Bull sbab151. https://doi.org/10.1093/schbul/sbab151
Holzman PS (2000) Eye movements and the search for the essence of schizophrenia. Brain Res Brain Res Rev 31:350–356. https://doi.org/10.1016/s0165-0173(99)00051-x
Hong LE, Turano KA, O'Neill HB et al (2009) Is motion perception deficit in schizophrenia a consequence of eye-tracking abnormality? Biol Psychiatry 65:1079–1085. https://doi.org/10.1016/j.biopsych.2008.10.021
Hubel DH, Wiesel TN (1959) Receptive fields of single neurones in the cat's striate cortex. J Physiol 148:574–591. https://doi.org/10.1113/jphysiol.1959.sp006308
Humphreys GW (2003) Conscious visual representations built from multiple binding processes: evidence from neuropsychology. Prog Brain Res 142:243–255. https://doi.org/10.1016/S0079-6123(03)42017-7
Humphreys GW, Romani C, Olson A et al (1994) Non-spatial extinction following lesions of the parietal lobe in humans. Nature 372:357–359. https://doi.org/10.1038/372357a0
Humphreys GW, Yoon EY, Kumar S et al (2010) The interaction of attention and action: from seeing action to acting on perception. Br J Psychol 101:185–206. https://doi.org/10.1348/000712609X458927
James M, Warrington E (1991) Visual object and space perception battery (VOSP) Pearson, Oxford
Jardri R, Denève S (2013) Circular inferences in schizophrenia. Brain 136:3227–3241. https://doi.org/10.1093/brain/awt257
Javitt DC (2009) When doors of perception close: bottom-up models of disrupted cognition in schizophrenia. Annu Rev Clin Psychol 5:249–275. https://doi.org/10.1146/annurev.clinpsy.032408.153502
Joos E, Giersch A, Hecker L et al (2020) Large EEG amplitude effects are highly similar across Necker cube, smiley, and abstract stimuli. PLoS One 15:e0232928. https://doi.org/10.1371/journal.pone.0232928
Kaliuzhna M, Stein T, Sterzer P, Seymour KJ (2020) Examining motion speed processing in schizophrenia using the flash lag illusion. Schizophr Res Cogn 19:100165. https://doi.org/10.1016/j.scog.2019.100165
Kantrowitz JT, Butler PD, Schecter I et al (2009) Seeing the world dimly: the impact of early visual deficits on visual experience in schizophrenia. Schizophr Bull 35:1085–1094. https://doi.org/10.1093/schbul/sbp100

Keane BP, Silverstein SM, Barch DM et al (2012) The spatial range of contour integration deficits in schizophrenia. Exp Brain Res 220:251–259. https://doi.org/10.1007/s00221-012-3134-4

Keane BP, Silverstein SM, Wang Y et al (2016a) Seeing more clearly through psychosis: depth inversion illusions are normal in bipolar disorder but reduced in schizophrenia. Schizophr Res 176:485–492. https://doi.org/10.1016/j.schres.2016.06.015

Keane BP, Paterno D, Kastner S, Silverstein SM (2016b) Visual integration dysfunction in schizophrenia arises by the first psychotic episode and worsens with illness duration. J Abnorm Psychol 125:543–549. https://doi.org/10.1037/abn0000157

Keane BP, Cruz LN, Paterno D, Silverstein SM (2018) Self-reported visual perceptual abnormalities are strongly associated with core clinical features in psychotic disorders. Front Psych 9:69

Keane BP, Erlikhman G, Serody M, Silverstein SM (2022) A brief psychometric test reveals robust shape completion deficits in schizophrenia that are less severe in bipolar disorder. Schizophr Res 240:78–80. https://doi.org/10.1016/j.schres.2021.12.015

Keesey UT (1972) Flicker and pattern detection: a comparison of thresholds. J Opt Soc Am 62:446–448. https://doi.org/10.1364/josa.62.000446

Kéri S, Benedek G (2007) Visual contrast sensitivity alterations in inferred magnocellular pathways and anomalous perceptual experiences in people at high-risk for psychosis. Vis Neurosci 24: 183–189. https://doi.org/10.1017/S0952523807070253

Kéri S, Kelemen O, Benedek G, Janka Z (2001) Different trait markers for schizophrenia and bipolar disorder: a neurocognitive approach. Psychol Med 31:915–922. https://doi.org/10.1017/s0033291701004068

Kéri S, Kiss I, Kelemen O et al (2005) Anomalous visual experiences, negative symptoms, perceptual organization and the magnocellular pathway in schizophrenia: a shared construct? Psychol Med 35:1445–1455. https://doi.org/10.1017/S0033291705005398

Kéri S, Kelemen O, Benedek G (2009) Attentional modulation of perceptual organisation in schizophrenia. Cogn Neuropsychiatry 14:77–86. https://doi.org/10.1080/13546800902757936

Keshavan MS, Diwadkar VA, Montrose DM et al (2005) Premorbid indicators and risk for schizophrenia: a selective review and update. Schizophr Res 79:45–57. https://doi.org/10.1016/j.schres.2005.07.004

King DJ, Hodgekins J, Chouinard PA et al (2017) A review of abnormalities in the perception of visual illusions in schizophrenia. Psychon Bull Rev 24:734–751. https://doi.org/10.3758/s13423-016-1168-5

Kiss I, Fábián A, Benedek G, Kéri S (2010) When doors of perception open: visual contrast sensitivity in never-medicated, first-episode schizophrenia. J Abnorm Psychol 119:586–593. https://doi.org/10.1037/a0019610

Klosterkötter J, Hellmich M, Steinmeyer EM, Schultze-Lutter F (2001) Diagnosing schizophrenia in the initial prodromal phase. Arch Gen Psychiatry 58:158–164. https://doi.org/10.1001/archpsyc.58.2.158

Knight RA, Silverstein SM (2001) A process-oriented approach for averting confounds resulting from general performance deficiencies in schizophrenia. J Abnorm Psychol 110:15–30. https://doi.org/10.1037//0021-843x.110.1.15

Koch C, Tsuchiya N (2007) Attention and consciousness: two distinct brain processes. Trends Cogn Sci 11:16–22. https://doi.org/10.1016/j.tics.2006.10.012

Kok P, de Lange FP (2015) Predictive coding in sensory cortex. In: Forstmann BU, Wagenmakers E-J (eds) An introduction to model-based cognitive neuroscience. Springer, New York, pp 221–244

Kok P, Failing MF, de Lange FP (2014) Prior expectations evoke stimulus templates in the primary visual cortex. J Cogn Neurosci 26:1546–1554. https://doi.org/10.1162/jocn_a_00562

Krishnan GP, Vohs JL, Hetrick WP et al (2005) Steady state visual evoked potential abnormalities in schizophrenia. Clin Neurophysiol 116:614–624. https://doi.org/10.1016/j.clinph.2004.09.016

Kulikowski JJ, Tolhurst DJ (1973) Psychophysical evidence for sustained and transient detectors in human vision. J Physiol 232:149–162. https://doi.org/10.1113/jphysiol.1973.sp010261

Kurylo DD, Pasternak R, Silipo G et al (2007) Perceptual organization by proximity and similarity in schizophrenia. Schizophr Res 95:205–214. https://doi.org/10.1016/j.schres.2007.07.001
Kwon JS, O'Donnell BF, Wallenstein GV et al (1999) Gamma frequency-range abnormalities to auditory stimulation in schizophrenia. Arch Gen Psychiatry 56:1001–1005. https://doi.org/10.1001/archpsyc.56.11.1001
Lalanne L, Dufour A, Després O, Giersch A (2012a) Attention and masking in schizophrenia. Biol Psychiatry 71:162–168. https://doi.org/10.1016/j.biopsych.2011.09.018
Lalanne L, van Assche M, Giersch A (2012b) When predictive mechanisms go wrong: disordered visual synchrony thresholds in schizophrenia. Schizophr Bull 38:506–513. https://doi.org/10.1093/schbul/sbq107
Lalanne L, Van Assche M, Wang W, Giersch A (2012c) Looking forward: an impaired ability in patients with schizophrenia? Neuropsychologia 50:2736–2744. https://doi.org/10.1016/j.neuropsychologia.2012.07.023
Lamme VA, Roelfsema PR (2000) The distinct modes of vision offered by feedforward and recurrent processing. Trends Neurosci 23:571–579. https://doi.org/10.1016/s0166-2236(00)01657-x
Lefaucheur J-P, André-Obadia N, Antal A et al (2014) Evidence-based guidelines on the therapeutic use of repetitive transcranial magnetic stimulation (rTMS). Clin Neurophysiol 125:2150–2206. https://doi.org/10.1016/j.clinph.2014.05.021
Lencer R, Nagel M, Sprenger A et al (2005) Reduced neuronal activity in the V5 complex underlies smooth- pursuit deficit in schizophrenia: evidence from an fMRI study. Neuroimage 24:1256–1259. https://doi.org/10.1016/j.neuroimage.2004.11.013
Lencer R, Meyhöfer I, Triebsch J et al (2021) Saccadic suppression in schizophrenia. Sci Rep 11:13133. https://doi.org/10.1038/s41598-021-92531-2
Leroux E, Poirel N, Dollfus S (2020) Anatomical connectivity of the visuospatial attentional network in schizophrenia: a diffusion tensor imaging tractography study. J Neuropsychiatry Clin Neurosci 32:266–273. https://doi.org/10.1176/appi.neuropsych.19040101
Li W, Piëch V, Gilbert CD (2004) Perceptual learning and top-down influences in primary visual cortex. Nat
Lieder F, Stephan KE, Daunizeau J et al (2013) A neurocomputational model of the mismatch negativity. PLoS Comput Biol 9:e1003288. https://doi.org/10.1371/journal.pcbi.1003288
Limanowski J, Friston K (2020) Attentional modulation of vision versus proprioception during action. Cereb Cortex 30:1637–1648. https://doi.org/10.1093/cercor/bhz192
Liu D, Fan HZ, Zhao WX et al (2020) Deficits of tactile passive perception acuity in patients with schizophrenia. Front Psych 11:519248. https://doi.org/10.3389/fpsyt.2020.519248
Livingstone MS, Hubel DH (1987) Psychophysical evidence for separate channels for the perception of form, color, movement, and depth. J Neurosci 7:3416–3468. https://doi.org/10.1523/JNEUROSCI.07-11-03416.1987
MacQueen GM, Grof P, Alda M et al (2004) A pilot study of visual backward masking performance among affected versus unaffected offspring of parents with bipolar disorder. Bipolar Disord 6:374–378. https://doi.org/10.1111/j.1399-5618.2004.00133.x
Marques-Carneiro JE, Polgári P, Koning E et al (2020) Where and when to look: sequential effects at the millisecond level. Atten Percept Psychophys 82:2821–2836. https://doi.org/10.3758/s13414-020-01995-3
Marques-Carneiro JE, Krieg J, Duval CZ et al (2021) Paradoxical sensitivity to sub-threshold asynchronies in schizophrenia: a behavioural and EEG approach. Schizophr Bull Open. https://doi.org/10.1093/schizbullopen/sgab011
Martin B, Giersch A, Huron C, van Wassenhove V (2013) Temporal event structure and timing in schizophrenia: preserved binding in a longer "now". Neuropsychologia 51:358–371. https://doi.org/10.1016/j.neuropsychologia.2012.07.002
Martin B, Wittmann M, Franck N et al (2014) Temporal structure of consciousness and minimal self in schizophrenia. Front Psychol 5:1175. https://doi.org/10.3389/fpsyg.2014.01175

Martin B, Franck N, Cermolacce M et al (2017) Fragile temporal prediction in patients with schizophrenia is related to minimal self disorders. Sci Rep 7:8278. https://doi.org/10.1038/s41598-017-07987-y

Martínez A, Hillyard SA, Dias EC et al (2008) Magnocellular pathway impairment in schizophrenia: evidence from functional magnetic resonance imaging. J Neurosci 28:7492–7500. https://doi.org/10.1523/JNEUROSCI.1852-08.2008

Martínez A, Hillyard SA, Bickel S et al (2012) Consequences of magnocellular dysfunction on processing attended information in schizophrenia. Cereb Cortex 22:1282–1293. https://doi.org/10.1093/cercor/bhr195

Mashour GA, Roelfsema P, Changeux J-P, Dehaene S (2020) Conscious processing and the global neuronal workspace hypothesis. Neuron 105:776–798. https://doi.org/10.1016/j.neuron.2020.01.026

McClure RK (1999) Backward masking in bipolar affective disorder. Prog Neuropsychopharmacol Biol Psychiatry 23:195–206. https://doi.org/10.1016/s0278-5846(98)00105-5

Meyer L, Lakatos P, He Y (2021) Language dysfunction in schizophrenia: assessing neural tracking to characterize the underlying disorder(s)? Front Neurosci 15:640502

Mikanmaa E, Grent-'t-Jong T, Hua L et al (2019) Towards a neurodynamical understanding of the prodrome in schizophrenia. Neuroimage 190:144–153. https://doi.org/10.1016/j.neuroimage.2017.11.026

Moran J, Desimone R (1985) Selective attention gates visual processing in the extrastriate cortex. Science 229:782–784. https://doi.org/10.1126/science.4023713

Moseley P, Alderson-Day B, Ellison A et al (2015) Non-invasive brain stimulation and auditory verbal hallucinations: new techniques and future directions. Front Neurosci 9:515. https://doi.org/10.3389/fnins.2015.00515

Muckli L, Kohler A, Kriegeskorte N, Singer W (2005) Primary visual cortex activity along the apparent- motion trace reflects illusory perception. PLoS Biol 3:e265. https://doi.org/10.1371/journal.pbio.0030265

Myles JB, Rossell SL, Phillipou A et al (2017) Insights to the schizophrenia continuum: a systematic review of saccadic eye movements in schizotypy and biological relatives of schizophrenia patients. Neurosci Biobehav Rev 72:278–300. https://doi.org/10.1016/j.neubiorev.2016.10.034

Neuhaus AH, Karl C, Hahn E et al (2011) Dissection of early bottom-up and top-down deficits during visual attention in schizophrenia. Clin Neurophysiol 122:90–98. https://doi.org/10.1016/j.clinph.2010.06.011

Neuhaus AH, Brandt ESL, Goldberg TE et al (2013) Evidence for impaired visual prediction error in schizophrenia. Schizophr Res 147:326–330. https://doi.org/10.1016/j.schres.2013.04.004

Nikitova N, Keane BP, Demmin D et al (2019) The audio-visual abnormalities questionnaire (AVAQ): development and validation of a new instrument for assessing anomalies in sensory perception in schizophrenia spectrum disorders. Schizophr Res 209:227–233. https://doi.org/10.1016/j.schres.2019.03.016

Northoff G, Duncan NW (2016) How do abnormalities in the brain's spontaneous activity translate into symptoms in schizophrenia? From an overview of resting state activity findings to a proposed spatiotemporal psychopathology. Prog Neurobiol 145–146:26–45. https://doi.org/10.1016/j.pneurobio.2016.08.003

Notredame C-E, Pins D, Deneve S, Jardri R (2014) What visual illusions teach us about schizophrenia. Front Integr Neurosci 8:63. https://doi.org/10.3389/fnint.2014.00063

O'Donnell BF, Hetrick WP, Vohs JL et al (2004) Neural synchronization deficits to auditory stimulation in bipolar disorder. Neuroreport 15:1369–1372. https://doi.org/10.1097/01.wnr.0000127348.64681.b2

Parnas J, Raballo A, Handest P et al (2011) Self-experience in the early phases of schizophrenia: 5-year follow-up of the Copenhagen prodromal study. World Psychiatry 10:200–204

Phillips RC, Salo T, Carter CS (2015a) Distinct neural correlates for attention lapses in patients with schizophrenia and healthy participants. Front Hum Neurosci 9:502. https://doi.org/10.3389/fnhum.2015.00502

Phillips WA, Clark A, Silverstein SM (2015b) On the functions, mechanisms, and malfunctions of intracortical contextual modulation. Neurosci Biobehav Rev 52:1–20. https://doi.org/10.1016/j.neubiorev.2015.02.010

Place EJ, Gilmore GC (1980) Perceptual organization in schizophrenia. J Abnorm Psychol 89:409–418. https://doi.org/10.1037//0021-843x.89.3.409

Plomp G, Roinishvili M, Chkonia E et al (2013) Electrophysiological evidence for ventral stream deficits in schizophrenia patients. Schizophr Bull 39:547–554. https://doi.org/10.1093/schbul/sbr175

Pokorny J, Smith VC (1997) Psychophysical signatures associated with magnocellular and parvocellular pathway contrast gain. J Opt Soc Am A Opt Image Sci Vis 14:2477–2486. https://doi.org/10.1364/josaa.14.002477

Rao RP, Ballard DH (1999) Predictive coding in the visual cortex: a functional interpretation of some extra- classical receptive-field effects. Nat Neurosci 2:79–87. https://doi.org/10.1038/4580

Rassovsky Y, Green MF, Nuechterlein KH et al (2004) Paracontrast and metacontrast in schizophrenia: clarifying the mechanism for visual masking deficits. Schizophr Res 71:485–492. https://doi.org/10.1016/j.schres.2004.02.018

Rassovsky Y, Green MF, Nuechterlein KH et al (2005) Modulation of attention during visual masking in schizophrenia. Am J Psychiatry 162:1533–1535. https://doi.org/10.1176/appi.ajp.162.8.1533

Reavis EA, Lee J, Wynn JK et al (2017) Linking optic radiation volume to visual perception in schizophrenia and bipolar disorder. Schizophr Res 190:102–106. https://doi.org/10.1016/j.schres.2017.03.027

Reilly JL, Lencer R, Bishop JR et al (2008) Pharmacological treatment effects on eye movement control. Brain Cogn 68:415–435. https://doi.org/10.1016/j.bandc.2008.08.026

Remy I, Schwitzer T, Albuisson É et al (2022) Impaired P100 among regular cannabis users in response to magnocellular biased visual stimuli. Prog Neuropsychopharmacol Biol Psychiatry 113:110437. https://doi.org/10.1016/j.pnpbp.2021.110437

Rensink RA, Enns JT (1998) Early completion of occluded objects. Vision Res 38:2489–2505. https://doi.org/10.1016/s0042-6989(98)00051-0

Reuter F, Del Cul A, Audoin B et al (2007) Intact subliminal processing and delayed conscious access in multiple sclerosis. Neuropsychologia 45:2683–2691. https://doi.org/10.1016/j.neuropsychologia.2007.04.010

Revheim N, Butler PD, Schechter I et al (2006) Reading impairment and visual processing deficits in schizophrenia. Schizophr Res 87:238–245. https://doi.org/10.1016/j.schres.2006.06.022

Richards SE, Hughes ME, Woodward TS et al (2021) External speech processing and auditory verbal hallucinations: a systematic review of functional neuroimaging studies. Neurosci Biobehav Rev 131:663–687. https://doi.org/10.1016/j.neubiorev.2021.09.006

Riecher-Rössler A, Gschwandtner U, Borgwardt S et al (2006) Early detection and treatment of schizophrenia: how early? Acta Psychiatr Scand Suppl:73–80. https://doi.org/10.1111/j.1600-0447.2005.00722.x

Rivolta D, Castellanos NP, Stawowsky C et al (2014) Source-reconstruction of event-related fields reveals hyperfunction and hypofunction of cortical circuits in antipsychotic-naive, first-episode schizophrenia patients during Mooney face processing. J Neurosci 34:5909–5917. https://doi.org/10.1523/JNEUROSCI.3752-13.2014

Robson AG, Nilsson J, Li S et al (2018) ISCEV guide to visual electrodiagnostic procedures. Doc Ophthalmol 136:1–26. https://doi.org/10.1007/s10633-017-9621-y

Roinishvili M, Cappe C, Shaqiri A et al (2015) Crowding, grouping, and gain control in schizophrenia. Psychiatry Res 226:441–445. https://doi.org/10.1016/j.psychres.2015.01.009

Rolls ET, Loh M, Deco G, Winterer G (2008) Computational models of schizophrenia and dopamine modulation in the prefrontal cortex. Nat Rev Neurosci 9:696–709. https://doi.org/10.1038/nrn2462

Ruhrmann S, Schultze-Lutter F, Klosterkötter J (2003) Early detection and intervention in the initial prodromal phase of schizophrenia. Pharmacopsychiatry 36(Suppl 3):S162–S167. https://doi.org/10.1055/s-2003-45125

Rund BR (1993) Backward-masking performance in chronic and nonchronic schizophrenics, affectively disturbed patients, and normal control subjects. J Abnorm Psychol 102:74–81. https://doi.org/10.1037//0021-843x.102.1.74

Saccuzzo DP, Braff DL (1981) Early information processing deficit in schizophrenia. New findings using schizophrenic subgroups and manic control subjects. Arch Gen Psychiatry 38:175–179. https://doi.org/10.1001/archpsyc.1981.01780270061008

Samani NN, Proudlock FA, Siram V et al (2018) Retinal layer abnormalities as biomarkers of schizophrenia. Schizophr Bull 44:876–885. https://doi.org/10.1093/schbul/sbx130

Schechter I, Butler PD, Silipo G et al (2003) Magnocellular and parvocellular contributions to backward masking dysfunction in schizophrenia. Schizophr Res 64:91–101. https://doi.org/10.1016/s0920-9964(03)00008-2

Schellekens W, van Wezel RJA, Petridou N et al (2016) Predictive coding for motion stimuli in human early visual cortex. Brain Struct Funct 221:879–890. https://doi.org/10.1007/s00429-014-0942-2

Schmidt H, McFarland J, Ahmed M et al (2011) Low-level temporal coding impairments in psychosis: preliminary findings and recommendations for further studies. J Abnorm Psychol 120:476–482. https://doi.org/10.1037/a0023387

Schneider WX (1993) Space-based visual attention models and object selection: constraints, problems, and possible solutions. Psychol Res 56:35–43. https://doi.org/10.1007/BF00572131

Schultze-Lutter F (2001) Früherkennung der Schizophrenie anhand subjektiver eschwerdeschilderungen: Ein methodenkritischer Vergleich der Vorhersageleistung nonparametrischer statistischer und alternativer Verfahren zur Generierung von Vorhersagemodellen [Köln Universität]. http://www.deutsche-digitale-bibliothek.de/item/RJTAIO5G554Q2ZW7ED7UIZOUBGMOI2BA

Schultze-Lutter F (2009) Subjective symptoms of schizophrenia in research and the clinic: the basic symptom concept. Schizophr Bull 35:5–8. https://doi.org/10.1093/schbul/sbn139

Schultze-Lutter F, Klosterkötter J, Picker H, Steinmeyer EM, Ruhrmann S (2007) Predicting first-episode psychosis by basic symptom criteria. Clin Neuropsychiatry 4(1):11–22

Schultze-Lutter F, Ruhrmann S, Fusar-Poli P et al (2012) Basic symptoms and the prediction of first- episode psychosis. Curr Pharm Des 18:351–357. https://doi.org/10.2174/138161212799316064

Schwartz BD, McGinn T, Winstead DK (1987) Disordered spatiotemporal processing in schizophrenics. Biol Psychiatry 22:688–698. https://doi.org/10.1016/0006-3223(87)90200-9

Sears SM, Hewett SJ (2021) Influence of glutamate and GABA transport on brain excitatory/inhibitory balance. Exp Biol Med (Maywood) 246:1069–1083. https://doi.org/10.1177/1535370221989263

Sehatpour P, Dias EC, Butler PD et al (2010) Impaired visual object processing across an occipital-frontal- hippocampal brain network in schizophrenia: an integrated neuroimaging study. Arch Gen Psychiatry 67:772–782. https://doi.org/10.1001/archgenpsychiatry.2010.85

Senkowski D, Moran JK (2022) Early evoked brain activity underlies auditory and audiovisual speech recognition deficits in schizophrenia. Neuroimage Clin 33:102909. https://doi.org/10.1016/j.nicl.2021.102909

Sergent C, Dehaene S (2004) Neural processes underlying conscious perception: experimental findings and a global neuronal workspace framework. J Physiol Paris 98:374–384. https://doi.org/10.1016/j.jphysparis.2005.09.006

Shoshina II, Hovis JK, Felisberti FM et al (2021) Visual processing and BDNF levels in first-episode schizophrenia. Psychiatry Res 305:114200. https://doi.org/10.1016/j.psychres.2021.114200
Silverstein SM (2016) Visual perception disturbances in schizophrenia: a unified model. Neuropsychopathol Schizophr:77–132
Silverstein SM, Keane BP (2011) Perceptual organization impairment in schizophrenia and associated brain mechanisms: review of research from 2005 to 2010. Schizophr Bull 37:690–699. https://doi.org/10.1093/schbul/sbr052
Silverstein SM, Elliott CM, Feusner JD et al (2015a) Comparison of visual perceptual organization in schizophrenia and body dysmorphic disorder. Psychiatry Res 229:426–433. https://doi.org/10.1016/j.psychres.2015.05.107
Silverstein SM, Harms MP, Carter CS et al (2015b) Cortical contributions to impaired contour integration in schizophrenia. Neuropsychologia 75:469–480. https://doi.org/10.1016/j.neuropsychologia.2015.07.003
Silverstein SM, Fradkin SI, Demmin DL (2020) Schizophrenia and the retina: towards a 2020 perspective. Schizophr Res 219:84–94. https://doi.org/10.1016/j.schres.2019.09.016
Skottun BC, Skoyles JR (2007) Contrast sensitivity and magnocellular functioning in schizophrenia. Vision Res 47:2923–2933. https://doi.org/10.1016/j.visres.2007.07.016
Skottun B, Skoyles J (2013) Is vision in schizophrenia characterized by a generalized reduction? Front Psychol 4:999
Slaghuis WL (1998) Contrast sensitivity for stationary and drifting spatial frequency gratings in positive- and negative-symptom schizophrenia. J Abnorm Psychol 107:49–62. https://doi.org/10.1037//0021-843x.107.1.49
Slaghuis WL (2004) Spatio-temporal luminance contrast sensitivity and visual backward masking in schizophrenia. Exp Brain Res 156:196–211. https://doi.org/10.1007/s00221-003-1771-3
Slaghuis WL, Thompson AK (2003) The effect of peripheral visual motion on focal contrast sensitivity in positive- and negative-symptom schizophrenia. Neuropsychologia 41:968–980. https://doi.org/10.1016/s0028-3932(02)00321-4
Spencer KM (2008) Visual gamma oscillations in schizophrenia: implications for understanding neural circuitry abnormalities. Clin EEG Neurosci 39:65–68. https://doi.org/10.1177/155005940803900208
Spencer KM, Nestor PG, Niznikiewicz MA et al (2003) Abnormal neural synchrony in schizophrenia. J Neurosci 23:7407–7411
Spencer KM, Salisbury DF, Shenton ME, McCarley RW (2008a) Gamma-band auditory steady-state responses are impaired in first episode psychosis. Biol Psychiatry 64:369–375. https://doi.org/10.1016/j.biopsych.2008.02.021
Spencer KM, Niznikiewicz MA, Shenton ME, McCarley RW (2008b) Sensory-evoked gamma oscillations in chronic schizophrenia. Biol Psychiatry 63:744–747. https://doi.org/10.1016/j.biopsych.2007.10.017
Sperry RW (1950) Neural basis of the spontaneous optokinetic response produced by visual inversion. J Comp Physiol Psychol 43:482–489. https://doi.org/10.1037/h0055479
Stanghellini G, Ballerini M, Presenza S et al (2016) Psychopathology of lived time: abnormal time experience in persons with schizophrenia. Schizophr Bull 42:45–55. https://doi.org/10.1093/schbul/sbv052
Sterzer P, Adams RA, Fletcher P et al (2018) The predictive coding account of psychosis. Biol Psychiatry 84:634–643. https://doi.org/10.1016/j.biopsych.2018.05.015
Stevenson RA, Park S, Cochran C et al (2017) The associations between multisensory temporal processing and symptoms of schizophrenia. Schizophr Res 179:97–103. https://doi.org/10.1016/j.schres.2016.09.035
Stuke H, Kress E, Weilnhammer VA et al (2021) Overly strong priors for socially meaningful visual signals are linked to psychosis proneness in healthy individuals. Front Psychol 12:583637. https://doi.org/10.3389/fpsyg.2021.583637

Sun L, Castellanos N, Grützner C et al (2013) Evidence for dysregulated high-frequency oscillations during sensory processing in medication-naïve, first episode schizophrenia. Schizophr Res 150:519–525. https://doi.org/10.1016/j.schres.2013.08.023
Tallon-Baudry C (2003) Oscillatory synchrony and human visual cognition. J Physiol Paris 97: 355–363. https://doi.org/10.1016/j.jphysparis.2003.09.009
Thakkar KN, Rolfs M (2019) Disrupted corollary discharge in schizophrenia: evidence from the oculomotor system. Biol Psychiatry Cogn Neurosci Neuroimaging 4:773–781. https://doi.org/10.1016/j.bpsc.2019.03.009
Theeuwes J (2018) Visual selection: usually fast and automatic; seldom slow and volitional. J Cogn 1:29. https://doi.org/10.5334/joc.13
Thoenes S, Oberfeld D (2017) Meta-analysis of time perception and temporal processing in schizophrenia: differential effects on precision and accuracy. Clin Psychol Rev 54:44–64. https://doi.org/10.1016/j.cpr.2017.03.007
Thorpe S, Fize D, Marlot C (1996) Speed of processing in the human visual system. Nature 381: 520–522. https://doi.org/10.1038/381520a0
Tibber MS, Anderson EJ, Bobin T et al (2013) Visual surround suppression in schizophrenia. Front Psychol 4:88. https://doi.org/10.3389/fpsyg.2013.00088
Tibber MS, Anderson EJ, Bobin T et al (2015) Local and global limits on visual processing in schizophrenia. PLoS One 10:e0117951. https://doi.org/10.1371/journal.pone.0117951
Todorovic A, de Lange FP (2012) Repetition suppression and expectation suppression are dissociable in time in early auditory evoked fields. J Neurosci 32:13389–13395. https://doi.org/10.1523/JNEUROSCI.2227-12.2012
Tolhurst DJ (1973) Separate channels for the analysis of the shape and the movement of moving visual stimulus. J Physiol 231:385–402. https://doi.org/10.1113/jphysiol.1973.sp010239
Trillenberg P, Lencer R, Heide W (2004) Eye movements and psychiatric disease. Curr Opin Neurol 17:43–47. https://doi.org/10.1097/00019052-200402000-00008
Tschacher W, Giersch A, Friston K (2017) Embodiment and schizophrenia: a review of implications and applications. Schizophr Bull 43:745–753. https://doi.org/10.1093/schbul/sbw220
Ueda N, Tanaka K, Maruo K et al (2022) Perceptual inference, accuracy, and precision in temporal reproduction in schizophrenia. Schizophr Res Cogn 28:100229. https://doi.org/10.1016/j.scog.2021.100229
Uhlhaas PJ (2013) Dysconnectivity, large-scale networks and neuronal dynamics in schizophrenia. Curr Opin Neurobiol 23:283–290. https://doi.org/10.1016/j.conb.2012.11.004
Uhlhaas PJ, Singer W (2010) Abnormal neural oscillations and synchrony in schizophrenia. Nat Rev Neurosci 11:100–113. https://doi.org/10.1038/nrn2774
Uhlhaas PJ, Singer W (2012) Neuronal dynamics and neuropsychiatric disorders: toward a translational paradigm for dysfunctional large-scale networks. Neuron 75:963–980. https://doi.org/10.1016/j.neuron.2012.09.004
Uhlhaas PJ, Phillips WA, Mitchell G, Silverstein SM (2006a) Perceptual grouping in disorganized schizophrenia. Psychiatry Res 145:105–117. https://doi.org/10.1016/j.psychres.2005.10.016
Uhlhaas PJ, Linden DEJ, Singer W et al (2006b) Dysfunctional long-range coordination of neural activity during gestalt perception in schizophrenia. J Neurosci 26:8168–8175. https://doi.org/10.1523/JNEUROSCI.2002-06.2006
Umbricht D, Krljes S (2005) Mismatch negativity in schizophrenia: a meta-analysis. Schizophr Res 76:1–23. https://doi.org/10.1016/j.schres.2004.12.002
Vallesi A, Lozano VN, Correa Á (2013) Dissociating temporal preparation processes as a function of the inter-trial interval duration. Cognition 127:22–30. https://doi.org/10.1016/j.cognition.2012.11.011
van Assche M, Giersch A (2011) Visual organization processes in schizophrenia. Schizophr Bull 37:394–404. https://doi.org/10.1093/schbul/sbp084
van Kemenade BM, Wilbertz G, Müller A, Sterzer P (2022) Non-stimulated regions in early visual cortex encode the contents of conscious visual perception. Hum Brain Mapp 43:1394–1402. https://doi.org/10.1002/hbm.25731

Varela F, Lachaux JP, Rodriguez E, Martinerie J (2001) The brainweb: phase synchronization and large-scale integration. Nat Rev Neurosci 2:229–239. https://doi.org/10.1038/35067550
Vogel DHV, Beeker T, Haidl T et al (2019) Disturbed time experience during and after psychosis. Schizophr Res Cogn 17:100136. https://doi.org/10.1016/j.scog.2019.100136
Vogeley K, Kupke C (2007) Disturbances of time consciousness from a phenomenological and a neuroscientific perspective. Schizophr Bull 33:157–165. https://doi.org/10.1093/schbul/sbl056
Wachtmeister L (1981) Further studies of the chemical sensitivity of the oscillatory potentials of the electroretinogram (erg). Acta Ophthalmol 59:247–258. https://doi.org/10.1111/j.1755-3768.1981.tb02987.x
Wacongne C (2016) A predictive coding account of MMN reduction in schizophrenia. Biol Psychol 116:68–74. https://doi.org/10.1016/j.biopsycho.2015.10.011
Walther DB, Koch C (2007) Attention in hierarchical models of object recognition. Prog Brain Res 165:57–78. https://doi.org/10.1016/S0079-6123(06)65005-X
Warner R, Laugharne J, Peet M et al (1999) Retinal function as a marker for cell membrane omega-3 fatty acid depletion in schizophrenia: a pilot study. Biol Psychiatry 45:1138–1142. https://doi.org/10.1016/s0006-3223(98)00379-5
Weilnhammer V, Röd L, Eckert A-L et al (2020) Psychotic experiences in schizophrenia and sensitivity to sensory evidence. Schizophr Bull 46:927–936. https://doi.org/10.1093/schbul/sbaa003
Wells DS, Leventhal D (1984) Perceptual grouping in schizophrenia: replication of place and Gilmore. J Abnorm Psychol 93:231–234. https://doi.org/10.1037//0021-843x.93.2.231
Wilson TW, Rojas DC, Reite ML et al (2007) Children and adolescents with autism exhibit reduced MEG steady-state gamma responses. Biol Psychiatry 62:192–197. https://doi.org/10.1016/j.biopsych.2006.07.002
Winterer G, Weinberger DR (2004) Genes, dopamine and cortical signal-to-noise ratio in schizophrenia. Trends Neurosci 27:683–690. https://doi.org/10.1016/j.tins.2004.08.002
Wolpert DM, Ghahramani Z, Jordan MI (1995) An internal model for sensorimotor integration. Science 269:1880–1882. https://doi.org/10.1126/science.7569931
Wutz A, Zazio A, Weisz N (2020) Oscillatory bursts in parietal cortex reflect dynamic attention between multiple objects and ensembles. J Neurosci 40:6927–6937. https://doi.org/10.1523/JNEUROSCI.0231-20.2020
Wynn JK, Green MF, Engel S et al (2008) Increased extent of object-selective cortex in schizophrenia. Psychiatry Res 164:97–105. https://doi.org/10.1016/j.pscychresns.2008.01.005
Wynn JK, Mathis KI, Ford J et al (2013) Object substitution masking in schizophrenia: an event-related potential analysis. Front Psychol 4:30. https://doi.org/10.3389/fpsyg.2013.00030
Xu S, Humphreys GW, Mevorach C, Heinke D (2017) The involvement of the dorsal stream in processing implied actions between paired objects: a TMS study. Neuropsychologia 95:240–249. https://doi.org/10.1016/j.neuropsychologia.2016.12.021
Yang E, Tadin D, Glasser DM et al (2013) Visual context processing in schizophrenia. Clin Psychol Sci 1:5–15. https://doi.org/10.1177/2167702612464618
Yao B, Neggers SFW, Kahn RS, Thakkar KN (2020) Altered thalamocortical structural connectivity in persons with schizophrenia and healthy siblings. Neuroimage Clin 28:102370. https://doi.org/10.1016/j.nicl.2020.102370
Yung AR, Yuen HP, McGorry PD et al (2005) Mapping the onset of psychosis: the comprehensive assessment of at-risk mental states. Aust N Z J Psychiatry 39:964–971. https://doi.org/10.1080/j.1440-1614.2005.01714.x
Zopf R, Boulton K, Langdon R, Rich AN (2021) Perception of visual-tactile asynchrony, bodily perceptual aberrations, and bodily illusions in schizophrenia. Schizophr Res 228:534–540. https://doi.org/10.1016/j.schres.2020.11.038

Episodic Memory and Schizophrenia: From Characterization of Relational Memory Impairments to Neuroimaging Biomarkers

Delphine Raucher-Chéné, Katie M. Lavigne, and Martin Lepage

Contents

D. Raucher-Chéné
Cognition, Health, and Society Laboratory (EA 6291), University of Reims Champagne-Ardenne, Reims, France

Academic Department of Psychiatry, University Hospital of Reims, EPSM Marne, Reims, France

K. M. Lavigne
Douglas Research Centre, Verdun, QC, Canada

Department of Psychiatry, McGill University, Montréal, QC, Canada

McGill Centre for Integrative Neuroscience, Montreal Neurological Institute, McGill University, Montreal, Canada

M. Lepage (✉)
Douglas Research Centre, Verdun, QC, Canada

Department of Psychiatry, McGill University, Montréal, QC, Canada
e-mail: martin.lepage@mcgill.ca

Curr Topics Behav Neurosci (2023) 63: 115–136
https://doi.org/10.1007/7854_2022_379
Published Online: 29 July 2022

Abstract Episodic memory research in schizophrenia has a long history already which has clearly established significant impairments and strong associations with brain measures and functional outcome. The purpose of this chapter is not to make an exhaustive review of the recent literature but to highlight some relatively recent developments in the cognitive neuroscience field of episodic memory and schizophrenia. Hence, we present a contemporary view focusing specifically of relational memory which represents a form of episodic memory that refers to associations or binding among items or elements presented together. We describe the major tasks used and illustrate how their combination with brain imaging has: (1) favored the use of experimental memory tasks to isolate specific processes with specific neural correlates, (2) led to a distributed view of the neural correlates of memory impairments in schizophrenia where multiple regions are contributing, and (3) made possible the identification of fMRI biomarkers specific to episodic memory. We then briefly propose what we see as the next steps for memory research in schizophrenia so that the impact of this work can be maximized.

Keywords Brain imaging · Episodic memory · Functional Magnetic Resonance Imaging · Hippocampus · Psychosis · Schizophrenia

1 Preamble

Episodic memory is disproportionately impaired in schizophrenia compared to other cognitive domains (Erk et al. 2017). It is also a distinct Research Domain Criteria construct that has been associated with a genetic risk and altered brain activation in this population. This impairment is evident in all phases of illness: clinical high-risk (individuals presenting an elevated risk for psychosis; Valli et al. 2012), first-episode schizophrenia (Mesholam-Gately et al. 2009), and in enduring (chronic) schizophrenia (Heinrichs and Zakzanis 1998). Even when other cognitive impairments (e.g., executive functions, working memory, and IQ) are controlled, episodic memory remains significantly impaired (Egeland et al. 2003, Leeson et al. 2009, Kopald et al. 2012). Within the episodic memory system, more contemporary approaches have examined relational memory (RM), a form of episodic memory that refers to associations or binding among items or elements presented together (O'Keefe and Nadel 1978). RM may be the key element that drives episodic memory deficits in schizophrenia. Many studies have specifically examined relational memory across stages of psychotic disorders and found significant deficits compared to non-clinical controls (Achim and Lepage 2003; Lepage et al. 2005; Pelletier et al. 2005; Lepage et al. 2006; Luck et al. 2009; Hannula et al. 2010; Armstrong et al. 2018, 2012b; Greenland-White et al. 2017; Suh et al. 2020; Avery et al. 2021). We previously proposed relational memory as a unique neurocognitive marker for schizophrenia (Lepage et al. 2015). As Eichenbaum suggested (Eichenbaum et al. 1996), relational memory is subtended by the hippocampus, surrounding medial temporal lobe cortex, and connected cortical regions. One key characteristic linking the hippocampal system to relational memory is the flexibility of representations produced by this system, which can be dynamically reconfigured to reflect changing contexts. Anatomical and hippocampal lesion studies have confirmed the key role of the hippocampus and the surrounding cortex in binding together different elements of a memory trace to form a rich representation (Eichenbaum 1999; Hannula et al. 2006; Watson et al. 2013). Functional MRI studies in healthy individuals have revealed a significant contribution of hippocampal and prefrontal areas to normal relational memory (Lepage et al. 2003; Davachi 2006; Blumenfeld et al. 2011; Zeithamova et al. 2012; Hawco et al. 2017; Reagh and Ranganath 2018; Spalding et al. 2018) and abnormal activity in those areas has been observed in people with schizophrenia (Lepage et al. 2006; Hawco et al. 2015; Ragland et al. 2015; Guimond et al. 2017). In the rest of this chapter, we review RM tasks that have been used in schizophrenia memory research and how they have driven the identification of neuroimaging biomarkers of episodic memory impairment in schizophrenia.

2 Relational Memory Tasks in Schizophrenia Research

2.1 Associative Recognition Tasks

The boundaries of the concept of RM have long been determined in contrast to item-related memory, with tasks comparing the two (relational vs. item-related) in encoding and retrieval conditions to delineate specific features of each memory system. Indeed, item-related memory and RM correspond to two different types of retrieval. In the tasks built to explore RM, questions that promote forming an association between two items at the time of encoding can promote better recollection of relational information.

When considering the batteries that assess cognition in clinical populations, the Paired-Associates Learning (PAL) task developed in the Cambridge Neuropsychological Test Automated Battery (CANTAB® [Cognitive assessment software]. Cambridge Cognition (2019)) allows an easy assessment of visual associative learning and memory. In this task, boxes are displayed on the screen and are automatically opened in a randomized order to show a few patterns. Participants must learn to associate the patterns with locations on the screen. After all the boxes have been opened each pattern is then shown in the center of the screen and the participant must touch the box where that pattern was located. Despite its intent to quickly assess associative memory, the PAL is an abstract task that might underestimate or miss the memory difficulties encountered in daily life by patients living with schizophrenia. To explore more specifically, at a behavioral and neuroimaging level, the different processes that contribute to relational memory, some experimental tasks have been developed using different modalities: word pairs (Bartholomeusz et al. 2011) or associating visual and verbal items that we encounter in everyday life (e.g., face/name or object/scene), sometimes presented in a complex scene (e.g., Ragland et al. 2017).

The verbal tasks using pairs of words showed RM impairment in patients living with schizophrenia (Weinhold et al. 2022) but not in first-episode psychosis (FEP) patients (Bartholomeusz et al. 2011). The tasks with visual items have shown RM impairment for patients at all stages of the disorder: in people with a high level of negative schizotypy (Sahakyan et al. 2019) or clinical high-risk subjects (Cao et al. 2019), in early stages of psychosis (Avery et al. 2021) and schizophrenia-spectrum disorder patients (Ragland et al. 2017; Oertel et al. 2019; Baajour et al. 2020). More specifically, a study conducted in recent-onset patients demonstrated that they were more prone than healthy subjects to confidently provide incorrect recognition judgments (Seabury et al. 2021).

To measure RM more systematically in patients living with schizophrenia, consortia of experts have selected RM tasks to detect impairments in this population. The Cognitive Neuroscience Treatment Research to Improve Cognition in Schizophrenia (CNTRICS) initiative (Ragland et al. 2009a) and the Cognitive Neuroscience Test Reliability and Clinical Applications for Schizophrenia (CNTRACS) Consortium (Smucny et al. 2019) have selected the following two tasks to explore RM impairment in schizophrenia: the Relational and Item-Specific Encoding Task (Ragland et al. 2012) and the Associative Inference Paradigm (DeVito et al. 2010; Armstrong et al. 2012b).

2.2 The Relational and Item-Specific Encoding Task (RISE)

In the RISE task, item-specific encoding is operationally defined by presenting single items and prompting participants to decide whether each is living or nonliving, whereas relational encoding involves the presentation of pairs of items and prompting participants to decide whether, in real life, one of the items could fit inside the other (Ragland et al. 2012). In the retrieval part of the task, items are judged "old or new" requiring either familiarity or recollection, and relations are judged "intact or rearranged," relying more on recollection (Hockley and Consoli 1999; Ragland et al. 2012).

The RISE task was developed for clinical research. It is a reliable measure of RM that is well tolerated, with good psychometric characteristics (Ragland et al. 2012). From CHR to enduring schizophrenia-spectrum disorder via FEP patients, this task consistently reports impairment in patients when compared to controls (Ragland et al. 2015; Greenland-White et al. 2017; Smucny et al. 2019; Moran et al. 2020; Smucny et al. 2020). More specific RM tasks focus on the processes that might underlie this impairment and therefore could potentially help to develop focused cognitive remediation interventions.

2.3 *Associative Inference Paradigm (AIP)*

The second task proposed by the consortia relies on transitive inference, the ability to infer the relationship between two indirectly related items that have not been presented together, based on earlier acquired information (Heckers et al. 2004; DeVito et al. 2010). This capacity to build a hierarchically organized series is recognized as a fundamental feature of RM.

The first transitive inference tasks developed for humans showed impairments in schizophrenia-spectrum disorder patients (Titone et al. 2004; Öngür et al. 2006) but failed to demonstrate a significant difference in performance between early-stage patients and controls (Williams et al. 2012) while relatives had deficits (Onwuameze et al. 2016).

The initial version of the AIP, suggested by the CNTRICS initiative, showed alterations in RM but had limited feasibility due to the high attrition of subjects in the training phase (Armstrong et al. 2012a). A revised version was proposed with shorter training-test blocks to reduce memory load, feedback throughout the training period, and explicit instructions on how to solve the inference pairs that improved the feasibility. With this revised version, schizophrenia patients were more impaired on inferential pairs than non-inferential ones compared to healthy controls (Armstrong et al. 2012b). And in a recent 2-year follow-up of patients in the early phase of psychosis, patients were impaired at baseline and the ability to make inferences about trained relationships improved across time, although never reaching the level of healthy control performance (Avery et al. 2021).

2.4 *Transverse Patterning (TP) Tasks*

To remember two items, the ability to combine these improves encoding. It is the principle of the unitization strategy (Li et al. 2019; Sousa et al. 2021c). The TP tasks require learning of previously unknown relations between items as in the rock paper scissors game (i.e., the rock defeats the scissors, the scissors defeats the paper, the paper defeats the rock) and then assessing RM. For the relational learning TP condition, subjects have to learn the relationship between 3 pairs of overlapping stimuli (e.g., A > B, B > C, C > A) during training sessions. Only TP learners (i.e., participants who obtain a sufficient score after training) could then be assessed. For TP learners, they required more trials to learn the TP task (verbal or non-verbal) and performed worse after training than controls (Hanlon et al. 2012). The limitation of this task is that the performance of a subgroup of patients living with schizophrenia remains impaired despite the training (Spieker et al. 2013).

The Relational Trip Task (RTT) is a performance-based naturalistic task simulating real-life circumstances. It has been developed to display a strong degree of agreement between the task cognitive demands and everyday demands. The "winner/loser" relationship used in TP was replaced by those commonly found between people and places (going to/coming from) and between people and objects (like/dislike; Sousa et al. 2021b). This more ecological task showed similar performance to the TP tasks.

2.5 The Semantic Encoding Memory Task (SEMT)

RM impairments in schizophrenia could also be partly driven by a deficit to self-initiate efficient semantic encoding strategies. The self-initiation of semantic encoding strategies is a process through which individuals evaluate semantic relationships between information when such an evaluation is not prompted or directly required for the task. The Semantic Encoding Memory Task (SEMT) is an associative episodic memory task developed to target the self-initiation of these strategies. When prompted to use semantic encoding strategies, schizophrenia patients exhibited similar recognition performance as healthy controls. However, when required to self-initiate these strategies, patients had significant reduced recognition performance (Guimond and Lepage 2016; Guimond et al. 2017, 2018) (Fig. 1).

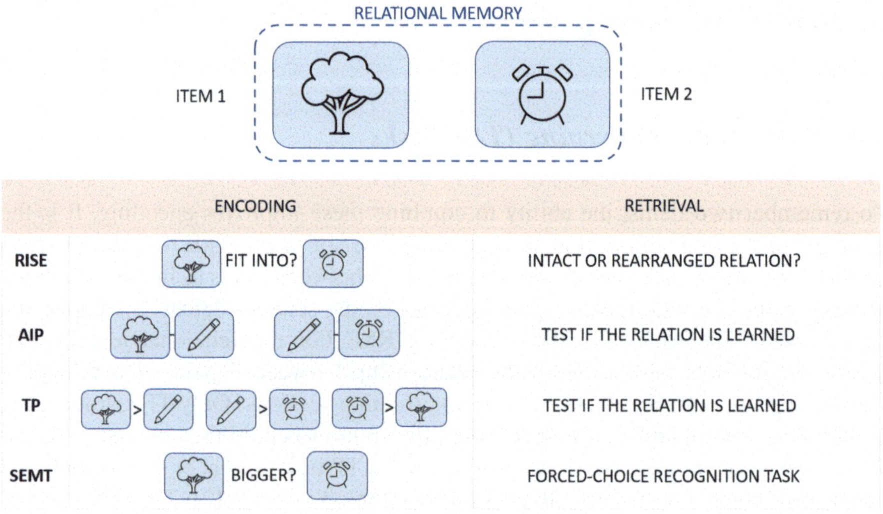

Fig. 1 Relational memory tasks: instructions for encoding the items and retrieval conditions for each type of task (*RISE* relational and item-specific encoding, *AIP* associative inference paradigm, *TP* transverse patterning, *SEMT* semantic encoding memory task)

2.6 Eye-Tracking Tasks

Novel procedures including eye movement tracking as a proxy for the measurement of RM are also becoming more common (Nickel et al. 2015). Unlike the traditional approach of memory, measuring eye movements does not require the comprehension of the instructions of a task nor the requirement to generate responses (Hannula et al. 2012). Additionally, this measure can be recorded at the same time as other behavioral measures. In the exploration of a visual scene, participants tend to prioritize regions that have been presented previously during the test and manipulated even when they cannot explain which changes have been made (Hannula and Ranganath 2009). This measure is sensitive to unconscious memory traces, and stored information can be captured immediately without reliance on verbal reports, even with subliminal cues (Williams et al. 2010; Nickel et al. 2015). This effect, mostly explored in the face-scene tasks, has been associated with early recollection and has been called the relational eye movement effect (Hannula and Ranganath 2009). Indeed, according to the two-stage model of recollection, explicit memory recollection is preceded by an early unconscious stage (Moscovitch 2008). The hypothesis was that this first stage, detected through the relational eye movement effect, was mandatory for relational retrieval (Hannula and Ranganath 2009; Hannula et al. 2012), but some recent studies observed recollection without this effect, suggesting that other routes might exist through the familiarity process (Nagy and Kiraly 2018).

Globally, the results of these eye-tracking studies demonstrate that eye movement behavior is affected in patients living with schizophrenia with delayed and reduced viewing of the matching face in patients when compared to controls or even to bipolar disorder patients (Sheffield et al. 2012). And this impairment is evident in the early stages of the disorder (Suh et al. 2020).

RM impairment is now well established in populations suffering from schizophrenia-spectrum disorders, and thanks to the development of tasks more precisely evaluating the different processes involved, some strategies can be tested to improve this domain of memory, such as Unitization (Li et al. 2019) or the Strategy for Semantic Association Memory training (Guimond et al. 2018). Neuroimaging studies can also improve the comprehension of this core feature of schizophrenia-spectrum disorders (Table 1).

3 Biomarkers of Episodic Memory Impairments in Schizophrenia

The search for neuroimaging biomarkers of episodic memory impairments in schizophrenia gained momentum with the advent of functional magnetic resonance imaging (fMRI), which allowed for unprecedented localization of brain activation (indirectly measured via the blood-oxygen-level-dependent signal) during the

Table 1 Studies assessing episodic memory in schizophrenia by task and clinical group

Reference	Clinical group	Patients (n)	Sex (M/F)	Mean age	Clinical characteristics	Medication (CPZ-equivalent)	EM task	fMRI
Associative recognition								
Sahakyan et al. (2019)	SZT	181	75/106	19.3 (1.6)	pos: 2.17 (2.38); neg: 2.28 (1.96); dis: 1.72 (2.44)		Object-scene pairs task	
Cao et al. (2019)	CHR	155 (18 converters; 137 non-converters)	10/8 81/56	17.22 ± 3.44 19.01 ± 4.19	Scale of prodromal symptoms cf. Table 1	107.08 (175.22) 39.44 (108.25)	Paired-associate episodic memory task	X
Bartholomeusz et al. (2011)	FEP	47	35/12	20.50 (3.29)	BPRS: 54.21 (16.88)	556.48 (683.93)	Verbal paired-associate learning task	
Avery et al. (2021)	eP	66	50/16	21 (3.19)	PANSS: 67 (20.60)	322 (142.04)	Face-scene binding	
Seabury et al. (2021)	eP	53	38/14	22.3 (3.4)	SAPS; SANS [subscores]		Computerized paired-associate memory task	
Ragland et al. (2017)	SZ	24	18/6	25.2 (4.2)	BPRS: 42.7 (13.3)		Item-spatial change	X
Oertel et al. (2019)	SZ REL	27 23	20/9 5/19	34.22 (11.38) 37.22 (9.14)	PANSS: 65.64 (15.22)	367 (12.34)	Face-name-association task	X
Baajour et al. (2020)	SZ	31	21/10	29.36 (7.99)	PANSS: pos: 12.84 (3.13); neg: 12.65 (3.52); gen: 23.52(4.95)		Object-location associative learning paradigm	X
Roes et al. (2021)	SZ	40	28/12	34.95 (8.90)	SAPS: 30.98 (20.70); SANS: 34.53 (20.52); BPRS: 51.54 (15.36)	523.56 (573.07)	Paired-associates encoding task	X

Weinhold et al. (2022)	SSD	18	12/6	33.6 (7.5)			Word pair learning task	
Relational and item-specific encoding (RiSE)								
Greenland-White et al. (2017)	FEP CHR	101 22	68/33 13/9	19.31 (3.90) 15.32 (3.03)	SAPS; SANS (no score)		RiSE	
Smucny et al. (2020)	FEP (+SSD; BD I)	28	18/10	18.82 (4.10)			RiSE	
Ragland et al. (2015)	SZ	52	40/12	33.8 (11.8)	BPRS: 42.4 (10.9)		RiSE	X
Smucny et al. (2020)	SZ SZaff	88 76	55/33 41/35	35.6 (10.7) 36.6 (10.9)	BPRS; CAINS	371.9 (301.0) 577.4 (778.2)	RiSE	
Moran et al. (2020)	SSD	148 medicated 48 unmedicated	84/64 28/20	37.93(10.38) 32.54(11.06)	BPRS; CAINS	432.79 (28.85)	RiSE	
Transitive inference								
Williams et al. (2012)	eP	41	30/11	20.85 (5.0)	PANSS: 56.64 (14.94)	290.79 (150.7)	Transitive inference task	X
Avery et al. (2021)	eP	66	50/16	21 (3.19)	PANSS: 67 (20.60)	322 (142.04)	AIP	
Adams et al. (2020)	SZ	18	15/3	31.3 (10.0)	PANSS: pos: 11.5 (5.4); neg: 13.7(6.5); gen: 25.9(7.3)		Memory integration task	MEG; PET
Titone et al. (2004)	SSD	29	18/11	39.5 (8.9)	BPRS: 44.4 (15.0)	641.6 (1000.5)	Transitive inference task	
Öngür et al. (2006)	SSD	15	11/4	39.7 (11.1)	PANSS: 57.2 (9.6)		Transitive inference task	X
Armstrong et al. (2012a)	SSD	37	17/20	38.43 (11.5)	PANSS: 56.22 (12.40)	589.06 (350.53)	Associative inference paradigm (AIP)	

(continued)

Table 1 (continued)

Reference	Clinical group	Patients (n)	Sex (M/F)	Mean age	Clinical characteristics	Medication (CPZ-equivalent)	EM task	fMRI
Armstrong et al. (2012b)	SSD	34	15/19	44.59 ± 9.70	PANSS: 58.53 ± 13.87	615.08 ± 307.32	Revised AIP	
Onwuameze et al. (2016)	REL (1st; 2nd)	22 26	12/10 10/16	20.3 (2.66) 19.8 (3.13)			Transitive inference task	
Transverse patterning								
Rowland et al. (2010)	SZ	17	9/8	41.9 (11)	BPRS; SANS		Transverse patterning	X
Hanlon et al. (2012)	SZ	21	15/6	38 (11.6)	PANSS: 52 (12)		Transverse patterning	DWI
Spieker et al. (2013)	SZ	20	10/10	43	BPRS: 34.2(6.8)		Transverse patterning	
Sousa et al. (2021a)	SZ	45 (21 TP learners; 24 TP non-learners)	15/6 11/13	36.6(12.4) 42.2(11.5)		455.2(509.5) 484.4(406.3)	Relational trip task (RTT)	
Semantic encoding memory task (SEMT)								
Guimond et al. (2017)	SZ	35 (18 good self-initiation; 17 poor self-initiation)	16/2 14/3	32.22 (7.01) 33.06 (8.8)	SAPS: 17.94 (21.66); 12.59 (8.94); SANS: 17.5 (10.05); 23 (11.66)	717.16 (624.28) 617.84 (390.09)	SEMT	X
Guimond et al. (2018)	SSD	15	12/3	32.13 (8.58)	SAPS: 11.93 (9.25); SANS: 22.53 (12.39)	611.44 (385.80)	SEMT	X
Eye-tracking tasks								
Avery et al. (2019)	eNAP	89	71/18	21 (3.1)	PANSS: 69 (20.5)	283 (200.6)	Face-scene pairs task	
Suh et al. (2020)	eNAP	69	55/14	21.27 (3.36)	PANSS: 69.17 (21.14)	265.14 (182.60)	Face-scene pairs task	

Hannula et al. (2010)	SZ	16	11/5	28.4 (8.2)	BPRS: 40.6 (8.7)	NR	Item-spatial change	
Sheffield et al. (2012)	BD SZ	25 28	8/17 13/15	35.0 (12.47) 39.1 (11.76)	46.9 (7.94) 57.2 (14.72)	450.7 (266.79) 416.8 (233.34)	Face-scene pair task	
Williams et al. (2010)	SSD	35	18/17	38.9 (11.13)	PANSS: 57.1(13.75)	366 (310.59)	Face-scene pair task	
Avery et al. (2018)	SSD	45	32/13	31 (13)	PANSS: 68(18)	458 (283)	Face-scene pair task	Resting-state

Note: *BD* bipolar disorder, *BPRS* Brief Psychotic Rating Scale, *CHR* clinical high-risk, *PZ* Chlorpromazine, *DWI* diffusion-weighted imaging, *eP* early psychosis, *EM* episodic memory, *F* female, *FEP* first-episode psychosis, *fMRI* functional magnetic resonance imaging, *M* male, *MEG* magnetoencephalography, *PANSS* Positive and Negative Syndrome Scale, *PET* positron emission tomography, *SANS* Scale for the Assessment of Negative Symptoms, *SAPS* Scale for the Assessment of Positive Symptoms, *SSD* schizophrenia-spectrum disorder, *SZ* schizophrenia, *SZT* Schizotypy performance of memory tasks. With the hippocampus and medial temporal lobe already established as key memory regions from animal and lesion studies and seminal case studies, such as patient H.M. (Scoville and Milner 1957), these were the main regions of interest in early fMRI studies, which found evidence of decreased hippocampal activation and increased parahippocampal activation during episodic memory tasks in schizophrenia (for a review, see Achim and Lepage 2005). Whole-brain fMRI studies also strongly implicated the prefrontal cortex (PFC), with robust findings of decreased PFC activation in schizophrenia (Achim and Lepage 2005; Ragland et al. 2009b). While informative, these early meta-analyses were limited by few studies and relatively simple fMRI paradigms that could not fully capture the complexities of encoding and retrieval processes in the brain or distinguish between distinct constructs of episodic memory, particularly item and relational memory. Since then, advances in neuroimaging techniques and fMRI task development, including neuroimaging adaptations of tasks described in the previous section, have allowed for more fine-grained investigation of the neural correlates of episodic memory impairments in schizophrenia, as we review below. Notably, we restricted our discussion to fMRI studies, as this is a more active area of research, but refer the reader to previous reviews for an overview of findings from other neuroimaging modalities, including positron emission tomography (Achim and Lepage 2005, Ragland et al. 2009b) and electroencephalography (Tang and Niznikiewicz 2020; Kwok et al. 2021).

3.1 Paired-Associates Tasks

fMRI studies employing paired-associates tasks across various stimulus modalities (verbal, visual, spatial) have consistently implicated the hippocampus and PFC in relational memory impairments in schizophrenia during both encoding and recognition. During *encoding*, Oertel et al. (2019) showed decreased bilateral hippocampal and left PFC activity with a face-name association task in schizophrenia patients and to a lesser degree in the hippocampus in relatives even in the absence of performance deficits in this latter group. Functional connectivity studies have also highlighted the importance of the hippocampus and PFC during relational memory encoding within distributed brain networks. Using directional functional connectivity, Baajour et al. (2020) observed decreased activation within a hippocampal–dorsolateral PFC (DLPFC)-fusiform network in schizophrenia in an object-location task. Through later trials of the task, patients showed decreased directional connectivity toward the DLPFC during encoding. Similarly, Roes et al. (2021) identified a verbal paired-associates task-specific network involving bilateral hippocampal, fusiform, and left PFC hypoactivity in schizophrenia during encoding. Hyper-activation during encoding has also been noted within "lower-level" processing regions (e.g., fusiform-SPL-ITG; Baajour et al. 2020) and in a failure to suppress regions of the default-mode network (Roes et al. 2021), which may point to over-reliance on bottom-up processing of stimulus features rather than top-down encoding strategies in schizophrenia, possibly as a compensatory mechanism.

Inefficient use of strategies and reliance on insufficient compensatory mechanisms are commonly proposed following evidence of hypo-/hyper-activation during paired-associates recognition in schizophrenia. Oertel et al.'s (2019) findings of hippocampal and PFC hypoactivity during encoding in schizophrenia patients and relatives were also observed during recognition, with the addition of parahippocampal hyperactivity in both groups, pointing to compensatory measures consistent with the meta-analysis by Achim and Lepage (2005). Baajour et al. (2020) implicated the dACC in early retrieval (increased bidirectional connectivity in schizophrenia) and DLPFC in late retrieval (increased toward, decreased away) supporting reliance on bottom-up processes. Hyperactivity in temporal, frontal, and parietal regions is also evident in individuals at high-risk for psychosis, particularly in those who later convert to psychosis (Cao et al. 2019).

Thus, schizophrenia is reliably associated with hippocampal and prefrontal cortex hypoactivity during paired-associates tasks, with more distributed hyper/hypoconnectivity likely depending on stimulus modality, task design, and potential use of compensatory strategies. Notably, even within the hippocampus, there is evidence that activation differences between patients and controls depend on task-related factors. Ragland et al. (2017) demonstrated a dissociation between anterior and posterior hippocampal activation related to item versus spatial recognition in schizophrenia. Individuals with schizophrenia showed reduced posterior activity during spatial but not item recognition, and increased anterior hippocampal activity during item but not spatial recognition.

3.2 RISE

The fMRI RiSE task (Ragland et al. 2015) probes item versus associative recognition following either item or relational encoding and can distinguish brain mechanisms underlying item and relational memory and the role of different encoding strategies in each. Schizophrenia patients demonstrated impaired item and associative recognition, but item recognition was disproportionately impaired following relational encoding, suggesting a relational encoding deficit. Indeed, patients showed DLPFC hypoactivity during relational encoding, a region which was associated with better associative recognition in controls. In contrast, ventrolateral PFC activation (which did not differ between groups) during relational encoding was associated with impaired associative recognition in patients, indicating a preference for item-level encoding strategies in schizophrenia. Altered hippocampal activity was also found in schizophrenia following relational encoding, with left and right lateralized activation for item and associative recognition, respectively, as well as reduced activation relative to controls during item recognition. This comprehensive task provides evidence of distinct alterations in brain function underlying item (VLPFC) and relational (DLPFC) encoding in schizophrenia and the specificity of hippocampal function to relational encoding strategies.

3.3 Transitive Inference

Transitive inference has been shown to recruit distributed frontal, parietal, and temporal regions with less widespread activation in patients with schizophrenia (Öngür et al. 2006; Williams et al. 2012). The role of the hippocampus in transitive inference remains a matter of debate, with evidence of increased hippocampal activity during challenging transitive inference in controls not seen in patients (Öngür et al. 2006) and associations between transitive inference and hippocampal activity in controls but not in first-episode psychosis (Williams et al. 2012). However, in the latter study, hippocampal volume reductions were noted in patients who failed to meet training criteria on the transitive inference paradigm, suggesting a key role for this region.

3.4 Transverse Patterning

During a transverse patterning task, Rowland et al. (2010) found that, compared to a simple discrimination task, controls recruited a distributed network of frontal, temporal, and parietal regions prior to learning the task that focalized post-training. In schizophrenia patients, no activations were noted for transverse patterning over and above a simple discrimination task though bilateral parietal activation was observed post-training. In contrast, some negative activations were noted both pre- and post-training, suggesting hyperactivity during the control condition versus TP. Relative to controls, patients showed decreased activity in right inferior frontal, precentral, inferior parietal, left MTG, and posterior hippocampus during pre-training and right middle cingulate, temporal, anterior hippocampus, and left parietal post-training. The hippocampal findings echo those in paired-associates task which found some lateralization of hippocampal activation (left = encoding, right = retrieval).

3.5 SEMT

The semantic encoding memory task (SEMT; Guimond et al. 2017) experimentally manipulates the use of semantic encoding strategies (probed or self-initiated) known to improve recognition performance. Schizophrenia patients' recognition was unimpaired when guided to use semantic encoding strategies, but suffered when self-initiating such strategies. Functional brain activity did not differ between patients and controls when prompted to use semantic encoding strategies. However, when self-initiating, patients showed decreased activity in left DLPFC, left superior parietal lobule, left inferior temporal gyrus, and subcortical regions. Semantic encoding deficits were also associated with decreased left DLPFC activity and more severe negative symptoms. A follow-up study demonstrated the benefit of training self-initiation of semantic strategies in improving recognition performance and brain function (bilateral DLPFC, right inferior parietal lobule) when self-initiating semantic encoding strategies, suggesting these behavioral and neurobiological deficits are amenable to treatment (Guimond et al. 2018).

3.6 Overview of fMRI Biomarker Findings

fMRI studies of episodic memory in schizophrenia have cemented the role of the hippocampus and prefrontal cortex, particularly in relational memory, which is disproportionately impaired in this group. Contemporary research has now taken a network perspective to consider biomarkers of episodic memory impairments in schizophrenia and, along with carefully designed experimental tasks, this work points toward inefficient strategies and less effective compensatory mechanisms underlying such deficits, possibly due to fundamental dysfunction in essential memory processes relying on the hippocampus and prefrontal cortex. Targeted interventions promoting the use of efficient strategies have shown promise in "normalizing" brain activity during episodic memory tasks in schizophrenia and are exciting areas of future research.

4 Conclusion: Outstanding Questions on Memory Research in Schizophrenia and Related Psychoses

This review has provided a brief and selective overview of the relatively long history on memory research in schizophrenia and related psychoses. As we can see, memory impairments have consistently received attention owing to the magnitude of the impairment observed relative to other domains and to the presence of strong associations with sociodemographic variables, clinical outcome and trajectories and ultimately, functioning and quality of life. Research in the last two decades has examined several aspects of episodic memory ranging from emotional memory (Herbener 2008) to autobiographical memory (Berna et al. 2015) and recollection/familiarity (Libby et al. 2013). We have focused our review on relational memory for several reasons described earlier. Having sophisticated and validated relational memory tasks for research in schizophrenia can play an important role in future studies examining pharmacological (Harvey and Bowie 2012; Koola et al. 2020; Sumiyoshi 2020) and behavioral factors spearheading interventions to improve episodic memory in the last few years (Guimond and Lepage 2016; Guimond et al. 2018; Sousa et al. 2021a, c). In addition, such refined tasks can help elucidate several unresolved questions. We briefly propose three of these below.

- *Linking episodic memory to social cognition and negative symptoms*. The relationship between social cognition and the neurocognitive domains has been an area of growing interest in the past few years (Oliver et al. 2019). Social cognition involves drawing inferences about others' beliefs and intentions and comprises social perception, social knowledge, attributional bias, emotional processing, and theory of mind (ToM) (Green et al. 2008). ToM refers to the ability to interpret others' speech and actions in terms of their intentions, knowledge, and beliefs (Corcoran et al. 1995) and is the most impaired social cognitive domain in schizophrenia (Bertrand et al. 2007, 2008; Beland and Lepage 2017). ToM performance is related to verbal episodic memory (Thibaudeau et al. 2020) as well as to negative symptoms' severity (Piskulic and Addington 2011; Lin et al. 2013; Mike et al. 2019; Green 2020) and might mediate the relationship between the two (Raucher-Chéné et al. 2021). Laurita and Spreng (2017) propose that our relational memory ability influences how we perceive, construct, interact, and ultimately connect with our social world. So, a better and more systematic assessment of these related domains (e.g., through combining RM tasks with the newly validated Brief battery of the Social Cognition Psychometric Evaluation study; Halverson et al. (2022)) would offer a more accurate representation of each patient's impairment that could inform a more focused treatment approach.
- *Proposing a conceptual model including the neuroanatomical level*. Eichenbaum's updated relational memory theory (Eichenbaum 2004) proposed that the hippocampus is responsible for computing an associative scaffold, linking items and events in "memory space." Tying in the social cognitive impairments discussed above, Schafer and Schiller (2019) propose an association between the hippocampus and social impairments in clinical populations, suggesting the hippocampus is involved in general relational processes. Similarly, Montagrin et al. (2018) suggested hippocampal representations combine multiple continuous dimensions and require dynamic navigation through social contexts; that is, we must continuously form and update relations within the social world to make sense of it. Thus, the hippocampus may organize social information into relational maps to guide social decision-making. As such, while some social impairments may be secondary to psychotic symptoms, others may be rooted in faulty hippocampal-based representations of social maps. As such, the hippocampal system is thought to play a crucial hub role in constructing and navigating a complex memory space, underlying flexible cognition as well as social behavior (Eichenbaum and Cohen 2014; Rubin et al. 2014). Altogether, the evolving view of the hippocampus is one that not only contributes to relational memory but also supports many other complex cognitive and social behaviors (e.g., empathy (Beadle et al. 2013), social discourse, and language (Duff and Brown-Schmidt 2012)) through its connectivity with widespread cortical regions. Studies on hippocampal–cortical connectivity are essential in light of this

cognitive model to improve our understanding of the pathophysiology of these impairments.

- *Improving functional outcomes.* Across different stages of schizophrenia, VM impairment has a detrimental impact on social functioning (Jordan et al. 2018; Karambelas et al. 2019). Specific cognitive interventions have been developed to improve RM impairment, such as Unitization (Li et al. 2019) or the Strategy for Semantic Association Memory training (Guimond et al. 2018). These two interventions incorporate up-to-date knowledge on the pathophysiology of RM to promote alternative ways to memorize information (Guimond et al. 2018). ToM also shows the strongest relation to functioning relative to other domains (Fett et al. 2011) and psychosocial interventions targeting ToM improve functional outcomes in schizophrenia (Javed and Charles 2018). So, based on a combined cognitive assessment and clarification of the cortical pathways involved, an adjusted psychosocial intervention taking all these elements into account might be more efficient in improving functional outcomes.

References

Achim AM, Lepage M (2003) Is associative recognition more impaired than item recognition memory in schizophrenia? A meta-analysis. Brain Cogn 53(2):121–124

Achim AM, Lepage M (2005) Episodic memory-related activation in schizophrenia: meta-analysis. Br J Psychiatry 187(6):500–509

Adams RA, Bush D, Zheng F, Meyer SS, Kaplan R, Orfanos S, Marques TR, Howes OD, Burgess N (2020) Impaired theta phase coupling underlies frontotemporal dysconnectivity in schizophrenia. Brain 143(4):1261–1277. https://doi.org/10.1093/brain/awaa035

Armstrong K, Kose S, Williams L, Woolard A, Heckers S (2012a) Impaired associative inference in patients with schizophrenia. Schizophr Bull 38(3):622–629

Armstrong K, Williams LE, Heckers S (2012b) Revised associative inference paradigm confirms relational memory impairment in schizophrenia. Neuropsychology 26(4):451–458

Armstrong K, Avery S, Blackford JU, Woodward N, Heckers S (2018) Impaired associative inference in the early stage of psychosis. Schizophr Res 202:86–90

Avery SN, Rogers BP, Heckers S (2018) Hippocampal network modularity is associated with relational memory dysfunction in schizophrenia. Biol Psychiatry Cogn Neurosci Neuroimaging 3(5):423–432. https://doi.org/10.1016/j.bpsc.2018.02.001

Avery SN, Armstrong K, Blackford JU, Woodward ND, Cohen N, Heckers S (2019) Impaired relational memory in the early stage of psychosis. Schizophr Res 212:113–120

Avery SN, Armstrong K, McHugo M, Vandekar S, Blackford JU, Woodward ND, Heckers S (2021) Relational memory in the early stage of psychosis: a 2-year follow-up study. Schizophr Bull 47(1):75–86

Baajour SJ, Chowdury A, Thomas P, Rajan U, Khatib D, Zajac-Benitez C, Falco D, Haddad L, Amirsadri A, Bressler S, Stanley JA, Diwadkar VA (2020) Disordered directional brain network interactions during learning dynamics in schizophrenia revealed by multivariate autoregressive models. Hum Brain Mapp 41(13):3594–3607

Bartholomeusz CF, Proffitt TM, Savage G, Simpson L, Markulev C, Kerr M, McConchie M, McGorry PD, Pantelis C, Berger GE, Wood SJ (2011) Relational memory in first episode psychosis: implications for progressive hippocampal dysfunction after illness onset. Aust N Z J Psychiatry 45(3):206–213

Beadle JN, Tranel D, Cohen NJ, Duff MC (2013) Empathy in hippocampal amnesia. Front Psychol 4:69
Beland S, Lepage M (2017) The relative contributions of social cognition and self-reflectiveness to clinical insight in enduring schizophrenia. Psychiatry Res 258:116–123
Berna F, Potheegadoo J, Aouadi I, Ricarte JJ, Allé MC, Coutelle R, Boyer L, Cuervo-Lombard CV, Danion J-M (2015) A meta-analysis of autobiographical memory studies in schizophrenia spectrum disorder. Schizophr Bull 42(1):56–66
Bertrand MC, Sutton H, Achim AM, Malla AK, Lepage M (2007) Social cognitive impairments in first episode psychosis. Schizophr Res 95(1–3):124–133
Bertrand MC, Achim AM, Harvey PO, Sutton H, Malla AK, Lepage M (2008) Structural neural correlates of impairments in social cognition in first episode psychosis. Soc Neurosci 3(1):79–88
Blumenfeld RS, Parks CM, Yonelinas AP, Ranganath C (2011) Putting the pieces together: the role of dorsolateral prefrontal cortex in relational memory encoding. J Cogn Neurosci 23(1): 257–265
Cao H, McEwen SC, Chung Y, Chen OY, Bearden CE, Addington J, Goodyear B, Cadenhead KS, Mirzakhanian H, Cornblatt BA, Carrion RE, Mathalon DH, McGlashan TH, Perkins DO, Belger A, Seidman LJ, Thermenos H, Tsuang MT, van Erp TGM, Walker EF, Hamann S, Anticevic A, Woods SW, Cannon TD (2019) Altered brain activation during memory retrieval precedes and predicts conversion to psychosis in individuals at clinical high risk. Schizophr Bull 45(4):924–933
Corcoran R, Mercer G, Frith CD (1995) Schizophrenia, symptomatology and social inference: investigating “theory of mind” in people with schizophrenia. Schizophr Res 17(1):5–13
Davachi L (2006) Item, context and relational episodic encoding in humans. Curr Opin Neurobiol 16(6):693–700
DeVito LM, Lykken C, Kanter BR, Eichenbaum H (2010) Prefrontal cortex: role in acquisition of overlapping associations and transitive inference. Learn Mem 17(3):161–167
Duff MC, Brown-Schmidt S (2012) The hippocampus and the flexible use and processing of language. Front Hum Neurosci 6:69
Egeland J, Sundet K, Rund BR, Asbjornsen A, Hugdahl K, Landro NI, Lund A, Roness A, Stordal KI (2003) Sensitivity and specificity of memory dysfunction in schizophrenia: a comparison with major depression. J Clin Exp Neuropsychol 25(1):79–93
Eichenbaum H (1999) The hippocampus and mechanisms of declarative memory. Behav Brain Res 103(2):123–133
Eichenbaum H (2004) Hippocampus: cognitive processes and neural representations that underlie declarative memory. Neuron 44(1):109–120
Eichenbaum H, Cohen NJ (2014) Can we reconcile the declarative memory and spatial navigation views on hippocampal function? Neuron 83(4):764–770
Eichenbaum H, Schoenbaum G, Young B, Bunsey M (1996) Functional organization of the hippocampal memory system. Proc Natl Acad Sci U S A 93(24):13500–13507
Erk S, Mohnke S, Ripke S, Lett TA, Veer IM, Wackerhagen C, Grimm O, Romanczuk-Seiferth N, Degenhardt F, Tost H, Mattheisen M, Mühleisen TW, Charlet K, Skarabis N, Kiefer F, Cichon S, Witt SH, Nöthen MM, Rietschel M, Heinz A, Meyer-Lindenberg A, Walter H (2017) Functional neuroimaging effects of recently discovered genetic risk loci for schizophrenia and polygenic risk profile in five RDoC subdomains. Transl Psychiatry 7(1):e997
Fett A-KJ, Viechtbauer W, Dominguez M-d-G, Penn DL, van Os J, Krabbendam L (2011) The relationship between neurocognition and social cognition with functional outcomes in schizophrenia: a meta-analysis. Neurosci Biobehav Rev 35(3):573–588. https://doi.org/10.1016/j.neubiorev.2010.07.001
Green MF (2020) From social cognition to negative symptoms in schizophrenia: how do we get there from here? Schizophr Bull 46(2):225–226
Green MF, Penn DL, Bentall R, Carpenter WT, Gaebel W, Gur RC, Kring AM, Park S, Silverstein SM, Heinssen R (2008) Social cognition in schizophrenia: an NIMH workshop on definitions, assessment, and research opportunities. Schizophr Bull 34(6):1211–1220

Greenland-White SE, Ragland JD, Niendam TA, Ferrer E, Carter CS (2017) Episodic memory functions in first episode psychosis and clinical high risk individuals. Schizophr Res 188:151–157
Guimond S, Lepage M (2016) Cognitive training of self-initiation of semantic encoding strategies in schizophrenia: a pilot study. Neuropsychol Rehabil 26(3):464–479
Guimond S, Hawco C, Lepage M (2017) Prefrontal activity and impaired memory encoding strategies in schizophrenia. J Psychiatr Res 91:64–73
Guimond S, Beland S, Lepage M (2018) Strategy for semantic association memory (SESAME) training: effects on brain functioning in schizophrenia. Psychiatry Res Neuroimaging 271:50–58
Halverson TF, Pinkham AE, Harvey PD, Penn DL (2022) Brief battery of the social cognition psychometric evaluation study (BB-SCOPE): development and validation in schizophrenia spectrum disorders. J Psychiatr Res 150:307–316
Hanlon FM, Houck JM, Klimaj SD, Caprihan A, Mayer AR, Weisend MP, Bustillo JR, Hamilton DA, Tesche CD (2012) Frontotemporal anatomical connectivity and working-relational memory performance predict everyday functioning in schizophrenia. Psychophysiology 49(10): 1340–1352
Hannula DE, Ranganath C (2009) The eyes have it: hippocampal activity predicts expression of memory in eye movements. Neuron 63(5):592–599
Hannula DE, Tranel D, Cohen NJ (2006) The long and the short of it: relational memory impairments in amnesia, even at short lags. J Neurosci 26(32):8352–8359
Hannula DE, Ranganath C, Ramsay IS, Solomon M, Yoon J, Niendam TA, Carter CS, Ragland JD (2010) Use of eye movement monitoring to examine item and relational memory in schizophrenia. Biol Psychiatry 68(7):610–616
Hannula DE, Baym CL, Warren DE, Cohen NJ (2012) The eyes know: eye movements as a veridical index of memory. Psychol Sci 23(3):278–287
Harvey PD, Bowie CR (2012) Cognitive enhancement in schizophrenia: pharmacological and cognitive remediation approaches. Psychiatr Clin North Am 35(3):683–698
Hawco C, Buchy L, Bodnar M, Izadi S, Dell'Elce J, Messina K, Joober R, Malla A, Lepage M (2015) Source retrieval is not properly differentiated from object retrieval in early schizophrenia: an fMRI study using virtual reality. Neuroimage Clin 7:336–346
Hawco C, Armony JL, Daskalakis ZJ, Berlim MT, Chakravarty MM, Pike GB, Lepage M (2017) Differing time of onset of concurrent TMS-fMRI during associative memory encoding: a measure of dynamic connectivity. Front Hum Neurosci 11:404
Heckers S, Zalesak M, Weiss AP, Ditman T, Titone D (2004) Hippocampal activation during transitive inference in humans. Hippocampus 14(2):153–162
Heinrichs RW, Zakzanis KK (1998) Neurocognitive deficit in schizophrenia: a quantitative review of the evidence. Neuropsychology 12(3):426–445
Herbener ES (2008) Emotional memory in schizophrenia. Schizophr Bull 34(5):875–887
Hockley WE, Consoli A (1999) Familiarity and recollection in item and associative recognition. Mem Cogn 27(4):657–664
Javed A, Charles A (2018) The importance of social cognition in improving functional outcomes in schizophrenia. Front Psych 9:157
Jordan G, Veru F, Lepage M, Joober R, Malla A, Iyer SN (2018) Pathways to functional outcomes following a first episode of psychosis: the roles of premorbid adjustment, verbal memory and symptom remission. Aust N Z J Psychiatry 52(8):793–803
Karambelas GJ, Cotton SM, Farhall J, Killackey E, Allott KA (2019) Contribution of neurocognition to 18-month employment outcomes in first-episode psychosis. Early Interv Psychiatry 13(3):453–460
Koola MM, Looney SW, Hong H, Pillai A, Hou W (2020) Meta-analysis of randomized controlled trials of galantamine in schizophrenia: significant cognitive enhancement. Psychiatry Res 291: 113285

Kopald BE, Mirra KM, Egan MF, Weinberger DR, Goldberg TE (2012) Magnitude of impact of executive functioning and IQ on episodic memory in schizophrenia. Biol Psychiatry 71(6): 545–551
Kwok SC, Xu X, Duan W, Wang X, Tang Y, Allé MC, Berna F (2021) Autobiographical and episodic memory deficits in schizophrenia: a narrative review and proposed agenda for research. Clin Psychol Rev 83:101956
Laurita AC, Spreng RN (2017) The hippocampus and social cognition. In: Hannula DE, Duff MC (eds) The hippocampus from cells to systems: structure, connectivity, and functional contributions to memory and flexible cognition. Springer International Publishing, Cham, pp 537–558
Leeson VC, Robbins TW, Franklin C, Harrison M, Harrison I, Ron MA, Barnes TR, Joyce EM (2009) Dissociation of long-term verbal memory and fronto-executive impairment in first-episode psychosis. Psychol Med 39(11):1799–1808
Lepage M, Brodeur M, Bourgouin P (2003) Prefrontal cortex contribution to associative recognition memory in humans: an event-related functional magnetic resonance imaging study. Neurosci Lett 346(1–2):73–76
Lepage M, Blondin F, Achim AM, Menear M, Brodeur M (2005) The interfering effect of related events on recognition memory discriminability: a functional magnetic resonance imaging study. Brain Res Cogn Brain Res 22(3):429–437
Lepage M, Montoya A, Pelletier M, Achim AM, Menear M, Lal S (2006) Associative memory encoding and recognition in schizophrenia: an event-related fMRI study. Biol Psychiatry 60(11):1215–1223
Lepage M, Hawco C, Bodnar M (2015) Relational memory as a possible neurocognitive marker of schizophrenia. JAMA Psychiat 72(9):946–947
Li B, Han M, Guo C, Tibon R (2019) Unitization modulates recognition of within-domain and cross-domain associations: evidence from event-related potentials. Psychophysiology 56(11): e13446
Libby LA, Yonelinas AP, Ranganath C, Ragland JD (2013) Recollection and familiarity in schizophrenia: a quantitative review. Biol Psychiatry 73(10):944–950
Lin CH, Huang CL, Chang YC, Chen PW, Lin CY, Tsai GE, Lane HY (2013) Clinical symptoms, mainly negative symptoms, mediate the influence of neurocognition and social cognition on functional outcome of schizophrenia. Schizophr Res 146(1–3):231–237
Luck D, Montoya A, Menear M, Achim AM, Lal S, Lepage M (2009) Selective pair recognition memory impairment with no response bias in schizophrenia. Psychiatry Res 169(1):39–42
Mesholam-Gately RI, Giuliano AJ, Goff KP, Faraone SV, Seidman LJ (2009) Neurocognition in first-episode schizophrenia: a meta-analytic review. Neuropsychology 23(3):315–336
Mike L, Guimond S, Kelly S, Thermenos H, Mesholam-Gately R, Eack S, Keshavan M (2019) Social cognition in early course of schizophrenia: exploratory factor analysis. Psychiatry Res 272:737–743
Montagrin A, Saiote C, Schiller D (2018) The social hippocampus. Hippocampus 28(9):672–679
Moran EK, Gold JM, Carter CS, MacDonald AW, Ragland JD, Silverstein SM, Luck SJ, Barch DM (2020) Both unmedicated and medicated individuals with schizophrenia show impairments across a wide array of cognitive and reinforcement learning tasks. Psychol Med. https://doi.org/10.1017/S003329172000286X
Moscovitch M (2008) The hippocampus as a "stupid," domain-specific module: implications for theories of recent and remote memory, and of imagination. Can J Exp Psychol 62(1):62–79
Nagy M, Kiraly I (2018) Evidence of relational retrieval, even in the absence of the relational eye movement effect (REME). Conscious Cogn 66:40–53
Nickel AE, Henke K, Hannula DE (2015) Relational memory is evident in eye movement behavior despite the use of subliminal testing methods. PLoS One 10(10):e0141677
O'Keefe J, Nadel L (1978) The hippocampus as a cognitive map. Oxford University Press, Oxford
Oertel V, Kraft D, Alves G, Knöchel C, Ghinea D, Storchak H, Matura S, Prvulovic D, Bittner RA, Linden DEJ, Reif A, Stäblein M (2019) Associative memory impairments are associated with

functional alterations within the memory network in schizophrenia patients and their unaffected first-degree relatives: an fMRI study. Front Psych 10. https://doi.org/10.3389/fpsyt.2019.00033
Oliver LD, Haltigan JD, Gold JM, Foussias G, DeRosse P, Buchanan RW, Malhotra AK, Voineskos AN, SPINS Group (2019) Lower- and higher-level social cognitive factors across individuals with schizophrenia spectrum disorders and healthy controls: relationship with neurocognition and functional outcome. Schizophr Bull 45(3):629–638
Öngür D, Cullen TJ, Wolf DH, Rohan M, Barreira P, Zalesak M, Heckers S (2006) The neural basis of relational memory deficits in schizophrenia. Arch Gen Psychiatry 63(4):356–365
Onwuameze OE, Titone D, Ho BC (2016) Transitive inference deficits in unaffected biological relatives of schizophrenia patients. Schizophr Res 175(1–3):64–71
Pelletier M, Achim AM, Montoya A, Lal S, Lepage M (2005) Cognitive and clinical moderators of recognition memory in schizophrenia: a meta-analysis. Schizophr Res 74(2–3):233–252
Piskulic D, Addington J (2011) Social cognition and negative symptoms in psychosis. Psychiatry Res 188(2):283–285
Ragland JD, Cools R, Frank M, Pizzagalli DA, Preston A, Ranganath C, Wagner AD (2009a) CNTRICS final task selection: long-term memory. Schizophr Bull 35(1):197–212
Ragland JD, Laird AR, Ranganath C, Blumenfeld RS, Gonzales SM, Glahn DC (2009b) Prefrontal activation deficits during episodic memory in schizophrenia. Am J Psychiatr 166(8):863–874
Ragland JD, Ranganath C, Barch DM, Gold JM, Haley B, MacDonald AW, Silverstein SM, Strauss ME, Yonelinas AP, Carter CS (2012) Relational and item-specific encoding (RISE): task development and psychometric characteristics. Schizophr Bull 38(1):114–124
Ragland JD, Ranganath C, Harms MP, Barch DM, Gold JM, Layher E, Lesh TA, MacDonald AW 3rd, Niendam TA, Phillips J, Silverstein SM, Yonelinas AP, Carter CS (2015) Functional and neuroanatomic specificity of episodic memory dysfunction in schizophrenia: a functional magnetic resonance imaging study of the relational and item-specific encoding task. JAMA Psychiat 72(9):909–916
Ragland JD, Layher E, Hannula DE, Niendam TA, Lesh TA, Solomon M, Carter CS, Ranganath C (2017) Impact of schizophrenia on anterior and posterior hippocampus during memory for complex scenes. NeuroImage Clin 13:82–88
Raucher-Chéné D, Thibaudeau E, Sauvé G, Lavigne KM, Lepage M (2021) Understanding others as a mediator between verbal memory and negative symptoms in schizophrenia-spectrum disorder. J Psychiatr Res 143:429–435
Reagh ZM, Ranganath C (2018) What does the functional organization of cortico-hippocampal networks tell us about the functional organization of memory? Neurosci Lett 680:69–76
Roes MM, Chinchani AM, Woodward TS (2021) Reduced functional connectivity in brain networks underlying paired associates memory encoding in schizophrenia. Biol Psychiatr Cogn Neurosci Neuroimaging. https://doi.org/10.1016/j.bpsc.2021.07.003
Rowland LM, Griego JA, Spieker EA, Cortes CR, Holcomb HH (2010) Neural changes associated with relational learning in schizophrenia. Schizophr Bull 36(3):496–503
Rubin RD, Watson PD, Duff MC, Cohen NJ (2014) The role of the hippocampus in flexible cognition and social behavior. Front Hum Neurosci 8:742
Sahakyan L, Kwapil TR, Lo Y, Jiang L (2019) Examination of relational memory in multidimensional schizotypy. Schizophr Res 211:36–43
Schafer M, Schiller D (2019) The hippocampus and social impairment in psychiatric disorders. Cold Spring Harb Symp Quant Biol. https://doi.org/10.1101/sqb.2018.83.037614
Scoville WB, Milner B (1957) Loss of recent memory after bilateral hippocampal lesions. J Neurol Neurosurg Psychiatry 20(1):11
Seabury RD, Bearden CE, Ventura J, Subotnik KL, Nuechterlein KH, Cannon TD (2021) Confident memory errors and disrupted reality testing in early psychosis. Schizophr Res 238:170–177
Sheffield JM, Williams LE, Cohen N, Heckers S (2012) Relational memory in psychotic bipolar disorder. Bipolar Disord 14(5):537–546
Smucny J, Iosif A-M, Eaton NR, Lesh TA, Ragland JD, Barch DM, Gold JM, Strauss ME, MacDonald AW III, Silverstein SM, Carter CS (2019) Latent profiles of cognitive control,

episodic memory, and visual perception across psychiatric disorders reveal a dimensional structure. Schizophr Bull 46(1):154–162
Smucny J, Zarubin VC, Ragland J, Carter CS (2020) Are visual memory deficits in recent-onset psychosis degenerative? Am J Psychiatry 177(4):355–356
Sousa AE, Mahdid Y, Brodeur M, Lepage M (2021a) A feasibility study on the use of the method of loci for improving episodic memory performance in schizophrenia and non-clinical subjects. Front Psychol 12:612681
Sousa AE, Pochiet G, Ryan JD, Lepage M (2021b) The relational trip task, a novel ecological measure of relational memory: data from a schizophrenia sample. Cogn Neuropsychiatry 26(6): 421–440
Sousa AE, Ryan JD, Lepage M (2021c) A feasibility pilot study on using unitization to circumvent relational memory impairments in schizophrenia. Schizophr Res 231:98–99
Spalding KN, Schlichting ML, Zeithamova D, Preston AR, Tranel D, Duff MC, Warren DE (2018) Ventromedial prefrontal cortex is necessary for normal associative inference and memory integration. J Neurosci 38(15):3767–3775
Spieker EA, Griego JA, Astur RS, Holcomb HH, Rowland LM (2013) Facilitation of relational learning in schizophrenia. Behav Sci (Basel) 3(2):206–216
Suh DY, Vandekar SN, Heckers S, Avery SN (2020) Visual exploration differences during relational memory encoding in early psychosis. Psychiatry Res 287:112910
Sumiyoshi T (2020) Cognitive enhancement in schizophrenia by buspirone: role of serotonin1A receptor agonism. Schizophr Res 215:455–456
Tang Y, Niznikiewicz MA (2020) Event related potential studies and findings: schizophrenia as a disorder of cognition. In: Kubicki M, Shenton ME (eds) Neuroimaging in schizophrenia. Springer International Publishing, Cham, pp 241–300
Thibaudeau E, Achim AM, Parent C, Turcotte M, Cellard C (2020) A meta-analysis of the associations between theory of mind and neurocognition in schizophrenia. Schizophr Res 216:118–128
Titone D, Ditman T, Holzman PS, Eichenbaum H, Levy DL (2004) Transitive inference in schizophrenia: impairments in relational memory organization. Schizophr Res 68(2–3):235–247
Valli I, Tognin S, Fusar-Poli P, Mechelli A (2012) Episodic memory dysfunction in individuals at high-risk of psychosis: a systematic review of neuropsychological and neurofunctional studies. Curr Pharm Des 18(4):443–458
Watson PD, Voss JL, Warren DE, Tranel D, Cohen NJ (2013) Spatial reconstruction by patients with hippocampal damage is dominated by relational memory errors. Hippocampus 23(7): 570–580
Weinhold SL, Lechinger J, Ittel J, Ritzenhoff R, Drews HJ, Junghanns K, Goder R (2022) Dysfunctional overnight memory consolidation in patients with schizophrenia in comparison to healthy controls: disturbed slow-wave sleep as contributing factor? Neuropsychobiology 81(2):104–115
Williams LE, Must A, Avery S, Woolard A, Woodward ND, Cohen NJ, Heckers S (2010) Eye-movement behavior reveals relational memory impairment in schizophrenia. Biol Psychiatry 68(7):617–624
Williams LE, Avery SN, Woolard AA, Heckers S (2012) Intact relational memory and normal hippocampal structure in the early stage of psychosis. Biol Psychiatry 71(2):105–113
Zeithamova D, Dominick AL, Preston AR (2012) Hippocampal and ventral medial prefrontal activation during retrieval-mediated learning supports novel inference. Neuron 75(1):168–179

Working Memory in People with Schizophrenia

James M. Gold and Steven J. Luck

Contents

Abstract Working memory (WM) refers to the ability to maintain a small number of representations in an activated, easily accessible state for a short period of time in the service of ongoing cognitive processing and behavior. Because WM is a resource critical for multiple forms of complex cognition and executive control of behavior, it is of central interest in the study of disorders such as schizophrenia that involve a broad compromise of cognitive function and in the regulation of goal-directed behavior. There is now robust evidence that WM impairment is characteristic of people with schizophrenia. The impairment includes both elementary storage capacity as well as more complex forms of WM that involve the manipulation and updating of WM representations. These impairments appear to underlie a substantial portion of the generalized cognitive deficit in schizophrenia. Neuroimaging studies have implicated widespread abnormalities in the broad neural system that subserves

J. M. Gold (✉)
Maryland Psychiatric Research Center, Department of Psychiatry, University of Maryland School of Medicine, Baltimore, MD, USA
e-mail: JGold@som.umaryland.edu

S. J. Luck
Center for Mind & Brain and Department of Psychology, University of California, Davis, CA, USA

Curr Topics Behav Neurosci (2023) 63: 137–152
https://doi.org/10.1007/7854_2022_381
Published Online: 2 August 2022

WM performance, consistent with the evidence of broad cognitive impairment seen in PSZ.

Keywords Ability · Capacity · Executive control · General cognitive · Working memory

1 What Is Working Memory

Working memory (WM) has been a major focus of basic and clinical cognitive neuroscience research since the early use of the term by Miller, Galanter, and Pribram in 1960 (Miller et al. 1960). A Google Scholar search in January 2022 using working memory as a search term yielded 1,580,000 citations with 143,000 since 2021. While precise definitions of working memory differ somewhat across theorists (see 2 for recent comprehensive review), the major models, including the National Institute of Mental Health Research Domain Operational Criteria definition of WM (https://www.nimh.nih.gov/research/research-funded-by-nimh/rdoc/definitions-of-the-rdoc-domains-and-constructs), all emphasize that WM refers to the ability to maintain a small number of representations in an activated, easily accessible state for a short period of time in the service of ongoing cognitive processing and behavior. These representations may have originated from the perception of a stimulus/event in the external environment or from the activation of a representation from long-term memory. WM representations are held in a somewhat "privileged" state where they are easily retrieved and are relatively immune, temporarily, to the impact of potentially distracting information. The information maintained in working memory is needed for most aspects of complex cognition such as language comprehension, reasoning, decision-making, and cognitive control (Logie et al. 2021). Indeed, it can be difficult to know where (or if) to draw the line between working memory, attention, executive control, and other cognitive functions given the dense interaction and functional integration of these processes.

Working memory representations are also critical for the ability to over-ride prepotent response tendencies that are based in long-term and procedural memory systems. Consider the example of needing to go to the pharmacy to pick up a prescription on the way to work. The goal of completing this errand, which requires turning in the opposite direction out of the driveway than when going to work, must be kept activated in order to overcome the prepotent response that has been built up over years of making the same turn to go to work each day. Once the correct turn is made on the way to the pharmacy, the WM representation is no longer relevant, and the LTM representation of how to go to work should remain unchanged and available to guide action the following day. As seen in this example, WM representations interact with perceptual, attentional, LTM, and response selection processes and are central to the ability to guide behavior based on information that is not in the immediate environment. Because WM is a resource critical for multiple forms of complex cognition and executive control of behavior, it is of central interest in the study of disorders such as schizophrenia that involve a broad compromise of cognitive function and in the regulation of goal-directed behavior. In principle, a focal impairment of the working memory system could provide an integrated account of the impairments seen in people with schizophrenia (PSZ).

2 How Is WM Measured?

Given the breadth of the definition of WM, it is not surprising that a wide range of measurement approaches have been developed in the basic experimental and clinical literatures that emphasize different aspects of the construct ranging from initial encoding of perceptual representations to the ability to manipulate and update information held in WM. In spatial working memory measures, modeled closely after procedures used to study nonhuman primates (Funahashi et al. 1989, 1993; Starc et al. 2017), a target location is briefly highlighted, followed by a delay interval, and then a response cue that prompts the subject to make either an eye movement or a manual response to the target location (See Fig. 1a). This approach offers a measure of the precision of the WM representation and varying the delay interval provides for an assessment of the stability of maintenance activity. In contrast, span tasks, such as digit span, or its visual analog, spatial span, require the serial recall of a series of digits (or spatial locations), an approach which provides an assessment of the amount of information that can encoded and retrieved from WM. In the experimental literature, a large body of work has utilized visual change detection paradigms (see Fig. 1b) which offer a means/method of measuring WM capacity while minimizing the role of retrieval processes. In these paradigms, participants are first shown an encoding array (typically including 2–8 items), followed by a delay, and then a test array that either matches or mismatches (by one item) the encoding array and participants are asked to make unspeeded same or different judgements on each trial (Luck and Vogel 1997).

Other approaches to WM assessment emphasize the ability to manipulate information stored in WM, maintain information in WM in the face of distraction, or in the ability to dynamically update the information stored in WM. The Letter-Number Sequencing task, shown in panel C, involves the demand to simultaneously maintain

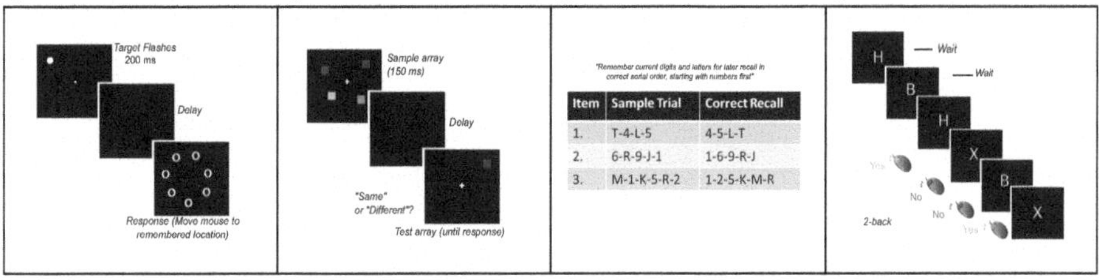

Fig. 1 Working memory tasks. (**a**) Spatial delayed response task, (**b**) change detection, (**c**) letter-number sequencing, (**d**) N-back

and manipulate information (Gold et al. 1997). Here participants are presented with a mixed alphanumeric series and are asked to first report the numbers in ascending order followed by the letters in alphabetical order. Complex span tasks such as Operation Span require that participants answer a series of arithmetic problems and then report the letter that appeared with each arithmetic problem (Turner and Engle 1989). Thus, participants need to maintain the letters in WM as they answer additional arithmetic problems. This demand for simultaneous storage and processing in operation span is similar to that imposed by Letter-Number sequencing. The N-back task presents a somewhat different mix of storage and processing (Kirchner 1958). Here, participants are presented with a series of numbers (or letter, objects, etc.) and are asked to respond when the same item appears on consecutive trials (one-back), when the same item appears separated by an additional intervening item (two back), or appear separated by two intervening items (three back) (see Fig. 1d). Thus, to perform the task, participants must dynamically "flush" and update the information being held in WM. While these tasks differ substantially from one another, they are substantially correlated with one another. For example, as seen in Fig. 2a, performance on visual change detection measures correlates significantly with performance on complex span tasks as well as other WM measures that involve simultaneous storage and processing in large groups of people with schizophrenia (PSZ) and healthy controls (HCs) studied at the Maryland Psychiatric Research Center (Gold et al. 2019).

PSZ show deficits on WM tasks ranging from tasks that involve simple storage to those that involve more complex manipulation and updating of information held in WM. An example of performance deficits on a task involving simple storage is seen in Fig. 3a, which shows the performance of large groups of PSZ and HCs on a

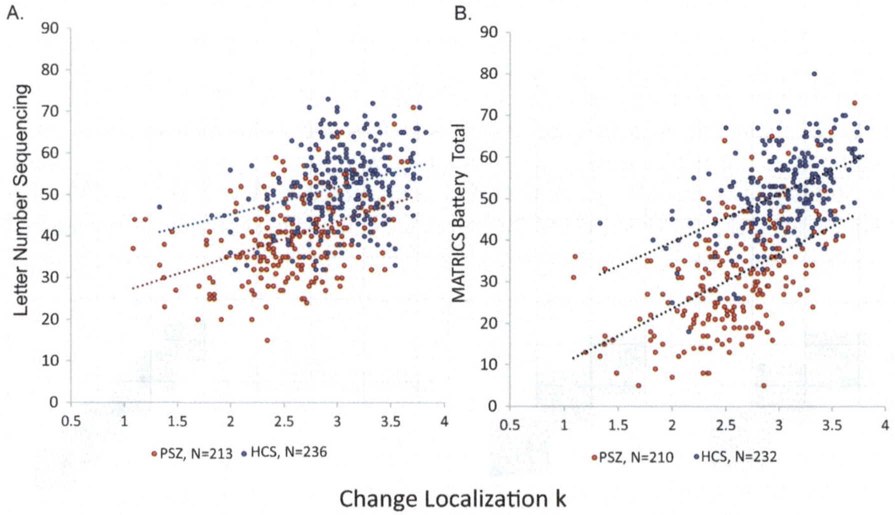

Fig. 2 Correlations between WM capacity and letter number sequencing and MCCB

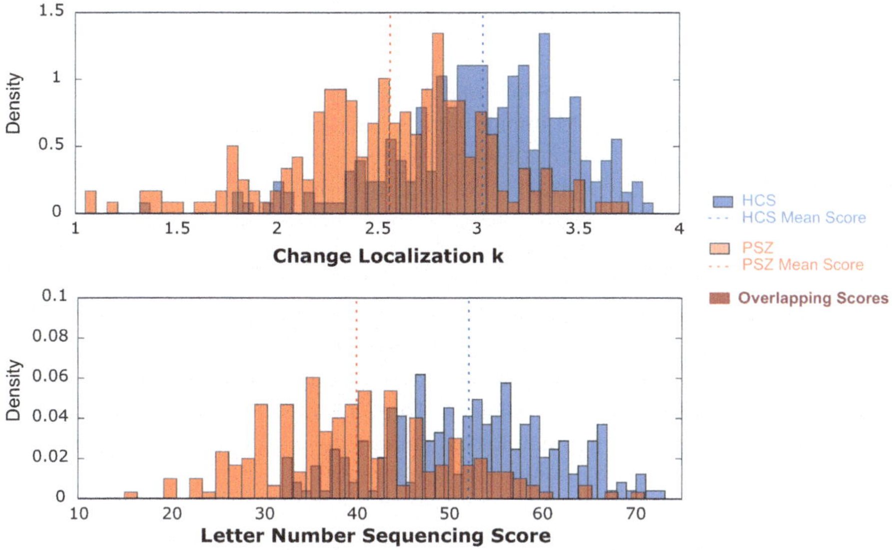

Fig. 3 WM test score distributions

variant of visual change detection called change localization where there is a single change from the encoding of four colored rectangles to the test array on every trial and the subject is asked to identify the change, a paradigm which offers a measure of WM capacity. Performance on task that involves simultaneous maintenance and manipulation of material stored in WM, Letter-number Sequencing is shown in Fig. 3b. On both tasks, the distribution of PSZ is sharply shifted toward lower performance levels, with relatively few patients found within the range of where 50% or more of HCs perform. The between group effect size is large and broadly similar on both measures ($d = 1.00$ and $d = 1.23$, for change localization and Letter-Number Sequencing), suggesting that the extent of impairment for simple storage capacity approximates that observed from a much more complex task that requires simultaneous storage and processing. Interestingly, both measures significantly contributed to successful group classification in a linear discriminant function analysis (of the data included in Fig. 2) that yielded an overall correct classification rate of 72%. WM impairment is a robust, widely replicated deficit, observed on a wide array of WM paradigms that assess different aspects of WM performance (Barnes-Scheufler et al. 2021; Lee and Park 2005; Piskulic et al. 2007).

Importantly WM impairments have been observed on several WM paradigms in the first-degree relatives of people with schizophrenia, albeit typically at a milder impairment level than is seen in patients suggesting that WM impairment may be related to genetic risk for the illness (Goldberg et al. 2003; Horan et al. 2008; Park and Gooding 2014; Pirkola et al. 2005). Perhaps, even more importantly, evidence of impairment in clinically unaffected first-degree relatives is clear evidence that the impairment seen in patients cannot be fully attributed to the consequences of the illness including persistent symptoms, distress, medication, and social disadvantage.

3 WM and Broad Cognitive Performance

As discussed above, WM is a crucial limited resource that is required by many other cognitive processes. Thus, WM impairments should be expected to have important consequences for broad aspects of cognitive performance. As seen in Fig. 2b, measures of WM capacity correlate significantly with the composite score from the MATRICS consensus cognitive battery which includes measures of processing speed, working memory, verbal and visual episodic memory, vigilance, reasoning, and social cognition (Nuechterlein and Green 2006). This relationship is observed at similar levels in both PSZ and in HCs (r's = 0.51 and 0.49 in PSZ and HCs, respectively). Johnson and colleagues (Johnson et al. 2013) reported that covarying for WM capacity accounts for 40% of the between group variance observed between HCs and PSZ on the MATRICS Battery. Thus, a simple measure of visual WM capacity appears to provide a principled explanation for a very substantial proportion of the general cognitive deficit seen in schizophrenia.

3.1 Origins of Impairment

There is a substantial research literature addressing the specific cognitive processes that are implicated in the origins of WM impairment in PSZ. As discussed below, it appears unlikely that a single mechanism can explain the variety of WM impairments that have been documented in the literature, and different processes may be maximally relevant for performance on specific paradigms, or in specific subpopulations of PSZ.

Different aspects of encoding, the process of transforming a perceptual representation into a durable WM representation have been extensively investigated. While long under-appreciated, there is now substantial evidence for early visual and auditory perceptual processing abnormalities in PSZ, abnormalities that are not surprising considering evidence for alterations in retinal function, and in the structure and function of primary auditory and visual cortex (Fish et al. 2021; Javitt et al. 1999; Javitt and Sweet 2015; Silverstein et al. 2020). Such abnormalities would be expected to impact the ability to encode high-fidelity WM representations. Not surprisingly, a number of studies have shown that patients need much longer exposure durations in order to successfully encode visual stimuli to match the level achieved by HCs with much shorter exposure durations (Badcock et al. 2008; Fuller et al. 2009; Hartman et al. 2002; Lencz et al. 2003; Tek et al. 2002). Similarly, PSZ require a much larger frequency difference between auditory tones than do HCs in order to successfully discriminate between pairs of tones (Javitt et al. 1999; Javitt and Sweet 2015). Some of these behavioral effects could be a result, at least in part, of lapses in attention (see Luck and Gold, this volume). These perceptual deficits are also reflected in EEG abnormalities during the performance of basic auditory and visual processing tasks (Friedman et al. 2012). With fMRI, there are multiple reports of reduced activation in early visual processing areas, consistent with the EEG reports, suggesting impairment in the formation of high-fidelity perceptual representations (Bittner et al. 2015; Haenschel et al. 2007; Martínez et al. 2008). In our view, the evidence that perceptual deficits may substantially contribute to performance in paradigms that require highly precise WM representations is convincing. However, such impairments are unlikely to provide a full explanation for WM deficits in PSZ as impairments are observed in paradigms that use highly discriminable stimuli where such perceptual limitations are unlikely to underlie impaired WM performance. For example, in the change localization data shown in Fig. 3, each color was categorically distinct from the other colors, so fine perceptual discriminations were not needed to perform the task. There is also suggestive evidence that such perceptual impairments are most characteristic of highly disabled, chronically ill patients and may not explain impairments seen in the broader population of PSZ (Dondé et al. 2019). Thus, the role of perceptual limitations in the genesis of WM impairment is more relevant for some WM tasks than others, depending on the importance of precise encoding in mediating task success.

Given that WM capacity is sharply limited, it is critical that task relevant information is efficiently prioritized for storage. Indeed, in HCs, failures of selective attention, the ability to filter out distractors so that task relevant information gains priority for further processing, are strongly associated with WM capacity reduction (Vogel and Machizawa 2004). That is, HCs who are unable to efficiently prioritize the storage of task relevant information and prevent the storage of task-irrelevant information show lower "effective" WM capacity. Thus, in HCs, individual differences in the operation of selective attention are implicated in individual differences in WM capacity. The idea that impairments of attention could underle the WM deficits in PSZ is an attractive hypothesis because abnormalities of attention have been considered to be central to schizophrenia since the original clinical descriptions by Krapelin and Bleuler (Bleuler 1911; Krapelin 1919). Here, surprisingly, multiple studies suggest that PSZ show fully normal ability to select relevant information and exclude irrelevant items from WM, yet still show reductions in overall WM capacity (Erickson et al. 2015; Gold et al. 2006; Mayer and Park 2012; Smith et al. 2011). However, there are also examples showing that selection may fail in PSZ when challenged by irrelevant information that has a salience advantage relative to relevant to-be-remembered information (Hahn et al. 2010; Mayer et al. 2012). These data suggest that the deficit is in the control of attention rather than in operation of selective attention per se (See Luck and Gold this volume). The fact that such failures in attentional selection occurs in highly specific experimental conditions suggests that this mechanism does not appear to offer a general explanation for the broad array of WM impairments seen in PSZ.

The fact that PSZ showed intact operation of selective attentional control over working memory encoding was initially quite surprising. Reasoning that an impairment in selection might emerge if challenged by a need to update the contents of WM, we did an experiment where people saw a series of seven pictures of everyday objects, and then were shown a test array and were asked to identify the item that had been presented previously (Hahn et al. 2012a). On some trials, a single cue-tone accompanied one picture in the stream, indicating it was most likely item to be tested, and therefore warranted the investment of extra attention in order to ensure precise encoding. On a subset of trials, a second item was also presented with a cue-tone cue, indicating that it was now the most likely item to be tested whereas the first cued item was now least likely to be tested. We hypothesized that PSZ would have difficulty updating attentional priority of the second item relative to the first. Surprisingly, PSZ not only showed intact updating of the second cued item, but they also showed more optimal inhibition of the initial cued item, further evidence of intact operation of selective attention for WM storage. The fact that PSZ were more efficient than HCs in restricting attentional priority to the second of the cued items raised the possibility that the focus of attention in PSZ might be unusually narrow.

Multiple subsequent experiments provided results consistent with this idea including evidence that PSZ had difficulty dividing spatial attention (attend to stimuli at two or more spatial locations), and that the ability to do so was highly correlated with WM capacity (Gray et al. 2014). Another experiment revealed that PSZs were able to use spatial cues to narrow attention to a single potential target location but had difficulty using cues to broaden and spread spatial attention (Hahn et al. 2012b). Further, with EEG, we found that contralateral delay activity, a neurophysiological marker of WM storage was greater in PSZ than controls when attending to a single lateralized item but reduced when attending to three or five items (Leonard et al. 2013). Further, the more patients showed lateralized activity for a single item, the less they were able to increase activation for multiple items. Similar evidence of excessive activation while storing a single item and reduced activation while storing multiple items has also been documented and replicated with fMRI suggesting that this is a robust, generalizable result (Hahn et al. 2018, 2020).

This pattern of results led us to the "hyperfocusing hypothesis" which suggests that patients focus their attentional resources in an overly narrow and intense fashion which makes it difficult to encode multiple items into WM (Luck et al. 2019), also see Luck and Gold this volume. This narrow attentional focus explains WM capacity reduction by suggesting that PSZ fail to attend to all the available items. However, this ability to focus attention narrowly facilitates selectively encoding relevant items and adaptively filtering irrelevant items. That is, hyperfocusing may be disadvantageous for some tasks, but this tendency to narrowly focus attention provides a potential explanation for the surprising evidence of intact operation of selective attention in WM encoding. As with the perceptual deficit account discussed above, hyperfocusing does not provide an account for all the WM deficits in PSZ. For example, hyperfocusing does not provide an explanation for why PSZ show less precise memory for the location of a single spatial working memory target (Starc et al. 2017). However, the hyperfocusing hypothesis provides an integrated account of multiple aspects of visual attention and visual WM in PSZ. Importantly, this framework also leads to the prediction of normal and "better than normal" performance in specific experimental environments, predictions that are inconsistent with accounts emphasizing poor perceptual processing or impairments in top-down cognitive control.

3.2 Delay-Dependent Deficits?

The idea that impairments might increase as a function of the length of a delay interval between encoding and retrieval/test almost seems inherent in the use of the term "memory." That is, we think of memory as extending over time, and it therefore seems natural to think that an impairment of memory would be amplified by increasing the passage of time. In the domain of WM, the question is whether impairments are magnified over an increasing number of seconds as opposed to over the minutes, hours, days, and years that are the domain of episodic memory.

The early literature examining this issue was quite mixed, some studies showing evidence of delay amplification, many others failing to show such evidence (Badcock et al. 2008; Carter et al. 1996; Gold et al. 2010; Snitz et al. 1999). Furthermore, when deficits are amplified by delay, it is difficult to determine if such performance declines are the result of a subject losing track of the task at hand and becoming distracted versus having increasing loss of memory fidelity over time. Thus, the boundaries between WM failure and loss of task set can become difficult to distinguish as unfilled delay intervals increase in length.

With that qualification in mind, earlier meta-analysis suggested that WM impairments were evident at the shortest delays that were tested and did not appear to increase at longer intervals, strongly suggesting that the primary locus of impairment in schizophrenia was at the encoding stage, and not at maintenance (Lee and Park 2005). While this conclusion was based on available evidence, there is reason to question if the methods employed in many of the early studies were likely sensitive to subtle changes in memory fidelity. For example, if participants were presented with a SWM task where targets could appear at one of a dozen or fewer marked locations, it is possible that some combination of verbal encoding and a relatively imprecise memory might suffice for identifying the original target location. In contrast, more recent SWM paradigms have used continuous report response formats where participants are asked to indicate precisely where a target appeared without the use of marked, fixed locations. Verbal encoding is less likely to suffice to guide a precise response with continuous report rather than fixed, marked locations. This indeed, appears to be the case, where there are now multiple studies using continuous report measures that have found reproducible evidence of increasing degrees of impairment in PSZ as a function of increasing delay intervals (Gold et al. 2020; Starc et al. 2017). Consistent with prior meta-analysis, impairment is seen at the shortest interval tested as well – so that the newer results suggest a combination of imprecise initial encoding, with increasing drift of the memory representation over time. The evidence favoring this view comes from studies of SWM, and the issue of delay dependence using other types of stimuli with a continuous report response format awaits future research. All that can be concluded on the basis of current evidence is that SWM shows delay-dependent increases in the extent of impairment from the level observed at the shortest delay interval tested.

Increasing drift of WM representations over time is consistent with predictions that come from neuro-computational models that suggest an alteration in the balance of excitatory–inhibitory processes characterized by a relative loss of inhibition

(Murray et al. 2014; Starc et al. 2017). That is, the loss of inhibition causes the excitatory processes that represent the target feature to spread over time, thereby becoming less precise. This is the pattern that has been documented in PSZ and is thought to be consistent with reports of alterations in inhibitory neurons seen in post-mortem neuropathology (Lewis 2014). Interestingly, these same computational models also make the prediction that distractors presented near the target during memory delay intervals should create a form of attraction between the target and distractor representations: absent normal levels of inhibition, the target and distractor representations are prone to drift toward one another leading to behavioral responses that are somewhere in-between the target and distractor locations. The same logic applies to tasks where two targets are presented in serial fashion: loss of inhibition should lead to attraction between representations that are maintained by neuronal populations that have overlapping receptive fields.

Interestingly, we have observed the precise opposite pattern of results in three recent experiments. In a SWM experiment where we manipulated the length of delay interval and the closeness of target and distractor representations, we found that PSZ, unlike controls, showed a bias to report targets as being farther away from the location of near-by distractors (Gold et al. 2020). That is, rather than being "attracted" toward distractors, patients showed "repulsion," specifically away from distractors appearing closest in space to previously presented targets. In a second experiment, we observed the same pattern of effects when we presented a target location at varying distances away from the vertical midline meridian: PSZs showed greater repulsion from the midline compared to HCs (Bansal et al. 2020). Additionally, PSZ also showed a greater repulsion bias than did HCs when asked to remember the orientation of two consecutively presented stimuli that resembled the hour hand on a clock face: PSZ reported the orientations as being farther apart from one another than did HCs (Bansal et al. 2020).

How to reconcile the evidence that single locations "drift," suggesting that the representation might be, in some sense, abnormally weak, with the evidence that WM representations are repelled away from one another, from the location of a distractor, or from the location of a landmark which might suggest that the representations are overly "strong." In our view, rather than characterizing representations as weak or strong, it may be more accurate to characterize the representations as being unstable, with the behavior of the representations being impacted by the experimental context that elicits them. Such contextual effects are not a feature of current computational models, and these data provide new information that future modeling efforts need to accommodate and explain.

4 Neural Systems Implicated in WM Dysfunction in Schizophrenia

The initial interest in the study of WM in schizophrenia was stimulated by Patricia Goldman-Rakic's elegant research in nonhuman primates looking at ocular-motor SWM performance which revealed that prefrontal neurons showed a pattern of sustained firing during delay intervals that appeared to carry information about the target spatial location (Funahashi et al. 1989, 1993; Goldlman-Rakic 1987, 1994). This emphasis on the role of the prefrontal cortex in WM was consistent with early functional imaging studies in PSZ that showed task related hypofrontality during the performance of the Wisconsin Card Sorting test (Weinberger et al. 1986). Indeed, the role of prefrontal cortex in the executive function and cognitive control deficits seen in PSZ has remained a central focus of schizophrenia research and a straight line can be drawn from the studies of Goldman-Rakic to the early studies of Weinberger and colleagues, to the early theoretical model of Cohen and Servan-Schreiber (1992), to the recent work of Carter and colleagues on the centrality of deficits in cognitive control (Smuncy et al. 2022).

However, the PFC has come to play a different role in our understanding of the neural system that underlies WM. In particular, a number of studies have shown that WM involves a widely distributed neural system, challenging the view proposed by Goldman-Rakic that sustained firing of prefrontal neurons mediated WM maintenance (Curtis and Sprague 2021; Logie et al. 2021). More importantly in the present context, there is consistent fMRI and EEG evidence that posterior parietal cortex, not the PFC, shows sensitivity to the amount of information that is being maintained in WM (Luria et al. 2016; Todd and Marois 2004). Note in any WM task, there are actually two types of information that are being maintained: (1) information about the goals of the task (i.e., "remember the location of this stimulus so that you can respond after the delay"), and (2) the actual stimulus to be remembered. It seems likely that WM storage for stimuli like colored squares and oriented bars is primarily reflected in the degree of activation of posterior parietal cortex, whereas it seems likely that activity observed in the PFC may be related to maintaining the goal (or the rule) of the task (Wallis et al. 2001).

In PSZ, there is replicated evidence of posterior parietal cortical hyperactivity for remembering a single feature item, with hypoactivity seen with increasing levels of load, conceptually consistent with expectations based on the hyperfocusing hypothesis (Coffman et al. 2020; Hahn et al. 2018). Interestingly these studies using variants of visual change detection paradigm have not documented robust evidence of abnormal PFC physiology. In contrast, evidence of PFC hypoactivity is most evident with tasks that involve manipulating the information in WM (Van Snellenberg et al. 2016; Wu and Jiang 2020). Thus, the neural circuitry involved in WM varies as a function of task demand, as does the locus of impairment observed in PSZ relative to HCs. Thus, it appears that the function and connectivity of the broad network that subserves WM that is implicated in PSZ rather than being localized to a single node (Cassidy et al. 2016; Chari et al. 2019; Hearne et al. 2021). As seen with the variety of behavioral paradigms shown in Fig. 1, the constant appears to be that PSZ will demonstrate differences and deficits relative to HCs during the performance of WM tasks, and these differences and deficits are evident both at the level of behavior and at the level of neurophysiology. Whereas earlier research sought to determine the primary locus of impairment both at the level of specific cognitive processes and anatomy, more recent literature has highlighted that WM is a complex cognitive/neural system that involves widely distributed processes that are dynamically configured to meet the demands of specific tasks.

The functioning of this system is compromised in PSZ, compromises that are implicated in the broad cognitive impairment that is a characteristic of the illness.

4.1 Summary and Future Directions

There is now robust evidence that WM impairment is a characteristic of PSZ. The impairment includes both elementary storage capacity and more complex forms of WM that involve the manipulation and updating of WM representations. These impairments appear to underlie a substantial portion of the generalized cognitive deficit in schizophrenia. Neuroimaging studies have implicated widespread abnormalities in the broad neural system that subserves WM performance, consistent with the evidence of broad cognitive impairment seen in PSZ.

Several questions remain for future research. While there is recent replicated evidence suggesting deficits in the maintenance of spatial WM representations, it remains unknown if the use of more optimal methods might reveal similar delay-dependent impairments with other kinds of to-be-remembered information such as object form and color. Recent studies suggesting qualitative alterations in the interaction between WM representations have opened a new area of investigation. Recent work has also highlighted the potential importance of lapses of attention during the maintenance period in healthy controls, a topic that has yet to be investigated in PSZ using optimal methods (Hakim et al. 2020). Despite extensive study and impressive progress, there are new questions to answer to come to a more complete understanding of WM in PSZ.

Acknowledgements Preparation of this chapter was made possible by NIH grant R01MH065034 to J.M.G. and S.J.L.

References

Badcock JC, Badcock DR, Read C, Jablensky A (2008) Examining encoding imprecision in spatial working memory in schizophrenia. Schizophr Res 100:144–152

Bansal S, Bae G-Y, Frankovich K, Robinson RM, Leonard CJ, Gold JM, Luck SJ (2020) Increased repulsion of working memory representations in schizophrenia. J Abnorm Psychol 129(8): 845–857

Barnes-Scheufler CV, Passow C, Rösler L, Mayer JS, Oertel V, Kittel-Schneider S, Matura S, Reif A, Bittner RA (2021) Transdiagnostic comparison of visual working memory capacity in bipolar disorder and schizophrenia. Int J Bipolar Disord 9:12

Bittner RA, Linden DEJ, Roebroeck A, Härtling F, Rotarska-Jagiela A, Maurer K, Goebel R, Singer W, Haenschel C (2015) The when and where of working memory dysfunction in early-onset schizophrenia—a functional magnetic resonance imaging study. Cereb Cortex 25:2494–2506

Bleuler E (1911) Dementia praecox or the Group of Schizophrenias (Zinkin L, trans). International Universities Press, New York

Carter C, Robertson L, Nordahl T, Chaderjian M, Kraft L, O'Shora-Celaya L (1996) Spatial working memory deficits and their relationship to negative symptoms in unmedicated schizophrenia patients. Biol Psychiatry 40:930–932

Cassidy CM, Van Snellenberg JX, Benavides C, Slifstein M, Wang Z, Moore H, Abi-Dargham A, Horga G (2016) Dynamic connectivity between brain networks supports working memory: relationships to dopamine release and schizophrenia. J Neurosci 36(15):4377–4388

Chari S, Minzenberg M, Solomon M, Ragland JD, Nguyen Q, Carter CS, Yoon JH (2019) Impaired prefrontal functional connectivity associated with working memory task performance and disorganization despite intact activations in schizophrenia. Psychiatr Res Neuroimaging 287: 10–18

Coffman BA, Murphy TK, Haas G, Olson C, Cho R, Ghuman AS, Sailsbury DF (2020) Lateralized evoked responses in parietal cortex demonstrate visual short-term memory deficits in first-episode schizophrenia. J Psychiatr Res 130:292–299

Cohen JD, Servan-Schreiber D (1992) Context, cortex, and dopamine: a connectionist approach to behavior and biology in schizophrenia. Psychol Rev 99(1):45–77

Curtis CE, Sprague TC (2021) Persistent activity during working memory from front to back. Front Neural Circ 15:696060

Dondé C, Martínez A, Kantrowitz JT, Silipo G, Dias EC, Patel GH, Sanchez-Peña J, Corcoran CM, Medalia A, Saperstein A, Vail B, Javitt DC (2019) Bimodal distribution of tone-matching deficits indicates discrete pathophysiological entities within the syndrome of schizophrenia. Transl Psychiatry 9(1):221

Erickson MA, Hahn B, Leonard CJ, Robinson B, Gray B, Luck SJ, Gold J (2015) Impaired working memory capacity is not caused by failures of selective attention in schizophrenia. Schizophr Bull 41(2):366–373

Fish KN, Rocco BR, DeDionisio AM, Dienel SJ, Sweet RA, Lewis DA (2021) Altered parvalbumin basket cell terminals in the cortical visuospatial working memory network in schizophrenia. Biol Psychiatry 90(1):47–57

Friedman T, Sehatpour P, Dias E, Perrin M, Javitt DC (2012) Differential relationships of mismatch negativity and visual p1 deficits to premorbid characteristics and functional outcome in schizophrenia. Biol Psychiatry 71(6):521–529

Fuller RL, Luck SJ, Braun EL, Robinsion BM, McMahon RP, Gold JM (2009) Impaired visual working memory consolidation in schizophrenia. Neuropsychology 23:71–80

Funahashi S, Bruce CJ, Goldman-Rakic PS (1989) Mnemonic coding of visual space in the monkey's dorsolateral prefrontal cortex. J Neurophysiol 61:1–19

Funahashi S, Bruce CJ, Goldman-Rakic PS (1993) Dorsolateral prefrontal lesions and oculomotor delayed-response performance: evidence for mnemonic "scotomas". J Neurosci 13:1479–1497

Gold JM, Carpenter C, Randolph C, Goldberg TE, Weinberger DR (1997) Auditory working memory and Wisconsin card sorting test performance in schizophrenia. Arch Gen Psychiatry 54(2):159–165

Gold JM, Fuller RL, Robinson BM, McMahon RP, Braun EL, Luck SJ (2006) Intact attentional control of working memory encoding in schizophrenia. J Abnorm Psychol 115(4):658–673

Gold JM, Hahn B, Zhang WW, Robinson BM, Kappenman ES, Beck VM, Luck SJ (2010) Reduced capacity but spared precision and maintenance of working memory representations in schizophrenia. Arch Gen Psychiatry 67(6):570–577

Gold JM, Barch DM, Feuerstahler LM, Carter CS, MacDonald AW, Ragland JD, Silverstein SM, Strauss ME, Luck SJ (2019) Working memory impairment across psychotic disorders. Schizophr Bull 45(4):804–812

Gold JM, Bansal S, Anticevic A, Cho YT, Repovs G, Murray JD, Hahn B, Robinson BM, Luck SJ (2020) Refining the empirical constraints on computational models of spatial working memory in schizophrenia. Biol Psychiatr Cogn Neurosci Neuroimaging 5(9):913–922

Goldberg TE, Egan MF, Gscheidle T, Coppola R, Weickert T, Kolachana BS, Goldman D, Weinberger DR (2003) Executive subprocesses in working memory: relationship to catechol-

O-methyltransferase Val158M et genotype and schizophrenia. Arch Gen Psychiatry 60(9): 889–896
Goldlman-Rakic PS (1987) Circuitry of the prefrontal cortex and the regulation of behavior by representational knowledge. In: Plum F, Mountcastle V (eds) Handbook of physiology, vol 5. American Physiological Society, Bethesda, pp 373–417
Goldman-Rakic PS (1994) Working memory dysfunction in schizophrenia. J Neuropsychiatr 6(4): 348–357
Gray BE, Hahn B, Robinson B, Harvey A, Leonard CJ, Luck SJ, Gold JM (2014) Relationships between divided attention and working memory impairment in people with schizophrenia. Schizophr Bull 40(6):1462–1471
Haenschel C, Bittner RA, Haertling F, Rotarska-Jagiela A, Maurer K, Singer W, Liinden DEJ (2007) Contribution of impaired early-stage visual processing to working memory dysfunction in adolescents with schizophrenia: a study with event-related potentials and functional magnetic resonance imaging. Arch Gen Psychiatry 64(11):1229–1240
Hahn B, Robinson BM, Kaiser ST, Harvey AN, Beck VM, Leonard CJ, Kappenman ES, Luck SJ, Gold JM (2010) Failure of schizophrenia patients to overcome salient distracters during working memory encoding. Biol Psychiatry 68(7):603–609. Comment in: Biol Psychiatr 2010;68(7): 603–609
Hahn B, Hollingworth A, Robinson BM, Kaiser ST, Leonard CJ, Beck VM, Kapperman ES, Luck SJ, Gold JM (2012a) Control of working memory content in schizophrenia. Schizophr Res 134(1):70–75
Hahn B, Robinson BM, Harvey AN, Kaiser ST, Leonard CJ, Luck SJ, Gold JM (2012b) Visuospatial attention in schizophrenia: deficits in broad monitoring. J Abnorm Psychol 121(1): 119–128
Hahn B, Robinson BM, Leonard CJ, Luck SJ, Gold JM (2018) Posterior parietal cortex dysfunction is central to working memory storage and broad cognitive deficits in schizophrenia. J Neurosci 38(39):8378–8387
Hahn B, Bae G-Y, Robinson BM, Leonard CJ, Luck SJ, Gold JM (2020) Cortical hyperactivation at low working memory load: a primary processing abnormality in people with schizophrenia? Neuroimage Clin 26:102270
Hakim N, deBettencourt MT, Awh E, Vogel ET (2020) Attention fluctuations impact ongoing maintenance of information in working memory. Psychon Bull Rev 27:1269–1278
Hartman M, Stekette MC, Silva S, Lanning K, McCann H (2002) Working memory and schizophrenia: evidence for slowed encoding. Schizophr Res 59:99–113
Hearne LJ, Mill RD, Keane BP, Repovš G, Anticevic A, Cole MW (2021) Activity flow underlying abnormalities in brain activations and cognition in schizophrenia. *Science*. Advances 7(29): eabf2513
Horan WP, Braff DL, Nuechterlein KH, Sugar CA, Cadenhead KS, Calkins ME, Dobie DJ, Freedman R, Greenwood TA, Gur RE, Gur RC, Light GA, Mintz J, Olincy A, Radant AD, Schork NJ, Seidman LJ, Siever LJ, Silverman JM, Stone WS, Swerdlow NR, Tsuang DW, Tsuang MT, Turetsky BI, Green MF (2008) Verbal working memory impairments in individuals with schizophrenia and their first-degree relatives: findings from the consortium on the genetics of schizophrenia. Schizophr Res 103(1–3):218–228
Javitt DC, Sweet RA (2015) Auditory dysfunction in schizophrenia: integrating clinical and basic features. Nat Rev Neurosci 16(9):535–550
Javitt DC, Liederman E, Cienfuegos A, Shelley A-M (1999) Panmodal processing imprecision as a basis for dysfunction of transient memory storage systems in schizophrenia. Schizophr Bull 25(4):763–775
Johnson MK, McMahon RP, Robinson BM, Harvey AN, Hahn B, Leonard CJ, Luck SJ, Gold JM (2013) The relationship between working memory capacity and broad measures of cognitive ability in healthy adults and people with schizophrenia. Neuropsychology 27:220–229
Kirchner WK (1958) Age difference in short-term retention of rapidly changing information. J Exp Psychol 55:352–358

Krapelin E (1919) Dementia praecox and paraphrenia (Mary Barclay R, trans), vol 3, 8th edn. Livingstone, Edinburgh
Lee J, Park S (2005) Working memory impairments in schizophrenia: a meta-analysis. J Abnorm Psychol 114(4):599–611
Lencz T, Bilder RM, Turkel E, Goldman RS, Robinson D, Kane JM, Lieberman JA (2003) Impairments in perceptual competency and maintenance on a visual delayed match-to-sample test in first-episode schizophrenia. Arch Gen Psychiatry 60(3):238–243
Leonard CJ, Kaiser ST, Robinson BM, Kappenman ES, Hahn B, Gold JM, Luck SJ (2013) Toward the neural mechanisms of reduced working memory capacity in schizophrenia. Cereb Cortex 23(7):1582–1592
Lewis DA (2014) Inhibitory neurons in human cortical circuits: substrate for cognitive dysfunction in schizophrenia. Curr Opin Neurobiol 26:22–26
Logie RH, Camos V, Cowan N (eds) (2021) Working memory. State of the science. Oxford University Press, New York
Luck SJ, Vogel EK (1997) The capacity of visual working memory for features and conjunctions. Nature 390:279–281
Luck SJ, Hahn B, Leonard CJ, Gold JM (2019) The hyperfocusing hypothesis: a new account of cognitive dysfunction in schizophrenia. Schizophr Bull 45(5):991–1000
Luria R, Balaban H, Awh E, Vogel EK (2016) The contralateral delay activity as a neural measure of visual working memory. Neurosci Behav Rev 62:100–108
Martínez A, Hillyard SA, Dias EC, Hagler DJ Jr, Butler PD, Guilfoyle DN, Jalbrzikowski M, Silipo G, Javitt DC (2008) Magnocellular pathway impairment in schizophrenia: evidence from functional magnetic resonance imaging. J Neurosci 28(30):7492–7500
Mayer JS, Park S (2012) Working memory encoding and false memory in schizophrenia and bipolar disorder in a spatial delayed response task. J Abnorm Psychol 121(3):784–794
Mayer JS, Fukuda K, Vogel EK, Park S (2012) Impaired contingent attentional capture predicts reduced working memory capacity in schizophrenia. PLoS One 7(11):e48586
Miller GA, Galanter E, Pribram KH (1960) Plans and the structure of behavior. Holt, Rinehart and Winston Inc, New York
Murray JD, Anticevic A, Gancsos M, Ichinose M, Corlett PR, Krystal JH, Wang XJ (2014) Linking microcircuit dysfunction cognitive impairment effects disinhibition associated with schizophrenia in cortical working memory model. Cereb Cortex 24(4):859–872
Nuechterlein KH, Green MF (2006) MATRICS consensus cognitive battery, manual. MATRICS Assessment Inc, Los Angeles
Park S, Gooding DC (2014) Working memory impairment as an endophenotypic marker of a schizophrenia diathesis. Schizophr Res Cogn 1(3):127–136
Pirkola T, Tuulio-Henriksson A, Glahn D, Kieseppä T, Haukka J, Kapiro J, Lönnqvist J, Cannon TD (2005) Spatial working memory function in twins with schizophrenia and bipolar disorder. Biol Psychiatry 58:930–936
Piskulic D, Oliver JS, Norman TR, Maruff P (2007) Behavioural studies of spatial working memory of dysfunction in schizophrenia: a quantitative literature review. Psychiatry Res 150(2):111–121
Silverstein SM, Fradkin SI, Demmin DL (2020) Schizophrenia and the retina: towards a 2020 perspective. Schizophr Res 219:84–94
Smith EE, Eich TS, Cebenoyan D, Malapani C (2011) Intact and impaired cognitive-control processes in schizophrenia. Schizophr Res 126:132–137
Smuncy J, Dienel SJ, Lewis DA, Carter CS (2022) Mechanisms underlying dorsolateral prefrontal cortex contributions to cognitive dysfunction in schizophrenia. Neuropsychopharmacology 47(1):292–308
Snitz BE, Curtis CE, Zald DH, Katsanis J, Iacono WG (1999) Neuropsychological and oculomotor correlates of spatial working memory performance in schizophrenia patients and controls. Schizophr Res 38:37–50

Starc M, Murray JD, Santamauro N, Savic A, Diehl C, Cho YT, Srihari V, Morgan PT, Krystal JH, Wang XJ, Repovs G, Anticevic A (2017) Schizophrenia is associated with a pattern of spatial working memory deficits consistent with cortical disinhibition. Schizophr Res 181:107–116
Tek C, Gold J, Blaxton T, Wilk C, Buchanan RW (2002) Visual perceptual and working memory impairments in schizophrenia. Arch Gen Psychiatry 59(2):146–153
Todd JJ, Marois R (2004) Capacity limit of visual short-term memory in human posterior parietal cortex. Nature 428(6984):751–754. https://doi.org/10.1038/nature02466
Turner ML, Engle RW (1989) Is working memory capacity task dependent? J Mem Lang 28:127–154
Van Snellenberg JX, Girgis RR, Horga G, van de Giessen E, Slifstein M, Ojeil N, Weinstein JJ, Moore H, Lieberman JA, Shohamy D, Smith EE, Abi-Dargham A (2016) Mechanisms of working memory impairment in schizophrenia. Biol Psychiatry 80:617–626
Vogel EK, Machizawa MG (2004) Neural activity predicts individual differences in visual working memory capacity. Nature 428(6984):748–751
Wallis JD, Anderson KC, Miller EK (2001) Single neurons in prefrontal cortex encode abstract rules. Nature 411:953–956
Weinberger DR, Berman KF, Zec R (1986) Physiologic dysfunction of dorsolateral prefrontal cortex in schizophrenia. I. Regional cerebral blood flow evidence. Arch Gen Psychiatry 43(2): 114–124
Wu D, Jiang T (2020) Schizophrenia-related abnormalities in the triple network: a meta-analysis of working memory studies. Brain Imaging Behav 14:971–980

Targeting Frontal Gamma Activity with Neurofeedback to Improve Working Memory in Schizophrenia

I-Wei Shu, Eric L. Granholm, and Fiza Singh

Contents

Abstract Optimal working memory (WM), the mental ability to internally maintain and manipulate task-relevant information, requires coordinated activity of dorsal-lateral prefrontal cortical (DLPFC) neurons. More specifically, during delay periods of tasks with WM features, DLPFC microcircuits generate persistent, stimulus-specific higher-frequency (e.g., gamma) activity. This activity largely depends on recurrent connections between parvalbumin positive inhibitory interneurons and pyramidal neurons in more superficial DLPFC layers. Due to the size and organization of pyramidal neurons (especially apical dendrites), local field potentials generated by DLPFC microcircuits are strong enough to pass outside the skull and can be detected using electroencephalography (EEG). Since patients with schizophrenia (SCZ) exhibit both DLPFC and WM abnormalities, EEG markers of DLPFC microcircuit activity during WM may serve as effective biomarkers or treatment targets. In this review, we summarize converging evidence from primate and human studies for a critical role of DLPFC microcircuit activity during WM and in the pathophysiology of SCZ. We also present a meta-analysis of studies available in PubMed specifically comparing frontal gamma activity between participants with SCZ and healthy controls, to determine whether frontal gamma activity may be a valid biomarker or treatment target for patients with SCZ. We summarize the complex cognitive and neurophysiologic processes contributing to neural oscillations during tasks with WM features, and how such complexity has stalled the

I.-W. Shu, E. L. Granholm, and F. Singh (✉)
Department of Psychiatry, University of California San Diego, La Jolla, CA, USA
e-mail: ishu@ucsd.edu; egranholm@ucsd.edu; fsingh@ucsd.edu

Curr Topics Behav Neurosci (2023) 63: 153–172
https://doi.org/10.1007/7854_2022_377
Published Online: 22 August 2022

development of neurophysiologic biomarkers and treatment targets. Finally, we summarize promising results from early reports using neuromodulation to target DLPFC neural activity and improve cognitive function in participants with SCZ, including a study from our team demonstrating that gamma-EEG neurofeedback increases frontal gamma power and WM performance in participants with SCZ. From the evidence discussed in this review, we believe the emerging field of neuromodulation, which includes extrinsic (electrical or magnetic stimulation) and intrinsic (EEG neurofeedback) modalities, will, in the coming decade, provide promising treatment options targeting specific neurophysiologic properties of specific brain areas to improve cognitive and behavioral health for patients with SCZ.

Keywords Cortical microcircuit · DLPFC · EEG · Gamma · Neurofeedback · Schizophrenia · Working memory

1 Introduction

Working memory (WM), our mental ability to internally maintain and manipulate task-relevant information, is critical for complex, goal-directed behaviors, and is closely related to other executive functions, including sustained attention, planning, and cognitive control – a set of cognitive processes largely mapping onto frontal, parietal, and limbic/paralimbic (e.g., cingulate) brain areas (Niendam et al. 2012). The basic information processing function of WM can be roughly divided into three stages: (1) encoding, i.e., uploading information to internal storage; (2) active maintenance of information in storage; and, (3) retrieval, i.e., accessing or downloading information from storage (Baddeley 1996; Roux and Uhlhaas 2014). In addition to its importance for complex behaviors in humans and animal models, WM is significantly impaired at varying levels across multiple neuropsychiatric disorders including schizophrenia (SCZ), major depression, dementia, and posttraumatic stress disorder (Banich et al. 2009; Menon 2011). In fact, given its critical role in both healthy brain function and the pathophysiology of neuropsychiatric disorders, WM is considered a core construct linking varying levels of analysis (e.g., cortical microcircuitry, cognitive performance) within the Cognitive Systems Domain of the National Institute of Mental Health's (NIMH) Research Domain Criteria (RDoC) initiative – which aims to, in the coming decades, develop a neurobiologically informed, personalized, precision-medicine diagnostic system for neuropsychiatric disorders (Cuthbert and Insel 2013).

Our current understanding of WM originated in the 1960s, from efforts to apply information processing theory to cognitive models of human behavior (Atkinson and Shiffrin 1968; Miller et al. 1960). These largely conceptual models were heavily influenced by empirical evidence supporting functional differentiation among brain areas (Milner 1971). For example, among patients with brain lesions (e.g., following surgical removal of epileptogenic tissue), left temporal lobe lesions produced primarily semantic memory deficits; right temporal lobe lesions, primarily visual and non-semantic memory deficits; bilateral temporal lobe lesions, profound and global memory deficits. In contrast, patients with frontal lobe lesions exhibited deficits primarily related to task-relevant information processing. Within the frontal lobe, the dorsal-lateral prefrontal cortex (DLPFC) emerged as an area of specific functional importance, as even relatively focal DLPFC lesions significantly impaired executive function (e.g., Wisconsin Card Sorting Task) and performance on tasks requiring recall of information after a delay period (a period generally on the order of seconds), i.e. delayed recall/response tasks.

That DLPFC lesions can specifically impair the basic information processing stages of WM, i.e., encoding, maintenance, retrieval, was also supported by lesion studies in non-human primates. For example, in contrast to primates with pre-central motor lesions, those with DLPFC lesions were unable to internally maintain information presented only seconds earlier, even though performance on tests of primarily attention was largely unaffected (Pribram et al. 1952). Conversely, if internal maintenance of information was not required (e.g., in the presence of external cues), primates with bilateral DLPFC lesions were capable of relatively complex tasks (Jacobsen et al. 1936).

Intracranial recordings of DLPFC neural activity in primates subsequently demonstrated that internal maintenance of information likely involves persistent, stimulus-specific spike activity during delay periods of WM tasks (Fuster and Alexander 1971; Kubota and Niki 1971). During these periods, persistent (e.g., absent external stimulus) spike activity by DLPFC neurons largely arises from extensive, mutually reinforcing connections between layer 2/3 pyramidal neurons (Kritzer and Goldman-Rakic 1995). This activity is further regulated by extensive inhibitory inputs from interneurons – more specifically, parvalbumin (PV) positive, GABA (gamma-aminobutyric acid)-ergic basket cells – to produce high-frequency bursts on the order of 30–60 bursts/s, i.e., gamma frequency activity (Buzsaki and Wang 2012; Gray 1994).

Due to the size of pyramidal neurons, and their parallel organization and synchronous activity within cortical microcircuits (Douglas and Martin 2004), local electromagnetic field potentials generated by assemblies of synchronous pyramidal neurons are strong enough to pass to the cortical surface and beyond, enabling direct recording by intracranial electrodes on the cortical surface (electrocorticography, or ECoG), or electrodes or magnetic sensors on the scalp surface, i.e., electroencephalography (EEG) or magnetoencephalography (MEG), respectively (Buzsaki et al. 2012; Jackson and Bolger 2014; Lopes da Silva 2013). For example, during a task involving self-paced movements of hands or feet, planning or initiating a movement was associated with EEG markers of activation at electrodes over cortical motor areas representing the corresponding hand or feet; furthermore, hand movement was associated with EEG markers of inhibition at electrodes over cortical motor areas corresponding to feet, and vice versa (Pfurtscheller et al. 1997). Synchronous neural activity from deeper cortical areas can also be detected under specific conditions. For example, greater synchronous low-frequency (e.g., theta) neural activity from

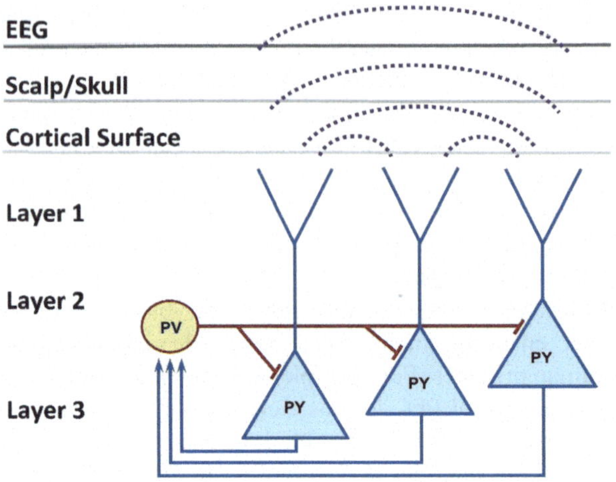

Fig. 1 Schematic summarizing current models of generation of LFPs, including higher-frequency (e.g., gamma) oscillatory activity, by apical dendrites in superficial layers (1/2) of layer 2/3 pyramidal neurons (PY) and transmission of electromagnetic potentials (dotted purple lines) through cortical/cranial/scalp tissue to EEG sensors. During delay periods of behavioral tasks with WM features, extensive, mutually reinforcing connections (not shown) between layer 2/3 PY neurons generate persistent, stimulus-specific spike activity. Layer 2/3 PY neurons project excitatory axons (blue arrows) to and stimulate layer 2/3 parvalbumin (PV) positive inhibitory interneurons, which further regulate layer 2/3 PY neurons through inhibitory projections (red lines) to produce high-frequency bursts on the order of 30–60 bursts/s (i.e., gamma frequency activity). Please see main text for detailed discussion of studies supporting above model

medial-frontal cortical microcircuits during conflict detection can be directly and reliably recorded by midline-frontal EEG electrodes (Cohen 2014).

Synchronous high-frequency neural activity (e.g., gamma) from DLPFC microcircuits during WM tasks can similarly be directly and reliably recorded by frontal EEG electrodes. More specifically, consistent with their routine use as locations for assessing or targeting DLPFC activity (e.g., during near-infrared spectroscopy and transcranial magnetic stimulation, respectively), the electrode sites F3 and F4 (from the International 10-20 System for EEG electrode placement) are estimated to be approximately 14 mm directly above the left and right DLPFC in 81% and 98% of individuals, respectively, with standard deviation of alignment being on the order of 8 mm (Okamoto et al. 2004). The limited simultaneous EEG–ECoG studies available have also reported high correlation between DLPFC and F3/F4 neurophysiologic activity (Ball et al. 2009). Thus, despite the limited anatomic resolution of EEG in general, specifically during delay periods of WM tasks, gamma activity recorded at frontal electrodes (e.g., F3, F4) can directly measure persistent, high-frequency activity of DLPFC neural assemblies (Fig. 1).

While the properties of magnetic fields enable MEG to provide greater anatomic resolution than EEG (e.g., less signal drop through tissue), the above evidence supports F3/F4 gamma activity being a valid marker of DLPFC microcircuit activity, specifically during delay periods of WM tasks. Furthermore, in addition to the feasibility of EEG acquisition (e.g., mobile/portable functionality, equipment and operating costs several orders-of-magnitude less than other neuroimaging modalities), recent computational and technological advances (which have vastly improved the predictive power of EEG) have established EEG as the biosignal of choice for clinical brain–computer interface (BCI) applications, including for monitoring cognitive and emotional states in real time (Abiri et al. 2019; Yan et al. 2021). Given this review's focus on translating our understanding of DLPFC microcircuit activity into clinically feasible targets for neurofeedback, we focus here on EEG measures of optimal DLPFC function during working memory, and their impairment in patients with SCZ.

More specifically, in the following discussion, we first present evidence supporting a critical role for DLPFC microcircuit activity during WM and in the pathophysiology of SCZ. From this evidence, and from a meta-analysis of studies specifically comparing frontal gamma activity between participants with SCZ and healthy controls (presented below), we discuss the potential role for EEG markers of DLPFC microcircuit activity during WM as effective biomarkers or treatment targets for patients with SCZ. We review the complex cognitive and neurophysiologic processes contributing to neural oscillations during tasks with WM features, and how such complexity has stalled the development of neurophysiologic biomarkers and treatment targets. Finally, we summarize promising results from early reports using neuromodulation to target DLPFC neural activity and improve cognitive function in participants with SCZ, including a study from our team demonstrating that gamma-EEG neurofeedback increases frontal gamma power and WM performance in participants with SCZ.

2 Schizophrenia-Related DLPFC Microcircuit Abnormalities

As models mapping brain areas to specific cognitive functions gained prominence in the 1970s, applying such models to clinical populations suggested that the pathophysiology of schizophrenia (SCZ) likely involves frontal/prefrontal dysfunction – e.g., given similarities in neurocognitive profiles between patients with SCZ and frontal lesions (Levin 1984). In addition to impairments to executive function and WM (Goldberg and Weinberger 1988), frontal cortical dysfunction in patients with SCZ was further supported by early neuroimaging studies demonstrating decreased frontal cerebral perfusion at rest and during cognitive testing (Franzen and Ingvar 1975; Ingvar and Franzen 1974; Weinberger et al. 1986). Meta-analyses of studies published in subsequent decades comparing cognitive performance of patients with SCZ to healthy controls have confirmed deficits with medium to large effect sizes in cognitive functions driven by frontal/prefrontal areas, e.g. attention, verbal/visual WM, executive function (Fatouros-Bergman et al. 2014). Meta-analyses of studies comparing functional brain activity between patients with SCZ and healthy controls during tasks involving WM or executive functions such as cognitive control have identified decreased activation of a cortical network that includes bilateral DLPFC, right dorsal anterior cingulate, pre-motor and posterior temporal/parietal areas in patients with SCZ (Minzenberg et al. 2009). While DLPFC dysfunction in patients with SCZ likely arises from multiple related abnormalities, e.g., neural morphology/structure, local and distant network connectivity/structure, neurotransmitter signaling, neural/network activity (Lewis et al. 2012; Smucny et al. 2022), abnormalities to the above-described DLPFC microcircuit responsible for greater pyramidal gamma synchronization during WM would offer the opportunity to directly monitor specific DLPFC microcircuit abnormalities using EEG, and target such abnormalities using EEG-guided interventions.

Consistent with this possibility, post-mortem studies of samples from patients with SCZ demonstrate decreased DLPFC pyramidal size and dendritic density (Garey et al. 1998; Glantz and Lewis 2000; Rajkowska et al. 1998), which would be expected to decrease synchronous neural responses during WM. While the general structure and morphology of DLPFC PV+ GABA-ergic (i.e., inhibitory) basket interneurons are not altered in patients with SCZ (Woo et al. 1997), the expression of activation-dependent genes by prefrontal PV+ inhibitory basket interneurons (including in ventral-posterior parts of the DLPFC) is deficient in post-mortem samples from patients with SCZ (Hashimoto et al. 2003), consistent with reduced activation by DLPFC pyramidal neurons with SCZ-related abnormalities. Consistent with these SCZ-related DLPFC microcircuit abnormalities in post-mortem samples, Chen and colleagues observed that L DLPFC GABA levels most significantly and strongly correlated with F3 gamma activity (versus gamma activity from other 10–20 electrode positions), and that (1) compared to healthy controls, participants with SCZ exhibited significantly lower F3 gamma activity during WM, and (2) L DLPFC GABA levels positively correlated with both WM performance and F3 gamma activity in all subjects – i.e., individual participants with SCZ exhibiting lower DLPFC GABA levels also exhibited lower F3 gamma activity and more impaired WM (Chen et al. 2014).

To further confirm lower frontal gamma activity as a marker of impaired WM in patients with SCZ, we conducted a meta-analysis of all studies available in PubMed comparing *frontal gamma* activity during *WM* between patients with SCZ and healthy controls. In brief, entering the following search terms – schizophrenia AND EEG AND "working memory" – on Nov 2021 produced 61 results. After excluding ten non-human studies, ten non-research articles (e.g., reviews, conference proceedings), and 35 studies not meeting inclusion criteria (e.g., no participants with SCZ, no healthy controls, non-WM task, no analysis of frontal gamma activity, duplicated datasets), we identified six studies comparing gamma activity at frontal electrodes during WM between participants with SCZ and healthy controls (Table 1).

For each study, effect sizes of differences in frontal gamma power between participants with SCZ and healthy controls (in terms of standardized mean difference, or SMD) were calculated from reported T or F statistics as described by Lipsey

Table 1 Summary of studies available in PubMed comparing frontal gamma activity during WM in patients with SCZ and healthy controls

Reference	Task	Neurophysiology	Electrodes	Time window	SMD (SCZ minus HC)	95% CI	
						Lower limit	Upper limit
Missonnier et al. (2020)	N-Back	EEG: Phase-synchronized power (35–45 Hz)	F3, Fz, F4	50–150 ms post-stimulus	−0.91	−1.41	−0.41
Chen et al. (2014)	Modified Stern-berg WM	EEG: Event-synchronized power (30–56 Hz)	F3	Encoding, retention, retrieval (12 s total)	−1.28	−2.03	−0.54
Koychev et al. (2012)	Delayed visual discrimination	EEG: Phase-synchronized power (30–50 Hz)	FC1, FC2, FCz, C1, C2, Cz	100–250 ms post-stimulus	−0.83	−1.29	−0.38
Barr et al. (2010)	N-Back	EEG: Phase-synchronized power (30–50 Hz)	AF3, AF4, F3, F4, Fz, F5, F6	0–100 ms post-stimulus	0.62	0.21	1.03
Haenschel et al. (2009)	Delayed visual discrimination	EEG: Phase-synchronized power (55–100 Hz)	F1, FZ, F2, FC1, FCZ, FC2, C1, CZ, C2	2,500–4,500 ms post-stimulus	−1.28	−1.83	−0.73
Basar-Eroglu et al. (2007)	N-Back	EEG: Event-synchronized power (28–48 Hz)	Fz (equivalent results at Cz, Pz, oz)	0–500 ms post-stimulus	0.89	0.23	1.55
				All studies (n = 185)	*−0.39*	*−0.60*	*−0.19*

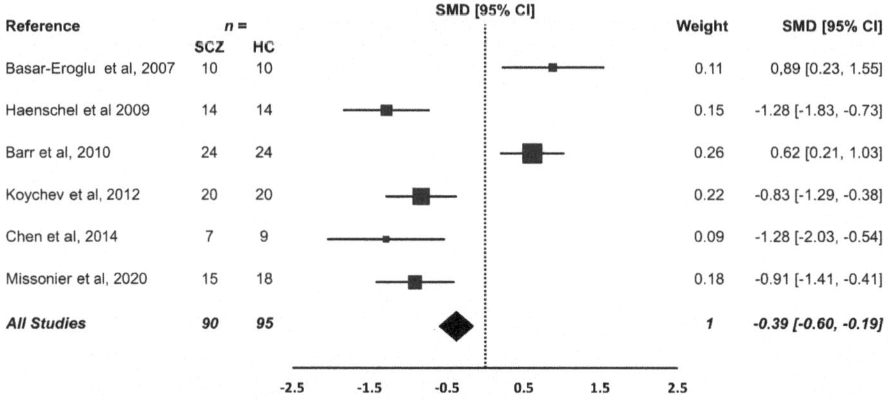

Fig. 2 Forest plot summarizing individual and weighted average effects sizes (SMD) and 95% confidence intervals (95% CI) of six studies available in PubMed comparing frontal gamma activity during WM in patients with SCZ and healthy controls. Originally, 61 results were identified in PubMed Nov 2021 using search terms: schizophrenia AND EEG AND "working memory." Fifty-five studies excluded as follows: ten non-human studies, ten non-research articles (e.g., reviews, conference proceedings), and 35 studies not meeting inclusion criteria (e.g., no participants with SCZ, no healthy controls, non-WM task, no analysis of frontal gamma activity, duplicated datasets). Meta-analysis of six included studies ($n = 90$ participants with SCZ; 95, healthy controls; 185, total) demonstrates a statistically significant medium effect size of −0.39 (participants with SCZ exhibiting decreased frontal gamma power compared to healthy controls) with 95% CI of [−0.60, −0.19]. Please see main text for full analysis and discussion of six included studies

and Wilson (Lipsey and Wilson 2001). Ninety-percent confidence intervals (95% CI) for each study, as well as weighted average of SMD (and 95% CI) for all studies were then calculated as described by Higgins and colleagues (Higgins and Cochrane Collaboration 2020). As summarized in Table 1 and Fig. 2, a meta-analysis of six included studies ($n = 90$ participants with SCZ; 95, healthy controls; 185, total) demonstrates a statistically significant medium effect size of −0.39 (participants with SCZ exhibiting decreased frontal gamma power compared to healthy controls) with 95% CI of [−0.60, −0.19] – consistent with a model where the above-described SCZ-related DLPFC microcircuit abnormalities produce lower frontal gamma activity during WM.

This significant effect was robust against choice of task, electrode(s), or method for gamma power extraction. More specifically, three different tasks with WM features were represented across the six included studies. Three of the six studies utilized the N-Back – where participants are presented with series of stimuli (e.g., white letter on black background) and instructed to evaluate whenever the current stimulus was presented generally 1, 2, or 3 trials (on the order of 5–15 s) earlier. The second most common task, utilized in two of the six studies, was a visual delayed match-to-sample (DMS) task requiring recall of whether a visual design was presented 12 s earlier. One study utilized a modified Sternberg task requiring recall of whether a letter was presented 7 s earlier. Choice of task was not associated with trends in effect sizes.

With regard to method for gamma power extraction, two studies extracted all gamma power in time windows set to stimulus onset (e.g., event-synchronized power), and four studies attempted to extract power only from gamma oscillations in phase with stimulus onset (e.g., phase-synchronized power, which includes evoked power). There is currently no consensus on how best to extract phase-synchronized power, and whether phase-synchronized power generally provides more valid information than event-synchronized power (Herrmann et al. 2010; Roach and Mathalon 2008). Extracting phase-versus event-synchronized gamma was not associated with trends in effect sizes across the six studies. With regard to choice of electrode(s), two studies extracted gamma power from a single electrode – F3 (Chen et al. 2014) and Fz (Basar-Eroglu et al. 2007), while four studies averaged gamma power extracted from frontal (Barr et al. 2010; Missonnier et al. 2020) or frontal-central electrodes (Haenschel et al. 2009; Koychev et al. 2012). Choice of electrodes was not associated with trends in effect sizes.

In contrast to task, phase- versus event-synchronized gamma power or electrode location, time window was associated with trends in effect sizes. More specifically, the two studies demonstrating the largest expected effect sizes (lower frontal gamma power in participants with SCZ compared to healthy controls) both analyzed gamma power over time windows that either mostly covered the delay period on the order of seconds (Haenschel et al. 2009) or the entirety of the trial on the order of 12 s (Chen et al. 2014). In contrast, the two studies demonstrating the opposite effects (greater frontal gamma power in participants with SCZ) both analyzed gamma power over time windows on the order of 100 (Barr et al. 2010) and 500 (Basar-Eroglu et al. 2007) ms after, and including, stimulus onset – a time window mostly devoted to encoding and retrieval during the N-Back tasks used. Thus, while our meta-analysis supports patients with SCZ generally exhibiting decreased WM-related frontal gamma activity compared to healthy controls – a significant effect fairly robust against choice of task, frontal electrode(s), or method for gamma power extraction, the effect appears closely associated with internal maintenance during delay periods and becomes difficult to localize during other stages of WM, e.g. encoding, retrieval (please see Sect. 3 for detailed discussion of neural oscillations during separate stages of WM).

3 Neural Oscillations During WM

As a conserved mechanism for processing incoming information by local neural assemblies, gamma oscillations have been observed throughout multiple brain areas under various cognitive and behavioral conditions, including during multiple stages of WM (Herrmann et al. 2010). Consistent with the evidence reviewed above, however, studies focusing on delay periods have generally observed a primary role for frontal gamma activity during internal maintenance; for example, using high-density EEG while participants completed the N-Back, Semprini and colleagues demonstrate that, in contrast to theta and beta (see below), gamma activity (relatively attenuated during encoding and retrieval) was most active during maintenance, especially in frontal, including DLPFC, areas (Semprini et al. 2021). Tallon-Baudry and colleagues similarly observed significant gamma responses at frontal electrodes, including F3 and F4, in trials requiring maintenance during a visual DMS task, compared to control trials where maintenance was not required (Tallon-Baudry et al. 1998). Similarly, in a combined MEG/EEG study of participants performing a DMS task requiring higher-order visual processing of shape, color, and location, Honkanen and colleagues, using a whole-brain, data-driven analytic approach, observed expected gamma and beta responses in visual processing areas; however, only gamma synchronization was significantly increased in prefrontal areas during the delay period (Honkanen et al. 2015). Intriguingly, in an MEG study of participants performing a DMS with varying loads, Roux and colleagues observed that only gamma activity localized to Brodmann Area 9 (medial and DL PFC) correlated with and predicted load (0, 3, or 6 items) in a load-dependent manner (Roux et al. 2012).

In contrast to gamma activity, synchronous activity in lower frequencies, e.g., theta (3–7 Hz), alpha (8–14 Hz), and beta (15–30 Hz), is less specifically associated with internal maintenance during delay periods of WM tasks. For example, in the above-described study by Semprini and colleagues, in contrast to gamma activity (which was most active during maintenance, especially in frontal, including DLPFC, areas), theta activity (from prefrontal, pre-motor, and posterior parietal areas) was most active during encoding and retrieval (Semprini et al. 2021), suggesting that transfer of information between encoding, maintenance, and retrieval stages involves coordinated theta and gamma responses. Consistent with such a model, intracranial recordings from epilepsy patients demonstrate that, during cognitive control and WM tasks, in multiple brain areas including frontal and temporal, peak bursts of gamma power are synchronized to phase of theta oscillations (Axmacher et al. 2010; Canolty et al. 2006). This theta-gamma phase-amplitude coupling (PAC) has been demonstrated in multiple brain areas in multiple species during information processing and is likely a conserved neural mechanism for communicating and maintaining task-relevant information (Canolty and Knight 2010).

Intriguingly, the phase of theta oscillations can be entrained, or reset/shifted, by external or internal stimuli. For example, in contrast to garbled sentences, the onset of intelligible speech is associated with shifts in phase of temporal theta consistent with the recognition of intelligible syllables (Luo and Poeppel 2007). Specific to WM, onset of probe for retrieval is associated with shifts in phase of frontal and temporal theta consistent with recognition and retrieval (Rizzuto et al. 2003). Thus, with a temporal resolution, or a "refresh rate," approximating 200 ms, i.e., about 5 "frames per second," theta entrainment has likely evolved as a conserved information processing mechanism, as many naturalistic behaviors and stimuli, e.g., vocalizations/speech, saccades, motor responses, occur at similar frequencies of about 4–7 Hz (Cohen 2014). Furthermore, theta-gamma cross-frequency coupling (CFC) has likely emerged as a conserved mechanism for distributed processing of such stimuli, including during WM (Canolty and Knight 2010).

While the above evidence supports active roles for theta and gamma in "task-relevant" information processing during WM tasks, alpha synchronization, while equally active during WM tasks, appears more involved in the inhibition of "task-irrelevant" processes. For example, during a visual WM task where contralateral visual hemifields received differing task-relevant versus irrelevant stimuli, posterior parietal theta-gamma CFC increased in a load-dependent manner only in the hemisphere corresponding to task-relevant hemifield (Sauseng et al. 2009). In contrast, posterior parietal alpha activity increased in a load-dependent manner only in the hemisphere corresponding to task-irrelevant hemifield. Using transcranial magnetic stimulation (TMS) to further increase posterior parietal alpha activity in the task-irrelevant hemisphere improved WM performance, while using TMS to increase posterior parietal alpha activity in the task-relevant hemisphere impaired WM performance (Sauseng et al. 2009). This detrimental effect of alpha synchronization on task-relevant processing was confirmed and further refined by Riddle and colleagues who observed that using TMS to activate frontal areas (by increasing theta activity) and inhibit posterior parietal areas (by increasing alpha activity) improved WM performance (and produced expected increases in frontal, and decreases in posterior parietal, blood oxygen level dependent, or BOLD, signal); conversely, increasing frontal alpha activity and posterior parietal theta activity impaired WM performance (Riddle et al. 2020; Sauseng and Liesefeld 2020).

While alpha synchronization appears largely associated with the inhibition of task-irrelevant processes in task-irrelevant brain areas, beta synchronization appears to play a more modulatory role during WM tasks, including on task-relevant processes in task-relevant areas. For example, Michail and colleagues demonstrate that, during the N-Back, as load increases, increased frontal-central theta and gamma activity was accompanied by decreased frontal-central beta activity, in a manner suggesting that lowering beta (i.e., beta suppression) lowers inhibition of, and thus promotes, theta and gamma activation (Michail et al. 2021). Furthermore, in an intriguing modification of the N-Back used in their study, Michail and colleagues added a sound-induced flash illusion (SIFI) at the end of every trial, and observed that, as beta activity decreased, inhibition of not only theta and gamma activity but also of sensory discrimination decreased, producing greater vulnerability to perception of illusory flashes. Semprini and colleagues in the study discussed above similarly observed modulatory effects of beta on both task-relevant and task-irrelevant processes. More specifically, frontal, pre-motor, and posterior parietal beta activity were lower during encoding and retrieval (to promote greater theta activity in these areas during these stages), while, during maintenance, beta activity was increased in posterior parietal areas (to promote inhibition of task-irrelevant activity) but remained lower in frontal areas, in order to promote greater gamma activity during maintenance (Semprini et al. 2021).

From the above, we can observe that, as we broaden our focus from DLPFC gamma activity during internal maintenance, to lower-frequency oscillations in other brain areas, additional cognitive and neurophysiologic processes begin to confound the specificity of extracted neurophysiologic features; e.g., role of theta synchronization in the processing of external and internal stimuli, including through entrainment or phase shift/resetting; or, the generally inhibitory effects of alpha synchronization on task-irrelevant processes and more modulatory effects of beta synchronization on both task-relevant and task-irrelevant processes. Even in the focused set of studies included in the meta-analyses above, studies utilizing earlier, shorter time windows (which likely captured activity more related to stimulus processing, including encoding and retrieval) produced results opposite to those utilizing later, longer time windows, which were likely more specific to internal maintenance.

Furthermore, in addition to the complex relationship between cognitive and neurophysiologic processes described above, additional challenges when assessing neural oscillations in patients with SCZ – e.g., heterogeneity with regard to pathophysiology, including developmental pathophysiology, as well as co-morbidities and the immediate- and long-term effects of heterogeneous forms and levels of treatment – have stalled the development of biomarkers and treatment targets (Uhlhaas and Singer 2015). Despite these challenges, however, motivated by the evidence presented earlier, we review in the following section additional clinical evidence indicating that the relative specificity of DLPFC gamma activity in relation to WM may provide a promising path forward.

4 Targeting DLPFC Gamma Activity to Improve WM in Patients with SCZ

In contrast to the complex, overlapping cognitive and neurophysiologic sources of most neural oscillations (see previous section), delay period frontal gamma activity, as discussed above, may be sufficiently specific to DLPFC microcircuit activity to serve as a feasible biomarker or treatment target for patients with SCZ. Early reports are consistent with this hypothesis and suggest that larger clinical trials testing potential benefits of treatments targeting DLPFC neural activity to cognitive function for patients with SCZ may be indicated. For example, in a double-blind, sham-controlled, randomized cross-over study of 18 participants with SCZ, a single 2 mA dose of transcranial direct current stimulation (TDCS) with anode applied to F3 scalp location for 20 min significantly improved accuracy during N-Back performance 40 min after stimulation (Hoy et al. 2014). In contrast, sham or 1 mA stimulation led to lower N-Back performance 40 min later. A follow-up study demonstrated that F3 gamma power increased 40 min after 2 mA stimulation, but decreased 40 min after sham or 1 mA stimulation; furthermore, increases in F3 gamma power were significantly correlated with increases in N-Back performance (Hoy et al. 2015). These effects were recently confirmed by Boudewyn and colleagues who demonstrated that, in a double-blind, sham-controlled, randomized cross-over study of 27 participants with SCZ, compared to sham stimulation, a single 2 mA dose of TDCS with anode applied to F3 scalp location for 20 min (while participants performed N-Back in order to enhance DLPFC engagement) significantly improved performance during a cognitive control task which included WM features, and significantly increased frontal gamma power during the delay period (Boudewyn et al. 2020). While promising, these TDCS studies were not designed to assess the longer-term effects of a course of TDCS treatment, e.g. multiple sessions per week for periods on the order of several weeks. With regard to longer treatment studies using neuromodulation to target DLPFC neural activity in patients with SCZ, Güleken and colleagues, in a pilot randomized, double-blind, sham-controlled clinical trial of bilateral DLPFC stimulation, observed a positive effect of TMS on cognitive performance (Guleken et al. 2020). More specifically, participants receiving bilateral 20 Hz DLPFC stimulation daily for 4 weeks (20 sessions total, $n = 11$) exhibited significantly improved cognitive control (Stroop Task) and WM (Digit Span) performance by end-of-treatment, compared to participants ($n = 10$) receiving sham TMS, who exhibited no change in cognitive performance.

While the above-discussed early reports suggest that larger clinical trials of TDCS and TMS targeting DLPFC neural activity to improve WM in patients with SCZ may be indicated, concerns about safety (e.g., seizure risk with TMS) and cost of equipment, staff, and facilities have limited efficient testing of potentially therapeutic TDCS and TMS protocols. A safer and more clinically feasible way to target DLPFC neural activity may be through EEG neurofeedback (EEG-NFB), a form of operant conditioning where an EEG signal of interest (e.g., frontal gamma activity) is coupled, in real time, to positive and negative reinforcement signals – e.g., the playing or pausing of, or other modulations to, auditory and visual features of content running on a desktop computer (Singh et al. 2020a). While EEG-NFB is a well-tolerated, non-invasive, non-pharmacologic treatment modality that can be rapidly disseminated at low cost, widespread institutional acceptance has, to date, been limited due to concerns about specificity of observed effects and discrepancies with current models of brain function (Ros et al. 2020). With specific regard to DLPFC microcircuit activity, however, for reasons discussed above, using EEG-NFB to modulate frontal gamma activity would likely directly modulate DLPFC gamma activity.

In exploring the development of an EEG-NFB protocol for increasing frontal gamma activity to improve WM in patients with SCZ, we first reviewed studies of NFB and schizophrenia available in PubMed (Gandara et al. 2020). We demonstrate that, among EEG-NFB studies, none targeted frontal gamma activity, and, among NFB studies utilizing BOLD signals, none targeted prefrontal (including DLPFC) activity. To date, we are the first and only group to test frontal gamma EEG-NFB for patients with SCZ (Singh et al. 2020b). More specifically, to test whether EEG-NFB reinforcing increased frontal gamma activity improves SCZ-related WM impairments, we enrolled 31 participants with schizophrenia in an open-label pilot study, where participants presented for training twice weekly for 12 weeks. To target frontal gamma synchronization during training, we selected gamma power coherence (Roach and Mathalon 2008) between F3 and F4 as the feature of interest:

$$|G_{F3-F4}(f)|^2/(G_{F3-F3}(f) \times G_{F4-F4}(f))$$

where $G_{X\text{-}Y}(f)$ indicates cross-spectral density between EEG signals from channels X and Y, $G_{X\text{-}X}(f)$ indicates the auto-spectral density of X, f indicates gamma band frequency, and F3/F4 indicating data source. Thus, coherence is primarily a function of cross-spectral densities between power from two sources, normalized by spectral power of each source, and exhibits the following advantages. First, power from a single source is especially vulnerable to artifacts (e.g., muscle or line noise), whereas such interference is attenuated when considering cross-spectral densities between two sources. Secondly, while F3-F4 coherence is still primarily a function of power (the neural signal of interest), by synchronously targeting both F3 and F4 gamma power, F3-F4 gamma coherence increases the engagement of bilateral DLPFC assemblies in a more physiologic manner. Clinical results from this study were previously reported (Singh et al. 2020b). In brief, we observe that estimates of EEG-NFB performance were positively correlated with WM performance. NFB training was also associated with improved clinical and neuropsychological outcomes, as measured by the Positive and Negative Syndrome Scale (PANSS) and the Measurement and Treatment Research to Improve Cognition in Schizophrenia (MATRICS) Consensus Cognitive Battery (MCCB), including at follow-up one-month post-treatment. Specifically for this review, we present here a new follow-up analysis from this study, focusing on the effects of F3/F4 gamma coherence EEG-NFB on 2-Back WM performance and event-synchronized frontal gamma power (Fig. 3).

More specifically, consistent with the above discussion, participants with SCZ exhibited robust, early (0–500 ms latency) event-related synchronization in lower frequencies prior to EEG-NFB training (Fig. 3a). Compared to lower frequencies, pre-treatment event-related gamma synchronization was relatively weaker (Fig. 3a). EEG-NFB training increased event-related gamma synchronization, especially at latencies following the early (about 0–250 ms) stimulus-processing/encoding interval (Fig. 3b). For completeness, we extracted total event-synchronized gamma (30–50 Hz) between 0 and 1.5 s post-stimulus (gray, rectangular dashed outline in Fig. 3b) from assessments at Weeks 0 (pre-treatment baseline), 4, 8, and 12 (end-of-treatment) and observed a significant effect of time for frontal gamma power ($\gamma = 0.04$, $t(29) = 3.35$, $p = 0.003$; data not shown). To better characterize the relationship between NFB performance, frontal gamma activity, and WM, we tested strengths of correlation between training-related changes in NFB performance, frontal gamma power, and WM performance. If training-related improvements in NFB performance produced greater increases in frontal gamma power; and, if greater frontal gamma power improved WM performance; then, participants with the greatest training-related improvements in NFB performance would be expected to exhibit the greatest increases in frontal gamma power, and in 2-Back accuracy. Consistent with this hypothesis, we observed significant correlations between change in NFB performance (Week 12 minus Week 1) and change in frontal gamma power (Week 12 minus Week 0), $\rho = 0.378$, $p = 0.024$ (Fig. 3c).

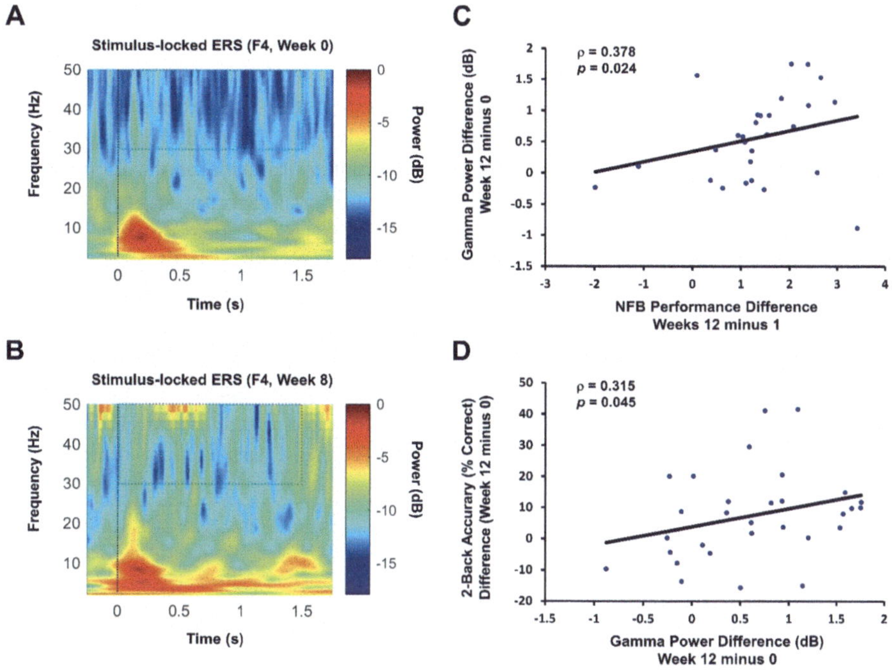

Fig. 3 On the left, representative event-related spectrograms from an individual participant of oscillatory EEG activity (from frontal channel F4 during 2-Back trials) in the 1,500 ms time window after stimulus (letter) onset: Week 0 (**a**), Week 8 (**b**). Frequency of oscillatory activity (Hz) is plotted on the y-axis; and, latency (ms) along the x-axis. Color at each individual time–frequency point indicates the magnitude of oscillatory power in decibels (dB), with yellow to orange to red indicating increasing power, and lighter to darker blue indicating decreasing power. Gray boxes indicate spectral–temporal region of interest for frontal gamma power, i.e. total event-synchronized gamma (30–50 Hz) between 0 and 1.5 s post-stimulus. On the right, for all participants, scatter plots for correlations between training-related changes in NFB performance (Week 12 minus Week 1) and frontal gamma power (Week 12 minus Week 0), $\rho = 0.378$, $p = 0.024$ (**c**), and between training-related changes in frontal gamma power (Week 12 minus Week 0) and 2-Back performance (Week 12 minus Week 0), $\rho = 0.315$, $p = 0.045$ (**d**)

Furthermore, training-related change in frontal gamma power (Week 12 minus Week 0) was significantly correlated with training-related changes in 2-Back performance (Week 12 minus Week 0), $\rho = 0.315$, $p = 0.045$ (Fig. 3d). Age and level of education were not significantly correlated with training-related changes in NFB performance, WM performance, or frontal gamma power.

Since this study was designed as an open-label pilot study, neither participants nor investigators were blinded to frontal gamma-NFB being the active intervention (i.e., no control or sham intervention). Therefore, potentially confounding effects from expectations or bias from participants or investigators, or from non-specific effects such as practice or positive, interpersonal feedback, cannot be fully excluded. As we designed this treatment study specifically to target frontal gamma activity, our primary analysis did not include gamma activity at other electrodes or other neural oscillations; thus, the specificity of the relationships between frontal gamma activity and WM performance, e.g., compared to gamma activity from other brain areas or other neural oscillations, has not been established at this time, though secondary analyses related to these questions are currently under way. Nevertheless, significant correlations between training-related NFB performance improvements, increases in frontal gamma activity, and WM improvements support the hypothesis that frontal gamma-NFB likely helps local, functional DLPFC assemblies produce greater frontal gamma responses, which then likely helps improve WM performance. While possible, a non-neurobiologic mechanism producing the observed correlations between training-related changes in NFB performance, frontal gamma responses, and WM performance has yet to be well-defined and is, thus, in our opinion, less likely. Nevertheless, to overcome potential limitations, we are currently conducting a double-blind, sham-controlled randomized clinical trial (RCT) comparing frontal gamma-NFB with sham-NFB for participants with SCZ (ClinicalTrials.gov Identifier: NCT03260257).

5 Conclusions and Future Directions

The last two decades have witnessed exponential growth in our understanding of the fundamental aspects of memory, and it has become increasingly evident that WM, a flexible and fluid memory space necessary for everyday functioning, arises from coordinated activity of neurons in the DLPFC. Convergent evidence from primate and human studies suggests that specific cognitive demands, including WM, produce robust DLPFC activation, a phenomenon that is characterized by large, reproducible, electrical deflections, measurable with scalp EEG recordings. Specifically, high-frequency activity, or gamma oscillations, produced during WM tasks provide both a biomarker of DLPFC integrity and a potential treatment target. This discovery has been especially relevant for disorders such as SCZ, where cognitive deficits are a core feature with great functional significance, yet lack effective treatments. In this context, the emerging field of neuromodulation with approaches such as TDCS, TMS, as well as the re-emergence of EEG-NFB as a specific implementation of BCI, has been utilized to enhance DLPFC function, with positive effects on oscillatory activity and cognitive performance in individuals with SCZ. These studies demonstrate that DLPFC function can be influenced directly, both through extrinsic (TDCS, TMS) and intrinsic (NFB) neuromodulation, in contrast to psychotropics and psychotherapies, neither one of which targets a biomarker. Thus, neuromodulation treatments are uniquely suited to implement the NIMH's RDoC (Insel et al. 2010), since they inherently characterize neuropsychiatric disorders as circuit level impairments, with treatments that restore circuit function. We anticipate that the coming decade will continue to build on these early exciting findings in the field of neuromodulation and to provide treatments that can improve the lives of individuals living with SCZ.

Acknowledgments We thank Beverly Castillo, Yayu Lin, Sheng-Hsiou Hsu, Peter Link, Jaime Pineda, Veronica Gandara, Zinong Yang, and Alexiss Rivas for their contributions to this research. This study was supported by the National Institute of Mental Health (R61MH112793, R33MH112793) and the University of California San Diego (Chancellor's Research Excellence Scholarship; or, CRES), and was registered on ClinicalTrials.gov (NCT03260257). Drs. Shu, Granholm, and Singh have equity interests in BioSignal Solutions LLC. The terms of this arrangement have been reviewed and approved by the University of California, San Diego in accordance with its conflict of interest policies.

References

Abiri R, Borhani S, Sellers EW, Jiang Y, Zhao X (2019) A comprehensive review of EEG-based brain-computer interface paradigms. J Neural Eng 16(1):011001

Atkinson R, Shiffrin R (1968) Human memory: a proposed system and its control processes. Psychol Learn Motiv 2:89–195

Axmacher N, Henseler MM, Jensen O, Weinreich I, Elger CE, Fell J (2010) Cross-frequency coupling supports multi-item working memory in the human hippocampus. Proc Natl Acad Sci U S A 107(7):3228–3233

Baddeley A (1996) The fractionation of working memory. Proc Natl Acad Sci U S A 93(24):13468–13472

Ball T, Kern M, Mutschler I, Aertsen A, Schulze-Bonhage A (2009) Signal quality of simultaneously recorded invasive and non-invasive EEG. NeuroImage 46(3):708–716

Banich MT, Mackiewicz KL, Depue BE, Whitmer AJ, Miller GA, Heller W (2009) Cognitive control mechanisms, emotion and memory: a neural perspective with implications for psychopathology. Neurosci Biobehav Rev 33(5):613–630

Barr MS, Farzan F, Tran LC, Chen R, Fitzgerald PB, Daskalakis ZJ (2010) Evidence for excessive frontal evoked gamma oscillatory activity in schizophrenia during working memory. Schizophr Res 121(1–3):146–152

Basar-Eroglu C, Brand A, Hildebrandt H, Karolina Kedzior K, Mathes B, Schmiedt C (2007) Working memory related gamma oscillations in schizophrenia patients. Int J Psychophysiol 64(1):39–45

Boudewyn MA, Scangos K, Ranganath C, Carter CS (2020) Using prefrontal transcranial direct current stimulation (tDCS) to enhance proactive cognitive control in schizophrenia. Neuropsychopharmacology 45(11):1877–1883

Buzsaki G, Wang XJ (2012) Mechanisms of gamma oscillations. Annu Rev Neurosci 35:203–225

Buzsaki G, Anastassiou CA, Koch C (2012) The origin of extracellular fields and currents--EEG, ECoG, LFP and spikes. Nat Rev Neurosci 13(6):407–420

Canolty RT, Knight RT (2010) The functional role of cross-frequency coupling. Trends Cogn Sci 14(11):506–515

Canolty RT, Edwards E, Dalal SS, Soltani M, Nagarajan SS, Kirsch HE, Berger MS, Barbaro NM, Knight RT (2006) High gamma power is phase-locked to theta oscillations in human neocortex. Science 313(5793):1626–1628

Chen CM, Stanford AD, Mao X, Abi-Dargham A, Shungu DC, Lisanby SH, Schroeder CE, Kegeles LS (2014) GABA level, gamma oscillation, and working memory performance in schizophrenia. Neuroimage Clin 4:531–539

Cohen MX (2014) A neural microcircuit for cognitive conflict detection and signaling. Trends Neurosci 37(9):480–490

Cuthbert BN, Insel TR (2013) Toward the future of psychiatric diagnosis: the seven pillars of RDoC. BMC Med 11:126

Douglas RJ, Martin KA (2004) Neuronal circuits of the neocortex. Annu Rev Neurosci 27:419–451

Fatouros-Bergman H, Cervenka S, Flyckt L, Edman G, Farde L (2014) Meta-analysis of cognitive performance in drug-naive patients with schizophrenia. Schizophr Res 158(1–3):156–162
Franzen G, Ingvar DH (1975) Absence of activation in frontal structures during psychological testing of chronic schizophrenics. J Neurol Neurosurg Psychiatry 38(10):1027–1032
Fuster JM, Alexander GE (1971) Neuron activity related to short-term memory. Science 173(3997):652–654
Gandara V, Pineda JA, Shu IW, Singh F (2020) A systematic review of the potential use of neurofeedback in patients with schizophrenia. Schizophr Bull Open 1(1):sgaa005
Garey LJ, Ong WY, Patel TS, Kanani M, Davis A, Mortimer AM, Barnes TR, Hirsch SR (1998) Reduced dendritic spine density on cerebral cortical pyramidal neurons in schizophrenia. J Neurol Neurosurg Psychiatry 65(4):446–453
Glantz LA, Lewis DA (2000) Decreased dendritic spine density on prefrontal cortical pyramidal neurons in schizophrenia. Arch Gen Psychiatry 57(1):65–73
Goldberg TE, Weinberger DR (1988) Probing prefrontal function in schizophrenia with neuropsychological paradigms. Schizophr Bull 14(2):179–183
Gray CM (1994) Synchronous oscillations in neuronal systems: mechanisms and functions. J Comput Neurosci 1(1–2):11–38
Guleken MD, Akbas T, Erden SC, Akansel V, Al ZC, Ozer OA (2020) The effect of bilateral high frequency repetitive transcranial magnetic stimulation on cognitive functions in schizophrenia. Schizophr Res Cogn 22:100183
Haenschel C, Bittner RA, Waltz J, Haertling F, Wibral M, Singer W, Linden DE, Rodriguez E (2009) Cortical oscillatory activity is critical for working memory as revealed by deficits in early-onset schizophrenia. J Neurosci 29(30):9481–9489
Hashimoto T, Volk DW, Eggan SM, Mirnics K, Pierri JN, Sun Z, Sampson AR, Lewis DA (2003) Gene expression deficits in a subclass of GABA neurons in the prefrontal cortex of subjects with schizophrenia. J Neurosci 23(15):6315–6326
Herrmann CS, Frund I, Lenz D (2010) Human gamma-band activity: a review on cognitive and behavioral correlates and network models. Neurosci Biobehav Rev 34(7):981–992
Higgins JPT, Cochrane Collaboration (2020) Cochrane handbook for systematic reviews of interventions, 2nd edn. Wiley-Blackwell, Hoboken
Honkanen R, Rouhinen S, Wang SH, Palva JM, Palva S (2015) Gamma oscillations underlie the maintenance of feature-specific information and the contents of visual working memory. Cereb Cortex 25(10):3788–3801
Hoy KE, Arnold SL, Emonson MR, Daskalakis ZJ, Fitzgerald PB (2014) An investigation into the effects of tDCS dose on cognitive performance over time in patients with schizophrenia. Schizophr Res 155(1–3):96–100
Hoy KE, Bailey NW, Arnold SL, Fitzgerald PB (2015) The effect of transcranial direct current stimulation on gamma activity and working memory in schizophrenia. Psychiatry Res 228(2):191–196
Ingvar DH, Franzen G (1974) Distribution of cerebral activity in chronic schizophrenia. Lancet 2(7895):1484–1486
Insel T, Cuthbert B, Garvey M, Heinssen R, Pine DS, Quinn K, Sanislow C, Wang P (2010) Research domain criteria (RDoC): toward a new classification framework for research on mental disorders. Am J Psychiatry 167(7):748–751
Jackson AF, Bolger DJ (2014) The neurophysiological bases of EEG and EEG measurement: a review for the rest of us. Psychophysiology 51(11):1061–1071
Jacobsen C, Elder J, Haslerud G (1936) Studies of cerebral function in primates. Comp Psychol Monogr 13(3):1–60
Koychev I, El-Deredy W, Mukherjee T, Haenschel C, Deakin JF (2012) Core dysfunction in schizophrenia: electrophysiology trait biomarkers. Acta Psychiatr Scand 126(1):59–71
Kritzer MF, Goldman-Rakic PS (1995) Intrinsic circuit organization of the major layers and sublayers of the dorsolateral prefrontal cortex in the rhesus monkey. J Comp Neurol 359(1):131–143

Kubota K, Niki H (1971) Prefrontal cortical unit activity and delayed alternation performance in monkeys. J Neurophysiol 34(3):337–347
Levin S (1984) Frontal lobe dysfunctions in schizophrenia--II. Impairments of psychological and brain functions. J Psychiatr Res 18(1):57–72
Lewis DA, Curley AA, Glausier JR, Volk DW (2012) Cortical parvalbumin interneurons and cognitive dysfunction in schizophrenia. Trends Neurosci 35(1):57–67
Lipsey MW, Wilson DB (2001) Practical meta-analysis. Sage Publications, Thousand Oaks
Lopes da Silva F (2013) EEG and MEG: relevance to neuroscience. Neuron 80(5):1112–1128
Luo H, Poeppel D (2007) Phase patterns of neuronal responses reliably discriminate speech in human auditory cortex. Neuron 54(6):1001–1010
Menon V (2011) Large-scale brain networks and psychopathology: a unifying triple network model. Trends Cogn Sci 15(10):483–506
Michail G, Senkowski D, Niedeggen M, Keil J (2021) Memory load alters perception-related neural oscillations during multisensory integration. J Neurosci 41(7):1505–1515
Miller GA, Galanter E, Pribram KH (1960) Plans and the structure of behavior. Holt, Rinehart and Winston, Inc., New York
Milner B (1971) Interhemispheric differences in the localization of psychological processes in man. Br Med Bull 27(3):272–277
Minzenberg MJ, Laird AR, Thelen S, Carter CS, Glahn DC (2009) Meta-analysis of 41 functional neuroimaging studies of executive function in schizophrenia. Arch Gen Psychiatry 66(8):811–822
Missonnier P, Prevot A, Herrmann FR, Ventura J, Padee A, Merlo MCG (2020) Disruption of gamma-delta relationship related to working memory deficits in first-episode psychosis. J Neural Transm (Vienna) 127(1):103–115
Niendam TA, Laird AR, Ray KL, Dean YM, Glahn DC, Carter CS (2012) Meta-analytic evidence for a superordinate cognitive control network subserving diverse executive functions. Cogn Affect Behav Neurosci 12(2):241–268
Okamoto M, Dan H, Sakamoto K, Takeo K, Shimizu K, Kohno S, Oda I, Isobe S, Suzuki T, Kohyama K, Dan I (2004) Three-dimensional probabilistic anatomical cranio-cerebral correlation via the international 10-20 system oriented for transcranial functional brain mapping. NeuroImage 21(1):99–111
Pfurtscheller G, Neuper C, Andrew C, Edlinger G (1997) Foot and hand area mu rhythms. Int J Psychophysiol 26(1–3):121–135
Pribram KH, Mishkin M, Rosvold HE, Kaplan SJ (1952) Effects on delayed-response performance of lesions of dorsolateral and ventromedial frontal cortex of baboons. J Comp Physiol Psychol 45(6):565–575
Rajkowska G, Selemon LD, Goldman-Rakic PS (1998) Neuronal and glial somal size in the prefrontal cortex: a postmortem morphometric study of schizophrenia and Huntington disease. Arch Gen Psychiatry 55(3):215–224
Riddle J, Scimeca JM, Cellier D, Dhanani S, D'Esposito M (2020) Causal evidence for a role of theta and alpha oscillations in the control of working memory. Curr Biol 30(9):1748–1754. e1744
Rizzuto DS, Madsen JR, Bromfield EB, Schulze-Bonhage A, Seelig D, Aschenbrenner-Scheibe R, Kahana MJ (2003) Reset of human neocortical oscillations during a working memory task. Proc Natl Acad Sci U S A 100(13):7931–7936
Roach BJ, Mathalon DH (2008) Event-related EEG time-frequency analysis: an overview of measures and an analysis of early gamma band phase locking in schizophrenia. Schizophr Bull 34(5):907–926
Ros T, Enriquez-Geppert S, Zotev V, Young KD, Wood G, Whitfield-Gabrieli S, Wan F, Vuilleumier P, Vialatte F, Van De Ville D, Todder D, Surmeli T, Sulzer JS, Strehl U, Sterman MB, Steiner NJ, Sorger B, Soekadar SR, Sitaram R, Sherlin LH, Schonenberg M, Scharnowski F, Schabus M, Rubia K, Rosa A, Reiner M, Pineda JA, Paret C, Ossadtchi A, Nicholson AA, Nan W, Minguez J, Micoulaud-Franchi JA, Mehler DMA, Luhrs M, Lubar J,

Lotte F, Linden DEJ, Lewis-Peacock JA, Lebedev MA, Lanius RA, Kubler A, Kranczioch C, Koush Y, Konicar L, Kohl SH, Kober SE, Klados MA, Jeunet C, Janssen TWP, Huster RJ, Hoedlmoser K, Hirshberg LM, Heunis S, Hendler T, Hampson M, Guggisberg AG, Guggenberger R, Gruzelier JH, Gobel RW, Gninenko N, Gharabaghi A, Frewen P, Fovet T, Fernandez T, Escolano C, Ehlis AC, Drechsler R, Christopher deCharms R, Debener S, De Ridder D, Davelaar EJ, Congedo M, Cavazza M, Breteler MHM, Brandeis D, Bodurka J, Birbaumer N, Bazanova OM, Barth B, Bamidis PD, Auer T, Arns M, Thibault RT (2020) Consensus on the reporting and experimental design of clinical and cognitive-behavioural neurofeedback studies (CRED-nf checklist). Brain 143(6):1674–1685

Roux F, Uhlhaas PJ (2014) Working memory and neural oscillations: alpha-gamma versus theta-gamma codes for distinct WM information? Trends Cogn Sci 18(1):16–25

Roux F, Wibral M, Mohr HM, Singer W, Uhlhaas PJ (2012) Gamma-band activity in human prefrontal cortex codes for the number of relevant items maintained in working memory. J Neurosci 32(36):12411–12420

Sauseng P, Liesefeld HR (2020) Cognitive control: brain oscillations coordinate human working memory. Curr Biol 30(9):R405–R407

Sauseng P, Klimesch W, Heise KF, Gruber WR, Holz E, Karim AA, Glennon M, Gerloff C, Birbaumer N, Hummel FC (2009) Brain oscillatory substrates of visual short-term memory capacity. Curr Biol 19(21):1846–1852

Semprini M, Bonassi G, Barban F, Pelosin E, Iandolo R, Chiappalone M, Mantini D, Avanzino L (2021) Modulation of neural oscillations during working memory update, maintenance, and readout: an hdEEG study. Hum Brain Mapp 42(4):1153–1166

Singh F, Shu IW, Granholm E, Pineda JA (2020a) Revisiting the potential of EEG neurofeedback for patients with schizophrenia. Schizophr Bull 46(4):741–742

Singh F, Shu IW, Hsu SH, Link P, Pineda JA, Granholm E (2020b) Modulation of frontal gamma oscillations improves working memory in schizophrenia. Neuroimage Clin 27:102339

Smucny J, Dienel SJ, Lewis DA, Carter CS (2022) Mechanisms underlying dorsolateral prefrontal cortex contributions to cognitive dysfunction in schizophrenia. Neuropsychopharmacology 47(1):292–308

Tallon-Baudry C, Bertrand O, Peronnet F, Pernier J (1998) Induced gamma-band activity during the delay of a visual short-term memory task in humans. J Neurosci 18(11):4244–4254

Uhlhaas PJ, Singer W (2015) Oscillations and neuronal dynamics in schizophrenia: the search for basic symptoms and translational opportunities. Biol Psychiatry 77(12):1001–1009

Weinberger DR, Berman KF, Zec RF (1986) Physiologic dysfunction of dorsolateral prefrontal cortex in schizophrenia. I. Regional cerebral blood flow evidence. Arch Gen Psychiatry 43(2):114–124

Woo TU, Miller JL, Lewis DA (1997) Schizophrenia and the parvalbumin-containing class of cortical local circuit neurons. Am J Psychiatry 154(7):1013–1015

Yan W, Liu X, Shan B, Zhang X, Pu Y (2021) Research on the emotions based on brain-computer technology: a bibliometric analysis and research agenda. Front Psychol 12:771591

Cognitive Dysfunction as a Risk Factor for Psychosis

Nicole R. Karcher, Jaisal Merchant, Jacob Pine, and Can Misel Kilciksiz

Contents

Abstract The current chapter summarizes recent evidence for cognition as a risk factor for the development of psychosis, including the range of cognitive impairments that exist across the spectrum of psychosis risk symptoms. The chapter examines several possible theories linking cognitive deficits with the development of psychotic symptoms, including evidence that cognitive deficits may be an intermediate risk factor linking genetic and/or neural metrics to psychosis spectrum symptoms. Although there is not strong evidence for unique cognitive markers associated specifically with psychosis compared to other forms of psychopathology, psychotic disorders are generally associated with the greatest severity of cognitive deficits. Cognitive deficits precede the development of psychotic symptoms and may

N. R. Karcher (✉) and C. M. Kilciksiz
Department of Psychiatry, School of Medicine, Washington University in St. Louis, St. Louis, MO, USA
e-mail: nkarcher@wustl.edu

J. Merchant and J. Pine
Department of Brain and Psychological Sciences, Washington University in St. Louis, St. Louis, MO, USA

Curr Topics Behav Neurosci (2023) 63: 173–204
https://doi.org/10.1007/7854_2022_387
Published Online: 22 August 2022

be detectable as early as childhood. Across the psychosis spectrum, both the presence and severity of psychotic symptoms are associated with mild to moderate impairments across cognitive domains, perhaps most consistently for language, cognitive control, and working memory domains. Research generally indicates the size of these cognitive impairments worsens as psychosis symptom severity increases. The chapter points out areas of unclarity and unanswered questions in each of these areas, including regarding the mechanisms contributing to the association between cognition and psychosis, the timing of deficits, and whether any cognitive systems can be identified that function as specific predictors of psychosis risk symptoms.

Keywords Clinical high risk · Cognition · Cognitive systems · Neurocognitive · Psychosis risk · Psychotic-like experiences

1 Introduction

The current chapter will examine cognitive deficits as a risk factor for psychosis. Psychosis is commonly defined as the experience of delusions, hallucinations, and thought disorder symptoms, symptoms that can occur as a feature of disorders such as schizophrenia as well as bipolar disorders (American Psychiatric Association 2013). Although only about 3% of the population receives a lifetime diagnosis of a threshold psychotic disorder (Perälä et al. 2007), psychosis spectrum symptoms occur in a much higher percentage of the general population, with prevalence estimates ranging from ~17–67% in childhood (Kelleher et al. 2012; Laurens et al. 2012) to ~3–5% in adulthood (van Os et al. 2009).

Psychotic symptoms are associated with a range of impairments in behavioral domains such as functioning, behavior, thought, speech, affect, and cognition. Cognitive dysfunction is recognized as a core deficit of psychotic disorders, with debate about even including cognitive deficits as a diagnostic symptom of psychotic disorders (Green et al. 2019; Keefe and Fenton 2007), in part owing to evidence that cognition functioning is strongly associated with functional outcomes in psychotic disorders (McCleery and Nuechterlein 2019). Due to the degree of cognitive and functional impairment associated with psychotic disorders, there is a push to understand risk factors associated with psychosis in order to benefit from early identification and prevention efforts. Risk factors often refer to antecedent conditions that predispose to the development of an outcome, such as a physical or mental health disorder (Werner and Smith 1992). This chapter will outline the current state of evidence for cognition as a risk factor for psychosis.

Cognition spans a broad range of domains (Fig. 1), and the current chapter will focus on both broad and specific cognitive abilities. Studies examining associations with psychosis spectrum symptoms have often focused on relationships with metrics of general intelligence, including IQ. Other studies have examined associations with

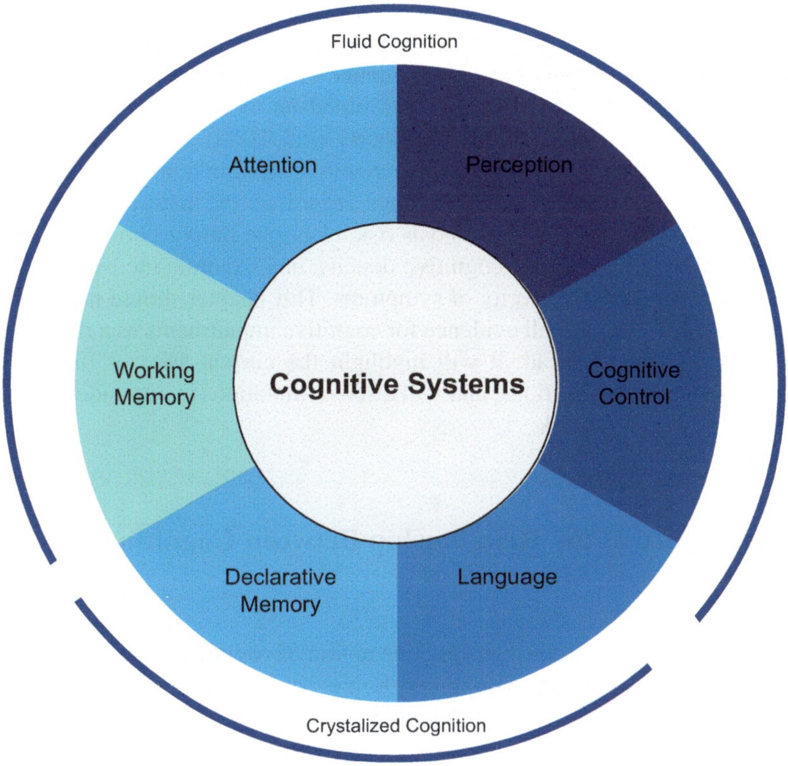

Fig. 1 Illustration of research domains of criteria (RDoC) cognitive domains discussed in the current chapter, including delineation of the overarching fluid and crystalized cognition domains

specific cognitive abilities. According to the Research Domains of Criteria (RDoC) initiative, cognitive systems include language abilities and declarative memory (also referred to as crystallized cognition; (Horn and Cattell 1967)), as well as attention, perception, working memory, and cognitive control (also referred to as fluid cognition). The current chapter will focus on associations between both general and specific cognitive abilities with psychosis risk.

Cognitive impairment in psychotic disorders is fairly ubiquitous. According to some evidence, approximately 80% of individuals diagnosed with a psychotic disorder exhibit marked cognitive deficits (Keefe and Fenton 2007). These deficits often begin well before the onset of the disorder, with some evidence for deficits occurring as early as childhood (Cannon et al. 2002; Mollon and Reichenberg 2017). However, despite the prevalence of cognitive deficits, there is substantial heterogeneity within the cognitive impairments exhibited by psychotic disorders. The heterogeneity found in psychotic disorders was in part the impetus behind RDoC efforts to better characterize these cognitive deficits (Cuthbert and Morris 2021). This research indicates that while the majority of individuals with cognitive disorders exhibit cognitive impairment, there is a subset of individuals with psychotic disorders who demonstrate cognitive performance within normal limits (Reichenberg et al. 2009). However, even in the absence of significant cognitive impairment, there is evidence that individuals with a primary psychotic disorder generally perform below what is expected based on their premorbid performance estimates (Reichenberg et al. 2005; Woodberry et al. 2008).

This chapter will outline evidence for cognitive dysfunction as a risk factor for psychotic disorders. It will detail findings regarding the nature of associations between cognition deficits and psychosis risk, elaborate on our current understanding of the scope and timing of cognitive deficits, and examine the extent to which cognitive deficits vary by severity of symptoms. This chapter should not be considered a systematic review of all evidence for cognitive impairments as a risk factor for psychosis risk states. Instead, it will highlight the current state of the evidence, several important considerations, and will discuss limitations in our understanding of cognition and psychosis risk.

2 The Nature of the Relationship Between Cognition and Psychosis Risk

There is a wealth of research supporting the notion of cognitive dysfunction as a risk factor for psychotic disorders (Kahn and Keefe 2013; McCleery and Nuechterlein 2019), although research has not fully elucidated whether the nature of this association is causal or correlational. The next section will detail several possible theories linking cognitive deficits with the development of psychotic symptoms. First, it is possible that cognitive deficits and psychosis may be causally linked (Fig. 2a; see Sect. 2.1). Second, the association between cognitive deficits and psychotic disorders may be correlational in nature, whereby genetic and/or pathophysiological markers may lead to both cognitive deficits and psychotic symptoms (Fig. 2b; see Sect. 2.3). Lastly, there is evidence indicating that cognition may be an intermediate risk factor linking genetic and/or pathophysiological markers to psychosis (Fig. 2c; see Sect. 2.2).

2.1 Cognitive Impairment as a Causal Mechanism for Psychosis

To constitute a causal factor or mechanism for psychosis, cognition would need to meet several requirements (Haynes et al. 2012). First, the two factors (psychosis and cognition) have to covary. There is a wealth of research supporting this tenet, much of which will be detailed in subsequent sections (Mollon and Reichenberg 2017; Sheffield et al. 2018). Second, there needs to be temporal precedence, such that cognitive impairments precede the development of psychosis. Evidence for

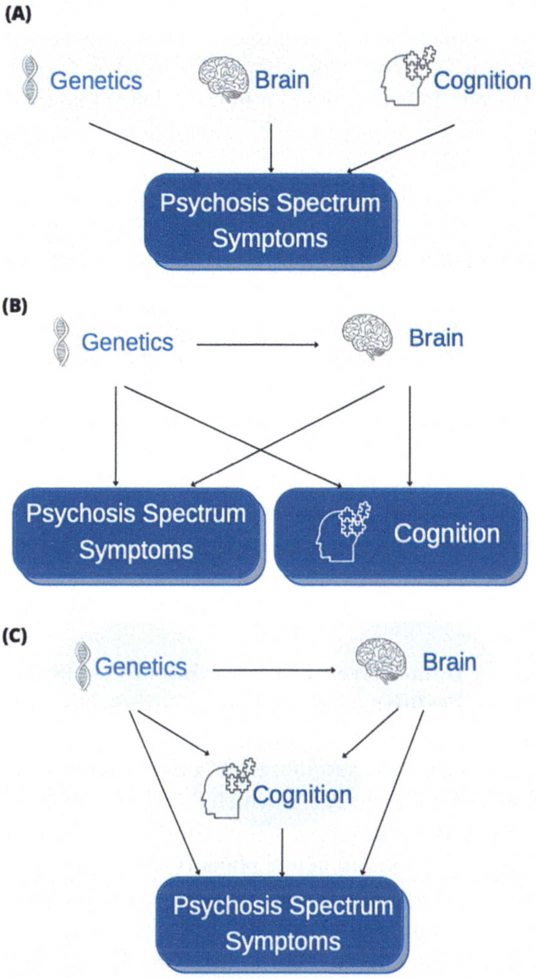

Fig. 2 Illustration of possible explanations for the link between cognition, neural and genetic metrics, and psychosis spectrum symptoms. At least three possibilities exist: (**a**) cognition, neural, and genetic metrics are each partially independently linked to psychosis spectrum symptoms. (**b**) Neural and genetic metrics are each linked to both cognition and psychosis spectrum symptoms. In this scenario, the associations between cognition and psychosis spectrum symptoms are attributable to shared mechanisms. (**c**) Cognition represents an intermediate phenotype, by which genetics and neural metrics lead to impairments in cognition, which then lead to psychosis spectrum symptoms

cognitive impairments preceding psychosis spectrum symptoms can be found in the form of premorbid cognitive deficits (Reichenberg et al. 2010; Sheffield et al. 2018) observable as early as childhood (Agnew-Blais et al. 2015; Kremen et al. 1998). Third, additional variables that may account for the relationship between cognition and psychosis must be ruled out. While those with psychotic symptoms tend to exhibit cognitive deficits, cognitive deficits in these populations frequently co-occur with other deficits and pathophysiological markers (Smeland and Andreassen 2018; Pruessner et al. 2017). Lastly, it is important to note that there are many disorders (e.g., behavioral, mood, anxiety disorders) that show evidence of impaired cognition (Abramovitch et al. 2021), making it unlikely that cognition is a causal factor specifically for psychosis. Thus, while there is evidence that cognition and psychosis have some elements required of a causal relationship (i.e., the two factors covary, there is evidence for temporal precedence of cognitive impairments), research generally fails to provide robust evidence that these associations are unique to either to cognition or psychotic disorders, thereby diminishing the likelihood of the causal hypothesis.

Additional potential evidence that cognition may not be directly related to psychotic symptoms comes from cognitive remediation literature. Several cognitive remediation interventions have been developed targeting cognitive deficits in psychotic disorders. A recent review of at-risk individuals found improvements in processing speed and verbal memory following cognitive remediation (Glenthøj et al. 2017). Although training was generally associated with functioning improvements, there were no significant improvements in symptoms, suggesting a lack of transference from improvement in cognition to improvement of psychotic symptoms. Further, there is other evidence that cognitive remediation does not result in improvements in at-risk individuals, findings that may be partially attributable to poor treatment adherence (Glenthøj et al. 2020). Thus, overall, while cognitive remediation therapies may improve cognitive deficits in psychotic disorders, these studies do not provide strong evidence for cognitive as a causal marker.

2.1.1 Data-Driven Classification of Psychosis Using Cognitive Performance

Recent research examining data-driven classifications of psychosis has also provided insight into the degree to which there is evidence for a causal link between cognition and psychosis risk. The search for data-driven classifications of psychotic disorders using cognitive and neural phenotypes arose as researchers have long recognized the heterogeneity of psychotic disorders. The creation of these classifications may be a potential solution for better organizing this heterogeneity, as well as better understanding the etiology of the disorder. These efforts are very much in line with the RDoC initiative, which posits that research should use tools such as neuroscience to re-examine the nature of psychiatric disorders, including schizophrenia. Much of the work developing new classifications using data from individuals with psychotic disorders has included broad cognitive batteries (e.g., the Measurement and Treatment Research to Improve Cognition in Schizophrenia [MATRICS] Consensus Cognitive Battery [MCCB]).

In general, these studies are consistent, finding a relatively "neuropsychologically normal" cluster, a globally and significantly impaired cluster, and a cluster (or two) of mixed or moderate impairment cognitive profiles (Crouse et al. 2018; Goldstein and Shemansky 1995; Lewandowski et al. 2018; Smucny et al. 2019). The first cluster generally consists of individuals diagnosed with psychotic disorders that lack impairments across cognitive system domains and exhibit average IQ scores (Green et al. 2020). The second cluster is generally defined as an intermediate cluster, consisting of individuals with mild impairments across cognitive system domains

(Green et al. 2020), with some evidence for larger, but still mild, impairments in cognitive control, language, attention, and working memory (Crouse et al. 2018). The last cluster is comprised of individuals showing significant cognitive deficits across cognitive domains (Green et al. 2020), with some evidence for particularly pronounced deficits in language and working memory (Crouse et al. 2018). Several of these studies have found evidence that these clusters transcend diagnostic boundaries (Seaton et al. 1999; Smucny et al. 2019). However, research finding a data-driven classification comprised of individuals with a psychotic disorder diagnosis but without significant cognitive impairments (i.e., the neuropsychologically normal' cluster; (Green et al. 2020)) makes the possibility that cognitive deficits represent a causal deficit more unlikely.

2.2 *Cognition as an Intermediate Risk Factor*

Another possibility is that cognitive deficits are the phenotypic manifestation of underlying genetic or neural abnormalities. In this scenario, cognition may not be a direct risk factor for psychosis, but instead may represent an intermediate phenotype, or a risk factor that lies between underlying genetic and neural abnormalities and the expression of psychosis spectrum symptoms (Fig. 2c) (Burdick et al. 2006; Ivleva et al. 2012). The following section will elaborate on evidence for cognitive deficits as intermediate phenotypic markers linking genetic and neural metrics with psychosis spectrum symptoms.

2.2.1 The Role of Genetics

Research is generally supportive of the notion that cognitive deficits may function as an intermediate phenotype between the symptoms of psychosis and more distal genetic variation (Mark and Toulopoulou 2016). First, decades of research support cognitive deficits reflecting underlying genetic variation in schizophrenia. Evidence indicates first-degree relatives of individuals with psychotic disorders show a variety of cognitive deficits (Hill et al. 2015; Hou et al. 2016; Keshavan et al. 2010). The majority of literature indicates evidence for some shared genetic risk between psychosis and cognitive impairments (Smeland and Andreassen 2018), although genomic studies have not fully elucidated the genetic architecture linking cognition to psychosis. Rare copy number variants (Genovese et al. 2016) are associated with both cognitive impairments (e.g., verbal recall deficits) and psychosis (Thygesen et al. 2020). Other evidence comes from a genome-wide association study finding evidence that higher cognitive test scores have a protective effect against the development of psychosis, with a smaller effect for psychotic symptoms predisposing individuals to impaired cognitive functioning (Savage et al. 2018). Overall, these studies highlight consistent evidence of genetic overlap of cognition and schizophrenia.

Recently, research has linked cognitive deficits and psychosis using polygenic risk scores (PRS), an index of genetic liability, with this research beginning to directly examine cognition as an intermediate phenotype between genetics and psychosis spectrum symptoms. There is evidence that genetic liability for educational attainment and IQ may be specifically associated with cognition in schizophrenia (Hubbard et al. 2016), even in comparison to major depressive disorder or bipolar disorder (Richards et al. 2020). In addition to schizophrenia, psychosis spectrum symptoms are also associated with polygenic liability for reduced educational attainment (Dwyer et al. 2020), and there is evidence in a childhood sample that this association is in part mediated by lower cognitive functioning (Karcher et al. 2020b). Other evidence in adults indicates that up to a third of the association between schizophrenia diagnosis and PRS is explained by cognitive functioning (Toulopoulou et al. 2019). Overall, research points to genetic overlap in cognition and schizophrenia, and signifies that the association between genetic liability and psychosis spectrum symptoms may be partially through cognitive impairments, providing support for the notion that cognitive impairments represent an intermediate phenotype of psychosis risk (Fig. 2c), as opposed to both cognitive impairments and psychosis risk sharing similar mechanisms (Fig. 2b).

2.2.2 The Role of Neural Metrics

Neural impairments in psychotic disorders are thought to derive from several sources, including the interplay of genetic factors and environmental sources, such as pre- and peri-natal complications (Cannon 2015; Davies et al. 2020). Neural impairments may progress across development as a function of neuromaturation, such as synaptic pruning, during adolescence (Uhlhaas 2011). There is also evidence that environmental factors, including toxins and stressful events, may progress neural impairments (Pruessner et al. 2017). There are a number of neural impairments associated with both cognitive impairments and psychosis that may at least partially explain the relationship between cognition and psychotic symptoms. Starting with structural evidence, there is evidence that psychosis spectrum symptoms are associated with widespread global brain volume and cortical thickness deficits (Cannon et al. 2015). There is also consistent evidence for lower volume and thickness in temporal regions (e.g., van Erp et al. 2018; Walton et al. 2017; Cullen et al. 2013). There is also consistent evidence for a decline in prefrontal cortical thickness, with evidence this occurs with increased severity of psychosis spectrum symptoms (Cannon et al. 2015; Chung et al. 2017; van Erp et al. 2018; Sun et al. 2009). Diffusion tensor imaging research also implicates alterations in white matter integrity, as measured by fractional anisotropy in psychosis risk (Kelly et al. 2018; Kubicki et al. 2007), including in anterior thalamic projections (Drakesmith et al. 2016). Resting-state functional connectivity research, which examines temporal correlations between spatially distinct brain regions, has also found widespread disruptions associated with psychosis spectrum symptoms. For example, research consistently finds decreased fronto-parietal network connectivity [e.g., involved in goal representation (Dosenbach et al. 2008)] in psychotic disorders (Dandash et al. 2014; Fornito et al. 2013; Horga et al. 2016; Yoon et al. 2014; Woodward and Heckers 2016). Research also generally implicates disrupted salience/cingulo-opercular network connectivity [e.g., information integration, salience attribution (Palaniyappan and Liddle 2012; Uddin 2015)] in psychosis spectrum symptoms (Peters et al. 2017; Raij et al. 2015; Karcher et al. 2019).

As with genetics, there are a number of studies linking these neural impairments to cognitive functioning in psychosis spectrum symptoms. Evidence links impaired executive functioning, including cognitive control and working memory abilities, to prefrontal volume in psychotic disorders (Broome et al. 2009; Eisenberg and Berman 2010; Tronchin et al. 2020). There is a wealth of evidence linking impaired relational memory to hippocampal function in psychosis (Avery et al. 2019; Mathew et al. 2014; Tamminga et al. 2010). Altered fronto-parietal network connectivity is associated with reduced cognitive functioning, perhaps specifically for verbal learning, in psychotic disorders (Woodward and Heckers 2016). There is also evidence that cognition may function as an intermediate phenotype between neural metrics and psychosis spectrum symptoms (Fig. 2c). Research finds impaired white matter integrity in regions relating to fronto-medial pathways (e.g., anterior thalamic projections) may partially mediate associations between childhood IQ and psychotic experiences (Drakesmith et al. 2016). For cingulo-opercular connectivity, there is evidence consistent with general cognitive ability partially mediating the association between connectivity and psychosis spectrum symptoms (Sheffield et al. 2016, 2017). Although future research will need to parse out associations specific to psychotic disorders compared to other forms of psychopathology (Friedman and Robbins 2021), this research generally supports the notion that cognitive functioning may act as an intermediate phenotype between neural impairments and psychosis spectrum symptoms.

2.3 Symptom Correlation Evidence

Although evidence exists that there are genetic and neural markers may partially produce the association between cognitive deficits and psychotic symptoms, alternative models may at least explain some of this association. It is likely that as psychosis spectrum symptoms worsen, cognitive performance may worsen in part as a function of the nature of the symptoms. By definition, psychotic symptoms involve a significant interference in thinking, and therefore any cognitive assessment performed while experiencing psychotic symptoms may be influenced by the severity of this interference (Moritz et al. 2021). This interference in thinking by psychotic symptoms may not be well captured by current assessments of symptom severity.

Other symptoms prevalent in psychotic disorders, including disorganized and negative symptoms, are also associated with cognitive impairments and likely contribute to associations between cognitive deficits and psychosis risk. Disorganized symptoms may be even more strongly associated with cognitive impairments than reality distortion (Ventura et al. 2010). As with positive symptoms, cognitive impairments may partly reflect the manifestation of disorganized symptoms during cognitive performance (e.g., disorganized speech making it challenging to perform certain cognitive tasks). There is strong evidence for associations between negative symptoms and cognitive performance, as well as evidence that negative symptoms may mediate the association between cognitive impairments and impairments in functioning (Meyer et al. 2014). Some have even theorized that cognitive impairments and some negative symptoms may be inextricably related (Pelletier-Baldelli and Holt 2020). For example, some deficits in task performance may reflect symptoms such as alogia (i.e., paucity of speech) and amotivation (i.e., paucity of motivation). Evidence indicates that motivation, including willingness to expend effort, may predict up to 24% of the variance in cognitive scores in schizophrenia (Bismark et al. 2018). To this end, there is some evidence that negative symptoms may be the downstream reflection of cognitive impairments, perhaps specifically impairments in social cognition (Pelletier-Baldelli and Holt 2020). However, there is other research suggesting the two concepts may be separable (Harvey et al. 2006). It is also likely that other symptoms contribute to cognitive deficits, including anxiety and depression (Moritz et al. 2021). Thus, it is likely that clinical symptoms, including disorganized symptoms, negative symptoms, depression, and anxiety, may contribute to associations between cognitive impairments and psychosis risk.

3 Specificity of Cognitive Deficits

Cognitive dysfunction is not unique to psychosis spectrum disorders. There is evidence that cognition may be a risk factor for general psychopathology. Evidence for this comes from research indicating that deficits in cognitive functioning are associated with a general factor for psychopathology, or p-factor (Castellanos-Ryan et al. 2016). Moreover, cognitive dysfunction is present in virtually all mental health conditions, from depression, anxiety, trauma disorders, ADHD, conduct, and substance use disorders (Abramovitch et al. 2021). Several indices, perhaps most strongly aspects of executive functioning including cognitive control and working memory, may represent transdiagnostic risk factors for the development of psychopathology (Huang-Pollock et al. 2017; McTeague et al. 2016). Although the current chapter does not cover cognitive deficits associated with these other disorders, it is critical to point out that research increasingly indicates that cognitive deficits are not specifically implicated in psychosis risk, but rather are considered a transdiagnostic risk factor for psychopathology (Abramovitch et al. 2021). Further, there is no cognitive impairment marker that has been consistently implicated in specifically psychosis spectrum disorders and is absent in other disorders (Moritz et al. 2021). However, it is often the case that these cognitive deficits are most strongly associated with psychosis spectrum symptoms (McCleery and Nuechterlein 2019). Thus, while cognitive deficits are present in a range of psychopathology, these deficits may be more pronounced and severe in psychosis spectrum symptoms.

4 Associations Between Cognitive Deficits with Symptom Severity

Research has accumulated that psychotic disorders are neurodevelopmental in nature (Weinberger 1987; McCleery and Nuechterlein 2019), with subtle cognitive deficits preceding the onset of psychotic symptoms. Decades of research on the timing of these deficits suggests that lesser abnormalities in neurocognitive domains precede the onset of psychotic symptoms by years or even decades (Mollon et al. 2018; Reichenberg et al. 2010). Evidence indicates that for children and adolescents who later develop schizophrenia, there are premorbid IQ deficits of approximately eight points (Woodberry et al. 2008). Research indicates large effect-sized premorbid cognitive deficits are evident in many cognition domains prior to the onset of psychotic disorders (McCleery and Nuechterlein 2019).

The following section will detail deficits associated with stages of psychotic symptom development—from early psychosis spectrum symptoms to the transition to threshold psychosis. Overall, research supports the idea that cognitive deficits increase with severity of symptoms, such that early psychosis spectrum symptoms are associated with the smallest magnitude of cognitive deficits, followed by attenuated psychotic symptoms, with transition to psychotic disorders associated with the largest magnitude cognitive deficits (Fig. 3).

However, the exact reason for this gradient is not entirely known. Neurodevelopmental theories posit that cognitive deficits are the result of factors (e.g., genetic) leading to neural impairments that then result in impairments in the acquisition of cognitive skills and abilities throughout development (Weinberger 1987). It is possible that cognitive deficits increase with severity of symptoms, with some evidence to support this notion. Longitudinal studies, for example, indicate declines in cognitive performance when comparing cognitive abilities prior to and after the onset of psychosis illness (Fig. 3a; (Meier et al. 2014; Reichenberg et al. 2010)). Evidence indicates that amongst those that later develop psychotic symptoms, overall cognitive performance declines through adolescence and early adulthood, although there is limited evidence for declines in declarative memory in early childhood (Mollon et al. 2018). There is also evidence that rather than declines, these increasing deficits compared to controls are the result of slower growth in cognitive abilities over time, resulting in lags in cognitive abilities. This delayed development may be especially the case for verbal reasoning and spatial processing abilities (Sheffield et al. 2018). It is also possible the association between symptom severity and greater cognitive impairments reflects that less severe groups, such as those with early psychosis spectrum symptoms, are more heterogeneous with respect to future clinical outcomes and that effect sizes increase as groups become increasingly distilled to those that are truly at risk for the development of psychosis (Fig. 3b). It is important to note that no studies to our knowledge have examined cognitive domain deficits across the entire psychosis symptom spectrum, research that is necessary to clarify some of these questions. Further, it will be important to focus

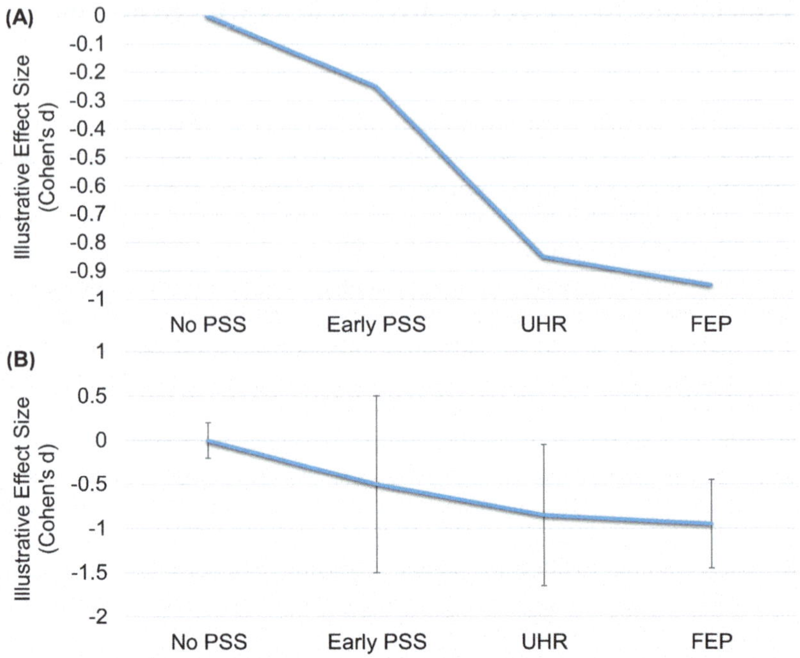

Fig. 3 Severity of cognitive impairments across the gradient of psychosis spectrum symptoms (PSS). (**a**) This gradient may reflect increasing cognitive impairments that correspond with symptom severity. (**b**) It is also possible that while cognitive impairment increases with symptom severity, differences between groups may be partially driven by heterogeneity of defined groups (as reflected in the error bars). Perhaps only those that are at-risk for the development of psychotic symptoms show marked cognitive deficits, with individuals why do not go on to develop significant PSS show lessened (or no) cognitive deficits. This would contribute to variability and therefore overall appearance of lessened cognitive deficits in these groups (especially for early PSS)

on cognitive tests more closely tied to neural function to help aid in the progression of our understanding of mechanisms underlying psychosis spectrum symptoms.

However, even if effect size differences between psychosis risk groups (Fig. 3) reflect an association between increased severity of cognitive deficits and increased severity of symptoms, the nature of this association is still unclear. There are several factors that may influence this association between cognitive deficits and symptom severity. As discussed above, possible explanations include that this may reflect the nature of the symptoms (i.e., increased psychotic symptoms leading to poorer test scores). There is some evidence psychosis may be associated with an exaggeration of the neuromaturation processes that occur over adolescence, such that psychosis may be associated with more pronounced synaptic pruning, structural changes, and alterations in hormonal functioning (Trotman et al. 2013; Walker and Bollini 2002). It is therefore possible that differences between groups are due to increased pathophysiological impairments over time worsening cognitive symptoms. It is also important to note that the timing of the onset of cognitive deficits is presumably variable across individuals. A number of factors may contribute to this variability of onset and degree of impairment, including the nature of these deficits (e.g., neural impairments) as well as buffering resiliency factors. The following sections will briefly discuss and summarize a review of the studies published over the past decade which have investigated changes in cognition among populations experiencing psychotic-like experiences, as well as high-risk populations, including those that transition to psychotic disorder.

4.1 Psychotic-Like Experiences

Cognitive deficits are present at a subclinical phase of the psychosis spectrum in early ages (Gur et al. 2014), although evidence indicates that these deficits are less pronounced compared to first episode psychosis and afterwards (Seidman et al. 2010). Investigating cognitive deficits among populations experiencing psychotic-like experiences (PLEs) may aid in helping clinicians detect vulnerable individuals in the general population prior to the development of a psychotic disorder. However, literature on cognitive deficits among early psychosis spectrum symptoms is limited (Sheffield et al. 2018).

Several studies have investigated the relationship between childhood and adolescent PLEs and cognition over the past decade. Although the number of studies examining associations between PLEs and cognition is dwarfed in comparison to those examining high-risk populations, there are a burgeoning number of studies examining these impairments. Research has found evidence for overall general cognitive deficits associated with increased PLEs (Laurens and Cullen 2016).

Overall, the majority of studies examining associations with PLEs and cognition have found impairments in a range of specific cognitive metrics. Of these metrics, the greatest support is for impairments in executive functioning abilities (Dickson et al. 2018; Hegarty et al. 2019; Karcher et al. 2020a; Laurens and Cullen 2016; O'Brien et al. 2020; Rossi et al. 2016; Ziermans 2013; Karcher et al. 2018), with a number of studies showing that specifically lower working memory is associated with increased PLEs (Hegarty et al. 2019; Laurens and Cullen 2016; O'Brien et al. 2020; Rossi et al. 2016; Ziermans 2013; Karcher et al. 2018). Further, a limited number of studies have found evidence for impairments in language abilities, including in tasks assessing receptive language (Karcher et al. 2020a; Dickson et al. 2018) and vocabulary (Dickson et al. 2018). To a lesser degree, deficits in other cognitive abilities have also been associated with PLEs, including episodic memory (Hegarty et al. 2019; Laurens and Cullen 2016), and attention (Hegarty et al. 2019; Kim et al. 2012). Studies have begun to delve into the nature of these associations, finding that working memory capacity is inversely associated with the presence of bizarre experiences and persecutory ideas (Ziermans 2013). There is also evidence that thought content disturbances may be associated with attentional deficits (Kim et al. 2012).

Although the number of studies examining PLEs has drastically increased over the past decade, there are still a number of limitations and future directions to this research. First, there is a great deal of variability to these studies, including in sample characteristics such as age, with some samples spanning into adulthood (e.g., (Hegarty et al. 2019; Ziermans 2013). In comparison to the research outlined above in childhood and adolescence, much of the work examining PLEs in adulthood demonstrates similar patterns of cognitive deficits (e.g., (Alderson-Day et al. 2019; de Leede-Smith et al. 2020; Dzafic et al. 2020; Evermann et al. 2020; Sheffield et al. 2016), although notably there is also evidence for processing speed impairments in adult populations (Rössler et al. 2015; Wallace et al. 2019)). Additionally, the vast majority of studies have examined cross-sectional investigations, with only two main studies that investigated longitudinal relationships between PLEs and cognition, information that informs how associations may change over time. For example, one longitudinal study found evidence indicating that the presence of PLEs at the age of 53 was significantly predicted by the lower cognitive scores at the age of 8, 11, and 15 (Barnett et al. 2012), potentially consistent with the neurodevelopmental hypothesis of psychosis. Another study (Dickson et al. 2018) showed evidence that individuals endorsing PLEs showed varied trajectories across cognitive domains, with some domains showing impairments that emerged early and remained stable in verbal working memory, verbal functioning, and executive functioning. Other domains showed evidence of early lagging deficits that eventually improved over time, including verbal memory and visual memory, information that furthers our understanding of changes in symptoms over time.

4.2 High-Risk Populations

In comparison to PLEs, there is a great deal of research examining cognitive deficits in clinical high-risk (CHR) populations. Clinical high-risk for psychosis, prodromal, and ultra-high-risk are terms utilized to describe elevated risk for the development of a first episode of psychosis, including experiencing attenuated psychotic symptoms. In terms of cognitive impairments, individuals at clinical high risk for psychosis often exhibit deficits in generalized neurocognitive function based on general IQ scores. The available evidence suggests that there is a small difference in IQ between CHR and otherwise healthy individuals, although this effect does not reliably demonstrate statistical significance. A number of studies find statistically significant differences between CHR and otherwise healthy individuals with regard to generalized IQ (Goghari et al. 2014; Kristensen et al. 2019; Lencz et al. 2006; Seidman et al. 2016; Tor et al. 2020), with others finding no significant differences (Addington et al. 2012; Corcoran et al. 2015; Gill et al. 2014; Ilonen et al. 2010; Lee et al. 2015; Magaud et al. 2014). Furthermore, analyses conducted as part of the Enhancing Neuro Imaging Genetics through Meta-Analysis (ENIGMA) consortium demonstrate statistically significant effects for IQ in less than half of all CHR HC study comparisons, based on a 0.05 alpha value (Jalbrzikowski et al. 2021). Nevertheless, meta-analyses of neurocognition in CHR individuals posit a small but present effect for IQ across comparisons of CHR and otherwise healthy individuals (hedges *G* ranging from −0.21 to −0.31 (Catalan et al. 2021; Fusar-Poli et al. 2012; Hauser et al. 2017)).

In terms of specific cognitive abilities, studies generally find small and inconsistent effects of cognitive abilities traditionally falling within the crystallized neurocognitive domain in CHR samples. Many studies find statistically significant differences between CHR and otherwise healthy individuals with respect to receptive language assessments (Brewer et al. 2003; Kristensen et al. 2019; Ohmuro et al. 2016, 2018; Seidman et al. 2016), although other studies do not find this effect (Becker et al. 2010; Koshiyama et al. 2018; Lepock et al. 2020; Simon et al. 2012). Along these lines, recent meta-analyses estimate the overall effect for crystallized neurocognition in CHR to be small-to-moderate in size, however, the confidence intervals for these estimates are noticeably larger than other neurocognitive indices, with some including zero (Hauser et al. 2017). Of the few studies that do report data on declarative knowledge assessments, these studies tend to find no differences between CHR and otherwise healthy individuals (Ilonen et al. 2010; Magaud et al. 2014).

In terms of other cognitive abilities traditionally falling under the fluid cognition domain, recent meta-analyses suggest that CHR individuals exhibit significant deficits in processing speed, attention, working memory, verbal learning, and executive function (Catalan et al. 2021; de Paula et al. 2015; Fusar-Poli et al. 2012; Giuliano et al. 2012; Hauser et al. 2017; Zheng et al. 2018). At present, there is limited evidence that CHR individuals exhibit deficits in any specific cognitive domain in particular. The most severe deficits, across studies, appear to be in the domains of processing speed (standardized mean difference (SMD) = −1.21 (Carrión et al. 2011; Zheng et al. 2018), hedge's $G = -0.427$ (Hauser et al. 2017)), visual-spatial working memory (mean weighted effect size = −0.71 (Bora et al. 2014)), and verbal memory (SMD = −0.5 (Giuliano et al. 2012)). Furthermore, to a lesser extent, other studies have found specific deficits in episodic memory (Greenland-White et al. 2017) and semantic verbal fluency (Hwang et al. 2019). Some work suggests that specific neurocognitive domains represent markers for psychosis risk or disease progression in CHR individuals, such as processing speed (Randers et al. 2021) and executive functioning (Frommann et al. 2011; Randers et al. 2021).

Overall, for CHR, there is robust evidence for impairments across cognitive domains, with some evidence for potentially stronger effects in the domains of visual-spatial working memory, verbal memory, and processing speed. However, there are several limitations to the extant literature, including variability in the definition of CHR. Individuals can meet the CHR category via differing paths, including experiencing Attenuated Psychotic Symptoms (APS), experiencing Brief (and Limited) Intermittent Psychotic Symptoms (BLIPS or BIPS), or by meeting criteria for Genetic Risk and Deterioration Syndrome (GRD). Research has not disentangled whether these different CHR categories vary in cognitive deficits.

4.3 Transition from CHR to First Episode

Understanding neurocognitive factors that predict whether CHR individuals will later convert to threshold psychosis is critical to efforts for early identification and prevention of psychotic disorders. There are mixed data regarding whether individuals at the prodromal phase show additional neurocognitive decline after conversion to psychosis. While some longitudinal studies have found a significant decline in certain neurocognitive domains from the CHR state to threshold psychosis (Jahshan et al. 2010; Wood et al. 2007), other work reports either no significant neurocognitive differences after conversion (Allott et al. 2013; Hawkins et al. 2008) or that CHR individuals who later transition to psychosis show similar cognitive performance to first-episode psychosis patients (Carrión et al. 2018; Eastvold et al. 2007; Liu et al. 2015; Wood et al. 2007). Similarly, one meta-analysis found no evidence of cognitive decline from high-risk to psychosis conversion states and suggested that cognitive decline is established at the prodromal phase of psychosis without a continued decrease at illness onset (Bora and Murray 2014). Overall, longitudinal research comparing baseline neuropsychological performance in CHR individuals who later convert to psychosis (CHR-C) versus those who not (CHR-NC) suggests a link between baseline neurocognition in CHR and a later psychotic disorder diagnosis (Addington et al. 2019; Hauser et al. 2017; Zaytseva et al. 2015). However, there are mixed findings, especially with regard to which specific cognitive domains are predictive of psychosis onset.

In terms of cognitive systems, there is some evidence for both generalized and specific cognitive domains implicated in the transition to psychosis. First, in terms of generalized cognitive abilities, there is limited evidence for premorbid IQ impairments, as assessed by receptive language (Wells et al. 2015), with transition to psychosis (Pukrop et al. 2007; Ziermans et al. 2014). Most research suggests that premorbid IQ does not differ between CHR-C and CHR-NC (Becker et al. 2010; Seidman et al. 2016). However, some work has found worse premorbid IQ in CHR-Cs than CHR-NCs (Metzler et al. 2016). There is also evidence that the level of decline in IQ from premorbid to CHR states may be predictive of increased psychotic symptoms or conversion to psychosis (Cosway et al. 2000; Woodberry et al. 2010).

There are several specific cognitive domains that have been implicated in CHR and later conversion to psychosis. A primary cognitive domain implicated in this distinction between CHR-C and CHR-NC involves language abilities traditionally falling within the fluid cognitive domain (e.g., verbal memory). Many studies find that verbal learning, memory, and/or fluency serve as primary significant predictors of conversion to psychosis or demonstrate significant differences between CHR-C and CHR-NC at baseline (Addington et al. 2016; Carrión et al. 2018; Kim et al. 2011; Lencz et al. 2006; Metzler et al. 2016; Mittal et al. 2010; Pukrop et al. 2007; Simon et al. 2012; Woodberry et al. 2010), differentiate between these groups at a trend-level (Brewer et al. 2005; Whyte et al. 2006), or show significantly worse performance compared to healthy controls in CHR-C but not CHR-NC (Becker et al.

2010; Eastvold et al. 2007). Still, as with every examined cognitive domain, there is research that has not replicated this relationship (De Herdt et al. 2013). Research has also suggested that baseline executive functioning, including cognitive control (Bolt et al. 2019; Koutsouleris et al. 2010; Guo et al. 2020) and working memory (Bolt et al. 2019; Carrión et al. 2018; Keefe et al. 2006; Kim et al. 2011; Metzler et al. 2016; Pukrop et al. 2007), as well as processing speed (Addington et al. 2016; Bolt et al. 2019; Metzler et al. 2016; Pukrop et al. 2007), and visual or spatial memory (Bang et al. 2015; Brewer et al. 2005; Kim et al. 2011; Lin et al. 2013) serve as predominant predictors of later psychosis conversion. There is also literature that indicates a distinction between CHR-C and CHR-NC on factors such as attention (Keefe et al. 2006), but these findings are more limited and mixed.

Further support for the importance of verbal abilities, as well as processing speed, in predicting risk for the development of psychosis comes from recent advances in the development of psychosis risk calculators. These calculators include demographic, clinical, functioning, and cognitive metrics to predict risk for the development of a psychotic disorder (Cannon et al. 2016; Carrion et al. 2016; Fusar-Poli et al. 2017). One such calculator consistently finds that both processing speed and verbal learning impairments contribute to the prediction of psychosis within a 2-year period (Cannon et al. 2016; Carrion et al. 2016). Although currently only validated in CHR populations, these calculators may represent a critical tool for early prediction efforts.

It is worth noting the variety of possible confounds in this literature that could contribute to the mixed results. First, across studies, there is a large range in the number of CHR individuals who convert to psychosis (CHR-C n range = ~5–93, with the majority falling on the lower end), with smaller studies having lower power to detect differences between groups. These studies also vary widely in the follow-up period for which the potential for conversion is tracked (follow-up range = ~6 months to >10 years). Additionally, differing diagnoses within psychosis conversion could affect findings. Some research limits CHR-C analyses to non-affective psychosis (Lencz et al. 2006; Metzler et al. 2016), while others include affective psychosis in the results (Walder et al. 2008; Woodberry et al. 2010). Similarly, differing inclusion criteria for high-risk individuals, from limiting to those at clinical ultra-high risk of psychosis (Ziermans et al. 2014) to also including those at genetic high risk (Eastvold et al. 2007) could confound results. Regardless of these limitations, overall, performance on measures of cognitive domains such as language abilities and executive functioning (e.g., working memory, cognitive control) in CHR individuals show the most robust evidence as predictors of transition to psychosis.

4.4 Overall Limitations and Considerations

Several limitations may generally contribute to differences across research examining associations between cognition and psychosis risk. Differing decisions about covariate use in predictive models could affect findings, as many of these studies reported distinct results with and without controlling for additional variables and studies varied on their covariates of choice. Additionally, the choice of which cognitive domains to assess and the specific tests within each of these domains likely contributes to heterogeneity in findings. Studies vary greatly in their conceptualization and measurement of cognition, making it challenging to compare across studies. While some studies included cognitive batteries (Cui 2020; Hegarty et al. 2019; Karcher et al. 2020a) or an array of cognitive tests (Barnett et al. 2012; Becker et al. 2010; Dickson et al. 2018; Laurens and Cullen 2016; Simon et al. 2012), many studies included one or a couple of cognitive measures of interest (e.g., Kristensen et al. 2019; Lepock et al. 2020; Seidman et al. 2016), making it unclear whether results would more broadly generalize if uniform measures of cognition had been administered. Utilizing the developing RDoC framework in future studies may minimize such confounds and tie more closely to neural mechanisms. Additionally, it is quite possible that results vary depending on the measures used to define psychosis spectrum symptoms. For PLEs, measures included the Schizotypal Personality Questionnaire (Rössler et al. 2015), Prodromal Questionnaire-Brief Child version (Karcher et al. 2018, 2020a; O'Brien et al. 2020), Psychosis-Like Symptom Interview (Rossi et al. 2016), Psychotic-Like Experiences Questionnaire (Dickson et al. 2018; Laurens and Cullen 2016), Community Assessment of Psychic Experiences (Evermann et al. 2020; Ziermans 2013), and the Eppendorf Schizophrenia Inventory (Kim et al. 2012). Along these lines, CHR research utilizes different measures (e.g., Structured Interview for Psychosis Risk Syndromes (Woods et al. 2019), CAARMS (Yung et al. 2005)) to measure whether participants meet CHR criteria.

5 Summary

Evidence indicates that neurocognitive deficits are an important risk factor for psychosis. The current chapter summarized this evidence, including that a range of cognitive impairments exists across the spectrum of psychosis risk. Evidence exists that cognitive impairments emerge early, often in childhood, and that these early cognitive impairments are generally milder and increase in severity in tandem with symptom severity. However, it is still unclear how early in development cognitive impairments emerge. It is also unclear whether some of the differences in effect sizes of cognitive impairments can be explained by the heterogeneity of risk groups. It is likewise unclear whether there are cognitive markers that can be utilized to differentiate psychosis risk compared to risk for other disorders. Third, the mechanisms for these cognitive impairments are also not fully elucidated. Consistent with Fig. 2c, it is likely that cognitive deficits act as an intermediate phenotype: genetic and neural impairments, perhaps in conjunction with other factors such as environment, may interact to exacerbate cognitive impairments, which in turn could lead to psychosis spectrum symptoms. Research is still elucidating these exact mechanisms, although they likely involve the combination of genetic and neural factors, including the prefrontal cortex and several subcortical structures (e.g., hippocampus, thalamus). Symptoms such as anxiety, depression, negative symptoms, disorganization, and distraction from positive symptoms, may also contribute to cognitive deficits either through similar or independent mechanisms.

To summarize cognitive deficits across symptom severity, the evidence provides support for both generalized cognitive deficits, as well as some specific cognitive systems that appear to be associated with more consistent impairments across symptom severity. Overall, across symptom severity, there are mild to moderate impairments in generalized cognition (Barnett et al. 2012; Fusar-Poli et al. 2012; Hauser et al. 2017; Karcher et al. 2020a). However, given that a number of studies use indices of receptive language abilities as metrics of premorbid IQ, it can be challenging to tease generalized deficits apart from specific deficits in language abilities. In terms of other specific cognitive domains, psychosis spectrum symptoms show deficits in indices of executive functioning, including working memory (Bolt et al. 2019; Bora and Murray 2014; Carrión et al. 2011; Hegarty et al. 2019; Ziermans 2013) and verbal fluency (Hwang et al. 2019; Metzler et al. 2016; Woodberry et al. 2010). Additionally, there is evidence for impairments in memory (Bang et al. 2015; Hegarty et al. 2019; J Giuliano et al. 2012; Lin et al. 2013) and processing speed (Addington et al. 2016; Bolt et al. 2019; Carrión et al. 2011; Metzler et al. 2016; Wallace et al. 2019; Zheng et al. 2018) across the psychosis spectrum, with the most severe deficits found for CHR and the transition to psychosis (Carrión et al. 2018; Metzler et al. 2016). There is also evidence that lower verbal abilities may be particularly predictive of the transition to psychosis (Addington et al. 2016; Carrión et al. 2018).

Although there is some evidence that these impairments may worsen with symptom severity, greater research is needed to determine the extent to which variation is due to symptom severity versus other possible confounding factors such as differences in cognitive tests used, heterogeneity of groups, and low sample sizes. Regardless of these unanswered questions, cognitive impairments constitute an important risk factor for psychosis. It is critical to better understand the exact nature, timing, and specificity of cognitive deficits in psychosis, in order to develop effective identification and remediation treatments to target these impairments. Future research should begin to develop and use cognitive tests that align with the RDoC framework of cognitive systems and are more closely tied to neural functions, in order to more comprehensively examine cognitive impairments across the psychosis symptom spectrum.

References

Abramovitch A, Short T, Schweiger A (2021) The c factor: cognitive dysfunction as a transdiagnostic dimension in psychopathology. Clin Psychol Rev:102007

Addington J, Piskulic D, Perkins D, Woods SW, Liu L, Penn DL (2012) Affect recognition in people at clinical high risk of psychosis. Schizophr Res 140(1–3):87–92

Addington J, Liu L, Perkins DO, Carrion RE, Keefe RS, Woods SW (2016) The role of cognition and social functioning as predictors in the transition to psychosis for youth with attenuated psychotic symptoms. Schizophr Bull:sbw152

Addington J, Farris M, Stowkowy J, Santesteban-Echarri O, Metzak P, Kalathil MS (2019) Predictors of transition to psychosis in individuals at clinical high risk. Curr Psychiatry Rep 21(6): 1–10

Agnew-Blais JC, Buka SL, Fitzmaurice GM, Smoller JW, Goldstein JM, Seidman LJ (2015) Early childhood IQ trajectories in individuals later developing schizophrenia and affective psychoses in the New England family studies. Schizophr Bull 41(4):817–823. https://doi.org/10.1093/schbul/sbv027

Alderson-Day B, Smailes D, Moffatt J, Mitrenga K, Moseley P, Fernyhough C (2019) Intentional inhibition but not source memory is related to hallucination-proneness and intrusive thoughts in a university sample. Cortex 113:267–278

Allott KA, Cotton SM, Chinnery GL, Baksheev GN, Massey J, Sun P, Collins Z, Barlow E, Broussard C, Wahid T (2013) The relative contribution of neurocognition and social cognition to 6-month vocational outcomes following individual placement and support in first-episode psychosis. Schizophr Res 150(1):136–143

American Psychiatric Association (2013) Diagnostic and statistical manual of mental disorders, 5th edn. https://doi.org/10.1176/appi.books.9780890425596

Avery SN, McHugo M, Armstrong K, Blackford JU, Woodward ND, Heckers S (2019) Disrupted habituation in the early stage of psychosis. Biol Psychiatry: Cogn Neurosci Neuroimaging 4(11):1004–1012

Bang M, Kim KR, Song YY, Baek S, Lee E, An SK (2015) Neurocognitive impairments in individuals at ultra-high risk for psychosis: who will really convert? Aust N Z J Psychiatry 49(5):462–470

Barnett JH, McDougall F, Xu MK, Croudace TJ, Richards M, Jones PB (2012) Childhood cognitive function and adult psychopathology: associations with psychotic and non-psychotic symptoms in the general population. Br J Psychiatry 201(2):124–130

Becker H, Nieman D, Wiltink S, Dingemans P, Van de Fliert J, Velthorst E, De Haan L, Van Amelsvoort T, Linszen D (2010) Neurocognitive functioning before and after the first psychotic episode: does psychosis result in cognitive deterioration? Psychol Med 40(10):1599–1606

Bismark AW, Thomas ML, Tarasenko M, Shiluk AL, Rackelmann SY, Young JW, Light GA (2018) Relationship between effortful motivation and neurocognition in schizophrenia. Schizophr Res 193:69–76

Bolt LK, Amminger GP, Farhall J, McGorry PD, Nelson B, Markulev C, Yuen HP, Schäfer MR, Mossaheb N, Schlögelhofer M (2019) Neurocognition as a predictor of transition to psychotic disorder and functional outcomes in ultra-high risk participants: findings from the NEURAPRO randomized clinical trial. Schizophr Res 206:67–74

Bora E, Murray RM (2014) Meta-analysis of cognitive deficits in ultra-high risk to psychosis and first-episode psychosis: do the cognitive deficits progress over, or after, the onset of psychosis? Schizophr Bull 40(4):744–755

Bora E, Lin A, Wood S, Yung A, McGorry P, Pantelis C (2014) Cognitive deficits in youth with familial and clinical high risk to psychosis: a systematic review and meta-analysis. Acta Psychiatr Scand 130(1):1–15

Brewer WJ, Wood SJ, McGorry PD, Francey SM, Phillips LJ, Yung AR, Anderson V, Copolov DL, Singh B, Velakoulis D (2003) Impairment of olfactory identification ability in individuals at ultra-high risk for psychosis who later develop schizophrenia. Am J Psychiatr 160(10): 1790–1794

Brewer WJ, Francey SM, Wood SJ, Jackson HJ, Pantelis C, Phillips LJ, Yung AR, Anderson VA, McGorry PD (2005) Memory impairments identified in people at ultra-high risk for psychosis who later develop first-episode psychosis. Am J Psychiatr 162(1):71–78

Broome MR, Matthiasson P, Fusar-Poli P, Woolley JB, Johns LC, Tabraham P, Bramon E, Valmaggia L, Williams SC, Brammer MJ (2009) Neural correlates of executive function and working memory in the 'at-risk mental state'. Br J Psychiatry 194(1):25–33

Burdick KE, Goldberg JF, Harrow M, Faull RN, Malhotra AK (2006) Neurocognition as a stable endophenotype in bipolar disorder and schizophrenia. J Nerv Ment Dis 194(4):255–260. https://doi.org/10.1097/01.nmd.0000207360.70337.7e

Cannon TD (2015) How schizophrenia develops: cognitive and brain mechanisms underlying onset of psychosis. Trends Cogn Sci 19(12):744–756

Cannon M, Caspi A, Moffitt TE, Harrington H, Taylor A, Murray RM, Poulton R (2002) Evidence for early-childhood, pan-developmental impairment specific to schizophreniform disorder: results from a longitudinal birth cohort. Arch Gen Psychiatry 59(5):449–456

Cannon TD, Chung Y, He G, Sun D, Jacobson A, van Erp TG, McEwen S, Addington J, Bearden CE, Cadenhead K, Cornblatt B, Mathalon DH, McGlashan T, Perkins D, Jeffries C, Seidman LJ, Tsuang M, Walker E, Woods SW, Heinssen R (2015) Progressive reduction in cortical thickness as psychosis develops: a multisite longitudinal neuroimaging study of youth at elevated clinical risk. Biol Psychiatry 77(2):147–157. https://doi.org/10.1016/j.biopsych.2014.05.023

Cannon TD, Yu C, Addington J, Bearden CE, Cadenhead KS, Cornblatt BA, Heinssen R, Jeffries CD, Mathalon DH, McGlashan TH, Perkins DO, Seidman LJ, Tsuang MT, Walker EF, Woods SW, Kattan MW (2016) An individualized risk calculator for research in prodromal psychosis. Am J Psychiatry 173(10):980–988. https://doi.org/10.1176/appi.ajp.2016.15070890

Carrión RE, Goldberg TE, McLaughlin D, Auther AM, Correll CU, Cornblatt BA (2011) Impact of neurocognition on social and role functioning in individuals at clinical high risk for psychosis. Am J Psychiatr 168(8):806–813

Carrion RE, Cornblatt BA, Burton CZ, Tso IF, Auther AM, Adelsheim S, Calkins R, Carter CS, Niendam T, Sale TG, Taylor SF, McFarlane WR (2016) Personalized prediction of psychosis: external validation of the NAPLS-2 psychosis risk calculator with the EDIPPP project. Am J Psychiatry 173(10):989–996. https://doi.org/10.1176/appi.ajp.2016.15121565

Carrión RE, Walder DJ, Auther AM, McLaughlin D, Zyla HO, Adelsheim S, Calkins R, Carter CS, McFarland B, Melton R (2018) From the psychosis prodrome to the first-episode of psychosis: no evidence of a cognitive decline. J Psychiatr Res 96:231–238

Castellanos-Ryan N, Brière FN, O'Leary-Barrett M, Banaschewski T, Bokde A, Bromberg U, Büchel C, Flor H, Frouin V, Gallinat J (2016) The structure of psychopathology in adolescence and its common personality and cognitive correlates. J Abnorm Psychol 125(8):1039

Catalan A, de Pablo GS, Aymerich C, Damiani S, Sordi V, Radua J, Oliver D, McGuire P, Giuliano AJ, Stone WS (2021) Neurocognitive functioning in individuals at clinical high risk for psychosis: a systematic review and meta-analysis. JAMA Psychiat 78(8):859–867

Chung Y, Haut KM, He G, van Erp TGM, McEwen S, Addington J, Bearden CE, Cadenhead K, Cornblatt B, Mathalon DH, McGlashan T, Perkins D, Seidman LJ, Tsuang M, Walker E, Woods SW, Cannon TD (2017) Ventricular enlargement and progressive reduction of cortical gray matter are linked in prodromal youth who develop psychosis. Schizophr Res 189:169–174. https://doi.org/10.1016/j.schres.2017.02.014

Corcoran C, Keilp J, Kayser J, Klim C, Butler P, Bruder G, Gur R, Javitt D (2015) Emotion recognition deficits as predictors of transition in individuals at clinical high risk for schizophrenia: a neurodevelopmental perspective. Psychol Med 45(14):2959–2973

Cosway R, Byrne M, Clafferty R, Hodges A, Grant E, Abukmeil S, Lawrie S, Miller P, Johnstone E (2000) Neuropsychological change in young people at high risk for schizophrenia: results from the first two neuropsychological assessments of the Edinburgh High Risk Study. Psychol Med 30(5):1111–1121

Crouse JJ, Moustafa AA, Bogaty SER, Hickie IB, Hermens DF (2018) Parcellating cognitive heterogeneity in early psychosis-spectrum illnesses: a cluster analysis. Schizophr Res 202:91–98. https://doi.org/10.1016/j.schres.2018.06.060

Cui H, Giuliano AJ, Zhang T, Xu L, Wei Y, Tang Y, Qian Z, Stone LM, Li H, Whitfield-Gabrieli S, Niznikiewicz M, Keshavan MS, Shenton ME, Wang J, Stone WS (2020) Cognitive dysfunction in a psychotropic medication-naïve clinical high-risk sample from the ShangHai-At-Risk-for-Psychosis (SHARP) study: associations with clinical outcomes. Schizophr Res 226:138–146. S0920996420303704. https://doi.org/10.1016/j.schres.2020.06.018

Cullen AE, De Brito SA, Gregory SL, Murray RM, Williams SC, Hodgins S, Laurens KR (2013) Temporal lobe volume abnormalities precede the prodrome: a study of children presenting antecedents of schizophrenia. Schizophr Bull 39(6):1318–1327. https://doi.org/10.1093/schbul/sbs128

Cuthbert BN, Morris SE (2021) Evolving concepts of the schizophrenia spectrum: a research domain criteria perspective. Front Psych 12:170

Dandash O, Fornito A, Lee J, Keefe RS, Chee MW, Adcock RA, Pantelis C, Wood SJ, Harrison BJ (2014) Altered striatal functional connectivity in subjects with an at-risk mental state for psychosis. Schizophr Bull 40(4):904–913. https://doi.org/10.1093/schbul/sbt093

Davies C, Segre G, Estradé A, Radua J, De Micheli A, Provenzani U, Oliver D, de Pablo GS, Ramella-Cravaro V, Besozzi M (2020) Prenatal and perinatal risk and protective factors for psychosis: a systematic review and meta-analysis. Lancet Psychiatry 7(5):399–410

De Herdt A, Wampers M, Vancampfort D, De Hert M, Vanhees L, Demunter H, Van Bouwel L, Brunner E, Probst M (2013) Neurocognition in clinical high risk young adults who did or did not convert to a first schizophrenic psychosis: a meta-analysis. Schizophr Res 149(1–3):48–55

de Leede-Smith S, Roodenrys S, Horsley L, Matrini S, Mison E, Barkus E (2020) Role for positive schizotypy and hallucination proneness in semantic processing. Front Psychol 11:2272

de Paula ALD, Hallak JEC, Maia-de-Oliveira JP, Bressan RA, Machado-de-Sousa JP (2015) Cognition in at-risk mental states for psychosis. Neurosci Biobehav Rev 57:199–208

Dickson H, Cullen AE, Jones R, Reichenberg A, Roberts RE, Hodgins S, Morris RG, Laurens KR (2018) Trajectories of cognitive development during adolescence among youth at-risk for schizophrenia. J Child Psychol Psychiatry 59(11):1215–1224. https://doi.org/10.1111/jcpp.12912

Dosenbach NU, Fair DA, Cohen AL, Schlaggar BL, Petersen SE (2008) A dual-networks architecture of top-down control. Trends Cogn Sci 12(3):99–105. https://doi.org/10.1016/j.tics.2008.01.001

Drakesmith M, Dutt A, Fonville L, Zammit S, Reichenberg A, Evans CJ, Lewis G, Jones DK, David AS (2016) Mediation of developmental risk factors for psychosis by white matter microstructure in young adults with psychotic experiences. JAMA Psychiat 73(4):396–406

Dwyer DB, Kalman JL, Budde M, Kambeitz J, Ruef A, Antonucci LA, Kambeitz-Ilankovic L, Hasan A, Kondofersky I, Anderson-Schmidt H, Gade K, Reich-Erkelenz D, Adorjan K, Senner F, Schaupp S, Andlauer TFM, Comes AL, Schulte EC, Klöhn-Saghatolislam F, Gryaznova A, Hake M, Bartholdi K, Flatau-Nagel L, Reitt M, Quast S, Stegmaier S, Meyers M, Emons B, Haußleiter IS, Juckel G, Nieratschker V, Dannlowski U, Yoshida T, Schmauß M, Zimmermann J, Reimer J, Wiltfang J, Reininghaus E, Anghelescu IG, Arolt V, Baune BT, Konrad C, Thiel A, Fallgatter AJ, Figge C, von Hagen M, Koller M, Lang FU, Wigand ME, Becker T, Jäger M, Dietrich DE, Scherk H, Spitzer C, Folkerts H, Witt SH, Degenhardt F, Forstner AJ, Rietschel M, Nöthen MM, Mueller N, Papiol S, Heilbronner U, Falkai P, Schulze TG, Koutsouleris N (2020) An investigation of psychosis subgroups with prognostic validation and exploration of genetic underpinnings: the PsyCourse Study. JAMA Psychiat 77(5):523–533. https://doi.org/10.1001/jamapsychiatry.2019.4910

Dzafic I, Randeniya R, Harris CD, Bammel M, Garrido MI (2020) Statistical learning and inference is impaired in the nonclinical continuum of psychosis. J Neurosci 40(35):6759–6769

Eastvold A, Heaton R, Cadenhead K (2007) Neurocognitive deficits in the (putative) prodrome and first episode of psychosis. Schizophr Res 93(1–3):266–277

Eisenberg DP, Berman KF (2010) Executive function, neural circuitry, and genetic mechanisms in schizophrenia. Neuropsychopharmacology 35(1):258–277

Evermann U, Gaser C, Besteher B, Langbein K, Nenadić I (2020) Cortical gyrification, psychotic-like experiences, and cognitive performance in nonclinical subjects. Schizophr Bull 46(6):1524–1534

Fornito A, Harrison BJ, Goodby E, Dean A, Ooi C, Nathan PJ, Lennox BR, Jones PB, Suckling J, Bullmore ET (2013) Functional dysconnectivity of corticostriatal circuitry as a risk phenotype for psychosis. JAMA Psychiat 70(11):1143–1151. https://doi.org/10.1001/jamapsychiatry.2013.1976
Friedman NP, Robbins TW (2021) The role of prefrontal cortex in cognitive control and executive function. Neuropsychopharmacology:1–18
Frommann I, Pukrop R, Brinkmeyer J, Bechdolf A, Ruhrmann S, Berning J, Decker P, Riedel M, Möller H-J, Wölwer W (2011) Neuropsychological profiles in different at-risk states of psychosis: executive control impairment in the early—and additional memory dysfunction in the late—prodromal state. Schizophr Bull 37(4):861–873
Fusar-Poli P, Deste G, Smieskova R, Barlati S, Yung AR, Howes O, Stieglitz RD, Vita A, McGuire P, Borgwardt S (2012) Cognitive functioning in prodromal psychosis: a meta-analysis. Arch Gen Psychiatry 69(6):562–571. https://doi.org/10.1001/archgenpsychiatry.2011.1592
Fusar-Poli P, Rutigliano G, Stahl D, Davies C, Bonoldi I, Reilly T, McGuire P (2017) Development and validation of a clinically based risk calculator for the transdiagnostic prediction of psychosis. JAMA Psychiat 74(5):493–500. https://doi.org/10.1001/jamapsychiatry.2017.0284
Genovese G, Fromer M, Stahl EA, Ruderfer DM, Chambert K, Landén M, Moran JL, Purcell SM, Sklar P, Sullivan PF (2016) Increased burden of ultra-rare protein-altering variants among 4,877 individuals with schizophrenia. Nat Neurosci 19(11):1433–1441
Gill KE, Evans E, Kayser J, Ben-David S, Messinger J, Bruder G, Malaspina D, Corcoran CM (2014) Smell identification in individuals at clinical high risk for schizophrenia. Psychiatry Res 220(1–2):201–204
Giuliano AJ, Li H, Mesholam-Gately RI, Sorenson SM, Woodberry KA, Seidman LJ (2012) Neurocognition in the psychosis risk syndrome: a quantitative and qualitative review. Curr Pharm Des 18(4):399–415
Glenthøj LB, Hjorthøj C, Kristensen TD, Davidson CA, Nordentoft M (2017) The effect of cognitive remediation in individuals at ultra-high risk for psychosis: a systematic review. NPJ Schizophr 3(1):1–8
Glenthøj LB, Mariegaard LS, Fagerlund B, Jepsen JR, Kristensen TD, Wenneberg C, Krakauer K, Medalia A, Roberts DL, Hjorthøj C (2020) Effectiveness of cognitive remediation in the ultra-high risk state for psychosis. World Psychiatry 19(3):401
Goghari VM, Brett C, Tabraham P, Johns L, Valmaggia L, Broome M, Woolley J, Bramon E, Howes O, Byrne M (2014) Spatial working memory ability in individuals at ultra high risk for psychosis. J Psychiatr Res 50:100–105
Goldstein G, Shemansky WJ (1995) Influences on cognitive heterogeneity in schizophrenia. Schizophr Res 18(1):59–69
Green MF, Horan WP, Lee J (2019) Nonsocial and social cognition in schizophrenia: current evidence and future directions. World Psychiatry 18(2):146–161
Green MJ, Girshkin L, Kremerskothen K, Watkeys O, Quidé Y (2020) A systematic review of studies reporting data-driven cognitive subtypes across the psychosis spectrum. Neuropsychol Rev 30(4):446–460. https://doi.org/10.1007/s11065-019-09422-7
Greenland-White SE, Ragland JD, Niendam TA, Ferrer E, Carter CS (2017) Episodic memory functions in first episode psychosis and clinical high risk individuals. Schizophr Res 188:151–157
Guo JY, Niendam TA, Auther AM, Carrión RE, Cornblatt BA, Ragland JD, Adelsheim S, Calkins R, Sale TG, Taylor SF (2020) Predicting psychosis risk using a specific measure of cognitive control: a 12-month longitudinal study. Psychol Med 50(13):2230–2239
Gur RC, Calkins ME, Satterthwaite TD, Ruparel K, Bilker WB, Moore TM, Savitt AP, Hakonarson H, Gur RE (2014) Neurocognitive growth charting in psychosis spectrum youths. JAMA Psychiat 71(4):366–374
Harvey PD, Koren D, Reichenberg A, Bowie CR (2006) Negative symptoms and cognitive deficits: what is the nature of their relationship? Schizophr Bull 32(2):250–258

Hauser M, Zhang J-P, Sheridan EM, Burdick KE, Mogil R, Kane JM, Auther A, Carrión RE, Cornblatt BA, Correll CU (2017) Neuropsychological test performance to enhance identification of subjects at clinical high risk for psychosis and to be most promising for predictive algorithms for conversion to psychosis: a meta-analysis. J Clin Psychiatry 78(1):0–0

Hawkins KA, Keefe RS, Christensen BK, Addington J, Woods SW, Callahan J, Zipursky RB, Perkins DO, Tohen M, Breier A (2008) Neuropsychological course in the prodrome and first episode of psychosis: findings from the PRIME North America Double Blind Treatment Study. Schizophr Res 105(1–3):1–9

Haynes SN, O'Brien WH, Keawe'aimoku J, Witteman C (2012) Concepts of causality in psychopathology: applications in clinical assessment, clinical case formulation and functional analysis. J Unified Psychother Clin Sci 1(1)

Hegarty CE, Jolles DD, Mennigen E, Jalbrzikowski M, Bearden CE, Karlsgodt KH (2019) Disruptions in white matter maturation and mediation of cognitive development in youths on the psychosis spectrum. Biol Psychiatry: Cogn Neurosci Neuroimaging 4(5):423–433

Hill SK, Buchholz A, Amsbaugh H, Reilly JL, Rubin LH, Gold JM, Keefe RS, Pearlson GD, Keshavan MS, Tamminga CA (2015) Working memory impairment in probands with schizoaffective disorder and first degree relatives of schizophrenia probands extend beyond deficits predicted by generalized neuropsychological impairment. Schizophr Res 166(1–3): 310–315

Horga G, Cassidy CM, Xu X, Moore H, Slifstein M, Van Snellenberg JX, Abi-Dargham A (2016) Dopamine-related disruption of functional topography of striatal connections in unmedicated patients with schizophrenia. JAMA Psychiat 73(8):862–870. https://doi.org/10.1001/jamapsychiatry.2016.0178

Horn JL, Cattell RB (1967) Age differences in fluid and crystallized intelligence. Acta Psychol 26: 107–129

Hou C-L, Xiang Y-T, Wang Z-L, Everall I, Tang Y, Yang C, Xu M-Z, Correll CU, Jia F-J (2016) Cognitive functioning in individuals at ultra-high risk for psychosis, first-degree relatives of patients with psychosis and patients with first-episode schizophrenia. Schizophr Res 174(1–3): 71–76

Huang-Pollock C, Shapiro Z, Galloway-Long H, Weigard A (2017) Is poor working memory a transdiagnostic risk factor for psychopathology? J Abnorm Child Psychol 45(8):1477–1490

Hubbard L, Tansey KE, Rai D, Jones P, Ripke S, Chambert KD, Moran JL, McCarroll SA, Linden DE, Owen MJ, O'Donovan MC, Walters JT, Zammit S (2016) Evidence of common genetic overlap between schizophrenia and cognition. Schizophr Bull 42(3):832–842. https://doi.org/10.1093/schbul/sbv168

Hwang WJ, Lee TY, Shin W-G, Kim M, Kim J, Lee J, Kwon JS (2019) Global and specific profiles of executive functioning in prodromal and early psychosis. Front Psych 10:356

Ilonen T, Heinimaa M, Korkeila J, Svirskis T, Salokangas RK (2010) Differentiating adolescents at clinical high risk for psychosis from psychotic and non-psychotic patients with the Rorschach. Psychiatry Res 179(2):151–156

Ivleva EI, Morris DW, Osuji J, Moates AF, Carmody TJ, Thaker GK, Cullum M, Tamminga CA (2012) Cognitive endophenotypes of psychosis within dimension and diagnosis. Psychiatry Res 196(1):38–44. https://doi.org/10.1016/j.psychres.2011.08.021

J Giuliano A, Li H, I Mesholam-Gately R, M Sorenson S, A Woodberry K, J Seidman L (2012) Neurocognition in the psychosis risk syndrome: a quantitative and qualitative review. Curr Pharm Des 18(4):399–415

Jahshan C, Heaton RK, Golshan S, Cadenhead KS (2010) Course of neurocognitive deficits in the prodrome and first episode of schizophrenia. Neuropsychology 24(1):109

Jalbrzikowski M, Hayes RA, Wood SJ, Nordholm D, Zhou JH, Fusar-Poli P, Uhlhaas PJ, Takahashi T, Sugranyes G, Kwak YB (2021) Association of structural magnetic resonance imaging measures with psychosis onset in individuals at clinical high risk for developing psychosis: an ENIGMA Working Group mega-analysis. JAMA Psychiat 78(7):753–766

Kahn RS, Keefe RS (2013) Schizophrenia is a cognitive illness: time for a change in focus. JAMA Psychiat 70(10):1107–1112
Karcher NR, Barch DM, Avenevoli S, Savill M, Huber RS, Simon TJ, Leckliter IN, Sher KJ, Loewy RL (2018) Assessment of the prodromal questionnaire-brief child version for measurement of self-reported psychoticlike experiences in childhood. JAMA Psychiat 75(8):853–861. https://doi.org/10.1001/jamapsychiatry.2018.1334
Karcher NR, O'Brien KJ, Kandala S, Barch DM (2019) Resting-state functional connectivity and psychotic-like experiences in childhood: results from the adolescent brain cognitive development study. Biol Psychiatry 86(1):7–15. https://doi.org/10.1016/j.biopsych.2019.01.013
Karcher NR, Loewy RL, Savill M, Avenevoli S, Huber RS, Simon TJ, Leckliter IN, Sher KJ, Barch DM (2020a) Replication of associations with psychotic-like experiences in middle childhood from the adolescent brain cognitive development (ABCD) study. Schizophrenia Bulletin Open 1:sgaa009. https://doi.org/10.1093/schizbullopen/sgaa009
Karcher NR, Paul SE, Johnson EC, Hatoum AS, Baranger DA, Agrawal A, Thompson WK, Barch DM, Bogdan R (2020b) Psychotic-like experiences and polygenic liability in the ABCD Study. medRxiv:2020.2007.2014.20153551. https://doi.org/10.1101/2020.07.14.20153551
Keefe RS, Fenton WS (2007) How should DSM-V criteria for schizophrenia include cognitive impairment? Schizophr Bull 33(4):912–920
Keefe RS, Perkins DO, Gu H, Zipursky RB, Christensen BK, Lieberman JA (2006) A longitudinal study of neurocognitive function in individuals at-risk for psychosis. Schizophr Res 88(1–3): 26–35
Kelleher I, Connor D, Clarke MC, Devlin N, Harley M, Cannon M (2012) Prevalence of psychotic symptoms in childhood and adolescence: a systematic review and meta-analysis of population-based studies. Psychol Med 42(9):1857–1863. https://doi.org/10.1017/S0033291711002960
Kelly S, Jahanshad N, Zalesky A, Kochunov P, Agartz I, Alloza C, Andreassen O, Arango C, Banaj N, Bouix S (2018) Widespread white matter microstructural differences in schizophrenia across 4322 individuals: results from the ENIGMA Schizophrenia DTI Working Group. Mol Psychiatry 23(5):1261–1269
Keshavan MS, Kulkarni SR, Bhojraj T, Francis A, Diwadkar V, Montrose DM, Seidman L, Sweeney J (2010) Premorbid cognitive deficits in young relatives of schizophrenia patients. Front Hum Neurosci 3:62
Kim HS, Shin NY, Jang JH, Kim E, Shim G, Park HY, Hong KS, Kwon JS (2011) Social cognition and neurocognition as predictors of conversion to psychosis in individuals at ultra-high risk. Schizophr Res 130(1–3):170–175
Kim SJ, Lee YJ, Jang JH, Lim W, Cho IH, Cho S-J (2012) The relationship between psychotic-like experiences and attention deficits in adolescents. J Psychiatr Res 46(10):1354–1358
Koshiyama D, Kirihara K, Tada M, Nagai T, Fujioka M, Koike S, Suga M, Araki T, Kasai K (2018) Association between mismatch negativity and global functioning is specific to duration deviance in early stages of psychosis. Schizophr Res 195:378–384
Koutsouleris N, Patschurek-Kliche K, Scheuerecker J, Decker P, Bottlender R, Schmitt G, Rujescu D, Giegling I, Gaser C, Reiser M (2010) Neuroanatomical correlates of executive dysfunction in the at-risk mental state for psychosis. Schizophr Res 123(2–3):160–174
Kremen WS, Buka SL, Seidman LJ, Goldstein JM, Koren D, Tsuang MT (1998) IQ decline during childhood and adult psychotic symptoms in a community sample: a 19-year longitudinal study. Am J Psychiatry 155(5):672–677. https://doi.org/10.1176/ajp.155.5.672
Kristensen TD, Mandl RC, Raghava JM, Jessen K, Jepsen JRM, Fagerlund B, Glenthøj LB, Wenneberg C, Krakauer K, Pantelis C (2019) Widespread higher fractional anisotropy associates to better cognitive functions in individuals at ultra-high risk for psychosis. Hum Brain Mapp 40(18):5185–5201
Kubicki M, McCarley R, Westin C-F, Park H-J, Maier S, Kikinis R, Jolesz FA, Shenton ME (2007) A review of diffusion tensor imaging studies in schizophrenia. J Psychiatr Res 41(1–2):15–30

Laurens KR, Cullen AE (2016) Toward earlier identification and preventative intervention in schizophrenia: evidence from the London Child Health and Development Study. Soc Psychiatry Psychiatr Epidemiol 51(4):475–491. https://doi.org/10.1007/s00127-015-1151-x

Laurens KR, Hobbs MJ, Sunderland M, Green MJ, Mould GL (2012) Psychotic-like experiences in a community sample of 8000 children aged 9 to 11 years: an item response theory analysis. Psychol Med 42(7):1495–1506. https://doi.org/10.1017/S0033291711002108

Lee SY, Bang M, Kim KR, Lee MK, Park JY, Song YY, Kang JI, Lee E, An SK (2015) Impaired facial emotion recognition in individuals at ultra-high risk for psychosis and with first-episode schizophrenia, and their associations with neurocognitive deficits and self-reported schizotypy. Schizophr Res 165(1):60–65

Lencz T, Smith CW, McLaughlin D, Auther A, Nakayama E, Hovey L, Cornblatt BA (2006) Generalized and specific neurocognitive deficits in prodromal schizophrenia. Biol Psychiatry 59(9):863–871

Lepock JR, Ahmed S, Mizrahi R, Gerritsen CJ, Maheandiran M, Drvaric L, Bagby RM, Korostil M, Light GA, Kiang M (2020) Relationships between cognitive event-related brain potential measures in patients at clinical high risk for psychosis. Schizophr Res 226:84–94

Lewandowski KE, Baker JT, McCarthy JM, Norris LA, Ongur D (2018) Reproducibility of cognitive profiles in psychosis using cluster analysis. J Int Neuropsychol Soc 24(4):382–390. https://doi.org/10.1017/s1355617717001047

Lin A, Yung A, Nelson B, Brewer W, Riley R, Simmons M, Pantelis C, Wood S (2013) Neurocognitive predictors of transition to psychosis: medium-to long-term findings from a sample at ultra-high risk for psychosis. Psychol Med 43(11):2349–2360

Liu C-C, Hua M-S, Hwang T-J, Chiu C-Y, Liu C-M, Hsieh MH, Chien Y-L, Lin Y-T, Hwu H-G (2015) Neurocognitive functioning of subjects with putative pre-psychotic states and early psychosis. Schizophr Res 164(1–3):40–46

Magaud E, Morvan Y, Rampazzo A, Alexandre C, Willard D, Gaillard R, Kazes M, Krebs M-O (2014) Subjects at ultra high risk for psychosis have 'heterogeneous' intellectual functioning profile: a multiple-case study. Schizophr Res 152(2–3):415–420

Mark W, Toulopoulou T (2016) Cognitive intermediate phenotype and genetic risk for psychosis. Curr Opin Neurobiol 36:23–30. https://doi.org/10.1016/j.conb.2015.08.008

Mathew I, Gardin TM, Tandon N, Eack S, Francis AN, Seidman LJ, Clementz B, Pearlson GD, Sweeney JA, Tamminga CA (2014) Medial temporal lobe structures and hippocampal subfields in psychotic disorders: findings from the Bipolar-Schizophrenia Network on Intermediate Phenotypes (B-SNIP) Study. JAMA Psychiat 71(7):769–777

McCleery A, Nuechterlein KH (2019) Cognitive impairment in psychotic illness: prevalence, profile of impairment, developmental course, and treatment considerations. Dialogues Clin Neurosci 21(3):239

McTeague LM, Goodkind MS, Etkin A (2016) Transdiagnostic impairment of cognitive control in mental illness. J Psychiatr Res 83:37–46

Meier MH, Caspi A, Reichenberg A, Keefe RS, Fisher HL, Harrington H, Houts R, Poulton R, Moffitt TE (2014) Neuropsychological decline in schizophrenia from the premorbid to the postonset period: evidence from a population-representative longitudinal study. Am J Psychiatry 171(1):91–101. https://doi.org/10.1176/appi.ajp.2013.12111438

Metzler S, Dvorsky D, Wyss C, Nordt C, Walitza S, Heekeren K, Rössler W, Theodoridou A (2016) Neurocognition in help-seeking individuals at risk for psychosis: prediction of outcome after 24 months. Psychiatry Res 246:188–194

Meyer EC, Carrión RE, Cornblatt BA, Addington J, Cadenhead KS, Cannon TD, McGlashan TH, Perkins DO, Tsuang MT, Walker EF (2014) The relationship of neurocognition and negative symptoms to social and role functioning over time in individuals at clinical high risk in the first phase of the North American Prodrome Longitudinal Study. Schizophr Bull 40(6):1452–1461

Mittal VA, Walker EF, Bearden CE, Walder D, Trottman H, Daley M, Simone A, Cannon TD (2010) Markers of basal ganglia dysfunction and conversion to psychosis: neurocognitive deficits and dyskinesias in the prodromal period. Biol Psychiatry 68(1):93–99

Mollon J, Reichenberg A (2017) Cognitive development prior to onset of psychosis. Psychol Med:1–12. https://doi.org/10.1017/s0033291717001970

Mollon J, David AS, Zammit S, Lewis G, Reichenberg A (2018) Course of cognitive development from infancy to early adulthood in the psychosis spectrum. JAMA Psychiat 75(3):270–279

Moritz S, Silverstein SM, Beblo T, Özaslan Z, Zink M, Gallinat J (2021) Much of the neurocognitive impairment in schizophrenia is due to factors other than schizophrenia itself: implications for research and treatment. Schizophrenia Bulletin Open 2(1):sgaa034

O'Brien KJ, Barch DM, Kandala S, Karcher NR (2020) Examining specificity of neural correlates of childhood psychotic-like experiences during an emotional n-back task. Biol Psychiatry: Cogn Neurosci Neuroimaging 5(6):580–590

Ohmuro N, Katsura M, Obara C, Kikuchi T, Sakuma A, Iizuka K, Hamaie Y, Ito F, Matsuoka H, Matsumoto K (2016) Deficits of cognitive theory of mind and its relationship with functioning in individuals with an at-risk mental state and first-episode psychosis. Psychiatry Res 243:318–325

Ohmuro N, Katsura M, Obara C, Kikuchi T, Hamaie Y, Sakuma A, Iizuka K, Ito F, Matsuoka H, Matsumoto K (2018) The relationship between cognitive insight and cognitive performance among individuals with at-risk mental state for developing psychosis. Schizophr Res 192:281–286

Palaniyappan L, Liddle PF (2012) Does the salience network play a cardinal role in psychosis? An emerging hypothesis of insular dysfunction. J Psychiatry Neurosci: JPN 37(1):17–27. https://doi.org/10.1503/jpn.100176

Pelletier-Baldelli A, Holt DJ (2020) Are negative symptoms merely the "real world" consequences of deficits in social cognition? Schizophr Bull 46(2):236–241

Perälä J, Suvisaari J, Saarni SI, Kuoppasalmi K, Isometsä E, Pirkola S, Partonen T, Tuulio-Henriksson A, Hintikka J, Kieseppä T (2007) Lifetime prevalence of psychotic and bipolar I disorders in a general population. Arch Gen Psychiatry 64(1):19–28

Peters H, Riedl V, Manoliu A, Scherr M, Schwerthoffer D, Zimmer C, Forstl H, Bauml J, Sorg C, Koch K (2017) Changes in extra-striatal functional connectivity in patients with schizophrenia in a psychotic episode. Br J Psychiatry 210(1):75–82. https://doi.org/10.1192/bjp.bp.114.151928

Pruessner M, Cullen AE, Aas M, Walker EF (2017) The neural diathesis-stress model of schizophrenia revisited: an update on recent findings considering illness stage and neurobiological and methodological complexities. Neurosci Biobehav Rev 73:191–218. https://doi.org/10.1016/j.neubiorev.2016.12.013

Pukrop R, Ruhrmann S, Schultze-Lutter F, Bechdolf A, Brockhaus-Dumke A, Klosterkötter J (2007) Neurocognitive indicators for a conversion to psychosis: comparison of patients in a potentially initial prodromal state who did or did not convert to a psychosis. Schizophr Res 92(1–3):116–125

Raij TT, Mantyla T, Kieseppa T, Suvisaari J (2015) Aberrant functioning of the putamen links delusions, antipsychotic drug dose, and compromised connectivity in first episode psychosis – preliminary fMRI findings. Psychiatry Res 233(2):201–211. https://doi.org/10.1016/j.pscychresns.2015.06.008

Randers L, Jepsen JRM, Fagerlund B, Nordholm D, Krakauer K, Hjorthøj C, Glenthøj B, Nordentoft M (2021) Generalized neurocognitive impairment in individuals at ultra-high risk for psychosis: the possible key role of slowed processing speed. Brain Behav 11(3):e01962

Reichenberg A, Weiser M, Rapp MA, Rabinowitz J, Caspi A, Schmeidler J, Knobler HY, Lubin G, Nahon D, Harvey PD (2005) Elaboration on premorbid intellectual performance in schizophrenia: premorbid intellectual decline and risk for schizophrenia. Arch Gen Psychiatry 62(12):1297–1304

Reichenberg A, Harvey PD, Bowie CR, Mojtabai R, Rabinowitz J, Heaton RK, Bromet E (2009) Neuropsychological function and dysfunction in schizophrenia and psychotic affective disorders. Schizophr Bull 35(5):1022–1029. https://doi.org/10.1093/schbul/sbn044

Reichenberg A, Caspi A, Harrington H, Houts R, Keefe RS, Murray RM, Poulton R, Moffitt TE (2010) Static and dynamic cognitive deficits in childhood preceding adult schizophrenia: a 30-year study. Am J Psychiatry 167(2):160–169. https://doi.org/10.1176/appi.ajp.2009.09040574

Richards AL, Pardiñas AF, Frizzati A, Tansey KE, Lynham AJ, Holmans P, Legge SE, Savage JE, Agartz I, Andreassen OA, Blokland GAM, Corvin A, Cosgrove D, Degenhardt F, Djurovic S, Espeseth T, Ferraro L, Gayer-Anderson C, Giegling I, van Haren NE, Hartmann AM, Hubert JJ, Jönsson EG, Konte B, Lennertz L, Olde Loohuis LM, Melle I, Morgan C, Morris DW, Murray RM, Nyman H, Ophoff RA, van Os J, Petryshen TL, Quattrone D, Rietschel M, Rujescu D, Rutten BPF, Streit F, Strohmaier J, Sullivan PF, Sundet K, Wagner M, Escott-Price V, Owen MJ, Donohoe G, O'Donovan MC, Walters JTR (2020) The relationship between polygenic risk scores and cognition in schizophrenia. Schizophr Bull 46(2):336–344. https://doi.org/10.1093/schbul/sbz061

Rossi R, Zammit S, Button KS, Munafò MR, Lewis G, David AS (2016) Psychotic experiences and working memory: a population-based study using signal-detection analysis. PLoS One 11(4): e0153148

Rössler W, Ajdacic-Gross V, Müller M, Rodgers S, Kawohl W, Haker H, Hengartner MP (2015) Association between processing speed and subclinical psychotic symptoms in the general population: focusing on sex differences. Schizophr Res 166(1–3):316–321

Savage JE, Jansen PR, Stringer S, Watanabe K, Bryois J, De Leeuw CA, Nagel M, Awasthi S, Barr PB, Coleman JR (2018) Genome-wide association meta-analysis in 269,867 individuals identifies new genetic and functional links to intelligence. Nat Genet 50(7):912–919

Seaton BE, Allen DN, Goldstein G, Kelley ME, van Kammen DP (1999) Relations between cognitive and symptom profile heterogeneity in schizophrenia. J Nerv Ment Dis 187(7): 414–419

Seidman LJ, Giuliano AJ, Meyer EC, Addington J, Cadenhead KS, Cannon TD, McGlashan TH, Perkins DO, Tsuang MT, Walker EF, Woods SW, Bearden CE, Christensen BK, Hawkins K, Heaton R, Keefe RS, Heinssen R, Cornblatt BA (2010) Neuropsychology of the prodrome to psychosis in the NAPLS consortium: relationship to family history and conversion to psychosis. Arch Gen Psychiatry 67(6):578–588. https://doi.org/10.1001/archgenpsychiatry.2010.66

Seidman LJ, Shapiro DI, Stone WS, Woodberry KA, Ronzio A, Cornblatt BA, Addington J, Bearden CE, Cadenhead KS, Cannon TD, Mathalon DH, McGlashan TH, Perkins DO, Tsuang MT, Walker EF, Woods SW (2016) Association of neurocognition with transition to psychosis: baseline functioning in the second phase of the North American Prodrome Longitudinal Study. JAMA Psychiat 73(12):1239–1248. https://doi.org/10.1001/jamapsychiatry.2016.2479

Sheffield JM, Kandala S, Burgess GC, Harms MP, Barch DM (2016) Cingulo-opercular network efficiency mediates the association between psychotic-like experiences and cognitive ability in the general population. Biol Psychiatry Cogn Neurosci Neuroimaging 1(6):498–506. https://doi.org/10.1016/j.bpsc.2016.03.009

Sheffield JM, Kandala S, Tamminga CA, Pearlson GD, Keshavan MS, Sweeney JA, Clementz BA, Lerman-Sinkoff DB, Hill SK, Barch DM (2017) Transdiagnostic associations between functional brain network integrity and cognition. JAMA Psychiat 74(6):605–613. https://doi.org/10.1001/jamapsychiatry.2017.0669

Sheffield JM, Karcher NR, Barch DM (2018) Cognitive deficits in psychotic disorders: a lifespan perspective. Neuropsychol Rev 28:509–533. https://doi.org/10.1007/s11065-018-9388-2

Simon AE, Grädel M, Cattapan-Ludewig K, Gruber K, Ballinari P, Roth B, Umbricht D (2012) Cognitive functioning in at-risk mental states for psychosis and 2-year clinical outcome. Schizophr Res 142(1–3):108–115

Smeland OB, Andreassen OA (2018) How can genetics help understand the relationship between cognitive dysfunction and schizophrenia? Scand J Psychol 59(1):26–31. https://doi.org/10.1111/sjop.12407

Smucny J, Iosif AM, Eaton NR, Lesh TA, Ragland JD, Barch DM, Gold JM, Strauss ME, MacDonald AW, Silverstein SM, Carter CS (2019) Latent profiles of cognitive control, episodic memory, and visual perception across psychiatric disorders reveal a dimensional structure. Schizophr Bull. https://doi.org/10.1093/schbul/sbz025

Sun D, Phillips L, Velakoulis D, Yung A, McGorry PD, Wood SJ, van Erp TG, Thompson PM, Toga AW, Cannon TD, Pantelis C (2009) Progressive brain structural changes mapped as psychosis develops in 'at risk' individuals. Schizophr Res 108(1–3):85–92. https://doi.org/10.1016/j.schres.2008.11.026

Tamminga CA, Stan AD, Wagner AD (2010) The hippocampal formation in schizophrenia. Am J Psychiatr 167(10):1178–1193

Thygesen JH, Presman A, Harju-Seppänen J, Irizar H, Jones R, Kuchenbaecker K, Lin K, Alizadeh BZ, Austin-Zimmerman I, Bartels-Velthuis A (2020) Genetic copy number variants, cognition and psychosis: a meta-analysis and a family study. Mol Psychiatry:1–13

Tor J, Dolz M, Sintes-Estevez A, de la Serna E, Puig O, Muñoz-Samons D, Pardo M, Rodríguez-Pascual M, Sugranyes G, Sánchez-Gistau V (2020) Neuropsychological profile of children and adolescents with psychosis risk syndrome: the CAPRIS Study. Eur Child Adolesc Psychiatry 29(9):1311–1324

Toulopoulou T, Zhang X, Cherny S, Dickinson D, Berman KF, Straub RE, Sham P, Weinberger DR (2019) Polygenic risk score increases schizophrenia liability through cognition-relevant pathways. Brain J Neurol 142(2):471–485

Tronchin G, Akudjedu TN, Kenney JP, McInerney S, Scanlon C, McFarland J, McCarthy P, Cannon DM, Hallahan B, McDonald C (2020) Cognitive and clinical predictors of prefrontal cortical thickness change following first-episode of psychosis. Psychiatry Res Neuroimaging 302:111100

Trotman HD, Holtzman CW, Ryan AT, Shapiro DI, MacDonald AN, Goulding SM, Brasfield JL, Walker EF (2013) The development of psychotic disorders in adolescence: a potential role for hormones. Horm Behav 64(2):411–419

Uddin LQ (2015) Salience processing and insular cortical function and dysfunction. Nat Rev Neurosci 16(1):55–61. https://doi.org/10.1038/nrn3857

Uhlhaas PJ (2011) The adolescent brain: implications for the understanding, pathophysiology, and treatment of schizophrenia. Schizophr Bull 37(3):480–483

van Erp TGM, Walton E, Hibar DP, Schmaal L, Jiang W, Glahn DC, Pearlson GD, Yao N, Fukunaga M, Hashimoto R, Okada N, Yamamori H, Bustillo JR, Clark VP, Agartz I, Mueller BA, Cahn W, de Zwarte SMC, Hulshoff Pol HE, Kahn RS, Ophoff RA, van Haren NEM, Andreassen OA, Dale AM, Doan NT, Gurholt TP, Hartberg CB, Haukvik UK, Jorgensen KN, Lagerberg TV, Melle I, Westlye LT, Gruber O, Kraemer B, Richter A, Zilles D, Calhoun VD, Crespo-Facorro B, Roiz-Santianez R, Tordesillas-Gutierrez D, Loughland C, Carr VJ, Catts S, Cropley VL, Fullerton JM, Green MJ, Henskens FA, Jablensky A, Lenroot RK, Mowry BJ, Michie PT, Pantelis C, Quide Y, Schall U, Scott RJ, Cairns MJ, Seal M, Tooney PA, Rasser PE, Cooper G, Shannon Weickert C, Weickert TW, Morris DW, Hong E, Kochunov P, Beard LM, Gur RE, Gur RC, Satterthwaite TD, Wolf DH, Belger A, Brown GG, Ford JM, Macciardi F, Mathalon DH, O'Leary DS, Potkin SG, Preda A, Voyvodic J, Lim KO, McEwen S, Yang F, Tan Y, Tan S, Wang Z, Fan F, Chen J, Xiang H, Tang S, Guo H, Wan P, Wei D, Bockholt HJ, Ehrlich S, Wolthusen RPF, King MD, Shoemaker JM, Sponheim SR, De Haan L, Koenders L, Machielsen MW, van Amelsvoort T, Veltman DJ, Assogna F, Banaj N, de Rossi P, Iorio M, Piras F, Spalletta G, McKenna PJ, Pomarol-Clotet E, Salvador R, Corvin A, Donohoe G, Kelly S, Whelan CD, Dickie EW, Rotenberg D, Voineskos AN, Ciufolini S, Radua J, Dazzan P, Murray R, Reis Marques T, Simmons A, Borgwardt S, Egloff L, Harrisberger F, Riecher-Rossler A, Smieskova R, Alpert KI, Wang L, Jonsson EG, Koops S, Sommer IEC, Bertolino A, Bonvino A, Di Giorgio A, Neilson E, Mayer AR, Stephen JM, Kwon JS, Yun JY, Cannon DM, McDonald C, Lebedeva I, Tomyshev AS, Akhadov T, Kaleda V, Fatouros-Bergman H, Flyckt L, Busatto GF, Rosa PGP, Serpa MH, Zanetti MV, Hoschl C, Skoch A, Spaniel F, Tomecek D, Hagenaars SP, McIntosh AM, Whalley HC, Lawrie SM, Knochel C, Oertel-Knochel V, Stablein M, Howells FM, Stein DJ, Temmingh HS, Uhlmann A, Lopez-Jaramillo C, Dima D, McMahon A, Faskowitz JI, Gutman BA, Jahanshad N, Thompson PM,

Turner JA (2018) Cortical brain abnormalities in 4474 individuals with schizophrenia and 5098 control subjects via the enhancing neuro imaging genetics through meta analysis (ENIGMA) consortium. Biol Psychiatry. https://doi.org/10.1016/j.biopsych.2018.04.023
van Os J, Linscott RJ, Myin-Germeys I, Delespaul P, Krabbendam L (2009) A systematic review and meta-analysis of the psychosis continuum: evidence for a psychosis proneness-persistence-impairment model of psychotic disorder. Psychol Med 39(2):179–195. https://doi.org/10.1017/S0033291708003814
Ventura J, Thames AD, Wood RC, Guzik LH, Hellemann GS (2010) Disorganization and reality distortion in schizophrenia: a meta-analysis of the relationship between positive symptoms and neurocognitive deficits. Schizophr Res 121(1–3):1–14
Walder D, Mittal V, Trotman H, McMillan A, Walker E (2008) Neurocognition and conversion to psychosis in adolescents at high-risk. Schizophr Res 101(1–3):161–168
Walker E, Bollini AM (2002) Pubertal neurodevelopment and the emergence of psychotic symptoms. Schizophr Res 54(1–2):17–23
Wallace S, Morton SE, Linscott RJ (2019) Relationships between intra-individual variability and subclinical psychosis. Psychiatry Res 281:112592
Walton E, Hibar DP, van Erp TG, Potkin SG, Roiz-Santianez R, Crespo-Facorro B, Suarez-Pinilla P, Van Haren NE, de Zwarte SM, Kahn RS, Cahn W, Doan NT, Jorgensen KN, Gurholt TP, Agartz I, Andreassen OA, Westlye LT, Melle I, Berg AO, Morch-Johnsen L, Faerden A, Flyckt L, Fatouros-Bergman H, Jonsson EG, Hashimoto R, Yamamori H, Fukunaga M, Preda A, De Rossi P, Piras F, Banaj N, Ciullo V, Spalletta G, Gur RE, Gur RC, Wolf DH, Satterthwaite TD, Beard LM, Sommer IE, Koops S, Gruber O, Richter A, Kramer B, Kelly S, Donohoe G, McDonald C, Cannon DM, Corvin A, Gill M, Di Giorgio A, Bertolino A, Lawrie S, Nickson T, Whalley HC, Neilson E, Calhoun VD, Thompson PM, Turner JA, Ehrlich S (2017) Positive symptoms associate with cortical thinning in the superior temporal gyrus via the ENIGMA Schizophrenia consortium. Acta Psychiatr Scand 135(5):439–447. https://doi.org/10.1111/acps.12718
Weinberger DR (1987) Implications of normal brain development for the pathogenesis of schizophrenia. Arch Gen Psychiatry 44(7):660–669
Wells R, Swaminathan V, Sundram S, Weinberg D, Bruggemann J, Jacomb I, Cropley V, Lenroot R, Pereira AM, Zalesky A (2015) The impact of premorbid and current intellect in schizophrenia: cognitive, symptom, and functional outcomes. NPJ Schizophr 1(1):1–8
Werner EE, Smith RS (1992) Overcoming the odds: high risk children from birth to adulthood. Cornell University Press
Whyte M-C, Brett C, Harrison LK, Byrne M, Miller P, Lawrie SM, Johnstone EC (2006) Neuropsychological performance over time in people at high risk of developing schizophrenia and controls. Biol Psychiatry 59(8):730–739
Wood SJ, Brewer WJ, Koutsouradis P, Phillips LJ, Francey SM, Proffitt TM, Yung AR, Jackson HJ, McGorry PD, Pantelis C (2007) Cognitive decline following psychosis onset: data from the PACE clinic. Br J Psychiatry 191(S51):s52–s57
Woodberry KA, Giuliano AJ, Seidman LJ (2008) Premorbid IQ in schizophrenia: a meta-analytic review. Am J Psychiatry 165(5):579–587. https://doi.org/10.1176/appi.ajp.2008.07081242
Woodberry KA, Seidman LJ, Giuliano AJ, Verdi MB, Cook WL, McFarlane WR (2010) Neuropsychological profiles in individuals at clinical high risk for psychosis: relationship to psychosis and intelligence. Schizophr Res 123(2–3):188–198
Woods SW, Walsh BC, Powers AR, McGlashan TH (2019) Reliability, validity, epidemiology, and cultural variation of the structured interview for psychosis-risk syndromes (SIPS) and the scale of psychosis-risk symptoms (SOPS). In: Handbook of attenuated psychosis syndrome across cultures. Springer, pp 85–113
Woodward ND, Heckers S (2016) Mapping thalamocortical functional connectivity in chronic and early stages of psychotic disorders. Biol Psychiatry 79(12):1016–1025. https://doi.org/10.1016/j.biopsych.2015.06.026

Yoon JH, Westphal AJ, Minzenberg MJ, Niendam T, Ragland JD, Lesh T, Solomon M, Carter CS (2014) Task-evoked substantia nigra hyperactivity associated with prefrontal hypofunction, prefrontonigral disconnectivity and nigrostriatal connectivity predicting psychosis severity in medication naive first episode schizophrenia. Schizophr Res 159(2–3):521–526. https://doi.org/10.1016/j.schres.2014.09.022

Yung AR, Yuen HP, McGorry PD, Phillips LJ, Kelly D, Dell'Olio M, Francey SM, Cosgrave EM, Killackey E, Stanford C, Godfrey K, Buckby J (2005) Mapping the onset of psychosis: the comprehensive assessment of at-risk mental states. Aust N Z J Psychiatry 39(11–12):964–971. https://doi.org/10.1080/j.1440-1614.2005.01714.x

Zaytseva Y, Bendova M, Garakh Z, Tintera J, Rydlo J, Spaniel F, Horacek J (2015) In search of neural mechanisms of mirror neuron dysfunction in schizophrenia: resting state functional connectivity approach. Psychiatr Danub 27:269–272

Zheng W, Zhang Q-E, Cai D-B, Ng CH, Ungvari GS, Ning Y-P, Xiang Y-T (2018) Neurocognitive dysfunction in subjects at clinical high risk for psychosis: a meta-analysis. J Psychiatr Res 103: 38–45

Ziermans T (2013) Working memory capacity and psychotic-like experiences in a general population sample of adolescents and young adults. Front Psych 4:161

Ziermans T, Wit S, Schothorst P, Sprong M, Hv E, Kahn R, Durston S (2014) Neurocognitive and clinical predictors of long-term outcome in adolescents at ultra-high risk for psychosis: a 6-year follow-up. PLoS One 9(4):e93994

Environmental Risk Factors and Cognitive Outcomes in Psychosis: Pre-, Perinatal, and Early Life Adversity

Emily Lipner, Kathleen J. O'Brien, Madeline R. Pike, Arielle Ered, and Lauren M. Ellman

Contents

Abstract Risk for psychosis begins to accumulate as early as the fetal period through exposure to obstetric complications like fetal hypoxia, maternal stress, and prenatal infection. Stressors in the postnatal period, such as childhood trauma, peer victimization, and neighborhood-level adversity, further increase susceptibility for psychosis. Cognitive difficulties are among the first symptoms to emerge in individuals who go on to develop a psychotic disorder. We review the relationship between pre-, perinatal, and early childhood adversities and cognitive outcomes in individuals with psychosis. Current evidence shows that the aforementioned environmental risk factors may be linked to lower overall intelligence and executive dysfunction, beginning in the premorbid period and persisting into adulthood in individuals with psychosis. It is likely that early life stress contributes to cognitive difficulties in

E. Lipner, K. J. O'Brien, M. R. Pike, A. Ered, and L. M. Ellman (✉)
Department of Psychology & Neuroscience, Temple University, Philadelphia, PA, USA
e-mail: ellman@temple.edu

Curr Topics Behav Neurosci (2023) 63: 205–240
https://doi.org/10.1007/7854_2022_378
Published Online: 2 August 2022

psychosis through dysregulation of the body's response to stress, causing changes such as increased cortisol levels and chronic immune activation, which can negatively impact neurodevelopment. Intersectional aspects of identity (e.g., sex/gender, race/ethnicity), as well as gene–environment interactions, likely inform the developmental cascade to cognitive difficulties throughout the course of psychotic disorders and are reviewed below. Prospective studies of birth cohorts will serve to further clarify the relationship between early-life environmental risk factors and cognitive outcomes in the developmental course of psychotic disorders. Specific methodological recommendations are provided for future research.

Keywords Childhood trauma · Cognition · Obstetric complications · Psychosis

1 Introduction

Although psychotic disorders, such as schizophrenia, tend to emerge during later adolescence/early adulthood, substantial evidence points to its neurodevelopmental origins beginning as early as the fetal period. Specifically, repeated studies have linked pre- and perinatal complications (Davies et al. 2020) and postnatal childhood adversity (Varese et al. 2012) to increased risk of psychosis (Brown 2011), and worsened course (Walker et al. 2008), and earlier onset of illness (Verdoux et al. 1997; Cannon et al. 2002a; Neill et al. 2020). Furthermore, signs of brain compromise in a large subgroup of patients with psychosis have been observed well before the onset of the disorder, with premorbid cognitive difficulties in approximately 40–50% of cases (Khandaker et al. 2011; Mollon and Reichenberg 2018). Cumulatively, these findings suggest that disruptions in neurodevelopment, particularly from pre- and postnatal adverse events, can lead to observable changes in behavior before any symptoms of the disorder emerge.

This review summarizes human literature linking prenatal, perinatal, and early childhood risk factors for cognitive outcomes across the developmental course of psychosis spectrum disorders. Furthermore, this review examines the relationship between these early environmental risk factors, cognition, and intermediate phenotypes of these disorders. Various mechanistic underpinnings of these relationships, including dysregulation of the hypothalamic-pituitary adrenal (HPA) axis, inflammation, and structural and functional brain changes, are explored. Specificity of these relationships to psychosis spectrum disorders is also considered.

2 Obstetric Complications and Cognition in Psychosis

Obstetric complications (OCs) refer to a broad range of difficulties during pregnancy and at birth and are among the most well-replicated environmental risk factors for psychosis (Cannon et al. 2002a; Ellman and Cannon 2008; Mittal et al. 2008). Namely, prenatal infection (Brown and Derkits 2010), maternal stress (Lipner et al. 2019), and fetal hypoxia (Mittal et al. 2008) are among the most well-studied OCs associated with psychosis risk. Maternal health behaviors (e.g., nutrition, nicotine use) have also been linked with psychosis outcomes (Brown and Susser 2008; Scott et al. 2018), and act transactionally with other co-occurring OCs linked to psychosis, including stress (Lipner et al. 2019). Subtle neurodevelopmental changes conferred by these prenatal adversities can prime offspring to be more susceptible to postnatal challenges and/or lead to a cascade of other cognitive, social, and behavioral outcomes. This paper will discuss the aforementioned OCs and their relationship to cognitive functioning in the course of psychotic disorders. Given recall bias evident in retrospective reporting of OCs (McIntosh et al. 2002), only studies that prospectively collected information about OCs were included.

2.1 *Prenatal Infection*

Exposure to infections during pregnancy (e.g., influenza, rubella, genital/reproductive infections) has been associated with an increased risk for psychotic disorders in offspring (Brown and Derkits 2010; Karlsson and Dalman 2020). Ecologic studies were among the first to establish this relationship. In one such study, offspring of women pregnant during the 1957 influenza epidemic were more likely to develop schizophrenia than those who were pregnant in a different time (Mednick et al. 1988). Although useful in preliminarily understanding the link between prenatal infection and psychosis risk, ecologic studies include mothers who did not actually incur the infection themselves and may not adequately demonstrate the strength of the relationship between exposure and psychosis outcomes (Brown 2011). Individual-level evidence from birth cohort studies or population-based studies from countries with national health registries provide more specific evidence about the relationship between prenatal infection and offspring outcomes utilizing prospectively collected measures of infection, such as serologic determination or physician diagnoses from medical records. Often using a nested case–control design, birth cohort studies have also compared outcomes between psychosis cases and controls, with or without exposure to various types of infections (Ellman and Susser 2009).

A handful of birth cohort studies examine the relationship between prenatal infection exposure and premorbid cognition within offspring who did and did not go on to develop a psychotic disorder. One such cohort, the Collaborative Perinatal Project (CPP), provided evidence of associations between serologically determined prenatal infection and impairments in cognitive function at age 7 (Ellman et al. 2009). Maternal influenza B infections during the third trimester, but not influenza A infections, were associated with significant decreases in verbal IQ and performance on the Information subtest of the Wechsler Intelligence Scale for Children (WISC) in those who went on to develop schizophrenia, but not controls (Ellman et al. 2009). Findings from the Rubella Birth Defects Evaluation Project also demonstrated a relationship between serologically determined prenatal rubella exposure and diminished IQ among those who went on to develop a schizophrenia spectrum disorder (Brown et al. 2001). Exposed offspring who developed schizophrenia spectrum disorders, but not rubella-exposed controls, also demonstrated a significant decline in IQ from childhood to adolescence. These studies demonstrate that prenatal infection may account for poorer cognitive performance prior to the onset of psychotic disorders and highlight that the type, and even strain, of infection may impact the cognitive difficulties that arise following infection exposure.

To our knowledge, only two additional studies examine the relationship between prenatal infection and cognitive deficits in adults with psychosis. In the Developmental Insult and Brain Anomaly in Schizophrenia (DIBS) cohort, prenatal exposure to genital/reproductive infections, confirmed by either medical records or seropositivity to immunoglobulin antibody for herpes simplex virus-2, was examined with respect to cognitive outcomes in adulthood (Brown et al. 2011). Significantly poorer verbal memory performance, measured by the California Verbal Learning Test (CVLT), was observed in exposed, compared to unexposed, offspring with schizophrenia. Verbal memory findings were only significant in offspring born to Black mothers (Brown et al. 2011). In the same cohort, cases with serologically documented exposure to influenza and toxoplasmosis showed impaired performance on the Wisconsin Card Sorting Test (WCST) and Trails B assessments in adulthood, indicating poorer executive functioning, specifically in cognitive set shifting (Brown et al. 2009). In sum, these findings suggest that prenatal infection is associated with both general and specific (e.g., verbal memory, executive function) cognitive difficulties beginning as early as age 7 that persist into the full disorder. Maternal and offspring demographics, and qualities of the infection, are also likely meaningful moderators of these relationships.

The mechanisms by which infection confers risk to the fetus vary by infection type and gestational timing. Some infections, like rubella, can cross the placenta and fetal blood-brain barrier, directly impacting neurodevelopment (Brown et al. 2001). Genital and reproductive infections may impact the fetus by way of microbes present in the placenta or vagina, proximal to the fetus itself (Engman et al. 2008; Brown 2011). Alternatively, most prenatal infections (e.g., influenza) do not appear to cross the placenta and likely impact the developing fetus by mechanisms co-occurring with infections, such as the maternal proinflammatory response (Fineberg and Ellman 2013). Human studies have identified that elevations in specific inflammatory biomarkers, such as interleukin (IL)-8, during pregnancy are associated with increased risk for psychotic disorders, moderated by both timing of the elevation and fetal sex (Buka et al. 2001; Brown et al. 2004; Goldstein et al. 2014). A study from the New England Family Study (NEFS) examined the relationship between prenatal maternal cytokine levels and cognitive and academic outcomes across all offspring, finding that higher levels of tumor necrosis factor-alpha (TNF-α) in the second and third trimesters were associated with lower IQ at age 7 (Ghassabian et al. 2018). Higher maternal C-reactive protein has also been associated with poorer teacher-judged academic achievement in adolescence, a risk factor for psychosis, in a recent study of the Northern Finland Birth Cohort (Ramsay et al. 2021). No studies to date examine the relationship between prenatal inflammation and cognition in individuals with psychosis.

Methodological hurdles exist in examining immune markers and specific offspring outcomes. As such, animal models of maternal immune activation provide an opportunity to experimentally induce timing-specific changes in prenatal inflammation via bacterial (polyinosinic:polycytidylic acid) and viral (lipopolysaccharide; LPS) agents (Meyer 2014) to explore cognitive outcomes in offspring (Estes and McAllister 2016). For example, rodent models show that higher IL-10 and IL-6 at mid-gestation are associated with deficits in spatial exploration, associative learning, and prepulse and latent inhibition in adult offspring (Smith et al. 2007; Meyer et al. 2008). Furthermore, LPS-induction has been associated with changes in the hippocampus and alterations in learning and memory in rodents (Golan et al. 2005). These findings suggest that fetal exposure to maternal inflammation during pregnancy can result in cognitive changes similar to those observed in schizophrenia.

Overall, prenatal infection is associated with poorer general and verbal intellectual functioning in the premorbid period and in adults with psychotic disorders. There is also evidence that infection may impact verbal memory and executive functioning in adults with schizophrenia. These findings should be taken with caution given small sample sizes in nested case–control designs. Additional studies examining the link between proinflammatory markers and cognitive outcomes in individuals with psychosis are needed. Importantly, exposure to maternal prenatal infection has been linked to a greater incidence of infections in childhood, an additional risk factor for the onset of psychotic disorders (Blomström et al. 2016). Furthermore, serious early childhood infections have been linked with poorer cognitive performance (e.g., lower IQ) in individuals who develop a psychotic disorder, independent of genetic risk (Karlsson and Dalman 2020).

As such, prenatal infection is associated with poorer neurocognitive development in individuals prior to the onset of, and within the course of, psychotic disorders. Prenatal adversity may also increase risk for additional "hits" later in development, conferring added risk to offspring. Because there is evidence that prenatal infection and inflammation, and childhood infection, are linked to a range of psychiatric outcomes, including autism and depression (Jiang et al. 2016; Murphy et al. 2017), the effects of prenatal infection on premorbid cognitive changes may be shared amongst psychological disorders. Although prenatal infection has been more extensively studied in the context of schizophrenia risk compared to other psychopathologies (Ellman et al. 2018), studies examining the link between prenatal infection and other diagnostic outcomes are growing (e.g., Simanek and Meier 2015). Preliminary findings from rodent and non-human primate models may provide insight into transdiagnostic premorbid neurological and cognitive outcomes following maternal immune activation that contribute to the course of neurodevelopmental disorders (Giovanoli et al. 2015; Vlasova et al. 2021).

2.2 *Prenatal Maternal Stress*

Prenatal maternal stress (PNMS) has been associated with risk for psychosis spectrum disorders, as well as several other adverse psychological (e.g., depression, attention deficit disorder, autism) and physical health outcomes (e.g., cardiovascular disease, obesity, asthma) in offspring (Van den Bergh et al. 2020). Ecologic (e.g., war, natural disaster) and individual level (e.g., traumatic life events, perceived stress) studies have linked PNMS to psychosis outcomes, in particular (Lipner et al. 2019). Operationalization of PNMS varies, sometimes including both objective and subjective measures of PMNS (Sutherland and Brunwasser 2018). Timing of PNMS and fetal sex are shown to impact vulnerability to the effects of PNMS on neurodevelopment (Lipner et al. 2019; Eyles 2021). Although the association between psychotic disorders and PNMS is well-replicated, to our knowledge, no study has examined the impact of PNMS on cognitive difficulties in the developmental course of psychotic disorders. As such, we can only hypothesize about how PNMS may impact cognitive development in individuals with psychotic disorders in both the premorbid period and in adulthood.

Studies from non-psychiatric, community samples provide insight into how PNMS may contribute to cognitive deficits in psychosis. PNMS is associated with several early cognitive outcomes typical of individuals who develop psychotic disorders (Beydoun and Saftlas 2008; Kingston et al. 2015; Lafortune et al. 2021). Researchers have demonstrated that 4.5-month-old infants exposed to high levels of PNMS had lower physical reasoning performance (e.g., ability to deduce physical causality; Merced-Nieves et al. 2020). As physical reasoning can be impaired in those with psychosis (Brunet et al. 2003), PNMS may contribute to this outcome. Cognitive delays associated with PNMS may become more pronounced with development, with one study documenting cognitive delays on both the mental and motor scales of the Bayley Scales of Infant Development upwards of three times greater in toddlers exposed to high levels of prenatal maternal anxiety than their non-affected counterparts (Brouwers et al. 2001). Several studies have documented an association between PNMS and decreased performance on cognitive tasks measuring: (1) regulating and shifting attention (Huizink et al. 2004), (2) language abilities (Laplante et al. 2008, 2018), (3) executive functioning (Buss et al. 2011), and (4) learning and memory (Gutteling et al. 2006). Each of these cognitive domains has been shown to be impaired during the premorbid period for psychotic disorders (Mollon and Reichenberg 2018). Notably, there are mixed findings on the relationship between PNMS and child IQ (Grizenko et al. 2015; Cortes Hidalgo et al. 2020), a documented intermediate phenotype for multiple psychological disorders (Koenen et al. 2009; Kremen et al. 1998, 2010; Lewis 2004).

PNMS may also exacerbate risk for other OCs associated with poorer cognitive performance in psychotic disorders, including infection, fetal hypoxia, and low birth weight (Lipner et al. 2019). PNMS can also elevate maternal glucocorticoids and inflammatory levels, altering the fetal environment during pregnancy and consequentially the fetal HPA axis (Coussons-Read 2013). Higher maternal cortisol levels during pregnancy have been associated with low birth weight in males who developed schizophrenia (Ellman et al. 2019). Male fetuses appear to be particularly vulnerable to the deleterious effects of PNMS and may be more likely to suffer from cognitive difficulties following PNMS exposure (Sandman et al. 2013; Sutherland and Brunwasser 2018). From research using community samples, higher maternal cortisol in late gestation has been associated with lower childhood IQ (LeWinn et al. 2009), poorer mental functioning, and delayed psychomotor development (Zijlmans et al. 2015), which are also associated with risk for multiple psychological disorders. Further evidence from both rodent and human studies demonstrates that higher levels of glucocorticoids are linked to brain abnormalities associated with cognitive deficits found in psychotic disorders, including increases in dopamine D2-like receptors in the striatum of rodents (Vidal and Pacheco 2020), higher incidence of dermatoglyphic asymmetry (Newell-Morris et al. 1989), and overall structural and cerebral asymmetry (Weinstock 2001).

Exposure to PNMS can have long-term implications on brain development and adult cognition (Charil et al. 2010). High levels of PNMS have been linked to smaller accessory basal and cortical nuclei volumes in the amygdala as well as larger bilateral amygdala volumes to total brain volume ratios (Jones et al. 2019; Mareckova et al. 2021), similar to changes observed in schizophrenia patients (Rasetti et al. 2009). Similarly, PNMS is shown to alter prefrontal cortex (PFC) and hippocampal-dependent cognitive functions in humans, including consolidation of memory and passive avoidance, which may contribute to the pathogenesis of schizophrenia (Negrón-Oyarzo et al. 2016). Human studies examining the consequences of PNMS on cognitive outcomes beyond childhood/adolescence are scarce; instead, current PNMS longitudinal literature favors rodent models (Beydoun and Saftlas 2008; Paquin et al. 2021). Animal studies demonstrate that early cognitive delays pave the way for more profound cognitive deficits related to psychosis risk in adulthood. For example, adult male rodents exposed to PNMS exhibit deficits in memory, including novel object recognition memory, spatial memory, and working memory (Markham et al. 2010). Male vulnerability to these worse cognitive outcomes may contribute to heightened male vulnerability to psychosis risk. As such, additional longitudinal research in humans is needed to clarify the relationships between PNMS and cognitive outcomes in individuals on the psychosis spectrum, with particular attention to both premorbid and adult outcomes and how fetal sex may moderate these relationships.

2.3 Hypoxia-Associated Obstetric Complications

Hypoxia-associated OCs, OCs related to decreased oxygen to the fetus, are found in the histories of about 20–30% of cases of schizophrenia (Mittal et al. 2008). Hypoxia-related OCs are often categorized as chronic placental hypoxia, occurring during the prenatal period, and acute perinatal hypoxia, occurring around delivery. Often, studies examine *probable* hypoxia-ischemic exposures, given that they utilize medical records to identify OCs that may have hypoxic effects. Fewer studies utilize biomarkers of hypoxic events, such as erythropoietin from umbilical cord serum, to define hypoxia exposure (Fineberg et al. 2013).

Low birth weight is also often a consequence of OCs and has been associated with an increased risk of psychosis, although some findings suggest that these associations are more prevalent among male offspring (Cannon et al. 2002a; Eide et al. 2013; Ellman et al. 2019). It is important to consider that low birth weight itself may not be a causal factor that leads to the onset of psychosis, but rather an observable and reliably measurable proxy for other perinatal adversity like fetal hypoxia, preterm birth, or placental dysfunction (Brown 2011). A study examining the CPP cohort provided evidence to further clarify these relationships, utilizing serologic determination for both influenza and hypoxia (Fineberg et al. 2013). Individuals with schizophrenia or affective psychoses with exposure to fetal hypoxia and/or influenza had lower birth weight compared to controls and unexposed cases (Fineberg et al. 2013). These findings suggest that exposure to these OCs associated with psychosis outcomes is linked to lower birth weight, particularly in individuals with vulnerability for psychosis. OC type may also impact vulnerability to particular types of psychotic disorders. While fetal hypoxia was associated with lower birth weight among individuals with schizophrenia, influenza B exposure was associated with lower birth weight among individuals with affective psychoses (Fineberg et al. 2013). Recent evidence demonstrates that other early life environmental risk factors (e.g., physical abuse, bullying, sleep quality) are differentially associated with dimensionally-assessed psychotic experiences (Cosgrave et al. 2021); as such, future prenatal research may unveil if/how certain OCs may differentially contribute to specific psychosis diagnoses and symptoms, as well as shared phenotypes with other mental disorders.

Birth cohort and population-based studies have examined the relationship between hypoxia-related OCs and premorbid cognitive outcomes generally. Studies from the CPP examining the entire cohort identified an association between antenatal hypoxia-related OCs and poorer IQ, verbal-perceptual abilities, achievement, and perceptual-motor abilities at age 7 (Naeye and Peters 1987; Seidman et al. 2000). An additional study from the CPP identified sex differences in these relationships, showing that chronic placental hypoxia was associated with lower verbal IQ and increased inhibition in female offspring only, whereas acute perinatal hypoxia was associated with diminished cognitive outcomes across sexes (Anastario et al. 2012).

Relationships between fetal hypoxia and premorbid cognitive outcomes vary slightly when examining offspring who go on to develop a schizophrenia spectrum disorder. Particularly, genetic risk appears to interact with hypoxia-related OCs in the pathway to neurodevelopmental changes. High-risk studies, utilizing at least one parent with psychotic disorder history as a marker of genetic risk, provide further insight into these pathways. An additional study of the CPP examined cases, siblings, and matched controls and IQ outcomes at ages 4 and 7 (measured by the Stanford-Binet Intelligence Scale and WISC, respectively; Cannon et al. 2000). Findings demonstrated that there was no significant relationship between hypoxia-related OCs or birth weight and IQ in individuals who went on to develop schizophrenia spectrum disorders. Given that there were also no differences between IQ outcomes between cases and their unaffected siblings, it is likely that genetic vulnerability drives this relationship. Relatedly, in a study of offspring of parents with schizophrenia spectrum disorders and controls also from the CPP, hypoxia exposure was not associated with lower IQ at age 7 in high-risk offspring (Goldstein et al. 2000). Although it is possible that these analyses were not sufficiently powered to identify significance in this subgroup, these data highlight the importance of examining gene-OC interactions in relationship to cognitive outcomes in offspring with diagnoses across the psychosis spectrum.

Mechanisms by which genetic risk may interact with OC exposure to result in cognitive outcomes have been explored. Firstly, evidence from high-risk studies demonstrate that genetic vulnerability-fetal hypoxia interactions may account for various neurological sequelae in individuals with schizophrenia also associated with cognitive differences, including smaller hippocampal volumes, reductions in gray matter, and periventricular damage (Cannon et al. 1989, 2002b; van Erp et al. 2002). Furthermore, a study of the CPP examined the expression of brain-derived neurotrophic factor (BDNF) in maternal cord blood in cases with psychotic disorders and controls exposed to hypoxia (Cannon et al. 2008). In cases with psychotic disorders, hypoxia exposure was associated with decreases in BDNF in cord serum, whereas in controls, BDNF increased after exposure. Finally, a recent study examined the interaction between OCs and expression of schizophrenia risk genes derived from genome-wide association studies (Ursini et al. 2018). Their findings corroborate and expand upon the aforementioned CPP studies, identifying that genetic risk moderates the relationship between OCs and schizophrenia outcomes, such that schizophrenia-related genes are upregulated in placental samples exposed to hypoxia-related OCs (pre-eclampsia and intrauterine growth restriction), particularly in male placentae. Furthermore, a follow-up study demonstrated schizophrenia risk genes were associated with smaller intracranial volumes in neonates, and poorer cognitive outcomes per the Mullen Scales of Early learning at ages 1 and 2, but these cognitive outcomes were only apparent in singleton pregnancies (Ursini et al. 2021). These associations were also stronger in males. Although these studies utilize a more sophisticated measurement of genetic risk, it is of note that these studies do measure OC severity via the McNeil–Sjöström Scale and assess OCs using a combination of maternal recall and medical records. As such, genetic vulnerability, perhaps differentially expressed in the placenta, and OC exposure may additively and/or interactively increase risk for cognitive outcomes in offspring who go on to develop psychosis, with increased vulnerability for males.

Moreover, individuals born with low birth weight or small for gestational age have been shown to have poorer cognitive outcomes in childhood and adolescence in the general population (Sacchi et al. 2020). A study from the CPP, examining all cohort members, demonstrated that the relationship between low birth weight and poorer performance across all cognitive domains assessed (verbal-perceptual abilities, achievement, and perceptual-motor abilities) in children was strongest in effect size compared to other OC categories examined, including probable hypoxic-ischemic events and chronic hypoxia (Seidman et al. 2000). In individuals with psychosis, low birth weight has been associated with differences in intelligence and executive functioning. In the DIBS cohort, low birth weight was associated with impairments in performance on executive function tasks (WCST and Trails) as well as lower IQ as measured by the Wechsler Adult Intelligence Scale (WAIS) in adult cases with schizophrenia spectrum disorders and not controls (Freedman et al. 2013). A population-based study of schizophrenia cases and their unaffected siblings showed that both low birth weight and high birth weight were associated with poorer visuospatial reasoning, processing speed, set-shifting, and verbal and visual memory in adulthood, compared to cases born at normative birth weight (Torniainen et al. 2013). Of note, high birth weight has been identified as a protective factor against schizophrenia risk (Davies et al. 2020). Finally, changes in cognitive performance associated with low birth weight, particularly in individuals with psychosis, may not be reflected in studies examining neurological changes, as one study found that low birth weight was associated with reduced cortical surface area in adulthood across both cases and controls (Haukvik et al. 2014).

Additional studies have examined the relationship between various other OCs and cognitive deficits in adults with psychosis. A study of the Thematically Organized Psychosis cohort examined OC incidence broadly by examining records from the Norwegian birth registry and creating OC severity ratings using the McNeil-Sjöström Scale (Wortinger et al. 2020). Schizophrenia cases with exposure to severe OCs demonstrated lower premorbid and adult IQ, compared to unexposed cases. Another Norwegian study examined the impact of OCs on executive outcomes (measured by the WCST and D-KEFS Color Word Interference Test) in early onset schizophrenia cases and controls (Teigset et al. 2020). Exposure to various specific OCs (e.g., emergency cesarean, higher birth length, lower 5-min Apgar scores) was associated with executive dysfunction in schizophrenia cases. Shortened gestational length, not necessarily at threshold of preterm birth, was associated with poorer performance on the WCST only in adults with schizophrenia but no associations were identified between birth weight and executive functioning in this sample. It is of note that some OCs associated with executive dysfunction in schizophrenia patients in this study have not been reliably associated with psychosis risk in other studies (e.g., cesarean delivery), but may be associated with earlier age at onset (Verdoux et al. 1997).

A number of methodological limitations should be considered when assessing studies that examine OCs and psychosis outcomes. First, many studies examining OCs suffer from small sample sizes and, consequently, insufficient statistical power, to identify small effects (Cannon et al. 2002a). Second, given that OCs are a broad category of various pre- and perinatal adversities, there is substantial variability in the way these adversities are measured, operationalized, and analyzed. As previously mentioned, maternal recall of incidence and timing of OCs is likely biased (McIntosh et al. 2002), highlighting the importance of prospective designs. Additionally, many studies conflate OCs, examining them broadly as a combination of adversities or creating an overall severity rating, using scales like the McNeil–Sjöström Scale. Utilizing broad categories of OCs may be problematic, given that specific OCs may differentially impact fetal development and because dimensions of OCs (e.g., severity, duration, timing) may moderate the relationship between OCs and offspring outcomes. As such, studies that prospectively assess prenatal adversity using medical record data and or serologic determination provide more specific accounts of these OCs.

2.4 Maternal Health Behaviors

Maternal health behaviors during pregnancy, including substance use and nutritional intake, can have direct and indirect impacts on fetal neurodevelopment. Maternal malnutrition has been associated with an increased risk for offspring psychotic disorders in ecologic studies of famine (Brown and Susser 2008). Lower levels of specific micronutrients (e.g., folic acid, iron, vitamin D) during pregnancy have also been associated with increased risk for schizophrenia among offspring (McGrath et al. 2011) A study of the DIBS cohort identified that, in adult offspring with schizophrenia, compared to controls, lower serum hemoglobin levels were associated with lower scores on the Information subtest of the WAIS-III and poorer neuromotor performance (Ellman et al. 2012). Higher levels of homocysteine, a reliable proxy used to measure folic acid levels in sera, are associated with an increased risk for psychosis among offspring (Brown et al. 2007). In a rodent model of schizophrenia, Canever et al. (2018) examined the impact of folic acid supplementation on cognition, in addition to other OCs related to cognitive dysregulation in psychosis patients, such as inflammation. Folic acid supplementation was associated with an anti-inflammatory effect in rodents and buffered against spatial memory deficits associated with a folic acid-deficient diet (Canever et al. 2018). Given that higher pre-pregnancy BMI also has been associated with increased risk for psychosis outcomes in offspring (Schaefer et al. 2000), inflammatory dysregulation may be one pathway by which nutritional deficits during pregnancy incur risk for neurocognitive changes in offspring who go on to develop psychotic disorders (Bordeleau et al. 2020).

Maternal smoking has also been linked to offspring outcomes of psychosis (Hunter et al. 2020). Although there is no research to date examining the relationship between prenatal nicotine use and cognitive outcomes in offspring with psychotic disorders, there is evidence that smoking during pregnancy is associated with other OCs linked to cognitive outcomes, such as low birth weight, prenatal hypoxia, and exposure to toxins like lead (Huizink and Mulder 2006; Ellman et al. 2007; Ko et al.

2014). PNMS (e.g., pregnancy-specific stress) may also increase engagement in adverse health behaviors like smoking (Lobel et al. 2008). Of note, a recent study utilizing sibling comparisons demonstrated that the link between smoking exposure and psychosis outcomes became insignificant when controlling for shared genetic and environmental factors (Quinn et al. 2017), highlighting the importance of examining gene–environment interactions in studies of OCs. Nonetheless, examinations of maternal health behaviors emphasize the transactional nature of possible insults to the fetus during the perinatal period and the utility of examining them in concert with one another.

2.5 Obstetric Complications and Cognition in Psychosis: Summary

There is preliminary evidence that demonstrates a relationship between prenatal infection, hypoxia-related OCs, and maternal nutrition on premorbid and adult cognitive outcomes in individuals with psychosis. Generally, these OCs are associated with declines in overall IQ and in verbal IQ in the premorbid period, and difficulties in overall intelligence persist into adulthood, alongside poorer verbal memory and executive functioning (particularly, set shifting). Although there is evidence that PNMS is associated with alterations in cognition in population-based samples, and with intermediate phenotypes linked to poorer cognitive performance in individuals with psychosis (e.g., low birth weight), no study to date has examined the impact of PNMS on cognitive function in the course of psychosis. Given that many birth cohort studies employ nested case–control designs to examine differences in cognitive function based on OC exposure and diagnostic outcome (psychosis versus control), it is difficult to discern the specificity of these risk factors to cognitive outcomes in psychosis compared with other disorders. These comparisons are necessary, given that many of these OCs have been linked to a variety of mental health outcomes (Pugliese et al. 2019; Mathewson et al. 2017; Han et al. 2021). Nevertheless, all of these OCs likely confer risk for shared phenotypes between mental disorders, such as cognitive outcomes, which future studies will need to parse apart. A dimensional approach examining transdiagnostic symptom clusters (e.g., anhedonia), and/or examining multiple mental disorders simultaneously, may clarify the specificity of OCs to alterations in cognitive functioning in offspring with psychiatric symptoms and a range of mental disorders, more generally.

With the exception of research on prenatal infection, most studies examining OCs conflate exposures to various prenatal adversities in analyses, further stymieing our understanding of their unique effects on cognitive outcomes in psychosis. With greater specificity in the measurement of prenatal risk factors, we may also be able to more effectively examine the interactive influences of various OCs on cognitive outcomes (e.g., infection x fetal hypoxia). Existing literature examining the role of genetic risk in the relationship between hypoxia-related OCs and cognitive and psychosis outcomes (Ursini et al. 2021) emphasizes the need to examine how genetic vulnerability (and other early vulnerabilities) factor in concert with other OCs. Furthermore, our research on outcomes of depressive symptomatology in offspring demonstrates that second trimester daily life stress, only in the presence of infection, is associated with greater depressive symptoms in adolescent offspring (Murphy et al. 2017). Perhaps unique combinations of pre- and perinatal adversities contribute to earlier deficits in cognitive functioning in individuals who go on to develop psychotic disorders. Given high rates of comorbidity between mood disorders and psychosis, it is also possible that these unique combinations of pre- and perinatal risk factors may be related to cognitive outcomes evident across disorders or shared symptom clusters.

3 Early Life Stress and Cognition in Psychosis

Notably, not all fetuses exposed to OCs will go on to develop psychosis; therefore, it has been suggested that OCs may act as a "primer," increasing susceptibility to the negative effects of other postnatal stressors (Estes and McAllister 2016). Furthermore, adversity occurring in childhood and early adolescence is, in itself, a significant contributing factor to the development of both psychosis and cognitive impairments found in those experiencing psychosis, as these are important periods for brain development (McCabe et al. 2012). In a sample of individuals with recent-onset psychosis, individuals who experienced childhood trauma had more severe symptoms and worse functional outcomes (Rosenthal et al. 2020). The impact of early trauma on individuals' neurocognitive and psychosocial development highlights the importance of understanding links between early life stress, cognitive impairments, and psychosis.

Several forms of early adversity, including childhood trauma, peer victimization, and neighborhood-level stressors, likely contribute to the development of cognitive difficulties in schizophrenia by dysregulating the body's response to stress and increasing risk for neurobiological changes that impact cognition (Raymond et al. 2018). For example, chronic activation of the immune system in response to stress can lead to increased microglial activation, a key component of neuroinflammation, which may be associated with structural (e.g., impaired white matter integrity, volume loss; Müller et al. 2015; Poletti et al. 2015) and functional (e.g., changes to dopaminergic systems; Müller et al. 2015) changes that contribute to both cognitive difficulties and risk for psychosis (Nettis et al. 2020). Therefore, the relationship between early life stress and cognitive functioning among individuals with psychosis, and the mechanisms underlying these relationships, will be explored here.

3.1 Childhood Trauma

Childhood trauma is linked to cognitive difficulties in individuals across the psychosis spectrum. A meta-analysis of 23 studies found childhood trauma was associated with poorer overall neurocognitive function, measured as a single composite score averaged across multiple neuropsychological batteries, in individuals diagnosed with psychosis (Vargas et al. 2019). These findings contrast with earlier studies which reported no association (Sideli et al. 2014; van Os et al. 2017) or linked childhood trauma to better cognitive functioning in psychosis patients (Campbell et al. 2013). Among individuals at clinical high risk for psychosis (CHR), those with a history of childhood trauma show better overall cognitive functioning than those without childhood trauma (Velikonja et al. 2021). These discrepant findings may be because the link between childhood trauma and poorer cognition is stronger for non-psychiatric controls compared to patients (Vargas et al. 2019). It is also possible that specific cognitive domains are more likely to be affected by trauma in psychosis populations, or that these associations vary depending on the stage of the disorder examined (e.g., CHR versus chronic psychosis).

Childhood trauma may be particularly deleterious to higher order cognitive processes, such as executive functioning (Johnson et al. 2021). In the aforementioned meta-analysis, childhood trauma was associated with lower scores on a range of executive functioning tasks among individuals with psychosis, even prior to psychosis onset (Vargas et al. 2019; see review for specific tasks examined). In a study of individuals at CHR, childhood trauma was associated with worse performance on tasks involving cognitive control and executive functioning, such as the Stroop Test and WCST (Üçok et al. 2015). Among individuals with a family history of psychosis, those exposed to any childhood abuse or neglect (as identified by a clinician, rather than self-report) showed poorer performance in executive functions of initiation, as well as more combinations of cognitive deficits associated with lower overall functioning (Berthelot et al. 2015). However, in a large non-clinical sample, it was found that traumatic life events, but not psychotic-like experiences (PLEs; subclinical, attenuated forms of positive symptoms), contributed to attentional biases (demonstrated by slower reaction time) on an emotional Stroop task (Gibson et al. 2019). Finally, in another non-clinical sample, childhood trauma fully explained the association between reduced inhibition on a Stroop task and higher levels of PLEs, suggesting that impairments in executive functions may constitute a causal mechanism through which childhood trauma leads to the later development of psychotic symptoms (Begemann et al. 2016). This may also explain why psychotic symptoms are directly related to poorer executive functioning later in the course of psychosis, but this relationship is accounted for by childhood trauma in earlier phases of the disorder. Evidence among non-clinical populations indicates that childhood trauma impacts executive functioning through dysregulation of the HPA-axis, which drives changes in cortisol levels that can affect the development of brain regions integral to executive functioning, such as the PFC (Feola et al. 2020); however, this has yet to be explored in individuals on the psychosis spectrum. Although childhood trauma has been associated with poorer executive functioning across the psychosis spectrum, future research is needed to determine if similar mechanisms (e.g., dysregulation of the HPA axis leading to structural changes in the PFC) are associated with these deficits across phases of illness.

Childhood trauma has also been associated with poorer working memory for individuals with psychosis. Of the domains examined by Vargas et al. (2019), working memory (including letter-number sequencing, digit span, N-back, and spatial working memory tasks) showed the largest negative association with childhood trauma. Childhood trauma also remains associated with scores on letter-number sequencing and digit span tests, even after controlling for premorbid IQ (Shannon et al. 2011; Campbell et al. 2013) and depressive symptoms (Shannon et al. 2011). Alternatively, some studies do not provide evidence of this relationship. One study of first-episode psychosis (FEP) patients and controls found no differences in performance on the MATRICS Consensus Cognitive Battery (MCCB) working memory subscale between the groups with comparable levels of childhood trauma (Kilian et al. 2018). Likewise, in a recent study of patients with schizophrenia and bipolar disorder (with and without psychotic features), verbal N-back scores did not mediate the relationship between early life stress and severity of psychotic symptoms (Corcoran et al. 2020). While it is possible this study was underpowered to detect a mediation effect, the findings are consistent with research reporting that the association between childhood trauma and cognition is stronger for non-clinical controls than for individuals with psychosis (Vargas et al. 2019). Therefore, it is possible discrepant findings may be due to a floor effect, in which individuals with psychosis already show poorer working memory performance compared to controls.

Poorer performance in additional cognitive domains has been associated with childhood trauma. Among individuals with psychosis, childhood trauma was associated with poor attentional functioning, measured by RBANS digit span and coding subtests (Kasznia et al. 2021) and MCCB attention domain (Schalinski et al. 2018). Furthermore, Ayesa-Arriola et al. (2020) reported that childhood trauma, particularly when combined with recent life stress, was associated with decreases in processing speed on the WAIS-III Digit-Symbol subtest. Similarly, for individuals at CHR, total childhood trauma exposure was associated with poorer performance on tasks involving attention and processing speed (Üçok et al. 2015; Velikonja et al. 2021). In a study of adult psychosis patients, childhood trauma was associated with increased activation of the inferior frontal gyrus (IFG), a region involved in attentional processing, during a response-inhibition task (Go/No Go; Quidé et al. 2018). Decreased gray matter in the IFG has been associated with exposure to childhood trauma (Lim et al. 2014). Therefore, over-activation of the IFG may represent a possible compensatory mechanism in which individuals with childhood trauma require stronger salience signals from the IFG to maintain inhibitory control (Quidé et al. 2018). Regardless, childhood trauma appears to be associated with attentional functioning difficulties across the psychosis spectrum.

Childhood trauma is also associated with deficits in various memory processes for individuals with psychosis. For example, childhood trauma is associated with poorer scores on the Rey Auditory Verbal Learning Test, a test of verbal memory, in individuals in the early course of schizophrenia (Ayesa-Arriola et al. 2020). Similarly, in a study of FEP patients, lower cortisol awakening response, an indicator of blunted HPA-axis functioning, was also associated with deficits in verbal memory, measured by the Wechsler Memory Scale (Aas et al. 2011). Additionally, blunted HPA-axis functioning has been associated with early trauma in psychosis patients (Mondelli et al. 2010). Furthermore, for individuals with psychosis, childhood trauma was associated with poorer episodic narrative memory, measured by the WAIS-III logical memory test (Shannon et al. 2011), as well as lower scores on a visual facial memory task (Carrilho et al. 2019). Childhood trauma was also associated with lower scores on a range of tasks assessing delayed memory, such as list recall, list recognition, story memory, and figure recall among patients with psychosis (Kasznia et al. 2021). Among non-clinical individuals, childhood trauma is associated with deficits in short-term memory continuing throughout adulthood and these deficits are associated with severity of abuse (Bremner et al. 1995). Childhood trauma and subsequent HPA-axis dysregulation have been associated with reductions in hippocampal volume (Bremner et al. 1997, 2003; Stein et al. 1997), which are also evident in individuals with psychosis (Read et al. 2001), indicating a potential mechanistic pathway. Because memory impacts multiple cognitive domains, it is possible these deficits play a role in the dysfunction of higher-order cognitive processes among individuals with psychosis and a history of childhood trauma.

It is crucial to note that measurements of childhood trauma often rely on retrospective reporting. One such assessment, the Childhood Trauma Questionnaire, assesses frequency of five domains of childhood trauma, as well as if the individual may be minimizing their experiences (Bernstein et al. 1994). While measures like this one are well-validated, studies have shown that only 52% of individuals who reported traumatic events in prospective studies reported having experienced trauma when asked retrospectively (Baldwin et al. 2019). Retrospective reporting of trauma also fails to thoroughly capture the timing of such adversities. Timing and chronicity of childhood adversity, relative to developmental milestones, may be meaningful in understanding the impact on resulting cognitive deficits and its related functioning. Prospective reporting of childhood trauma may serve to improve the validity and timing-specificity of reporting.

Examining specific types of childhood trauma, such as abuse or neglect, may also shed light on the heterogeneity in cognitive difficulties observable in individuals with psychosis. For example, in a study of patients with psychosis spectrum disorders, physical and emotional neglect significantly predicted poorer MCCB verbal learning and overall cognition composite score, whereas physical, sexual, and emotional abuse did not (Kilian et al. 2018). Similarly, neglect, but not abuse, was associated with poorer scores on a working memory composite for individuals with psychosis spectrum disorders (Mørkved et al. 2020) see paper for specific tasks). Consequently, while many studies report overall trauma exposure, evidence shows that trauma type differentially impacts individual outcomes (Dauvermann and Donohoe 2019). Findings in non-psychiatric controls also show differential outcomes following physical abuse versus neglect, such as atypical fear learning associated with abusive or threatening experiences and reduced executive function associated with neglect (McLaughlin and Sheridan 2016). Given the unique effect of different types of trauma and the fact that abuse and neglect typically co-occur, future studies should control for the effect of co-occurring traumas in statistical models to better understand the impact of trauma specificity on cognitive outcomes (Ered and Ellman 2019).

3.2 Neighborhood-Level Adversity

Neighborhood-level factors, such as urbanicity, have been identified as risk factors for the development of psychosis (Krabbendam and van Os 2005; Fett et al. 2011); however, it remains unclear which aspects of urban living (e.g., social/economic stress, environmental toxins/pollution, lack of green space) drive this relationship (Fett et al. 2011). For example, perception of the neighborhood's condition, including crime and physical or social disorder, was associated with longer duration of untreated psychosis, even after controlling for participant's socioeconomic status (SES; Ku et al. 2020). To our knowledge, only one study to date has examined the relationship between neighborhood-level factors and cognition in individuals on the psychosis spectrum. In a large prospective cohort of Swedish men at CHR or diagnosed with nonaffective psychosis, 23% of the association between neighborhood deprivation (measured by crime rates, unemployment, low income, and receipt of social benefits) and psychosis was accounted for by IQ (Lewis et al. 2020).

Notably, many adverse neighborhood-level factors disproportionately impact individuals from low SES. Individuals who develop psychosis may also be more susceptible to the negative effects of low SES (Yeo et al. 2014; Czepielewski et al. 2021). A study examining cognitive functioning in schizophrenia patients across five Latin American countries found patients performed worse on all MCCB domains compared to controls, and that SES was more strongly related to MCCB scores in patients than controls (Czepielewski et al. 2021). Similarly, a U.S. study reported an association between lower parental SES and poorer scores on tests of planning and inhibition in schizophrenia patients, but not non-psychiatric controls (Yeo et al. 2014). These findings also showed that lower parental SES was associated with reduced gray matter volume of the superior frontal gyrus in patients, but not controls, suggesting a potential mechanism through which SES can influence cognitive functioning in individuals with psychosis. However, further research is needed to elucidate which aspects of these environmental factors are driving the relationship between neighborhood-level adversity and cognitive difficulties, and why individuals with psychosis may be particularly susceptible.

Moreover, experiences of discrimination, particularly among racial/ethnic minority groups and individuals from low SES backgrounds, are associated with increased risk for psychosis (Oh et al. 2014; Anglin et al. 2021) and greater severity of psychotic symptoms (Anglin et al. 2014; Shaikh et al. 2016) While the relationship between discrimination and cognitive function in psychosis has yet to be examined, a recent longitudinal study reported that discriminatory experiences are associated with thinning of several cortical regions over time in CHR individuals (Collins et al. 2021). These findings were moderated by gender and race/ethnicity, indicating females and racial/ethnic minorities show steeper rates of cortical thinning associated with discrimination. Several of the cortical regions examined, such as the PFC, are integral to cognitive functioning. Therefore, future research should examine how experiences of discrimination, moderated by intersectional aspects of identity (e.g., gendered racism), may contribute to cognitive difficulties among individuals with psychosis.

3.3 Peer Victimization

Bullying and peer victimization have been linked to increased risk for both psychosis (Schreier et al. 2009; Varese et al. 2012) and impairments in cognitive flexibility, demonstrated by longer times on the Trail Making Test (Medeiros et al. 2016). Peer victimization may lead to cognitive impairments through dysfunction of the HPA-axis, as discussed previously (Lataster et al. 2006). This theory is supported by a study which found help-seeking youths who experienced high levels of bullying showed more intense negative affect and psychotic experiences in response to stress compared to non-help-seeking controls (Rauschenberg et al. 2021). These findings are consistent with the theory that stress reactivity, a key aspect of HPA-axis dysregulation, may constitute a marker of psychosis risk (Myin-Germeys et al. 2001), and a contributing factor to cognitive difficulties (Lataster et al. 2006).

Cognitive impairments associated with genetic and environmental (e.g., OCs) risk factors may precede experiences of victimization and precipitate increased risk of victimization (Danese et al. 2017). A large-scale longitudinal study reported that peer victimization mediated the relationship between developmental impairments (including OCs, low IQ, and motor impairments) and PLEs, suggesting that individuals with developmental impairments are more likely to be bullied, thereby increasing the risk for developing psychosis (Liu et al. 2020). Existing cognitive impairments may increase risk for peer victimization, further exacerbating the impairment; however, these transactional relationships require further investigation.

3.4 Early Life Stress and Cognition in Psychosis: Summary

Early life stress impacts a range of cognitive domains among individuals with psychosis, with pronounced effects on executive functions, including working memory, potentially underlying deficits in overall cognition (Vargas et al. 2019). Early life stress likely contributes to cognitive difficulties in psychosis by dysregulating the body's response to stress (e.g., increased cortisol levels, chronic immune activation) which can negatively impact the neurodevelopment of regions involved in cognitive functioning, such as the PFC and hippocampus. Given that early life stress increases risk for a range of psychological sequelae, it is difficult to discern the extent to which early life stress impacts cognition in psychotic disorders, specifically. Nonetheless, there is preliminary evidence that traumatic events are more strongly associated with PLEs, as well as PTSD and borderline personality disorder symptoms, than other symptom domains (Gibson et al. 2017). Importantly, when adjusting for these co-occurring symptoms, traumatic life events were no longer associated with depressive symptoms, anxiety, or substance use, which previously had been well-documented relationships (Green et al. 2010; van Nierop et al. 2015). Therefore, early life stress may be linked to specific symptom clusters, including psychotic symptoms, further exacerbating cognitive difficulties which are characteristic of psychotic disorders. Inconsistencies in findings may be due to variability in the methodologies used to measure trauma, lack of specificity of trauma type, timing, and chronicity, and failure to account for co-occurring symptoms.

4 Discussion

Overall, there is evidence that prenatal and early childhood environmental risk factors impact general intelligence, verbal intelligence, and executive functioning, often beginning in the premorbid period and continuing into adulthood, in individuals with psychosis. These risk factors align with the conceptualization of schizophrenia as a neurodevelopmental disorder in which cognitive deficits arise prior to illness onset and remain relatively stable (Reichenberg et al. 2010). However, it has been suggested that some individuals with psychosis exhibit average premorbid cognitive function which declines as the illness progresses (Weickert et al. 2000; Badcock et al. 2005). These cognitive subtypes, often referred to as "compromised" and "deteriorated," respectively, show differing neurodevelopmental profiles (Woodward and Heckers 2015) and may account for variability in findings. The principle of multifinality (i.e., one risk factor may contribute to various outcomes) complicates our understanding of findings related to the pre-, perinatal, and childhood origins of psychosis risk. OCs and early childhood trauma have been associated with a number of psychopathological outcomes in offspring; as such, it is challenging to clarify the extent to which certain risk factors are *specific* to a particular diagnostic outcome (Huizink and de Rooij 2018). Few prenatal studies have attempted to answer questions of multifinality; however, investigations into early cognitive deficits may provide insight into potential mechanisms. Utilizing a developmental framework to understand issues of multifinality may be crucial to future analyses. For example, individuals who go on to develop schizophrenia, in particular, show lower premorbid cognitive performance (e.g., global IQ) compared to those that develop bipolar disorder (Bortolato et al. 2015). Prenatal and childhood stress are likely involved in the cascade of risk to neuropsychological deficits across disorders, but perhaps at different stages of neurodevelopment. Nonetheless, the high level of comorbidity of psychosis with other psychological disorders (e.g., affective disorders) adds to the challenge of identifying the specificity of early life risk factors to the emergence of psychosis and its related cognitive profile.

We have highlighted the myriad limitations of the existing research on these early life risk factors, including variability in measurement, issues with retrospective reporting, small sample sizes, and challenges in examining the specificity of various adversities on cognitive outcomes. Moreover, literature that integrates the impact of pre- and perinatal adversity and early life stress on cognitive outcomes in individuals with psychosis is scarce. Figure 1 illustrates how environmental risk factors may work additively/interactively across development toward specific cognitive difficulties in psychotic disorders, underscoring the need for future studies integrating the impact of various pre- and postnatal adversities on cognitive outcomes in psychosis. It is likely that specific risk factors do not lead to cognitive difficulties in psychotic disorders, but that there may be myriad unique developmental cascades associated with such outcomes (Lipner et al. 2019; Ellman et al. 2018). As such, this underscores the importance of measuring the unique risk factors so more specific, longitudinal, and transactional analyses can be conducted.

Early intervention proximal to these perinatal and childhood risk factors may aid in preventing some of these cognitive difficulties from cascading into difficulties resulting in a psychotic disorder. As early as the prenatal period, there is preliminary evidence that micronutrient supplementation (e.g., folic acid, choline, and possibly Vitamin D) may buffer the effects of maternal nutritional deficiencies and other related OCs to decrease the risk for psychotic disorders (Freedman et al. 2021). Interestingly, there is evidence that fetal sex may moderate the relationship between Vitamin D supplementation and decreased risk for psychosis, such that this intervention was only associated with decreased risk for schizophrenia in male offspring in a Finnish study (McGrath et al. 2004). Physician monitoring of maternal mental well-being at prenatal visits may also allow for early identification of antenatal anxiety and depression, facilitating early intervention to decrease fetal exposure to PNMS (Bhat et al. 2017).

Postnatally, positive parenting may buffer the association between earlier adversities and cognitive difficulties. Previous work in a non-psychiatric sample demonstrated that sensitive parenting (defined as greater supportive scaffolding during play and challenging puzzle tasks), measured via clinician rating of maternal-child interactions, moderated the relationship between low birth weight and poorer executive functioning in children at ages 3 and 5 (Camerota et al. 2015). School-based interventions, such as adaptive training programs, have been shown to improve and sustain the enhancement of poor working memory in children (Holmes et al. 2009). An experimental early childhood intervention aimed to provide quality education to children from disadvantaged backgrounds was associated with significant improvements in both cognitive and non-cognitive skills, especially in children from the most disadvantaged backgrounds (Xie et al. 2020). Minimizing exposures to environmental contaminants (e.g., manganese, lead, plastics with BPAs, and air pollution) may also improve cognitive functioning across development (Clifford et al. 2016; Mhaouty-Kodja et al. 2018; Martin et al. 2021). Therefore, environmental

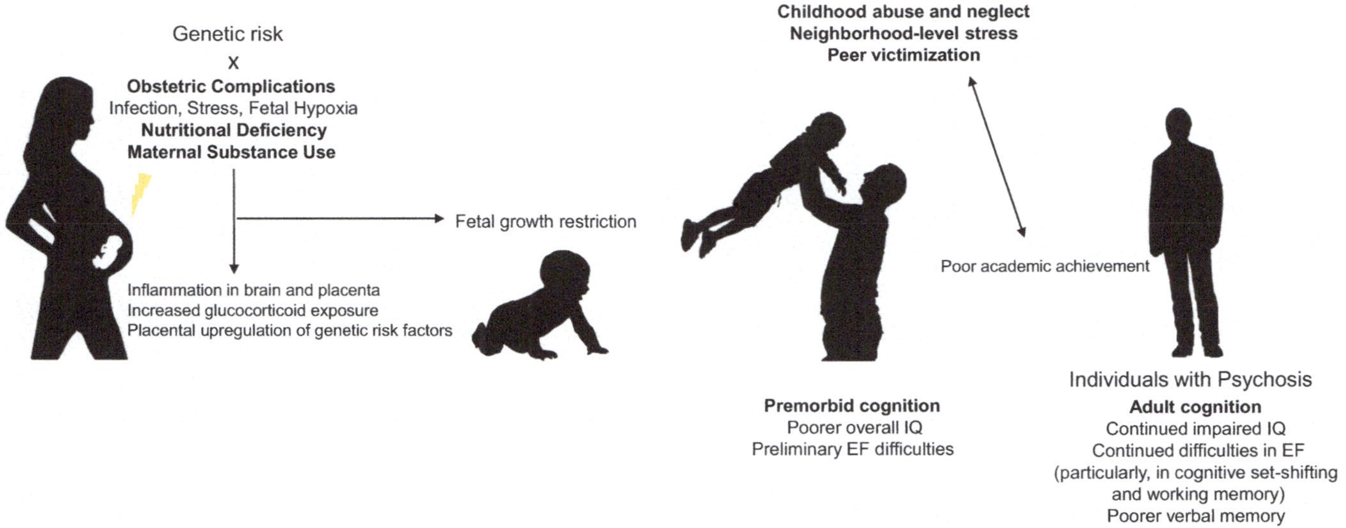

Fig. 1 Proposed developmental trajectory for the onset of cognitive difficulties from pre-, perinatal, and early childhood environmental risk factors in individuals with psychotic disorders. OCs confer changes on the brain beginning in-utero, which can persist into the postnatal period. These changes are evidenced in cognitive changes apparent as early as infancy that may extend through adulthood. While many women experience OCs over the course of their pregnancy, most offspring do not go on to develop neurodevelopmental disorders like schizophrenia; therefore, understanding the additional risk factors that combine with OCs to portend risk for schizophrenia is needed (Ellman et al. 2018). For example, there is evidence OCs can impact one another. PNMS has been associated with greater risk of infection, increased engagement in adverse health behaviors, and increased risk for gestational complications (Lipner et al. 2019). Individuals with a history of OCs are also more likely to experience stressful events during childhood, such as peer victimization, which may subsequently increase the risk for psychotic experiences in adulthood (Liu et al. 2020). Poorer cognitive functioning also likely impacts the way that individuals are treated within their childhood environment by parents, peers, and teachers (McIntosh et al. 1993; Haager and Vaughn 1995). As we strive to understand early environmental and genetic risk factors for cognitive impairments, we must consider transactional ways in which early "hits" or "primers" can work synergistically or additively with postnatal environmental factors (Estes and McAllister 2016). Sequelae resulting from perinatal adversities may be compounded by environmental risk factors in the postnatal period, including chronic stress and trauma during childhood. Figure adapted from Lipner et al. (2019)

stressors may have long-term effects on cognitive outcomes in psychotic disorders, but they are also identifiable and therefore treatable. Programs may aim to pay particular attention to the confluence of OCs and early life stressors as early cognitive complaints emerge and as an avenue for early intervention. Additional research on the utility of these various interventions on cognitive outcomes, specifically in those with psychotic disorders, is needed.

4.1 Considerations Pertaining to Intersectionality

Intersectional aspects of identity (e.g., sex/gender, race/ethnicity) likely also inform the developmental cascade to cognitive difficulties in the course of psychotic disorders. Firstly, males have demonstrated greater deficits in cognition and attention, specifically in verbal tasks, during the premorbid period (Goldstein et al. 1994) and sexual dimorphism persists into chronic schizophrenia (Goldstein et al. 1998). Pre- and perinatal risk factors likely set the stage for sex differences in cognitive performance, as studies have shown an increased risk for psychosis for male offspring after exposure to various OCs, including PNMS (Fineberg et al. 2016), and increased risk for intermediate phenotypes of psychosis, like low birth weight (Ellman et al. 2019). Increased psychosis risk for male offspring is likely regulated by the sex-moderated placenta (Bronson and Bale 2016), and recent findings demonstrate that males have higher placental expression of genetic risk factors for psychosis with stronger associations to poorer cognitive functioning in early life (Ursini et al. 2021). Sex differences in the inflammatory profile of the in-utero environment for male fetuses may also contribute to these differences, given that higher levels of proinflammatory cytokines are evident in males during the prenatal period, and male fetuses may be more sensitive to the impact of this inflammation (Kim-Fine et al. 2012; Hunter et al. 2021). Such findings support the theory that male and female fetuses are armed with different evolutionary strategies for survival, such that female fetuses are more equipped to adapt to environmental adversity whereas the male fetus more heavily invests resources in growth during adverse conditions (Sandman et al. 2013). These differences leave males at higher risk of prenatal environmental stressors and, consequentially, fetal neurodevelopmental deficits (Sutherland and Brunwasser 2018).

Sex differences also have been found in studies examining childhood trauma and cognitive deficits, such that females are more likely to be *protected* from the cognitive and neurological effects of childhood trauma, both for individuals with schizophrenia (Ruby et al. 2017) and in the general population (Samplin et al. 2013). Conversely, women with childhood trauma exhibit more positive and mood symptoms, as well as earlier age of onset of psychosis, compared to women without a history of childhood trauma, and this association is not present in men (Comacchio et al. 2019). As such, women may be protected from neurological effects (e.g., smaller hippocampi), but not the psychiatric effects, of childhood trauma exposure (Samplin et al. 2013). Examining sex differences in the trajectory from OCs to childhood trauma may serve to further clarify these trends in related cognitive difficulties.

Important to the discussion of the impact of environmental stressors on cognition is the disproportionate impact of these stressors on individuals of marginalized racial and ethnic groups due to systemic oppression. Mothers from marginalized racial groups in the US experience greater incidence of OCs overall, and perceived discrimination during pregnancy may account for increased risk for OCs, like low birth weight (Giscombé and Lobel 2005; Dominguez et al. 2008). In the postnatal period, individuals from marginalized racial groups are more likely to be exposed to childhood adversity such as physical abuse, sexual abuse, domestic violence, and low SES (Anglin et al. 2021). These stressors lead to HPA axis dysregulation and neural inflammation as early as the prenatal period (Glynn et al. 2007; Gillespie et al. 2016) and may lead to damage in stress-sensitive brain regions including the PFC and hippocampus, resulting in cognitive difficulties (Howes and McCutcheon 2017). The disproportionate impact of these stressors on individuals from marginalized racial groups, as well as the differential exposure to stressors based on an individual's racial/ethnic group and gender identity (e.g., police victimization of Black males), must be considered in studies of early life adversity and cognition on the psychosis spectrum.

4.2 Gene × Environment Interactions

Examination of OCs and genetic vulnerability for psychosis together will facilitate a clearer understanding of their relative contributions to cognitive sequelae. Findings suggest that fetal hypoxia exposure on its own is unlikely to result in cognitive changes; however, it likely interacts with genetic risk factors associated with psychosis, particularly expressed in the placenta of male fetuses, to incur damage to the developing brain (Cannon et al. 2000; Ursini et al. 2021). It is likely that this gene x environment interaction exists with other types of OCs. For example, genetic vulnerability to the teratogenic effects of particular infections during pregnancy may be of importance. Multiple immune-related genetic polymorphisms (e.g., genes from the IL-1 complex) have been associated with brain changes found in schizophrenia and polymorphisms in both the IL-1 complex and TNF-α have been shown to heighten inflammatory response to infection (Fineberg and Ellman 2013). Consequentially, carriers of these polymorphisms may exhibit an exaggerated inflammatory response, with the potential to hinder brain development, increase risk for other OCs associated with psychosis risk, and/or render the fetus more vulnerable to the adverse effects of maternal infection (Ellman and Cannon 2008; Mittal et al. 2008; Fineberg and Ellman 2013). Additional research examining the interaction between various OCs and genetic vulnerability for psychosis on cognitive outcomes in these disorders is needed.

Polymorphisms linked to schizophrenia risk have also been shown to interact with childhood stress to impact cognitive performance. Catechol-O-methyltransferase (COMT) Val(158)Met polymorphism is a common genetic variant that has been shown to influence executive functioning, as well as prefrontal physiology and dopamine levels (Egan et al. 2001; Meyer-Lindenberg et al. 2006).

Interestingly, a case–control study of participants from the Australian Schizophrenia Research Bank found that the COMT Val(158)Met polymorphism interacted with physical abuse to predict *better* executive functioning, despite a significant main effect of Val/Val homozygotes performing worse on tasks involving attention and immediate memory (Green et al. 2014). This suggests a pathway through which childhood trauma, namely physical abuse, downregulates Val/Val genotype expression and increases dopamine activity. Genetic variations implicated in stress response and glucocorticoid function (e.g., FKBP5, 5-HTTPLR) have also been shown to interact with childhood trauma to impart cognitive outcomes in patients with psychosis (Aas et al. 2012; Green et al. 2015). These findings highlight gene x environment interactions as potential mechanisms underlying the development of cognitive impairments associated with psychosis.

5 Conclusions and Recommendations

Further clarification of the role of early life adversity, beginning in the prenatal period, on cognition in disorders on the psychosis spectrum is needed. Methodological considerations for the future study of pre-, perinatal, and early childhood risk factors are outlined in Fig. 2. Comprehensive, prospective assessment of birth

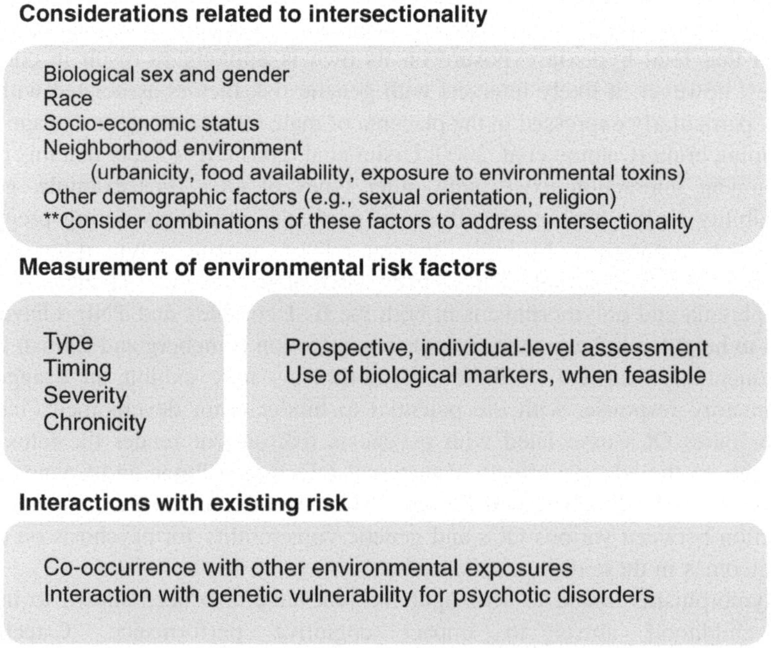

Fig. 2 Methodological considerations for future studies examining early life environmental risk factors and cognitive outcomes in individuals on the psychosis spectrum

cohorts will serve to further our developmental understanding of individual and contextual factors that impact cognitive outcomes. Further understanding of these risk factors earlier in development provides earlier opportunities for intervention. Additionally, greater understanding of the specificity of these cognitive difficulties associated with perinatal and early childhood stress to schizophrenia spectrum disorders, versus other neurodevelopmental disorders like autism, may be of interest.

References

Aas M, Dazzan P, Fisher HL et al (2011) Childhood trauma and cognitive function in first-episode affective and non-affective psychosis. Schizophr Res 129:12–19. https://doi.org/10.1016/j.schres.2011.03.017

Aas M, Djurovic S, Athanasiu L et al (2012) Serotonin transporter gene polymorphism, childhood trauma, and cognition in patients with psychotic disorders. Schizophr Bull 38:15–22. https://doi.org/10.1093/schbul/sbr113

Anastario M, Salafia CM, Fitzmaurice G, Goldstein JM (2012) Impact of fetal versus perinatal hypoxia on sex differences in childhood outcomes: developmental timing matters. Soc Psychiatry Psychiatr Epidemiol 47:455–464. https://doi.org/10.1007/s00127-011-0353-0

Anglin DM, Lighty Q, Greenspoon M, Ellman LM (2014) Racial discrimination is associated with distressing subthreshold positive psychotic symptoms among US urban ethnic minority young adults. Soc Psychiatry Psychiatr Epidemiol 49:1545–1555. https://doi.org/10.1007/s00127-014-0870-8

Anglin DM, Ereshefsky S, Klaunig MJ et al (2021) From womb to neighborhood: a racial analysis of social determinants of psychosis in the United States. Am J Psychiatry 178:599–610. https://doi.org/10.1176/appi.ajp.2020.20071091

Ayesa-Arriola R, Setién-Suero E, Marques-Feixa L et al (2020) The synergetic effect of childhood trauma and recent stressful events in psychosis: associated neurocognitive dysfunction. Acta Psychiatr Scand 141:43–51. https://doi.org/10.1111/acps.13114

Badcock JC, Dragović M, Waters FAV, Jablensky A (2005) Dimensions of intelligence in schizophrenia: evidence from patients with preserved, deteriorated and compromised intellect. J Psychiatr Res 39(1):11–19. https://doi.org/10.1016/j.jpsychires.2004.05.002

Baldwin JR, Reuben A, Newbury JB, Danese A (2019) Agreement between prospective and retrospective measures of childhood maltreatment: a systematic review and meta-analysis. JAMA Psychiat 76:584–593. https://doi.org/10.1001/jamapsychiatry.2019.0097

Begemann MJH, Heringa SM, Sommer IEC (2016) Childhood trauma as a neglected factor in psychotic experiences and cognitive functioning. JAMA Psychiat 73:875. https://doi.org/10.1001/jamapsychiatry.2016.0924

Bernstein DP, Fink L, Handelsman L et al (1994) Initial reliability and validity of a new retrospective measure of child abuse and neglect. Am J Psychiatry 151:1132–1136. https://doi.org/10.1176/ajp.151.8.1132

Berthelot N, Paccalet T, Gilbert E et al (2015) Childhood abuse and neglect may induce deficits in cognitive precursors of psychosis in high-risk children. J Psychiatry Neurosci 40:336–343. https://doi.org/10.1503/jpn.140211

Beydoun H, Saftlas AF (2008) Physical and mental health outcomes of prenatal maternal stress in human and animal studies: a review of recent evidence. Paediatr Perinat Epidemiol 22:438–466. https://doi.org/10.1111/j.1365-3016.2008.00951.x

Bhat A, Reed SD, Unützer J (2017) The obstetrician-gynecologist's role in detecting, preventing, and treating depression. Obstet Gynecol 129:157–163. https://doi.org/10.1097/AOG.0000000000001809

Blomström Å, Karlsson H, Gardner R et al (2016) Associations between maternal infection during pregnancy, childhood infections, and the risk of subsequent psychotic disorder--a Swedish cohort study of nearly 2 million individuals. Schizophr Bull 42:125–133. https://doi.org/10.1093/schbul/sbv112

Bordeleau M, Fernández de Cossío L, Chakravarty MM, Tremblay M-È (2020) From maternal diet to neurodevelopmental disorders: a story of neuroinflammation. Front Cell Neurosci 14:612705. https://doi.org/10.3389/fncel.2020.612705

Bortolato B, Miskowiak KW, Köhler CA et al (2015) Cognitive dysfunction in bipolar disorder and schizophrenia: a systematic review of meta-analyses. Neuropsychiatr Dis Treat 11:3111–3125

Bremner JD, Randall P, Scott TM et al (1995) Deficits in short-term memory in adult survivors of childhood abuse. Psychiatry Res 59:97–107. https://doi.org/10.1016/0165-1781(95)02800-5

Bremner JD, Randall P, Vermetten E et al (1997) Magnetic resonance imaging-based measurement of hippocampal volume in posttraumatic stress disorder related to childhood physical and sexual abuse--a preliminary report. Biol Psychiatry 41:23–32. https://doi.org/10.1016/s0006-3223(96)00162-x

Bremner JD, Vythilingam M, Vermetten E et al (2003) MRI and PET study of deficits in hippocampal structure and function in women with childhood sexual abuse and posttraumatic stress disorder. Am J Psychiatry 160:924–932. https://doi.org/10.1176/appi.ajp.160.5.924

Bronson SL, Bale TL (2016) The placenta as a mediator of stress effects on neurodevelopmental reprogramming. Neuropsychopharmacology 41:207–218. https://doi.org/10.1038/npp.2015.231

Brouwers EPM, van Baar AL, Pop VJM (2001) Maternal anxiety during pregnancy and subsequent infant development. Infant Behav Dev 24:95–106. https://doi.org/10.1016/S0163-6383(01)00062-5

Brown AS (2011) The environment and susceptibility to schizophrenia. Prog Neurobiol 93:23–58. https://doi.org/10.1016/j.pneurobio.2010.09.003

Brown AS, Derkits EJ (2010) Prenatal infection and schizophrenia: a review of epidemiologic and translational studies. Am J Psychiatry 167:261–280. https://doi.org/10.1176/appi.ajp.2009.09030361

Brown AS, Susser ES (2008) Prenatal nutritional deficiency and risk of adult schizophrenia. Schizophr Bull 34:1054–1063. https://doi.org/10.1093/schbul/sbn096

Brown AS, Cohen P, Harkavy-Friedman J et al (2001) A.E. Bennett research award. Prenatal rubella, premorbid abnormalities, and adult schizophrenia. Biol Psychiatry 49:473–486. https://doi.org/10.1016/s0006-3223(01)01068-x

Brown AS, Hooton J, Schaefer CA et al (2004) Elevated maternal interleukin-8 levels and risk of schizophrenia in adult offspring. Am J Psychiatry 161:889–895. https://doi.org/10.1176/appi.ajp.161.5.889

Brown AS, Bottiglieri T, Schaefer CA et al (2007) Elevated prenatal homocysteine levels as a risk factor for schizophrenia. Arch Gen Psychiatry 64:31–39. https://doi.org/10.1001/archpsyc.64.1.31

Brown AS, Vinogradov S, Kremen WS et al (2009) Prenatal exposure to maternal infection and executive dysfunction in adult schizophrenia. Am J Psychiatry 166:683–690. https://doi.org/10.1176/appi.ajp.2008.08010089

Brown AS, Vinogradov S, Kremen WS et al (2011) Association of maternal genital and reproductive infections with verbal memory and motor deficits in adult schizophrenia. Psychiatry Res 188:179–186. https://doi.org/10.1016/j.psychres.2011.04.020

Brunet E, Sarfati Y, Hardy-Baylé M-C (2003) Reasoning about physical causality and other's intentions in schizophrenia. Cogn Neuropsychiatry 8:129–139. https://doi.org/10.1080/13546800244000256

Buka SL, Tsuang MT, Torrey EF et al (2001) Maternal cytokine levels during pregnancy and adult psychosis. Brain Behav Immun 15:411–420. https://doi.org/10.1006/brbi.2001.0644

Buss C, Davis EP, Hobel CJ, Sandman CA (2011) Maternal pregnancy-specific anxiety is associated with child executive function at 6–9 years age. Stress 14:665–676. https://doi.org/10.3109/10253890.2011.623250

Camerota M, Willoughby MT, Cox M et al (2015) Executive function in low birth weight preschoolers: the moderating effect of parenting. J Abnorm Child Psychol 43:1551–1562. https://doi.org/10.1007/s10802-015-0032-9

Campbell C, Barrett S, Shannon C et al (2013) The relationship between childhood trauma and neuropsychological functioning in first episode psychosis. Psychosis 5:48–59. https://doi.org/10.1080/17522439.2012.660982

Canever L, Alves CSV, Mastella G et al (2018) The evaluation of folic acid-deficient or folic acid-supplemented diet in the gestational phase of female rats and in their adult offspring subjected to an animal model of schizophrenia. Mol Neurobiol 55:2301–2319. https://doi.org/10.1007/s12035-017-0493-7

Cannon TD, Mednick SA, Parnas J (1989) Genetic and perinatal determinants of structural brain deficits in schizophrenia. Arch Gen Psychiatry 46:883–889. https://doi.org/10.1001/archpsyc.1989.01810100025005

Cannon TD, Bearden CE, Hollister JM et al (2000) Childhood cognitive functioning in schizophrenia patients and their unaffected siblings: a prospective cohort study. Schizophr Bull 26: 379–393. https://doi.org/10.1093/oxfordjournals.schbul.a033460

Cannon M, Jones PB, Murray RM (2002a) Obstetric complications and schizophrenia: historical and meta-analytic review. AJP 159:1080–1092. https://doi.org/10.1176/appi.ajp.159.7.1080

Cannon TD, van Erp TGM, Rosso IM et al (2002b) Fetal hypoxia and structural brain abnormalities in schizophrenic patients, their siblings, and controls. Arch Gen Psychiatry 59:35–41. https://doi.org/10.1001/archpsyc.59.1.35

Cannon TD, Yolken R, Buka S et al (2008) Decreased neurotrophic response to birth hypoxia in the etiology of schizophrenia. Biol Psychiatry 64:797–802. https://doi.org/10.1016/j.biopsych.2008.04.012

Carrilho CG, Cougo SS, Bombassaro T et al (2019) Early trauma and cognitive functions of patients with schizophrenia. Front Psych 10:261. https://doi.org/10.3389/fpsyt.2019.00261

Charil A, Laplante DP, Vaillancourt C, King S (2010) Prenatal stress and brain development. Brain Res Rev 65:56–79. https://doi.org/10.1016/j.brainresrev.2010.06.002

Clifford A, Lang L, Chen R et al (2016) Exposure to air pollution and cognitive functioning across the life course – a systematic literature review. Environ Res 147:383–398. https://doi.org/10.1016/j.envres.2016.01.018

Collins MA, Chung Y, Addington J et al (2021) Discriminatory experiences predict neuroanatomical changes and anxiety among healthy individuals and those at clinical high risk for psychosis. Neuroimage Clin 31:102757. https://doi.org/10.1016/j.nicl.2021.102757

Comacchio C, Lasalvia A, Ruggeri M (2019) Current evidence of childhood traumatic experiences in psychosis - focus on gender differences. Psychiatry Res 281:112507. https://doi.org/10.1016/j.psychres.2019.112507

Corcoran M, Hawkins EL, O'Hora D et al (2020) Are working memory and glutamate concentrations involved in early-life stress and severity of psychosis? Brain Behav 10:e01616. https://doi.org/10.1002/brb3.1616

Cortes Hidalgo AP, Neumann A, Bakermans-Kranenburg MJ et al (2020) Prenatal maternal stress and child IQ. Child Dev 91:347–365. https://doi.org/10.1111/cdev.13177

Cosgrave J, Purple RJ, Haines R et al (2021) Do environmental risk factors for the development of psychosis distribute differently across dimensionally assessed psychotic experiences? Transl Psychiatry 11:1–13

Coussons-Read ME (2013) Effects of prenatal stress on pregnancy and human development: mechanisms and pathways. Obstet Med 6:52–57. https://doi.org/10.1177/1753495X12473751

Czepielewski LS, Alliende LM, Castañeda CP et al (2021) Effects of socioeconomic status in cognition of people with schizophrenia: results from a Latin American collaboration network with 1175 subjects. Psychol Med. https://doi.org/10.1017/S0033291721002403

Danese A, Moffitt TE, Arseneault L et al (2017) The origins of cognitive deficits in victimized children: implications for neuroscientists and clinicians. Am J Psychiatry 174:349–361. https://doi.org/10.1176/appi.ajp.2016.16030333

Dauvermann MR, Donohoe G (2019) The role of childhood trauma in cognitive performance in schizophrenia and bipolar disorder – a systematic review. Schizophr Res Cogn 16:1–11. https://doi.org/10.1016/j.scog.2018.11.001

Davies C, Segre G, Estradé A et al (2020) Prenatal and perinatal risk and protective factors for psychosis: a systematic review and meta-analysis. Lancet Psychiatry 7:399–410. https://doi.org/10.1016/S2215-0366(20)30057-2

Dominguez TP, Dunkel-Schetter C, Glynn LM et al (2008) Racial differences in birth outcomes: the role of general, pregnancy, and racism stress. Health Psychol 27:194–203. https://doi.org/10.1037/0278-6133.27.2.194

Egan MF, Goldberg TE, Kolachana BS et al (2001) Effect of COMT Val108/158 met genotype on frontal lobe function and risk for schizophrenia. Proc Natl Acad Sci U S A 98:6917–6922. https://doi.org/10.1073/pnas.111134598

Eide MG, Moster D, Irgens LM et al (2013) Degree of fetal growth restriction associated with schizophrenia risk in a national cohort. Psychol Med 43:2057–2066. https://doi.org/10.1017/S003329171200267X

Ellman LM, Cannon TD (2008) Environmental pre- and perinatal influences. In: Mueser KT, Jeste DV (eds) The clinical handbook of schizophrenia. Guilford Press, New York, pp 65–73

Ellman LM, Susser ES (2009) The promise of epidemiologic studies: neuroimmune mechanisms in the etiologies of brain disorders. Neuron 64:25–27. https://doi.org/10.1016/j.neuron.2009.09.024

Ellman LM, Huttunen M, Lönnqvist J, Cannon TD (2007) The effects of genetic liability for schizophrenia and maternal smoking during pregnancy on obstetric complications. Schizophr Res 93:229–236. https://doi.org/10.1016/j.schres.2007.03.004

Ellman LM, Yolken RH, Buka SL et al (2009) Cognitive functioning prior to the onset of psychosis: the role of Fetal exposure to serologically determined influenza infection. Biol Psychiatry 65:1040–1047. https://doi.org/10.1016/j.biopsych.2008.12.015

Ellman LM, Vinogradov S, Kremen WS et al (2012) Low maternal hemoglobin during pregnancy and diminished neuromotor and neurocognitive performance in offspring with schizophrenia. Schizophr Res 138:81–87. https://doi.org/10.1016/j.schres.2012.04.008

Ellman LM, Murphy SK, Maxwell SD (2018) Pre- and perinatal risk factors for serious mental disorders: ethical considerations in prevention and prediction efforts. J Ethics Mental Health 10:1–14

Ellman LM, Murphy SK, Maxwell SD et al (2019) Maternal cortisol during pregnancy and offspring schizophrenia: influence of fetal sex and timing of exposure. Schizophr Res 213:15–22. https://doi.org/10.1016/j.schres.2019.07.002

Engman M-L, Adolfsson I, Lewensohn-Fuchs I et al (2008) Neuropsychologic outcomes in children with neonatal herpes encephalitis. Pediatr Neurol 38:398–405. https://doi.org/10.1016/j.pediatrneurol.2008.02.005

Ered A, Ellman LM (2019) Specificity of childhood trauma type and attenuated positive symptoms in a non-clinical sample. J Clin Med 8:1537. https://doi.org/10.3390/jcm8101537

Estes ML, McAllister AK (2016) Maternal immune activation: implications for neuropsychiatric disorders. Science 353:772–777. https://doi.org/10.1126/science.aag3194

Eyles DW (2021) How do established developmental risk-factors for schizophrenia change the way the brain develops? Transl Psychiatry 11:1–15. https://doi.org/10.1038/s41398-021-01273-2

Feola B, Dougherty LR, Riggins T, Bolger DJ (2020) Prefrontal cortical thickness mediates the association between cortisol reactivity and executive function in childhood. Neuropsychologia 148:107636. https://doi.org/10.1016/j.neuropsychologia.2020.107636

Fett A-KJ, Viechtbauer W, Dominguez M-G et al (2011) The relationship between neurocognition and social cognition with functional outcomes in schizophrenia: a meta-analysis. Neurosci Biobehav Rev 35:573–588. https://doi.org/10.1016/j.neubiorev.2010.07.001

Fineberg AM, Ellman LM (2013) Inflammatory cytokines and neurological and neurocognitive alterations in the course of schizophrenia. Biol Psychiatry 73:951–966. https://doi.org/10.1016/j.biopsych.2013.01.001

Fineberg AM, Ellman LM, Buka S et al (2013) Decreased birth weight in psychosis: influence of prenatal exposure to serologically determined influenza and hypoxia. Schizophr Bull 39:1037–1044. https://doi.org/10.1093/schbul/sbs084

Fineberg AM, Ellman LM, Schaefer CA et al (2016) Fetal exposure to maternal stress and risk for schizophrenia spectrum disorders among offspring: differential influences of fetal sex. Psychiatry Res 236:91–97. https://doi.org/10.1016/j.psychres.2015.12.026

Freedman D, Bao Y, Kremen WS et al (2013) Birth weight and neurocognition in schizophrenia spectrum disorders. Schizophr Bull 39:592–600. https://doi.org/10.1093/schbul/sbs008

Freedman R, Hunter SK, Law AJ et al (2021) Choline, folic acid, vitamin D, and fetal brain development in the psychosis spectrum. Schizophr Res S0920-9964(21):00128–00126. https://doi.org/10.1016/j.schres.2021.03.008

Ghassabian A, Albert PS, Hornig M et al (2018) Gestational cytokine concentrations and neurocognitive development at 7 years. Transl Psychiatry 8:64. https://doi.org/10.1038/s41398-018-0112-z

Gibson LE, Cooper S, Reeves LE et al (2017) The association between traumatic life events and psychological symptoms from a conservative, transdiagnostic perspective. Psychiatry Res 252: 70–74. https://doi.org/10.1016/j.psychres.2017.02.047

Gibson LE, Cooper S, Reeves LE et al (2019) Attentional biases and trauma status: do psychotic-like experiences matter? Psychol Trauma 11:300–306. https://doi.org/10.1037/tra0000380

Gillespie SL, Porter K, Christian LM (2016) Adaptation of the inflammatory immune response across pregnancy and postpartum in black and White women. J Reprod Immunol 114:27–31. https://doi.org/10.1016/j.jri.2016.02.001

Giovanoli S, Notter T, Richetto J et al (2015) Late prenatal immune activation causes hippocampal deficits in the absence of persistent inflammation across aging. J Neuroinflammation 12:221. https://doi.org/10.1186/s12974-015-0437-y

Giscombé CL, Lobel M (2005) Explaining disproportionately high rates of adverse birth outcomes among African Americans: the impact of stress, racism, and related factors in pregnancy. Psychol Bull 131:662–683. https://doi.org/10.1037/0033-2909.131.5.662

Glynn LM, Schetter CD, Chicz-DeMet A et al (2007) Ethnic differences in adrenocorticotropic hormone, cortisol and corticotropin-releasing hormone during pregnancy. Peptides 28:1155–1161. https://doi.org/10.1016/j.peptides.2007.04.005

Golan HM, Lev V, Hallak M et al (2005) Specific neurodevelopmental damage in mice offspring following maternal inflammation during pregnancy. Neuropharmacology 48:903–917. https://doi.org/10.1016/j.neuropharm.2004.12.023

Goldstein JM, Seidman LJ, Santangelo S et al (1994) Are schizophrenic men at higher risk for developmental deficits than schizophrenic women? Implications for adult neuropsychological functions. J Psychiatr Res 28:483–498. https://doi.org/10.1016/0022-3956(94)90039-6

Goldstein G, Allen DN, Seaton BE (1998) A comparison of clustering solutions for cognitive heterogeneity in schizophrenia. J Int Neuropsychol Soc 4:353–362. https://doi.org/10.1017/S1355617798003531

Goldstein JM, Seidman LJ, Buka SL et al (2000) Impact of genetic vulnerability and hypoxia on overall intelligence by age 7 in offspring at high risk for schizophrenia compared with affective psychoses. Schizophr Bull 26:323–334. https://doi.org/10.1093/oxfordjournals.schbul.a033456

Goldstein JM, Cherkerzian S, Seidman LJ et al (2014) Prenatal maternal immune disruption and sex-dependent risk for psychoses. Psychol Med 44:3249–3261. https://doi.org/10.1017/S0033291714000683

Green JG, McLaughlin KA, Berglund PA et al (2010) Childhood adversities and adult psychiatric disorders in the national comorbidity survey replication I: associations with first onset of DSM-IV disorders. Arch Gen Psychiatry 67:113–123. https://doi.org/10.1001/archgenpsychiatry.2009.186

Green MJ, Chia T-Y, Cairns MJ et al (2014) Catechol-O-methyltransferase (COMT) genotype moderates the effects of childhood trauma on cognition and symptoms in schizophrenia. J Psychiatr Res 49:43–50. https://doi.org/10.1016/j.jpsychires.2013.10.018

Green MJ, Raudino A, Cairns MJ et al (2015) Do common genotypes of FK506 binding protein 5 (FKBP5) moderate the effects of childhood maltreatment on cognition in schizophrenia and healthy controls? J Psychiatr Res 70:9–17. https://doi.org/10.1016/j.jpsychires.2015.07.019

Grizenko N, Fortier M-È, Gaudreau-Simard M et al (2015) The effect of maternal stress during pregnancy on IQ and ADHD symptomatology. J Can Acad Child Adolesc Psychiatry 24:92–99

Gutteling BM, de Weerth C, Zandbelt N et al (2006) Does maternal prenatal stress adversely affect the child's learning and memory at age six? J Abnorm Child Psychol 34:787–796. https://doi.org/10.1007/s10802-006-9054-7

Haager D, Vaughn S (1995) Parent, teacher, peer, and self-reports of the social competence of students with learning disabilities. J Learn Disabil 28:205–215, 231. https://doi.org/10.1177/002221949502800403

Han VX, Patel S, Jones HF et al (2021) Maternal acute and chronic inflammation in pregnancy is associated with common neurodevelopmental disorders. Transl Psychiatry 11. https://doi.org/10.1038/s41398-021-01198-w

Haukvik UK, Rimol LM, Roddey JC et al (2014) Normal birth weight variation is related to cortical morphology across the psychosis spectrum. Schizophr Bull 40:410–419. https://doi.org/10.1093/schbul/sbt005

Holmes J, Gathercole SE, Dunning DL (2009) Adaptive training leads to sustained enhancement of poor working memory in children. Dev Sci 12:F9–F15. https://doi.org/10.1111/j.1467-7687.2009.00848.x

Howes OD, McCutcheon R (2017) Inflammation and the neural diathesis-stress hypothesis of schizophrenia: a reconceptualization. Transl Psychiatry 7:e1024. https://doi.org/10.1038/tp.2016.278

Huizink AC, de Rooij SR (2018) Prenatal stress and models explaining risk for psychopathology revisited: generic vulnerability and divergent pathways. Dev Psychopathol 30:1041–1062. https://doi.org/10.1017/S0954579418000354

Huizink AC, Mulder EJH (2006) Maternal smoking, drinking or cannabis use during pregnancy and neurobehavioral and cognitive functioning in human offspring. Neurosci Biobehav Rev 30:24–41. https://doi.org/10.1016/j.neubiorev.2005.04.005

Huizink AC, Mulder EJH, Buitelaar JK (2004) Prenatal stress and risk for psychopathology: specific effects or induction of general susceptibility. Psychol Bull 130:115–142. https://doi.org/10.1037/0033-2909.130.1.115

Hunter A, Murray R, Asher L, Leonardi-Bee J (2020) The effects of tobacco smoking, and prenatal tobacco smoke exposure, on risk of schizophrenia: a systematic review and meta-analysis. Nicotine Tob Res 22:3–10. https://doi.org/10.1093/ntr/nty160

Hunter SK, Hoffman MC, D'Alessandro A et al (2021) Male fetus susceptibility to maternal inflammation: c-reactive protein and brain development. Psychol Med 51:450–459. https://doi.org/10.1017/S0033291719003313

Jiang H, Xu L, Shao L et al (2016) Maternal infection during pregnancy and risk of autism spectrum disorders. Brain Behav Immun 58:165–172. https://doi.org/10.1016/j.bbi.2016.06.005

Johnson D, Policelli J, Li M et al (2021) Associations of early-life threat and deprivation with executive functioning in childhood and adolescence: a systematic review and meta-analysis. JAMA Pediatr 175:e212511. https://doi.org/10.1001/jamapediatrics.2021.2511

Jones SL, Dufoix R, Laplante DP et al (2019) Larger amygdala volume mediates the association between prenatal maternal stress and higher levels of externalizing behaviors: sex specific effects in project ice storm. Front Hum Neurosci 13:144. https://doi.org/10.3389/fnhum.2019.00144

Karlsson H, Dalman C (2020) Epidemiological studies of prenatal and childhood infection and schizophrenia. Curr Top Behav Neurosci 44:35–47. https://doi.org/10.1007/7854_2018_87

Kasznia J, Pytel A, Stańczykiewicz B et al (2021) Adverse childhood experiences and neurocognition in schizophrenia Spectrum disorders: age at first exposure and multiplicity matter. Front Psych 12:684099. https://doi.org/10.3389/fpsyt.2021.684099

Khandaker GM, Barnett JH, White IR, Jones PB (2011) A quantitative meta-analysis of population-based studies of premorbid intelligence and schizophrenia. Schizophr Res 132:220–227. https://doi.org/10.1016/j.schres.2011.06.017

Kilian S, Asmal L, Chiliza B et al (2018) Childhood adversity and cognitive function in schizophrenia spectrum disorders and healthy controls: evidence for an association between neglect and social cognition. Psychol Med 48:2186–2193. https://doi.org/10.1017/S0033291717003671

Kim-Fine S, Regnault TRH, Lee JS et al (2012) Male gender promotes an increased inflammatory response to lipopolysaccharide in umbilical vein blood. J Matern Fetal Neonatal Med 25:2470–2474. https://doi.org/10.3109/14767058.2012.684165

Kingston D, McDonald S, Austin M-P, Tough S (2015) Association between prenatal and postnatal psychological distress and toddler cognitive development: a systematic review. PLoS One 10: e0126929. https://doi.org/10.1371/journal.pone.0126929

Ko T-J, Tsai L-Y, Chu L-C et al (2014) Parental smoking during pregnancy and its association with low birth weight, small for gestational age, and preterm birth offspring: a birth cohort study. Pediatr Neonatol 55:20–27. https://doi.org/10.1016/j.pedneo.2013.05.005

Koenen KC, Moffitt TE, Roberts AL et al (2009) Childhood IQ and adult mental disorders: a test of the cognitive reserve hypothesis. Am J Psychiatry 166:50–57. https://doi.org/10.1176/appi.ajp.2008.08030343

Krabbendam L, van Os J (2005) Schizophrenia and urbanicity: a major environmental influence—conditional on genetic risk. Schizophr Bull 31:795–799. https://doi.org/10.1093/schbul/sbi060

Kremen WS, Buka SL, Seidman LJ et al (1998) IQ decline during childhood and adult psychotic symptoms in a community sample: a 19-year longitudinal study. AJP 155:672–677. https://doi.org/10.1176/ajp.155.5.672

Kremen WS, Vinogradov S, Poole JH et al (2010) Cognitive decline in schizophrenia from childhood to midlife: a 33-year longitudinal birth cohort study. Schizophr Res 118:1–5. https://doi.org/10.1016/j.schres.2010.01.009

Ku BS, Pauselli L, Manseau M, Compton MT (2020) Neighborhood-level predictors of age at onset and duration of untreated psychosis in first-episode psychotic disorders. Schizophr Res 218: 247–254. https://doi.org/10.1016/j.schres.2019.12.036

Lafortune S, Laplante DP, Elgbeili G et al (2021) Effect of natural disaster-related prenatal maternal stress on child development and health: a meta-analytic review. Int J Environ Res Public Health 18:8332. https://doi.org/10.3390/ijerph18168332

Laplante DP, Brunet A, Schmitz N et al (2008) Project ice storm: prenatal maternal stress affects cognitive and linguistic functioning in 5 1/2-year-old children. J Am Acad Child Adolesc Psychiatry 47:1063–1072. https://doi.org/10.1097/CHI.0b013e31817eec80

Laplante DP, Hart KJ, O'Hara MW et al (2018) Prenatal maternal stress is associated with toddler cognitive functioning: the Iowa Flood Study. Early Hum Dev 116:84–92. https://doi.org/10.1016/j.earlhumdev.2017.11.012

Lataster T, van Os J, Drukker M et al (2006) Childhood victimisation and developmental expression of non-clinical delusional ideation and hallucinatory experiences: victimisation and non-clinical psychotic experiences. Soc Psychiatry Psychiatr Epidemiol 41:423–428. https://doi.org/10.1007/s00127-006-0060-4

LeWinn KZ, Stroud LR, Molnar BE et al (2009) Elevated maternal cortisol levels during pregnancy are associated with reduced childhood IQ. Int J Epidemiol 38:1700–1710. https://doi.org/10.1093/ije/dyp200

Lewis R (2004) Should cognitive deficit be a diagnostic criterion for schizophrenia? J Psychiatry Neurosci 29:102–113

Lewis G, Dykxhoorn J, Karlsson H et al (2020) Assessment of the role of IQ in associations between population density and deprivation and nonaffective psychosis. JAMA Psychiat 77: 729–736. https://doi.org/10.1001/jamapsychiatry.2020.0103
Lim L, Radua J, Rubia K (2014) Gray matter abnormalities in childhood maltreatment: a voxel-wise meta-analysis. Am J Psychiatry 171:854–863. https://doi.org/10.1176/appi.ajp.2014.13101427
Lipner E, Murphy SK, Ellman LM (2019) Prenatal maternal stress and the cascade of risk to schizophrenia spectrum disorders in offspring. Curr Psychiatry Rep 21:99. https://doi.org/10.1007/s11920-019-1085-1
Liu Y, Mendonça M, Cannon M et al (2020) Testing the independent and joint contribution of exposure to neurodevelopmental adversity and childhood trauma to risk of psychotic experiences in adulthood. Schizophr Bull 47:776–784. https://doi.org/10.1093/schbul/sbaa174
Lobel M, Cannella DL, Graham JE et al (2008) Pregnancy-specific stress, prenatal health behaviors, and birth outcomes. Health Psychol 27:604–615. https://doi.org/10.1037/a0013242
Mareckova K, Marecek R, Andryskova L et al (2021) Impact of prenatal stress on amygdala anatomy in young adulthood: timing and location matter. Biol Psychiatr Cogn Neurosci Neuroimaging. https://doi.org/10.1016/j.bpsc.2021.07.009
Markham JA, Taylor AR, Taylor SB et al (2010) Characterization of the cognitive impairments induced by prenatal exposure to stress in the rat. Front Behav Neurosci 4:173. https://doi.org/10.3389/fnbeh.2010.00173
Martin KV, Sucharew H, Dietrich KN et al (2021) Co-exposure to manganese and lead and pediatric neurocognition in East Liverpool, Ohio. Environ Res 202:111644. https://doi.org/10.1016/j.envres.2021.111644
Mathewson KJ, Chow CHT, Dobson KG et al (2017) Mental health of extremely low birth weight survivors: a systematic review and meta-analysis. Psychol Bull 143:347–383. https://doi.org/10.1037/bul0000091
McCabe KL, Maloney EA, Stain HJ et al (2012) Relationship between childhood adversity and clinical and cognitive features in schizophrenia. J Psychiatr Res 46:600–607. https://doi.org/10.1016/j.jpsychires.2012.01.023
McGrath J, Saari K, Hakko H et al (2004) Vitamin D supplementation during the first year of life and risk of schizophrenia: a Finnish birth cohort study. Schizophr Res 67:237–245. https://doi.org/10.1016/j.schres.2003.08.005
McGrath J, Brown A, St Clair D (2011) Prevention and schizophrenia--the role of dietary factors. Schizophr Bull 37:272–283. https://doi.org/10.1093/schbul/sbq121
McIntosh R, Vaughn S, Schumm JS et al (1993) Observations of students with learning disabilities in general education classrooms. Except Child 60:249–261. https://doi.org/10.1177/001440299406000306
McIntosh AM, Holmes S, Gleeson S et al (2002) Maternal recall bias, obstetric history and schizophrenia. Br J Psychiatry 181:520–525. https://doi.org/10.1192/bjp.181.6.520
McLaughlin KA, Sheridan MA (2016) Beyond cumulative risk: a dimensional approach to childhood adversity. Curr Dir Psychol Sci 25:239–245. https://doi.org/10.1177/0963721416655883
Medeiros W, Torro-Alves N, Malloy-Diniz LF, Minervino CM (2016) Executive functions in children who experience bullying situations. Front Psychol 7:1197. https://doi.org/10.3389/fpsyg.2016.01197
Mednick SA, Machon RA, Huttunen MO, Bonett D (1988) Adult schizophrenia following prenatal exposure to an influenza epidemic. Arch Gen Psychiatry 45:189–192. https://doi.org/10.1001/archpsyc.1988.01800260109013
Merced-Nieves FM, Aguiar A, Dzwilewski KLC et al (2020) Association of prenatal maternal perceived stress with a sexually dimorphic measure of cognition in 4.5-month-old infants. Neurotoxicol Teratol 77:106850. https://doi.org/10.1016/j.ntt.2019.106850
Meyer U (2014) Prenatal poly(i:C) exposure and other developmental immune activation models in rodent systems. Biol Psychiatry 75:307–315. https://doi.org/10.1016/j.biopsych.2013.07.011

Meyer U, Engler A, Weber L et al (2008) Preliminary evidence for a modulation of fetal dopaminergic development by maternal immune activation during pregnancy. Neuroscience 154:701–709. https://doi.org/10.1016/j.neuroscience.2008.04.031

Meyer-Lindenberg A, Nichols T, Callicott JH et al (2006) Impact of complex genetic variation in COMT on human brain function. Mol Psychiatry 11:867–877. https://doi.org/10.1038/sj.mp.4001860

Mhaouty-Kodja S, Belzunces LP, Canivenc M-C et al (2018) Impairment of learning and memory performances induced by BPA: evidences from the literature of a MoA mediated through an ED. Mol Cell Endocrinol 475:54–73. https://doi.org/10.1016/j.mce.2018.03.017

Mittal VA, Ellman LM, Cannon TD (2008) Gene-environment interaction and covariation in schizophrenia: the role of obstetric complications. Schizophr Bull 34:1083–1094. https://doi.org/10.1093/schbul/sbn080

Mollon J, Reichenberg A (2018) Cognitive development prior to onset of psychosis. Psychol Med 48:392–403. https://doi.org/10.1017/S0033291717001970

Mondelli V, Dazzan P, Hepgul N et al (2010) Abnormal cortisol levels during the day and cortisol awakening response in first-episode psychosis: the role of stress and of antipsychotic treatment. Schizophr Res 116:234–242. https://doi.org/10.1016/j.schres.2009.08.013

Mørkved N, Johnsen E, Kroken RA et al (2020) Does childhood trauma influence cognitive functioning in schizophrenia? The association of childhood trauma and cognition in schizophrenia spectrum disorders. Schizophr Res Cogn 21:100179. https://doi.org/10.1016/j.scog.2020.100179

Müller N, Weidinger E, Leitner B, Schwarz MJ (2015) The role of inflammation in schizophrenia. Front Neurosci 9:372. https://doi.org/10.3389/fnins.2015.00372

Murphy SK, Fineberg AM, Maxwell SD et al (2017) Maternal infection and stress during pregnancy and depressive symptoms in adolescent offspring. Psychiatry Res 257:102–110. https://doi.org/10.1016/j.psychres.2017.07.025

Myin-Germeys I, van Os J, Schwartz JE et al (2001) Emotional reactivity to daily life stress in psychosis. Arch Gen Psychiatry 58:1137–1144. https://doi.org/10.1001/archpsyc.58.12.1137

Naeye RL, Peters EC (1987) Antenatal hypoxia and low IQ values. Obstet Anesth Dig 7:98

Negrón-Oyarzo I, Lara-Vásquez A, Palacios-García I et al (2016) Schizophrenia and reelin: a model based on prenatal stress to study epigenetics, brain development and behavior. Biol Res 49:16. https://doi.org/10.1186/s40659-016-0076-5

Neill E, Tan EJ, Toh WL et al (2020) Examining which factors influence age of onset in males and females with schizophrenia. Schizophr Res 223:265–270. https://doi.org/10.1016/j.schres.2020.08.011

Nettis MA, Pariante CM, Mondelli V (2020) Early-life adversity, systemic inflammation and comorbid physical and psychiatric illnesses of adult life. In: Khandaker GM, Meyer U, Jones PB (eds) Neuroinflammation and schizophrenia. Springer International Publishing, Cham, pp 207–225

Newell-Morris LL, Fahrenbruch CE, Sackett GP (1989) Prenatal psychological stress, dermatoglyphic asymmetry and pregnancy outcome in the pigtailed macaque (Macaca nemestrina). NEO 56:61–75. https://doi.org/10.1159/000243104

Oh H, Yang LH, Anglin DM, DeVylder JE (2014) Perceived discrimination and psychotic experiences across multiple ethnic groups in the United States. Schizophr Res 157:259–265. https://doi.org/10.1016/j.schres.2014.04.036

Paquin V, Lapierre M, Veru F, King S (2021) Early environmental upheaval and the risk for schizophrenia. Annu Rev Clin Psychol 17:285–311. https://doi.org/10.1146/annurev-clinpsy-081219-103805

Poletti S, Mazza E, Bollettini I et al (2015) Adverse childhood experiences influence white matter microstructure in patients with schizophrenia. Psychiatry Res Neuroimaging 234:35–43. https://doi.org/10.1016/j.pscychresns.2015.08.003

Pugliese V, Bruni A, Carbone EA et al (2019) Maternal stress, prenatal medical illnesses and obstetric complications: Risk factors for schizophrenia spectrum disorder, bipolar disorder and

major depressive disorder. Psychiatry Res 271:23–30. https://doi.org/10.1016/j.psychres.2018.11.023
Quidé Y, O'Reilly N, Watkeys OJ et al (2018) Effects of childhood trauma on left inferior frontal gyrus function during response inhibition across psychotic disorders. Psychol Med 48:1454–1463. https://doi.org/10.1017/S0033291717002884
Quinn PD, Rickert ME, Weibull CE et al (2017) Association between maternal smoking during pregnancy and severe mental illness in offspring. JAMA Psychiat 74:589–596. https://doi.org/10.1001/jamapsychiatry.2017.0456
Ramsay H, Surcel H-M, Björnholm L et al (2021) Associations between maternal prenatal C-reactive protein and risk factors for psychosis in adolescent offspring: findings from the northern Finland birth cohort 1986. Schizophr Bull 47:766–775. https://doi.org/10.1093/schbul/sbaa152
Rasetti R, Mattay VS, Wiedholz LM et al (2009) Evidence that altered amygdala activity in schizophrenia is related to clinical state and not genetic risk. Am J Psychiatry 166:216–225. https://doi.org/10.1176/appi.ajp.2008.08020261
Rauschenberg C, van Os J, Goedhart M et al (2021) Bullying victimization and stress sensitivity in help-seeking youth: findings from an experience sampling study. Eur Child Adolesc Psychiatry 30:591–605. https://doi.org/10.1007/s00787-020-01540-5
Raymond C, Marin M-F, Majeur D, Lupien S (2018) Early child adversity and psychopathology in adulthood: HPA axis and cognitive dysregulations as potential mechanisms. Prog Neuro-Psychopharmacol Biol Psychiatry 85:152–160. https://doi.org/10.1016/j.pnpbp.2017.07.015
Read J, Perry BD, Moskowitz A, Connolly J (2001) The contribution of early traumatic events to schizophrenia in some patients: a traumagenic neurodevelopmental model. Psychiatry 64:319–345. https://doi.org/10.1521/psyc.64.4.319.18602
Reichenberg A, Caspi A, Harrington H et al (2010) Static and dynamic cognitive deficits in childhood preceding adult schizophrenia: a 30-year study. Am J Psychiatry 167:160–169. https://doi.org/10.1176/appi.ajp.2009.09040574
Rosenthal A, Meyer MS, Mayo D et al (2020) Contributions of childhood trauma and atypical development to increased clinical symptoms and poor functioning in recent onset psychosis. Early Interv Psychiatry 14:755–761. https://doi.org/10.1111/eip.12931
Ruby E, Rothman K, Corcoran C et al (2017) Influence of early trauma on features of schizophrenia. Early Interv Psychiatry 11:322–333. https://doi.org/10.1111/eip.12239
Sacchi C, Marino C, Nosarti C et al (2020) Association of intrauterine growth restriction and small for gestational age status with childhood cognitive outcomes: a systematic review and meta-analysis. JAMA Pediatr 174:772–781. https://doi.org/10.1001/jamapediatrics.2020.1097
Samplin E, Ikuta T, Malhotra AK et al (2013) Sex differences in resilience to childhood maltreatment: effects of trauma history on hippocampal volume, general cognition and subclinical psychosis in healthy adults. J Psychiatr Res 47:1174–1179. https://doi.org/10.1016/j.jpsychires.2013.05.008
Sandman CA, Glynn LM, Davis EP (2013) Is there a viability-vulnerability tradeoff? Sex differences in fetal programming. J Psychosom Res 75:327–335. https://doi.org/10.1016/j.jpsychores.2013.07.009
Schaefer CA, Brown AS, Wyatt RJ et al (2000) Maternal prepregnant body mass and risk of schizophrenia in adult offspring. Schizophr Bull 26:275–286. https://doi.org/10.1093/oxfordjournals.schbul.a033452
Schalinski I, Teicher MH, Carolus AM, Rockstroh B (2018) Defining the impact of childhood adversities on cognitive deficits in psychosis: an exploratory analysis. Schizophr Res 192:351–356. https://doi.org/10.1016/j.schres.2017.05.014
Schreier A, Wolke D, Thomas K et al (2009) Prospective study of peer victimization in childhood and psychotic symptoms in a nonclinical population at age 12 years. Arch Gen Psychiatry 66:527–536. https://doi.org/10.1001/archgenpsychiatry.2009.23

Scott JG, Matuschka L, Niemelä S et al (2018) Evidence of a causal relationship between smoking tobacco and schizophrenia spectrum disorders. Front Psych 9:607. https://doi.org/10.3389/fpsyt.2018.00607

Seidman LJ, Buka SL, Goldstein JM et al (2000) The relationship of prenatal and perinatal complications to cognitive functioning at age 7 in the New England Cohorts of the National Collaborative Perinatal Project. Schizophr Bull 26:309–321. https://doi.org/10.1093/oxfordjournals.schbul.a033455

Shaikh M, Ellett L, Dutt A et al (2016) Perceived ethnic discrimination and persecutory paranoia in individuals at ultra-high risk for psychosis. Psychiatry Res 241:309–314. https://doi.org/10.1016/j.psychres.2016.05.006

Shannon C, Douse K, McCusker C et al (2011) The association between childhood trauma and memory functioning in schizophrenia. Schizophr Bull 37:531–537. https://doi.org/10.1093/schbul/sbp096

Sideli L, Fisher HL, Russo M et al (2014) Failure to find association between childhood abuse and cognition in first-episode psychosis patients. Eur Psychiatry 29:32–35. https://doi.org/10.1016/j.eurpsy.2013.02.006

Simanek AM, Meier HC (2015) Association between prenatal exposure to maternal infection and offspring mood disorders: a review of the literature. Curr Probl Pediatr Adolesc Health Care 45:325–364. https://doi.org/10.1016/j.cppeds.2015.06.008

Smith SEP, Li J, Garbett K et al (2007) Maternal immune activation alters fetal brain development through interleukin-6. J Neurosci 27:10695–10702. https://doi.org/10.1523/JNEUROSCI.2178-07.2007

Stein MB, Koverola C, Hanna C et al (1997) Hippocampal volume in women victimized by childhood sexual abuse. Psychol Med 27:951–959. https://doi.org/10.1017/s0033291797005242

Sutherland S, Brunwasser SM (2018) Sex differences in vulnerability to prenatal stress: a review of the recent literature. Curr Psychiatry Rep 20:102. https://doi.org/10.1007/s11920-018-0961-4

Teigset CM, Mohn C, Rund BR (2020) Perinatal complications and executive dysfunction in early-onset schizophrenia. BMC Psychiatry 20:103. https://doi.org/10.1186/s12888-020-02517-z

Torniainen M, Wegelius A, Tuulio-Henriksson A et al (2013) Both low birthweight and high birthweight are associated with cognitive impairment in persons with schizophrenia and their first-degree relatives. Psychol Med 43:2361–2367. https://doi.org/10.1017/S0033291713000032

Üçok A, Kaya H, Uğurpala C et al (2015) History of childhood physical trauma is related to cognitive decline in individuals with ultra-high risk for psychosis. Schizophr Res 169:199–203. https://doi.org/10.1016/j.schres.2015.08.038

Ursini G, Punzi G, Chen Q et al (2018) Convergence of placenta biology and genetic risk for schizophrenia. Nat Med 24:792–801. https://doi.org/10.1038/s41591-018-0021-y

Ursini G, Punzi G, Langworthy BW et al (2021) Placental genomic risk scores and early neurodevelopmental outcomes. Proc Natl Acad Sci U S A 118:e2019789118. https://doi.org/10.1073/pnas.2019789118

Van den Bergh BRH, van den Heuvel MI, Lahti M et al (2020) Prenatal developmental origins of behavior and mental health: the influence of maternal stress in pregnancy. Neurosci Biobehav Rev 117:26–64. https://doi.org/10.1016/j.neubiorev.2017.07.003

van Erp TGM, Saleh PA, Rosso IM et al (2002) Contributions of genetic risk and fetal hypoxia to hippocampal volume in patients with schizophrenia or schizoaffective disorder, their unaffected siblings, and healthy unrelated volunteers. AJP 159:1514–1520. https://doi.org/10.1176/appi.ajp.159.9.1514

van Nierop M, Viechtbauer W, Gunther N et al (2015) Childhood trauma is associated with a specific admixture of affective, anxiety, and psychosis symptoms cutting across traditional diagnostic boundaries. Psychol Med 45:1277–1288. https://doi.org/10.1017/S0033291714002372

van Os J, Marsman A, van Dam D et al (2017) Evidence that the impact of childhood trauma on IQ is substantial in controls, moderate in siblings, and absent in patients with psychotic disorder. Schizophr Bull 43:316–324. https://doi.org/10.1093/schbul/sbw177

Varese F, Smeets F, Drukker M et al (2012) Childhood adversities increase the risk of psychosis: a meta-analysis of patient-control, prospective- and cross-sectional cohort studies. Schizophr Bull 38:661–671. https://doi.org/10.1093/schbul/sbs050

Vargas T, Lam PH, Azis M et al (2019) Childhood trauma and neurocognition in adults with psychotic disorders: a systematic review and meta-analysis. Schizophr Bull 45:1195–1208. https://doi.org/10.1093/schbul/sby150

Velikonja T, Velthorst E, Zinberg J et al (2021) Childhood trauma and cognitive functioning in individuals at clinical high risk (CHR) for psychosis. Dev Psychopathol 33:53–64. https://doi.org/10.1017/S095457941900155X

Verdoux H, Geddes JR, Takei N et al (1997) Obstetric complications and age at onset in schizophrenia: an international collaborative meta-analysis of individual patient data. AJP 154:1220–1227. https://doi.org/10.1176/ajp.154.9.1220

Vidal PM, Pacheco R (2020) The cross-talk between the dopaminergic and the immune system involved in schizophrenia. Front Pharmacol 11:394. https://doi.org/10.3389/fphar.2020.00394

Vlasova RM, Iosif AM, Ryan AM et al (2021) Maternal immune activation during pregnancy alters postnatal brain growth and cognitive development in nonhuman primate offspring. J Neurosci 41:9971–9987. https://doi.org/10.1523/JNEUROSCI.0378-21.2021

Walker E, Mittal V, Tessner K (2008) Stress and the hypothalamic pituitary adrenal axis in the developmental course of schizophrenia. Annu Rev Clin Psychol 4:189–216. https://doi.org/10.1146/annurev.clinpsy.4.022007.141248

Weickert TW, Goldberg TE, Gold JM, Bigelow LB, Egan MF, Weinberger DR (2000) Cognitive impairments in patients with schizophrenia displaying preserved and compromised intellect. Arch Gen Psychiatry 57(9):907–913. https://doi.org/10.1001/archpsyc.57.9.907

Weinstock M (2001) Alterations induced by gestational stress in brain morphology and behaviour of the offspring. Prog Neurobiol 65:427–451. https://doi.org/10.1016/S0301-0082(01)00018-1

Woodward ND, Heckers S (2015) Brain structure in neuropsychologically defined subgroups of schizophrenia and psychotic bipolar disorder. Schizophr Bull 41(6):1349–1359. https://doi.org/10.1093/schbul/sbv048

Wortinger LA, Engen K, Barth C et al (2020) Obstetric complications and intelligence in patients on the schizophrenia-bipolar spectrum and healthy participants. Psychol Med 50:1914–1922. https://doi.org/10.1017/S0033291719002046

Xie Y, Near C, Xu H, Song X (2020) Heterogeneous treatment effects on Children's cognitive/non-cognitive skills: a reevaluation of an influential early childhood intervention. Soc Sci Res 86:102389. https://doi.org/10.1016/j.ssresearch.2019.102389

Yeo RA, Martinez D, Pommy J et al (2014) The impact of parent socio-economic status on executive functioning and cortical morphology in individuals with schizophrenia and healthy controls. Psychol Med 44:1257–1265. https://doi.org/10.1017/S0033291713001608

Zijlmans MAC, Riksen-Walraven JM, de Weerth C (2015) Associations between maternal prenatal cortisol concentrations and child outcomes: a systematic review. Neurosci Biobehav Rev 53:1–24. https://doi.org/10.1016/j.neubiorev.2015.02.015

Developmental Manipulation-Induced Changes in Cognitive Functioning

Sahith Kaki, Holly DeRosa, Brian Timmerman, Susanne Brummelte, Richard G. Hunter, and Amanda C. Kentner

Contents

S. Kaki and A. C. Kentner (✉)
School of Arts and Sciences, Health Psychology Program, Massachusetts College of Pharmacy and Health Sciences, Boston, MA, USA
e-mail: amanda.kentner@mcphs.edu

H. DeRosa
School of Arts and Sciences, Health Psychology Program, Massachusetts College of Pharmacy and Health Sciences, Boston, MA, USA

University of Massachusetts Boston, Boston, MA, USA

B. Timmerman
Department of Psychology, Wayne State University, Detroit, MI, USA

S. Brummelte
Department of Psychology, Wayne State University, Detroit, MI, USA

Translational Neuroscience Program, Wayne State University, Detroit, MI, USA

R. G. Hunter
University of Massachusetts Boston, Boston, MA, USA

Curr Topics Behav Neurosci (2023) 63: 241–290
https://doi.org/10.1007/7854_2022_389
Published Online: 28 August 2022

Abstract Schizophrenia is a complex neurodevelopmental disorder with as-yet no identified cause. The use of animals has been critical to teasing apart the potential individual and intersecting roles of genetic and environmental risk factors in the development of schizophrenia. One way to recreate in animals the cognitive impairments seen in people with schizophrenia is to disrupt the prenatal or neonatal environment of laboratory rodent offspring. This approach can result in congruent perturbations in brain physiology, learning, memory, attention, and sensorimotor domains. Experimental designs utilizing such animal models have led to a greatly improved understanding of the biological mechanisms that could underlie the etiology and symptomology of schizophrenia, although there is still more to be discovered. The implementation of the Research and Domain Criterion (RDoC) has been critical in taking a more comprehensive approach to determining neural mechanisms underlying abnormal behavior in people with schizophrenia through its transdiagnostic approach toward targeting mechanisms rather than focusing on symptoms. Here, we describe several neurodevelopmental animal models of schizophrenia using an RDoC perspective approach. The implementation of animal models, combined with an RDoC framework, will bolster schizophrenia research leading to more targeted and likely effective therapeutic interventions resulting in better patient outcomes.

Keywords RDoC · Development · Animal models · Schizophrenia · Cognition · Behavioral task

1 Overview

1.1 Diagnostic Considerations

Schizophrenia is a complex neurodevelopmental disorder that is characterized by delusions, hallucinations, disorganized speech, and behavior, as well as negative symptoms such as social withdrawal and/or blunted affect (American Psychiatric Association 2013; Substance Abuse and Mental Health Services Administration 2016; Patel et al. 2014). Schizophrenia is often first diagnosed in early adulthood and its chronic nature makes it a challenging disease to manage (Patel et al. 2014). The disease has a lifetime prevalence rate of approximately 0.5% (Simeone et al. 2015), and in addition to its high prevalence, schizophrenia is a leading cause of disability around the globe (Disease and Injury Incidence and Prevalence Collaborators 2016).

The Diagnostic and Statistical Manual of Mental Disorders (DSM) has been the flagship source for the nosology for mental illness; however, the diagnostic criterion of schizophrenia has changed considerably with each edition of the DSM – indicative of the complexity associated with the etiology, symptomology, and treatment of this disorder (Tandon et al. 2013). Despite a broadening of the clinical description of schizophrenia, especially with the advent of the DSM-5, it still sharply contrasts with much of the neurobiological research that demonstrates considerable heterogeneity among patients with schizophrenia, ultimately underscoring the need for a multidimensional approach (Potkin et al. 2020; Cariaga-Martinez et al. 2016).

In favor of this need for a dynamic and comprehensive understanding of schizophrenia and other psychiatric disorders, the National Institute of Mental Health (NIMH) created the Research Domain Criteria (RDoC). This framework, in conjunction with the DSM-5 and similar classification manuals, provides a foundation for simultaneous investigation of pathological behavior and cognition and the subsequent molecular mechanisms that drive them. These biological mechanisms could include aberrations at the genomic, cellular, or neural circuit level (Young et al. 2017).

The goals of RDoC are to establish an understanding of the essence of mental health and illnesses across several different degrees of dysfunction and to study psychological constructs that are relevant to psychopathology (National Institutes of Health n.d.). The six domains of human functioning that it aims to study are negative valence, positive valence, cognitive systems, systems for social processes, arousal/regulatory systems, and sensorimotor systems (Fig. 1; National Institutes of Health n.d.; Cuthbert and Morris 2021). Furthermore, RDoC's matrix of study is designed to evolve as novel constructs and domains are proposed and integrated (Carcone and Ruocco 2017; National Institutes of Health n.d.).

While there is still a strong preference for the use of DSM-5 in patient diagnoses, the evolution of the RDoC framework has fostered a movement to increase the types of transdiagnostic approaches used by providers (Cuthbert and Morris 2021). This movement has been bolstered by a general agreement within the scientific community that disorder classifications need to be revised (Kapadia et al. 2020; Cerveri et al. 2019; Cuthbert and Morris 2021). Furthermore, the implementation of RDoC has enabled the use of consistent methodologies in animal studies, allowing a more in-depth focus on the etiology and nature of dysfunction of those behaviors relevant to people with schizophrenia, and the direct assessment of their biological underpinnings (Cuthbert and Insel 2013; Young et al. 2017).

1.2 Developmental Origins

Despite the promising potential of RDoC, an important limitation to this framework is that its initial concept is testing adults, thus it lacks a developmental component

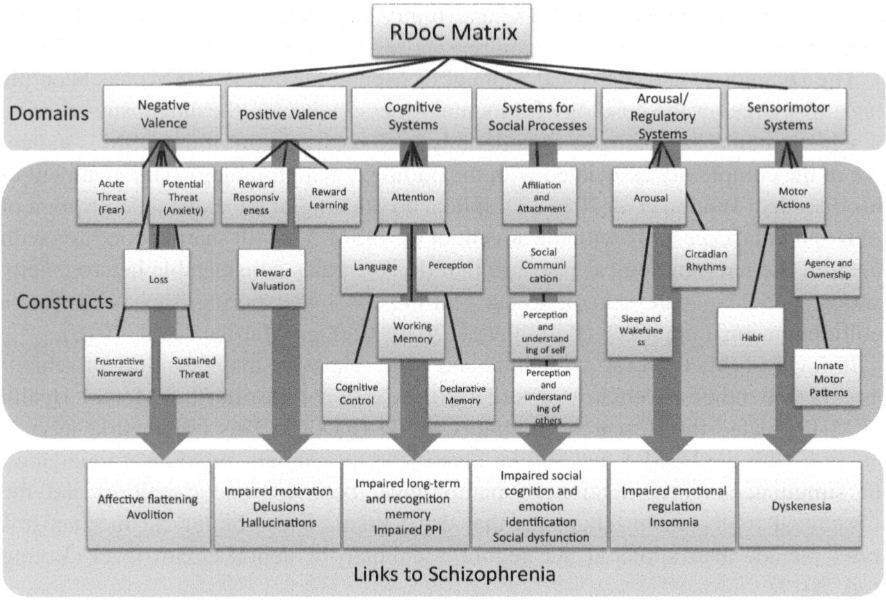

Source: https://www.nimh.nih.gov/research/research-funded-by-nimh/rdoc/definitions-of-the-rdoc-domains-and-constructs

Fig. 1 RDoC matrix relating constructs to schizophrenia

where external factors, such as early life adversity, interact with the trajectory of healthy brain development leading to psychiatric disease (Franklin et al. 2015). Indeed, adversity during early life is one major risk factor for developing schizophrenia. For example, epidemiological studies found that exposure to gestational infection increases offspring risk for developing psychiatric illnesses, including schizophrenia (Mahic et al. 2017; Meyer 2019; Estes and McAllister 2016) and there is an association between birth season and schizophrenia development risk; people born in the early spring have the highest risk (Konrath et al. 2016; Wang and Zhang 2017). In addition, exposure to stress after parturition (e.g., emotional, social, physical, or sexual) also increases the risk for developing schizophrenia (Fachim et al. 2021; Matheson et al. 2013). This evidence warrants the incorporation of a developmental perspective into the RDoC framework, which could offer tremendous insight on when certain populations are most vulnerable to environmental insults, or when treatment intervention is most effective (McLaughlin and Gabard-Durnam 2021).

A model is a representation of ideas or processes that are intended to be studied through the use of a manipulation and quantification of the manipulation's outcomes. Because many of the cognitive and behavioral symptoms seen in people with schizophrenia can be modeled in small laboratory rodents, particularly following exposure to insults experienced during early development, researchers are able to explore the biological mechanisms underlying the intersection of early life adversity and the development of schizophrenia. A good test of an animal model is to evaluate whether it provides construct, face, and predictive validity. Construct validity refers to the mechanistic similarities between the disease and the animal model, face validity is the extent that the animal model looks like it is modeling the disease of interest, and predictive validity is the degree that the response to a therapeutic treatment is similar between the disease and the animal model. Using an RDoC perspective, we will discuss and critique several developmental manipulations used in the generation of animal models for schizophrenia-related behaviors. We will also provide a review of several behavioral and cognitive tests commonly used in the laboratory to test the translational utility of these models.

2 Commonly Used Animal Models of Schizophrenia-Related Behaviors

There are several animal models that are used to understand mechanisms underlying the development of neuropsychiatric disorders such as schizophrenia. These animal models can be broken down into categories based on the timepoint in which the stressor is administrated. These include prenatal, neonatal, and combination models.

3 Prenatal Models

3.1 Maternal Immune Activation (MIA) Model

Epidemiological research suggests that *maternal immune activation (MIA)* in pregnant women can result in prolonged and permanent changes in the behavior and brain function of their offspring (Brown et al. 2009; Estes and McAllister 2016; Kentner et al. 2019a; Mednick et al. 1988). The immune responses that lead to these changes can be caused by a variety of pathogens and bacteria including *Toxoplasma gondii*, influenza, and rubella (Estes and McAllister 2016; Kentner et al. 2019a). Exposure to these pathogens *in utero* increases the risk for several disorders including autism and schizophrenia. In the animal laboratory, behaviors associated with schizophrenia and autism can be modelled by challenging pregnant rodents with immunogens. The two most commonly studied immunogens are lipopolysaccharide (LPS) and polyinosinic:polycytidylic acid [poly (I:C)] which are bacterial and viral mimetics, respectively (Brown et al. 2009; Arsenault et al. 2014). These MIA models are excellent for studying the mechanisms underlying the behavioral dysfunctions related to schizophrenia as they provide construct, face, and predictive validity (Estes and McAllister 2016; Kentner et al. 2019a). While the MIA manipulation does not recreate the exact profile that occurs in people, it does offer insights into the long-term impact of such MIA that can be compared to changes seen in people with schizophrenia.

People with schizophrenia show abnormal dopamine regulation and prefrontal cortex function and most pharmacological treatments target dopamine receptors (Meyer-Lindenberg et al. 2002; Purves-Tyson et al. 2021). In parallel, several studies have documented alterations in such dopaminergic and serotonin signaling among MIA-infected mouse offspring (Winter et al. 2009; Meyer et al. 2008; Csatlosova et al. 2021). In addition, elevated immune-related markers, such as interleukin (IL)-6, SERPINA3, and IL-8, seen in MIA mice are also observed in people with schizophrenia (Purves-Tyson et al. 2021; Knuesel et al. 2014; Reisinger et al. 2015; Fillman et al. 2013; Borovcanin et al. 2017). Additionally, medial prefrontal cortex functioning is disrupted in adult MIA-exposed mice, mediated through altered tyrosine hydroxylase expression and lowered spontaneous firing rate within this brain region (Purves-Tyson et al. 2021). MIA also results in reduced glutamate levels in the hippocampus of rats (Connors et al. 2014), also seen among people with schizophrenia (Howes et al. 2015). In fact, this observation is central to the glutamate hypothesis of schizophrenia and the premise of using glutamatergic-based treatments like bitopertin and minocycline which have shown some promise in clinical trials (Howes et al. 2015; Liu et al. 2014; Umbricht et al. 2014). Thus, despite some potential limitations, the MIA models recreate many of the structural abnormalities seen in people with schizophrenia.

Beyond structural changes, it has been consistently documented that MIA rodent offspring show many behaviors relating to schizophrenia and autism spectrum disorder. For example, offspring of rodents exposed to MIA exhibit decreased sensorimotor gating, increased amphetamine sensitivity, and disruptions in the latent inhibition task. Sensorimotor gating measures the animal's ability to process/filter out irrelevant information (Braff et al. 2001; Purves-Tyson et al. 2021). *Prepulse inhibition* (*PPI*; Fig. 2) is used to study sensorimotor gating and is conducted through an auditory, visual, or tactile modality (Basu and Ray 2016; Powell et al. 2012). It measures the response of the animal to a stimulus, called the pulse, after the presentation of a smaller pulse, called the prepulse. Frontal dopaminergic pathways are disrupted when decreased sensorimotor gating is observed (Tan et al. 2019; Powell et al. 2012). It is hypothesized that the prepulse induces an inhibitory mechanism which blocks the response of the subject to additional stimulation until the prepulse is processed completely in the brain (Basu and Ray 2016). MIA causes a decrease in PPI as MIA-treated offspring are not able to filter out the extraneous information thus disrupting the response (Scarborough et al. 2020; Shi et al. 2003). Similarly, people with schizophrenia have shown significant deficits in information processing as measured by PPI (Cadenhead et al. 2000). Moreover, the antipsychotic clozapine attenuates PPI deficits in rats prenatally exposed to MIA (Basta-Kaim et al. 2012). Attesting to this pharmacological predictive validity, antipsychotic medication also improves PPI in people with schizophrenia. However, PPI may be confounded by the class of antipsychotic prescribed in that typical antipsychotics such as haloperidol don't improve PPI in humans but the atypical antipsychotics such as clozapine do. Moreover, the duration of pharmacological treatment at the time the PPI task is administered matters as those who have been on antipsychotics longer show more improvement in PPI compared to those who just started taking them

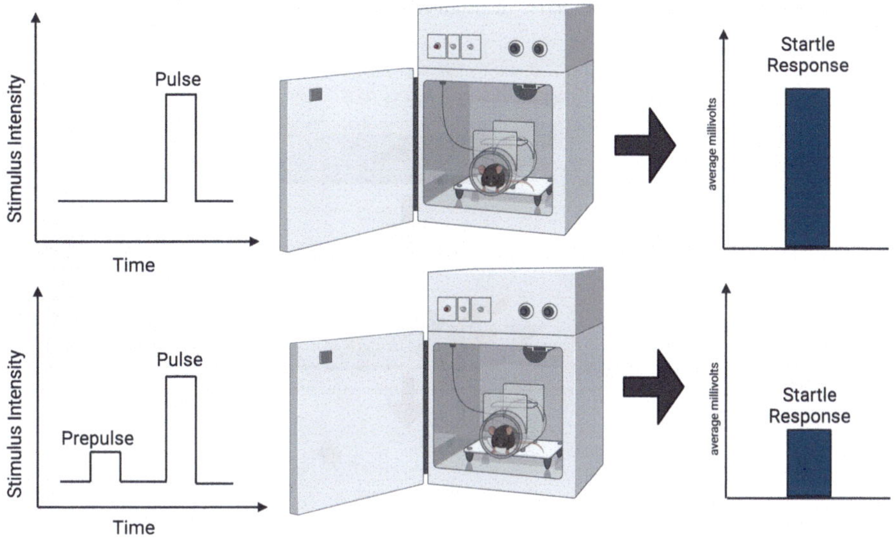

Fig. 2 Prepulse inhibition. An animal's startle response to a sound (pulse) is reduced by the presentation of a less intense sound (prepulse). Using an acoustic startle chamber, researchers can measure the animal's ability to inhibit its startle response (measured by average millivolts) during trials that contain a prepulse

(Kumari and Sharma 2002; Hedberg et al. 2021). Overall, PPI remains an inexpensive and potentially valuable tool to integrate into the RDoC matrix, given its transdiagnostic applicability and the abundance of research identifying its biological constituents (Pineles et al. 2016).

With *latent inhibition* (Fig. 3), previous exposure to a stimulus makes it more difficult to make new associations with that same stimulus (Castagné et al. 2009). MIA is generally associated with impairments in latent inhibition (Bikovsky et al. 2016; Haddad et al. 2020). In one experiment, researchers used white noise as the conditioned stimulus and an electric foot shock as the unconditioned stimulus (Bitanihirwe et al. 2010). Half of the rats received a preexposure to the white noise and the other half did not. On conditioning day, after administering the white noise, rats would avoid the shock if they *shuttled*, which is the process of moving to a different compartment, or area of the chamber to avoid the shock punishment. If animals did not shuttle (reduced response latency), they would immediately receive the shock. MIA-exposed animals showed impairments in social interaction and abnormal latent inhibition was seen in males (Bitanihirwe et al. 2010). There was also a sex-dependent effect on the male offspring from the poly (I:C)-treated mothers. In this two-way active avoidance procedure, the male offspring from poly (I:C)-treated mothers displayed significantly enhanced latent inhibition effects (Bitanihirwe et al. 2010). This effect shows heightened cognitive and behavioral inflexibility within the male, but not female, offspring (Bitanihirwe et al. 2010). Latent inhibition is a form of associative learning (Lubow and Moore 1959;

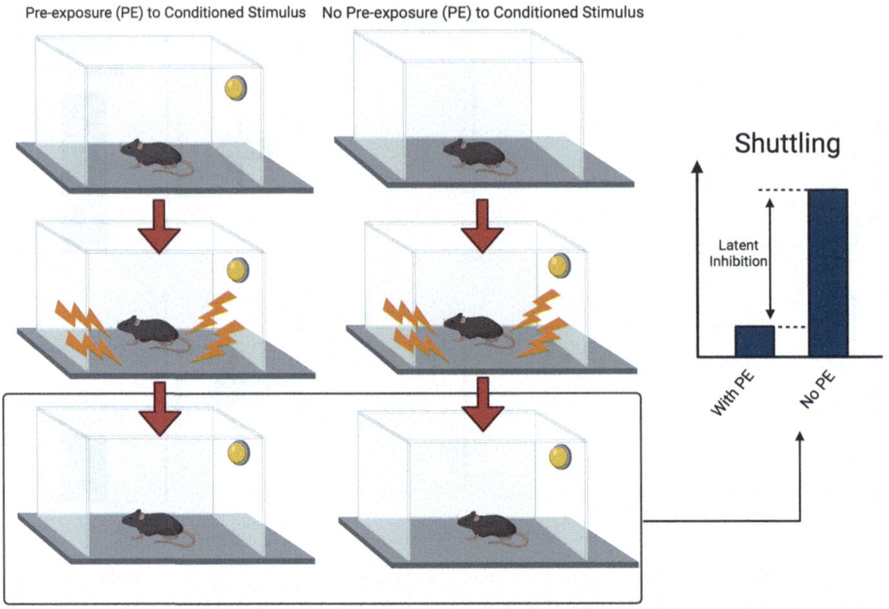

Fig. 3 Latent inhibition. Preexposure to the conditioned stimulus (light) before pairing with a conditioned stimulus (footshock) reduces the fear response compared to animals that receive the conditioned and unconditioned stimulus pairing without preexposure to the conditioned stimulus

Weiner 1985), although some have described it as a task of attention (Lubow 2005), making it closely applicable to the declarative memory subconstruct within the cognitive systems domain of RDoC.

Although reductions in PPI and latent inhibition are among the most consistent findings across studies that use the MIA model (Haddad et al. 2020), not all have demonstrated these deficits (Li et al. 2009; Meehan et al. 2017; Bitanihirwe et al. 2010). Some important factors that may contribute to this discrepancy include the timing of immune challenge, offspring sex, offspring age, drug dose, the source of immunogen, as well as the animal strain/genetic background. In addition (Table 1), most MIA model studies use nonvirulent agents that activate the immune system (poly (I:C) for example). However, these do not invoke the natural level of immune response caused by infectious pathogens experienced in nature (Mueller et al. 2019). An additional limitation of the MIA model is that it does not capture potential confounds, such as stressful environments, photoperiods, or stress brought on by navigating the world differently because of a triggered immune response. These limitations make it difficult to model the role of broader factors in contributing to altered offspring development. Epidemiological studies in this case are more robust as the human experience is built-in (Brown and Meyer 2018). Lastly, even with established protocols, immunogens may result in immune responses that are either too weak, too strong, or even potentially fatal which can lead to variability in this model (Kentner et al. 2019a; Roderick and Kentner 2019; Chow et al. 2016).

Table 1 Summary of developmental manipulations and cognitive effects

Developmental manipulation	Cognitive effects	References
Maternal immune activation (MIA)	PPI	(Scarborough et al. 2020; Shi et al. 2003; Cadenhead et al. 2000; Haddad et al. 2020)
	PPI (dose dependent)	(Meyer et al. 2005)
	No effect of MIA on PPI	(Li et al. 2009; Meehan et al. 2017)
	Latent inhibition	(Bikovsky et al. 2016; Haddad et al. 2020)
	Latent inhibition (males)	(Bitanihirwe et al. 2010)
Maternal methylazoxymethanol acetate exposure (MAM)	Performance on radial arm maze memory task	(Gourevitch et al. 2004)
	Attention set-shifting	(Featherstone et al. 2007a, b; Mar et al. 2017)
	Spatial navigation of water maze	(Leng et al. 2005)
	Premature responding on 5C-SRT	(Featherstone et al. 2007a, b; Mar et al. 2017)
	PPI	(Chalkiadaki et al. 2019; Hazane et al. 2009)
Prenatal psychosocial stress	Novel object recognition (males)	(Markham et al. 2010)
	PPI	(Koenig et al. 2005; Niu et al. 2020; Burton et al. 2006)
Maternal vitamin D deficiency	Memory in brightness discrimination task	(Becker et al. 2005)
	Performance on 5C-SRT and 5C-CPT	(Harms et al. 2012b; Turner et al. 2013)
Neonatal ventral hippocampal lesion (NVHL)	PPI	(Brady 2016)
	Spatial navigation of radial arm maze	(Brady 2016)
	Performance on the continuous spatial delayed alternation task	(Maruki et al. 2001; Brady et al. 2010; Lipska et al. 2002; Kim and Frank 2009)
	Performance on the discrete paired-trial variable-delay task (time dependent)	(Lipska et al. 2002)
Maternal separation (MS)	PPI	(Ellenbroek and Riva 2003; Garner et al. 2007)
	Reversal learning in Morris water maze	(Xue et al. 2013)
	Spatial navigation in Morris water maze	(Zhu et al. 2010; Garner et al. 2007)
	No effect of MS on Morris water maze	(Enthoven et al. 2008)
	Reversal learning in Morris water maze	(Mooney-Leber and Brummelte 2020)

(continued)

Table 1 (continued)

Developmental manipulation	Cognitive effects	References
Postnatal dopamine agonism	Spatial navigation in Morris water maze, elevated plus maze, and Cincinnati water maze	(Dawirs et al. 1996; Acevedo et al. 2007; Grace et al. 2010; Hrubá et al. 2010; Skelton et al. 2007; Vorhees et al. 2008, 2009)
	Novel location and object recognition	(Siegel et al. 2011; Acevedo et al. 2007)
	PPI	(Acevedo et al. 2007)
Postnatal NMDA receptor antagonism	PPI	(Mouri et al. 2013; Lim et al. 2012; Neill et al. 2010; Plataki et al. 2021)
	Fear conditioning	(Lim et al. 2012; Neill et al. 2010; Plataki et al. 2021)

3.2 Maternal Methylazoxymethanol Acetate Exposure (MAM) Model

In the *maternal methylazoxymethanol acetate exposure (MAM) model*, pregnant female rodents are treated with MAM, producing offspring that demonstrate schizophrenia-relevant behaviors (Flagstad et al. 2004; Featherstone et al. 2007a, b). MAM produces such effects in offspring because it is a neurotoxin that selectively targets neuroblasts and is typically administered on gestational day (GD) 16-17. GD17 in rodents coincides with the late second trimester in human gestation (Bitanihirwe et al. 2010). MAM treatment results in offspring with cognitive deficits as seen in people with schizophrenia, e.g., impairments in attention, long-term memory, working memory, and behavioral flexibility through the use of tests like the radial arm maze task and water maze experiments (Gourevitch et al. 2004; Featherstone et al. 2007a, b, Leng et al. 2005). In addition to affecting similar cognitive domains as schizophrenia, MAM treatment leads to abnormal hippocampal and cortical morphology and function (Featherstone et al. 2007a, b; Lavin et al. 2005). Importantly, the timing of MAM administration is critical to the effectiveness of this model. If given earlier, such as before GD15, MAM can produce widespread physiological changes in the brain, such as reduction in cortical thickness and overall brain weight (Di Fausto et al. 2007; Gourevitch et al. 2004). These neuroanatomical changes result in damage that is too drastic to serve as a valid model of schizophrenia, highlighting the importance of the timing of the neurodevelopmental manipulation.

To study effects of MAM exposure on the brain and cognitive function, two translationally relevant tests are the attentional set-shifting task and the 5-choice serial reaction time task (5-CSRTT; Pezze et al. 2007; Cope et al. 2016). The *attentional set-shifting task* (Fig. 4) requires the animal to discriminate between a relevant stimulus and an irrelevant stimulus to receive a reward, building the relevance of one dimension by repeated testing within that dimension driving the formation of an "attentional set." Next, animals are required to shift that attentional

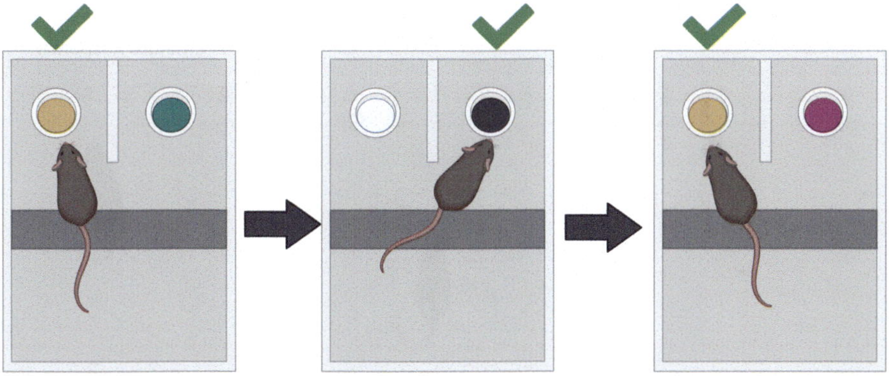

Fig. 4 Attentional set-shifting. An animal learns to discriminate between two stimuli to receive a food reward. Then the animal must learn to discriminate between two new stimuli to receive the reward. During the test trials, animals are required to "shift" their attention toward previously irrelevant stimuli

set, where the previously relevant dimension becomes irrelevant, and a stimulus from the originally irrelevant dimension must be chosen in order to receive the reward (Birrell and Brown 2000; Featherstone et al. 2007a, b; Heisler et al. 2015). This test was designed to assay cognitive flexibility and held as analogous to the Wisconsin Card Sort Task (WCST; Barcelo et al. 2000; Heisler et al. 2015), and more specifically the interdimensional/extradimensional task. The WCST reveals deficits in executive function in people with schizophrenia (Everett et al. 2001; Nieuwenstein et al. 2001; Singh et al. 2017), supporting the translational relevance of attentional set-shifting task in the study of the cognitive mechanisms related to schizophrenia. Offspring of MAM-treated dams require more trials than control, saline-treated groups to learn an extradimensional shift in the attentional set-shifting task (Featherstone et al. 2007a, b). Furthermore, they have difficulties in reversing discriminations that were previously acquired in the experiment (Featherstone et al. 2007a, b). As the attentional set-shifting task is used to study cognitive function and flexibility, naturally it fits into the cognitive systems domain of RDoC.

The *5-choice serial reaction time task* (*5-CSRT;* Fig. 5) is an analog of Leonard's (1959) choice reaction time task which was devised to test the impacts of stressors on human performance. Now, the 5-CSRT is widely used to study deficits in attention in animals (Robbins 2002). In this task, animals receive a visual light stimulus at one of the several locations. Animals must then go to the location while the light is on to receive a reward, generally a food reinforcement (Carli et al. 1983). The location of the light will change every trial. The 5-CSRT recruits several parts of the brain including the prefrontal cortex (Liu et al. 2019; Robbins 2002). Similar to the 5-CSRT in rodent models is the *5-choice continuous performance test* (*5C-CPT*; Fig. 6). In the 5C-CPT, animals are first trained in the 5-CSRT test (see Fig. 5), as above. When moved to the 5C-CPT, some trials will have all five light stimuli turned on (Bhakta and Young 2017), wherein the animal needs to inhibit from responding,

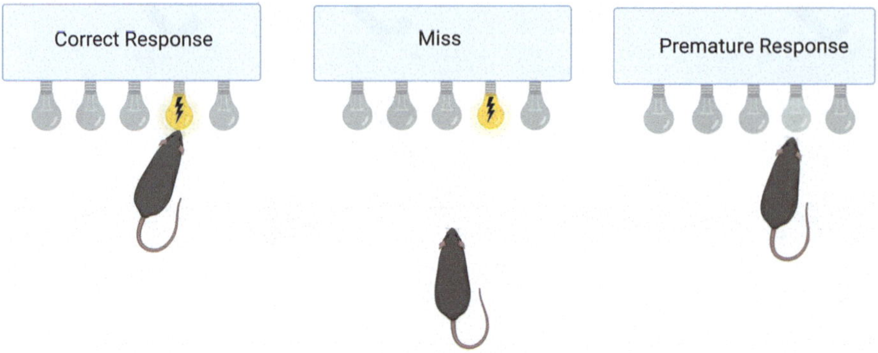

Fig. 5 5-choice serial reaction time task (5C-SRT). Animals are provided a food reward for entering a hole with a light illuminated. Misses and premature responses trigger a timeout

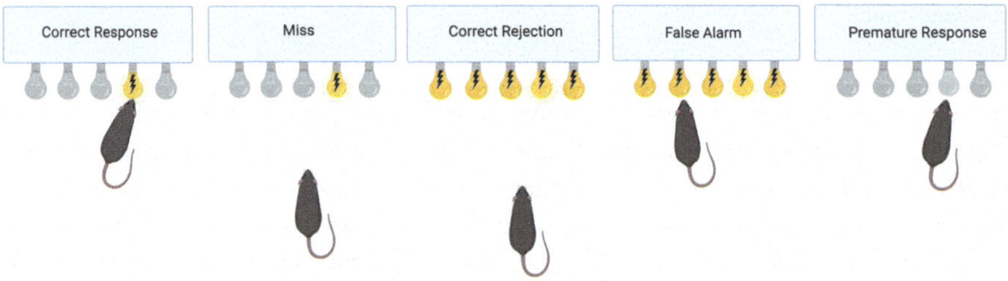

Fig. 6 5-choice continuous performance test (5C-CPT). Animals are first trained in the 5C-SRT test (see Fig. 5). In this task, animals must also demonstrate inhibition, by not approaching any of the lights when all of the lights are illuminated. This is recorded as a "correct rejection," which is rewarded

recorded as a correct rejection (response inhibition) and rewarded. A response to any of the five lights is recorded as a false alarm and punished. Like the 5-CSRT, if the animal responds before any lights appear (no stimulus present), it is recorded as a premature response. Essentially, the 5C-CPT task requires response inhibition, unlike the 5-CSRT (Young et al. 2009; Bhakta and Young 2017), because it includes non-target stimuli. As a result, researchers can better measure cognitive functions like response inhibition (Bhakta and Young 2017; McKenna et al. 2013; Young et al. 2009), and the recruitment of brain regions consistent with human CPTs like the parietal cortex (Young et al. 2020; McKenna et al. 2013), not needed in the 5-CSRT, recreating the core aspects of CPTs used to assess attention in people with schizophrenia.

In the attention set-shifting task, MAM-treated rats require more attempts to learn an extradimensional shift, have higher errors, and have more difficulty in reversing previously learned associations compared to the control group (Featherstone et al. 2007a, b; Mar et al. 2017). A higher error rate would mean that the animals display reduced cognitive flexibility. On the 5-CSRT, MAM-treated animals show increased premature responding compared to the control group (Featherstone et al. 2007a, b; Mar et al. 2017) suggestive of motor impulsivity and/or poor temporal perception (Cope et al. 2016), but no deficits in attentional measures – therefore assessment in the 5C-CPT is warranted. Given that people with schizophrenia do not show deficits in the 5-CSRT but do so in the 5C-CPT, the latter may provide more finite measurement of schizophrenia-relevant performance. In post-mortem analyses, MAM-treated animals had decreased tissue weight of the prefrontal cortex, dorsal striatum, parietal cortex, and the hippocampus (Featherstone et al. 2007a, b; Haijma et al. 2013; Nelson et al. 1998; Ohtani et al. 2014; Olabi et al. 2011; Veijola et al. 2014). These changes are analogous to post-mortem studies in humans with schizophrenia (Arnold et al. 2015; Gaser et al. 2004; Rajarethinam et al. 2007). Lastly, similar to the MIA model, MAM-treated rats display reduced PPI of the startle reflex (Chalkiadaki et al. 2019; Hazane et al. 2009). The MAM model is valuable for the study of behavioral and cognitive deficits that run in parallel to schizophrenia patients in terms of phenotypic expression (Table 1) and underlying mechanisms. However, to connect the experimental MAM-treated rodent data with human studies, complex effective connective modeling is required and the roles of neurotransmitters (GABA, dopamine, etc.) can generally only be inferred (Modinos et al. 2015a, b). Moreover, it should be noted that MAM is a potentially potent toxin and carcinogen and so researchers should exercise extreme caution and limit their exposure to MAM.

3.3 Prenatal Psychological Stress Models

Research shows that psychological stress experienced during gestation is a risk factor for impaired cognitive functioning and schizophrenia in offspring in later life (Khashan et al. 2008; Malaspina et al. 2008). In fact, exposure to prenatal psychological stressors, like natural disasters during pregnancy, can result in lower cognitive and language skills, increased risk for depression, and may increase the risk of developing schizophrenia (Antonelli et al. 2017; Laplante et al. 2008; Watson et al. 1999). In the animal laboratory, *prenatal psychological stressors* also lead to cognitive impairments in offspring (Lemaire et al. 2000; Markham et al. 2010; Szuran et al. 2000). Examples of prenatal stressors used in animal models include restraint or predator odor which are used to induce both *acute* (e.g., a short-term or single stressor) and *chronic* (e.g., multiple or long-term stress exposure) stress across gestation. In chronic stress paradigms, the stressors applied can be homotypic (e.g., using the same stressor repeatedly) or heterotrophic (e.g., using variable or different types of stressors). A commonly used test for evaluating cognitive function following prenatal stress is the *novel object recognition task* (Fig. 7). This task determines whether an animal can distinguish between a novel and familiar object. In this test, a rodent is placed inside of an arena with two different objects equidistant from each other. In the *introduction phase,* an animal is given a timed duration (e.g., 5 min or 10 min) to investigate both objects. Following this presentation, the animal is

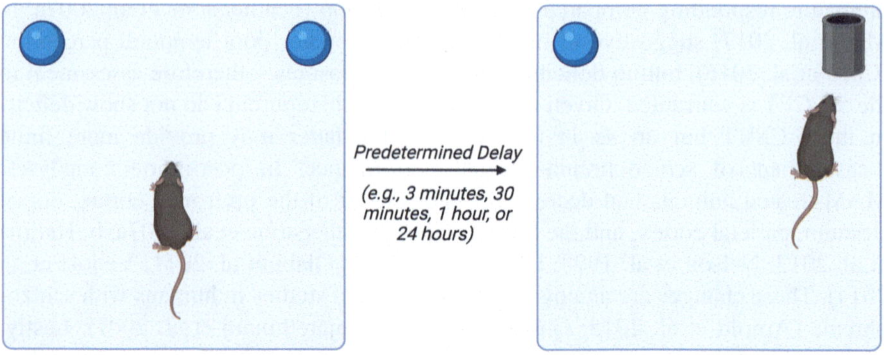

Fig. 7 Novel object recognition. The animal is first presented with two of the same stimuli for the duration of the habituation period (e.g., 5 or 10 min). One of these stimuli is then replaced with a novel object after a predetermined delay period (e.g., 3 min, 30 min, 1 h, 24 h) and the amount of time the animal spends exploring the novel object during the testing period is measured

removed from the arena and returned to its home cage. The investigators then replace one of the two familiar objects with a new (novel) one. After a timed delay (e.g., 3 min, 30 min, 1 h, 24 h), the animal is placed back into the arena and the amount of time they spend investigating the novel versus the familiar object is recorded, referred to as the *recognition* phase. When interpreting the results, if the animal spends more time investigating the new object than chance, it is thought to relate to memory and learning (Denninger et al. 2018; Markham et al. 2010). Using this task, male rodent offspring exposed to repeated variable stress during the final week of gestation were found to have an impaired ability to recognize objects, even as adults. Prenatal stress did not impair object recognition in female animals (Markham et al. 2010). This result differs from studies which show schizophrenia is present in men and women, however, schizophrenia prevalence is higher among men and merits further research (Li et al. 2016). While this task more broadly falls into the RDoC domain of cognitive systems (Vengeliene et al. 2017), it is important to acknowledge that the variation in time delays and lack of human counterpart for adults have made the translational validity of this task difficult to determine (Young et al. 2012).

In rodents, prenatal stress also impairs sensorimotor gating and development of the hypothalamic-pituitary-adrenal (HPA) axis, effects which are commonly found among schizophrenia patients (Kinnunen et al. 2003; Markham et al. 2010). The HPA axis is key in our bodies regulation to stress through secretions of corticotropin releasing factor, adrenal corticotropin releasing hormone, cortisol, and other hormones through a negative feedback process (Smith and Vale 2006). Cognitive disruptions in hippocampal processes following prenatal stress have been tied to reductions in hippocampal neurogenesis (Couch et al. 2021; Lemaire et al. 2000; Markham et al. 2010). In addition to damage to the hippocampus, impaired performance on *fear conditioning tests* (Fig. 8) points to damage or altered functioning in the amygdala (LeDoux 2003; Park and Chung 2020). These are associative learning tests where animals learn to associate a neutral conditioned stimulus (e.g., a light or a

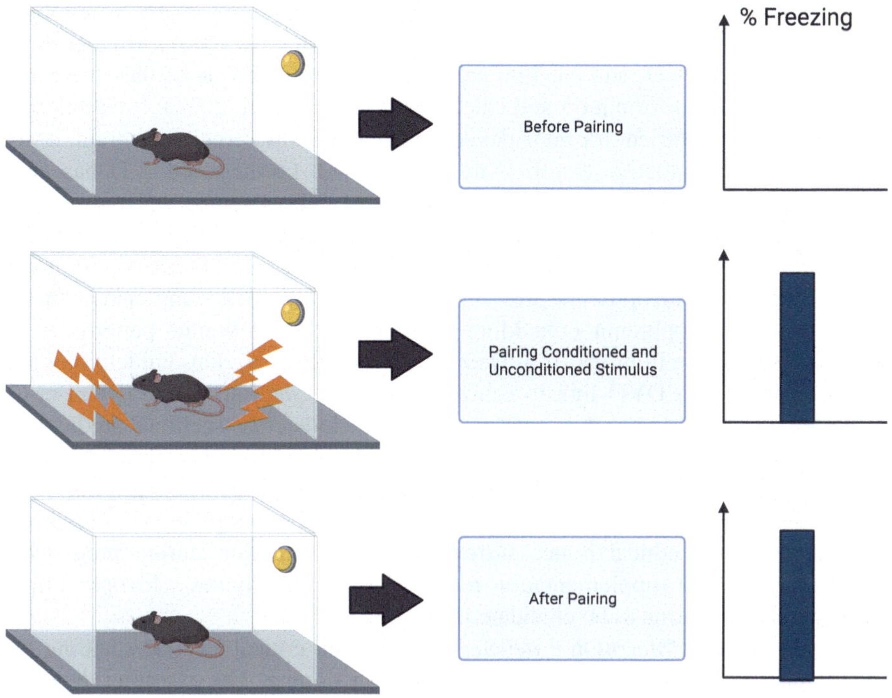

Fig. 8 Fear conditioning. A conditioned stimulus (light) does not trigger a fear response until after it is paired with an unconditioned stimulus (footshock). After this pairing, an animal learns to associate the light with the footshock and will demonstrate freezing behavior in response to the light only

tone) with an aversive unconditioned stimulus (e.g., a shock) to show a conditioned response (e.g., freezing behavior). Fear conditioning would most likely fall under the negative valence systems domain and acute threat construct of RDoC. Lastly, prenatal stress through restraint stress has been shown to decrease the PPI of acoustic startle responses in rodents (Koenig et al. 2005; Niu et al. 2020; Burton et al. 2006). Similarly, there has been a strong connection between HPA axis dysfunction (e.g., elevated cortisol secretion) and hippocampal function with schizophrenia severity (Walder et al. 2000). These findings speak to the validity of such prenatal stressors for relevance to schizophrenia.

3.4 Diet/Nutritional Deficiency

Nutrition is one of the most important factors contributing to the health and development of mothers and their offspring. There have been studies indicating that calcium and vitamin D deficiencies (DVD) in the mother may result in central nervous system disorders in offspring, including schizophrenia, multiple sclerosis, and type 1 diabetes (Bordeleau et al. 2021; Hyppönen et al. 2001; Mirzaei et al. 2011). Vitamin D (VD) and calcium are critical across gestation as they are foundational for skeleton formation and calcification (Curtis et al. 2014). In addition to being an essential nutrient for bone development, VD is also crucial for brain, heart, immune, and reproductive health (Xue et al. 2016). Furthermore, VD has anti-inflammatory properties, where the depletion of VD receptor or hydroxylase Cyp27b1 can increase placental inflammation (Liu et al. 2011). Concomitantly, VD receptor agonists reduce the expression of immune cells *in vitro* (Vojinovic 2014). Increased schizophrenia prevalence at higher latitudes, combined with the incidence of schizophrenia coinciding with summer and winter patterns (e.g., increased prevalence in births from December to March), provides epidemiological data in support of a DVD link to schizophrenia (McGrath et al. 2011; Cui et al. 2021). As a result of these observations – which include cross-sectional studies and longitudinal cohort studies – researchers have also been able to associate DVD to cognitive function, Parkinson's disease, multiple sclerosis, and autism (Cui et al. 2015). Directly testing the relationship between VD and schizophrenia in humans is difficult given the ethical issues surrounding VD restriction during pregnancy. Whether or not VD supplementation reduces risk of developing schizophrenia in this population remains to be elucidated.

Animal models of nutritional deficiency have been critical to understanding the underlying mechanisms of DVD to cognitive functioning. For example, developmentally DVD rodents exhibit enlarged lateral ventricles, smaller hippocampi, and altered expression of apoptosis compared to control groups (Harms et al. 2012a; Eyles et al. 2003), which are common physiological patterns seen in psychiatric patients (Del Re et al. 2016; Ershova et al. 2017). Developmental DVD may also lead to disruptions to glutamate and dopamine system functioning (McGrath et al. 2010) as these DVD rats are hypersensitive to the locomotor-stimulating effects of MK-801 and amphetamine, which are both psychotomimetic drugs (Kesby et al. 2006, 2010). Furthermore, prenatal DVD rats show impairments in learning and memory, as indicated by the *brightness discrimination task* (Fig. 9), along with damaged latent inhibition and attention, which are all features of schizophrenia (Becker et al. 2005; Harms et al. 2012b). For the brightness discrimination task, animals are trained to enter the illuminated alley of a Y-maze. Once the animal is trained, their ability to relearn this procedure is tested 24 h later. This measure of memory recall fits into the Declarative Memory construct within the cognitive systems domain of RDoC.

One notable experiment tested attentional processing among developmental DVD rats using both the 5-CSRT and 5C-CPT (Turner et al. 2013). While not impaired in the 5-CSRT, adult offspring of DVD dams made more false alarm responses in the 5C-CPT and had more premature responses compared to controls (Turner et al. 2013). This finding suggests that DVD rats have impaired inhibitory control and increased impulsivity resembling the impaired CPT of people with schizophrenia (Turner et al. 2013; Table 1). Concomitantly, 5C-CPT validly translates to human populations, can be fMRI assessed (McKenna et al. 2013). People with

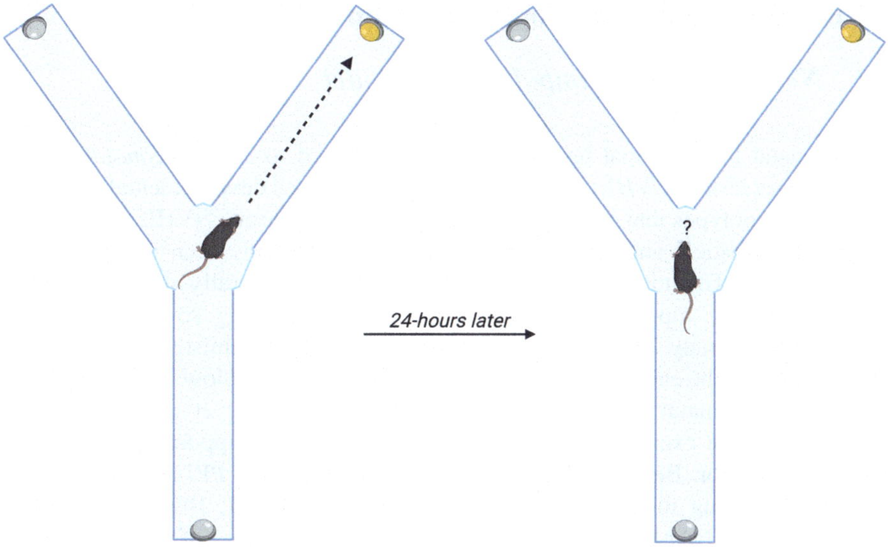

Fig. 9 Brightness discrimination task. Animals are trained to enter the illuminated alley of a Y-maze. Entering an unilluminated alley triggers a foot shock. Once the animal is trained, their ability to relearn to enter the illuminated alley is tested 24 h later

schizophrenia exhibit deficits in the human task with EEG biomarker deficits and these neural correlates associated with the task are conserved from mice to humans (Young et al. 2013; Cavanagh et al. 2021). This evidence further supports the integration of 5C-CPT into the attention construct within the cognitive systems domain of RDoC (Cope et al. 2016).

The 5C-CPT requires activation in several brain areas including the inferior frontal cortex, presupplementary motor area, premotor cortex, inferior parietal lobe, basal ganglia, and thalamus (McKenna et al. 2013; Young et al. 2020). Developmentally DVD exposed animals exhibit NMDA receptor and dopamine dysfunction within these brain regions in concert with increased motoric impulsivity and response disinhibition in the 5C-CPT (Kesby et al. 2006, 2017). Interestingly, DVD rats also exhibited deficits in novel object recognition (Overeem et al. 2019) and spatial navigation (Al-Harbi et al. 2017), but did not display altered PPI or delay-match-to-sample (Burne et al. 2014). Overall, developmental DVD may more reliably model symptoms of schizophrenia associated with deficits in locomotor function compared to those related to working memory or sensorimotor gating.

4 Early Postnatal Developmental Models

4.1 Neonatal Hippocampal Lesion Model

The neonatal hippocampal lesion model, also referred to as *the neonatal ventral hippocampal lesion (NVHL) model*, is a surgically induced developmental model for studying phenotypes that correlate to schizophrenia symptoms. NVHL recapitulates several neurological and anatomical impairments commonly seen in people with schizophrenia. To induce this model, an excitotoxin, generally ibotenic acid, is injected into the hippocampus of neonatal animals causing several behavioral abnormalities (Brady 2016). This excitotoxin is generally administered to the rodent hippocampus at the end of the first postnatal week, which is analogous with late third trimester or perinatal period of human development (Tseng et al. 2009). When administered, the excitotoxin disrupts the development of hippocampal pathways affecting behavior. Behavioral abnormalities include reduced PPI and impairments in spatial working memory of the *radial arm maze* (RAM; Brady et al. 2010; Fig. 10). In the RAM task, animals are trained to enter arms of a maze that are baited with a food reward. The un-baited arms are barricaded. After training, the test phase is followed by a predetermined delay (e.g., 1 min, 60 min). During the test, entrances to all of the arms of the maze are opened, and the animal is timed for how long it takes to navigate to all of the food rewards, with working memory errors equated to entering already visited arms (Brown and Giumetti 2006). NVHL results in decreased GAD67 mRNA expression, decreased NAA (N-acetylaspartate) levels,

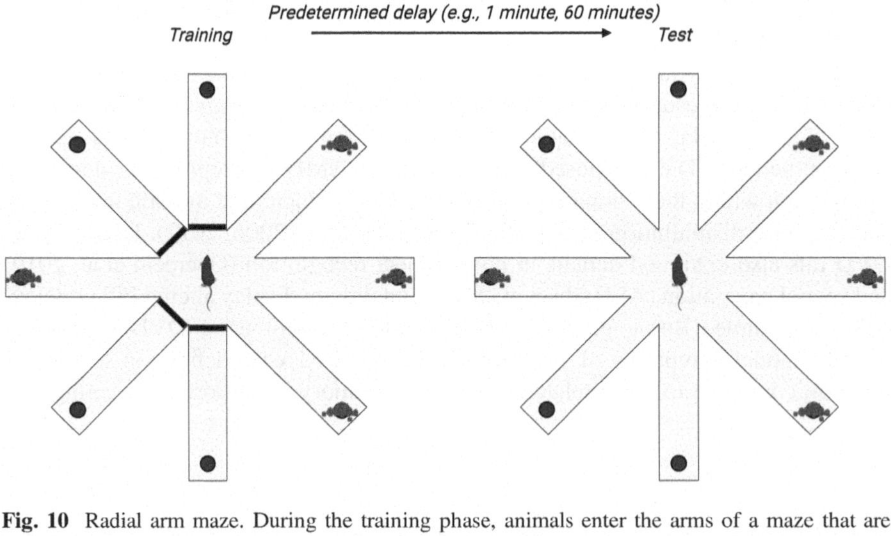

Fig. 10 Radial arm maze. During the training phase, animals enter the arms of a maze that are baited with a food reward. The un-baited arms are blocked. The test phase is followed by a predetermined delay (e.g., 1 min, 60 min). During the test, entrances to all of the arms of the maze are opened, and the latency to retrieve food rewards, number of incorrect, and correct entries are recorded

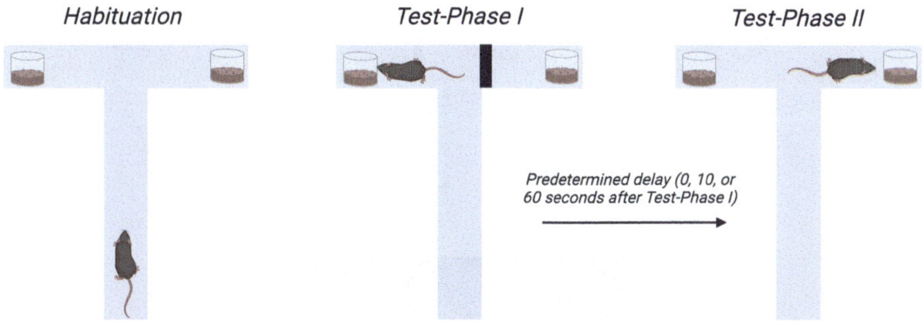

Fig. 11 Continuous spatial delayed alternation task. After habituation, one of the arms to the T-maze is closed off, forcing the animal to collect the food reward from the open arm. Next, following a predetermined delay (e.g., 0, 10, or 60 s) the closed arm is opened, and the animal must spatially recall that this arm contains the remaining reward. A correct response is recorded when the animal enters the previously closed arm after the forced run trial

and increased glutamatergic neurotransmission (Lipska et al. 2002; Lipska and Weinberger 2000; Modinos et al. 2015a, b; Roffman et al. 2000; Schroeder et al. 1999).

NVHL rats have impaired performance in the continuous spatial delayed alternation and the discrete paired-trial variable-delay tasks (Brito et al. 1983; Aultman and Moghaddam 2001; Lipska et al. 2002). In the *continuous spatial delayed alternation task* (Fig. 11), researchers employ a "T" shaped maze with food rewards located at the ends of both arms of the T-maze. At the start of this task, an animal is habituated to the maze with full access to the food rewards in each goal arms of the maze. During the test, one arm of the T-maze is blocked, forcing the animal to access the food reward in the opposite arm. After a delay (e.g., 0, 10, or 60 s) the animal is given full access to the previously blocked arm. If the animal demonstrates intact spatial working memory, they will enter the previously blocked arm to collect the food. When the delay between rounds is extended past one minute (typically the upper limit of working memory), animals with hippocampus inactivation perform significantly worse indicating impaired spatial working memory (Maruki et al. 2001). In the continuous spatial delayed alternation task, NVHL rats performed significantly worse compared to sham-operated rats (Brady et al. 2010; Lipska et al. 2002; Kim and Frank 2009). Interestingly, Lipska (2002) found control and NVHL rats had similar performance at the start of training until test day 11, however, the performance of control animals progressively improved over time. The inability for the neonatal lesion group to master this task shows an impaired acquisition and working memory (Lipska et al. 2002). Based on this pattern of deficits, the continuous spatial delayed alternation task would fall into the goal maintenance subdomain of the working memory construct.

In the *discrete paired-trial variable-delay task* (Fig. 12), the animal is placed into a discrete paired-trial variable-delay T-maze. Next, the animal is put through a randomly chosen forced run – a maze designed to force the animal to turn right or left after being placed inside the maze – following a delay in the home cage. Then,

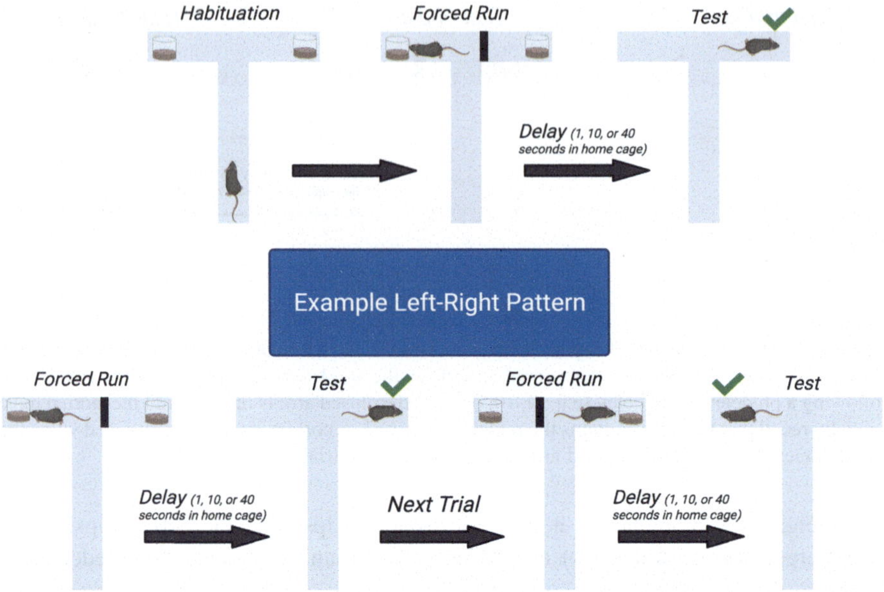

Fig. 12 Discrete paired-trial variable-delay task. This test runs like the continuous spatial delayed alternation task, except experimenters can evaluate the strength of an animal's memory over time. Animals are first trained to learn specific patterns of forced runs (e.g., left-right). Subjects are then tested on their memories of the patterns following varying lengths of delay (e.g., 1, 10, or 40 s)

the animal is placed back into the maze and allowed to go through the maze. Every day, the randomly chosen pattern changes but the pattern stays constant the whole day (Right-Right, Left-Right, Right-Left, or Left-Left). The delays are also variable at 1 s, 10 s, and 40 s (Papaleo et al. 2008; Leggio et al. 2020; Lipska et al. 2002). Although all the animals reached the 80% criterion of choice accuracy, NVHL animals performed worse than sham-operated rats during larger delay periods (Lipska et al. 2002), suggesting their goal-oriented working memory was compromised (Table 1). Both the continuous spatial delayed alternation task and discrete paired-trial variable-delay task fall under the goal maintenance working memory construct of the cognitive systems domain of the RDoC framework, and their mechanistic deconstruction could illuminate the biological constituents of schizophrenia symptomology.

Many of the anatomical changes related to cognitive disruptions that are induced by NVHL occur in the prefrontal cortex which is a key brain region implicated in schizophrenia (Brady et al. 2010; Placek et al. 2013). Thus, rather than inducing localized cell death, which lacks the ability to assess the role of cross-regional networks, the excitotoxin damages pathways to the prefrontal cortex and forebrain (Brady 2016). Furthermore, the cognitive effects of the NVHL model temporally matches the onset of schizophrenia in that abnormalities do not generally manifest until the adolescence or early adulthood (Brady 2016; Gogtay et al. 2011; Häfner 2019).

There are some disadvantages to the NVHL model. First, only 70–80% of all animals may produce a lesion and disorganization or cell loss following exposure to ibotenic acid (Brady 2016). This form of stereotaxic surgery requires heavy exposure to anesthetics and triggers an immune response which may explain the 70–80% success rate (Kirby et al. 2012). This model may also be influenced by environmental factors (Chambers and Sentir 2019), which can lead to variability between and within species. Lastly, the construct validity of all lesion models is questionable due to the lack of environmentally induced lesions present in people with schizophrenia (Modinos et al. 2015a, b).

4.2 *Psychosocial Stress in Neonates*

Childhood neglect and abuse are major predictors of schizophrenia in humans (Bennouna-Greene et al. 2011; Kraan et al. 2015; Rokita et al. 2020; Matheson et al. 2013). The *maternal separation (MS) model* is a commonly used method to induce early life stress in laboratory animals (Murthy and Gould 2018; Solas et al. 2010). In this model, a mother and her offspring are separated for a specified duration of time (e.g., minutes or hours) daily across several postnatal days or weeks (Kalinichev et al. 2002; Solas et al. 2010). MS impaired PPI and sensory gating (Ellenbroek and Riva 2003; Table 1) consistent to people with schizophrenia. MS also induced depressive-like behaviors, anxiety-like behaviors, and other cognitive impairments in offspring (Kalinichev et al. 2002; Romeo et al. 2003; Solas et al. 2010), suggesting that MS may not exclusively model schizophrenia and may be an effective model of other disorders. Indeed, some researchers have also used MS to model certain aspects of depression (Solas et al. 2010).

In the *Morris Water Maze* (*MWM;* Fig. 13), researchers utilize a rodents' aversion to water to test their spatial memory and learning (Bromley-Brits et al. 2011; Vorhees and Williams 2006). The MWM is the dominant form of testing to assess allocentric navigation, navigation using external cues and landmark in relation to each other to navigate, in animals (Vorhees and Williams 2016). A small pool is filled with water, made opaque, and a submerged platform is placed in a certain

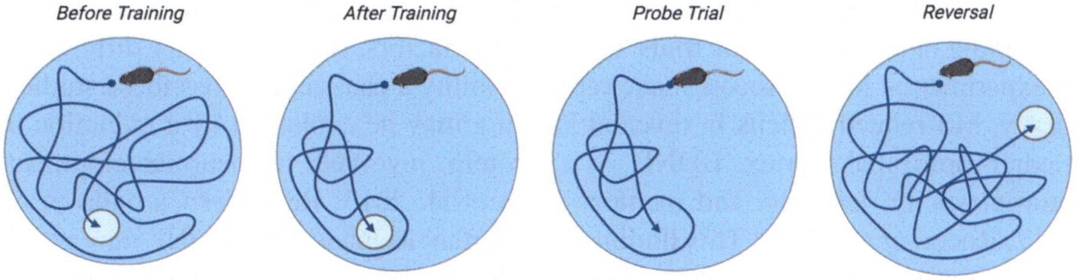

Fig. 13 Morris water maze. After several trials, the animal learns to swim to a platform it cannot see. For the test, the platform is removed and the experimenter times how long it takes the animal to swim to the relative location of where the platform was previously

location. Then, the rodent is brought to the environment where the pool is located to acclimate to the room. After acclimation, the animal is placed in the water, requiring a fixed time to locate and mount the platform (escaping the water). If the animal does not do this within the allotted time (around 60 s), the researcher places the animal on top of the platform and allows it to stand on the platform for several seconds. After this, the animal is returned to its cage. This training is repeated several times a day, for several days, wherein the animal gets faster at locating the platform. A probe trial is then conducted wherein the platform is removed from the pool and the time the animal spends in the quadrant of where the platform used to be is used as a measure of their memory (Vorhees and Williams 2006). The initial trials test the animal's acquisition ability while the probe trial assesses *reference memory*. For example, if the animal travels to the original location where the platform used to be relatively quickly, it may be presumed that the animal's reference memory is intact (Vorhees and Williams 2006). This test is relatively simple, inexpensive, and can provide results in as little as a week. As a result, it is commonly used to study learning and memory deficits in animal disease models including those for schizophrenia (Tian et al. 2019; Ning et al. 2017). There is even a virtual analog of the MWM that has been developed for humans (Fajnerová et al. 2014). The MWM falls into the declarative memory construct within the cognitive systems domain of the RDoC matrix, given the relational representation formed between the allocentric landmark and the location of the platform.

Repeated postnatal maternal separation leads to lasting impacts on rat performance on various tests, but initial learning is intact in the MWM (Xue et al. 2013). Impaired spatial reversal learning ability (e.g., when the platform is located in a new position and the rats are retested to determine how long it takes them to learn the new location of the platform) was observed in the MWM as MS-rats spent more time looking for the platform compared to the control group (Xue et al. 2013). There are ambiguous results regarding the impact of MS on spatial learning. Some studies have shown that MS impaired spatial learning and PPI (Garner et al. 2007; Zhu et al. 2010). Other work shows unaffected spatial learning and long-term memory (Enthoven et al. 2008) or even enhanced reversal learning when the platform was placed in a new quadrant, which indicates improved cognitive flexibility (Mooney-Leber and Brummelte 2020). These variations in results may be due to the frequency and length of time involved in the maternal separation, strain differences, variations in the MWM setup and experimental conditions (i.e., varying trial intervals, length of training or timing of probe trials, etc.) or other factors. Inter-laboratory differences in experimental MS protocols make reproducibility a challenge across these studies. Lastly, MS-related deficits in reversal learning may be explained by a reduction in medial prefrontal cortex BDNF – a protein involved in neurodevelopment, neuroplasticity, learning, and memory (Xue et al. 2013; Récamier-Carballo et al. 2017; Roceri et al. 2004). This finding is important as inadequate BDNF may play a role in the neurodevelopmental impairments and molecular mechanisms seen in people with schizophrenia (Nieto et al. 2013). Furthermore, schizophrenia patients also show impaired reversal learning which is similar with the MWM utilized in the animal models.

The cognitive deficits commonly seen among people with neurodevelopmental disorders, like schizophrenia, can be seen using the MS model in conjunction with tests like the MWM, forced swimming test, and object recognition testing (Table 1). While the MS model provides an inexpensive, simple, and effective way to invoke depressive- and cognitive deficit-like symptoms, it does come with a major drawback. As noted, there is not a singular, well-defined MS model. Most MS models have varied times of separation and varied frequencies, standardization across laboratories may help improve reproducibility of findings.

4.3 Postnatal Drug Challenges

Dopamine Agonist Models (Amphetamines): Animal models using postnatal drug administration have the ability to specifically target certain neurotransmitter systems that are implicated in schizophrenia-like phenotypes. Amphetamine-induced models of schizophrenia have been used for over 50 years, given that amphetamine overdose in humans can result in a stimulant-induced psychosis with a variety of behaviors consistent with schizophrenia (Snyder 1973; Featherstone et al. 2007a, b, Robinson and Becker 1986). Importantly, we need to distinguish between animal models of adult exposure that typically use chronic low doses to mimic drug-induced psychosis (for review, see: Grant et al. 2012; Jones et al. 2011) and models that use early life developmental exposures, often via a single high dose or brief exposures to disturb the maturation of essential monoamine neurotransmitter systems. Though one may argue that the postnatal administration of high doses of amphetamines has low construct validity, the resulting phenotype does indeed resemble many of the pathological and behavioral changes we observe in people with schizophrenia and thus these models have high face validity. Both amphetamine and methamphetamine (METH) are transporter inhibitors and dopamine releasers that cause an excess release of dopamine into the synaptic cleft, with METH being more potent and faster acting compared to amphetamine (Goodwin et al. 2009). Especially during development, the excessive presence of dopamine results in neurotoxicity and the formation of reactive oxygen species, which in turn cause the degeneration of synaptic terminals (Ricaurte et al. 1982; Cadet and Brannock 1998; Kita et al. 2003). In a gerbil model using a single high dose of METH on postnatal day 14 (PN14), dopaminergic innervation seems to decrease in prefrontal cortex areas while increasing in mesolimbic structures like the basolateral amygdala (Brummelte et al. 2008; Grund et al. 2007). This is in line with the "revised dopamine hypothesis" that suggests an imbalance in the dopaminergic systems with hyperactive dopamine transmission in the mesolimbic and reduced dopamine transmission in the prefrontal cortex (PFC) in people with schizophrenia (Brisch et al. 2014). Importantly, postnatal METH exposure in this gerbil model changed several other neurotransmitter systems including serotonin, acetylcholine, GABA, and glutamate (Brummelte et al. 2007; Bagorda et al. 2006; Busche et al. 2006; Lehmann et al. 2003, 2004). For instance, postnatal METH exposure resulted in a shift in

GABAergic innervation in the PFC with a reduction in somatic inhibition of pyramidal cells in layer V, but an increase in dendritic innervations in layers II/III (Brummelte et al. 2007; Nossoll et al. 1997). This pattern resembles reports of reduced GABAergic and parvalbumin-positive synapses on pyramidal cells in the post-mortem brains of people with schizophrenia (Blum and Mann 2002; Jahangir et al. 2021; Nahar et al. 2021; Pierri et al. 1999; Woo et al. 1998). Parvalbumin-positive interneurons are considered an essential RDoC element as they may be important for attention. In line with this, a decrease in parvalbumin-positive innervation and associated desynchronized activity in prefrontal cortices are commonly reported pathologies of schizophrenia, which may underlie issues with attention and related cognitive dysfunction such as working memory deficits (Spencer et al. 2004; Uhlhaas and Singer 2006; Mathalon and Sohal 2015).

In accordance with this, animal models of postnatal METH exposure frequently observe deficits in RDoC-relevant cognitive functions such as impairments in spatial learning and working memory in various mazes such as the elevated plus maze and water mazes (Dawirs et al. 1996; Acevedo et al. 2007; Grace et al. 2010; Hrubá et al. 2010; Skelton et al. 2007; Vorhees et al. 2009), novel location and novel object recognition (Siegel et al. 2011; Acevedo et al. 2007), and reduced sensorimotor gating in a pre-PPI tests (Acevedo et al. 2007). For instance, neonatal METH administration (with doses ranging from 10-25mg/kg, given 4/day) on PN6-15 or PN11–20 produced increased errors in the Cincinnati Water Maze at all doses with the earlier exposure having a stronger impact (i.e., more errors) (Vorhees et al. 2008, 2009). In conjunction with the behavioral similarities observed in cases of schizophrenia and METH-induced psychosis, MRI evidence has demonstrated comparable losses in hippocampal volume between these two groups (Orikabe et al. 2011). Therefore, METH-induced psychosis may function as a human pharmacological model of certain behavioral and physiological features of schizophrenia (Snyder 1973).

The Cincinnati water maze (*CWM;* Fig. 14) is a multiple T-maze that requires animals to use route-based egocentric navigation. Egocentric navigation in the CWM depends on striatal- and dopamine-dependent learning as well as internal cues and movement cues to find and remember the correct pathway. This contrasts with allocentric navigation, the main navigation strategy in the MWM, which depends on distal/spatial cues outside the organism and is thus more hippocampus-dependent (Vorhees and Williams 2016). The procedures for testing animals in the CWM are very similar to those described above for the MWM with some slight modifications. Before being tested in the CWM, rats undergo a pre-maze assessment by performing 4 consecutive trials in a separate straight tube to practice finding the submerged platform. On the test day, rats are placed in the start position in the maze containing room temperature water and are allowed for 5 min to find the platform at the end of the maze. Errors and latencies are recorded on each trial, with 2 trials a day for 5-6 days under normal light conditions or for 15-20 days in dark conditions (infrared light) (Vorhees and Williams 2016). In the CWM, animals do not receive any "help" from the researcher, i.e., they are not placed on the platform if they cannot find it by themselves. Interestingly, opposite sex differences in learning

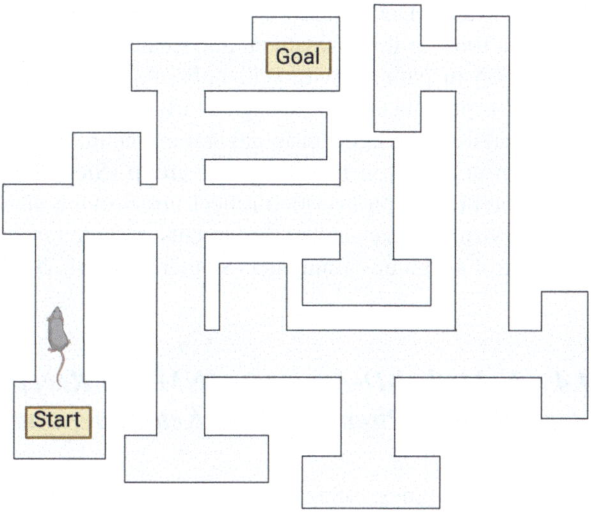

Fig. 14 Cincinnati water maze. The animal is given 5 min to find the goal platform. The amount of time it takes for the animal to find the platform and number of entries made into the incorrect maze arms are recorded for each trial

across the MWM and CWM are observed. Females learn to find the correct pathway faster than males in the CWM, while males learn to find the platform faster than females in the MWM (Vorhees and Williams 2016). This sex difference may reflect a dichotomy in the spatial strategy adopted to learn the tasks. Indeed, spatial learning strategy differs as a result of sex in rodents and gender in humans (Hawley et al. 2012). Together this supports the importance of considering sex and gender differences in task learning and performance which could confound results regarding task performance in the broader context of schizophrenia.

Interestingly, neonatal METH exposure from PN1-10 (i.e., right after birth) did not result in an increase in errors in the CWM (Vorhees et al. 2009), while later METH exposure (i.e., PN6-15 or PN11–20) did cause deficits in long-term path learning and spatial deficits (Vorhees et al. 2009). This difference suggests that the disturbances caused by METH depend on the development of the dopaminergic system and possibly the hippocampus (Siegel et al. 2011), which are slowly maturing during the postnatal period (Brummelte and Teuchert-Noodt 2006; Dawirs et al. 1993; Shin et al. 2019; Tarazi and Baldessarini 2000). Importantly, learning deficits in the CWM after postnatal METH exposure are somewhat preventable with pre-administration of a dopamine D1 receptor antagonist (SCH23390) (Jablonski et al. 2019) or other drugs that preferentially affect dopamine, while drugs that primarily affect serotonin (i.e., MDMA and fenfluramine) did not impact performance in the CWM (Vorhees et al. 2011). This underlines the idea that the dopaminergic system plays a crucial role in METH-induced learning deficits in the CWM. Taken together, the CWM is a complex water maze that tests a different aspect of *learning and memory (egocentric navigation*) than other spatial navigation tests, which may be particularly relevant for the RDoC framework. Egocentric navigation requires some form of self-recognition and perception (i.e., knowing where oneself is in a certain space) and could relate to the social processes and cognitive systems domain of the RDoC framework. In line with this, egocentric navigation has been used as a tool for the assessment and treatment of cognitive deficits related to self-recognition in patients with schizophrenia (Siemerkus et al. 2012). When people with schizophrenia are put through a virtual maze without topographic markings and are required to use egocentric navigation techniques, they had an impaired performance in comparison to the control group (Siemerkus et al. 2012). Furthermore, schizophrenia symptoms often reflect impairments in social interactions and social context; virtual mazes and environments provide researchers with the ability to test and control social environments (Siemerkus et al. 2012).

4.4 N-Methyl-D-Aspartate (NMDA) Receptor Antagonist Models (Phencyclidine, Ketamine, and MK-801)

Like amphetamines, schizophrenia research with *N-methyl-D-aspartate receptor (NMDA-R) antagonists* began from the observation that acute inhibition of the glutamatergic NMDA-R can exacerbate the positive and cognitive symptoms of schizophrenic patients and induce similar symptoms in healthy volunteers (Gilmour et al. 2012; Murray et al. 2013). Likewise, in rodents both NMDA-R antagonists and amphetamines can induce behaviors such as hyperlocomotion and increased stereotypic behavior which may be analogues of positive symptoms of schizophrenia in humans (Nakazawa et al. 2017). NMDA-R antagonists and amphetamines can promote cognitive-related symptoms, such as impaired PPI, working memory, cognitive flexibility, and attention (Mouri et al. 2013). However, NMDA-R antagonists are better able to model negative symptoms, such as social withdrawal, than amphetamines (Neill et al. 2010; Gilmour et al. 2012; Mouri et al. 2013; Lee and Zhou 2019). The capacity of NMDA-R antagonists to model the three main categories of schizophrenia symptoms (i.e., positive, cognitive, and negative) suggests that dysregulation of glutamatergic activity may play a major role in the pathology of schizophrenia (Coyle et al. 2012). Notably, the inhibition of NMDA-Rs in neonates alters dopaminergic, serotonergic, noradrenergic, and GABAergic neurotransmitter systems which are all implicated in schizophrenia (as reviewed by Lim et al. 2012; Lee and Zhou 2019).

In animal models of NMDA-R hypoactivity, subjects are injected with NMDA-R antagonists such as phencyclidine (PCP), ketamine, and MK-801. These compounds are often administered to subjects during the neonatal period (around postnatal days 1–15) to recreate the neurodevelopmental aspects of schizophrenia (Lee and Zhou 2019). Neonatal exposure to NMDA-R antagonists impairs learning and memory, PPI, fear conditioning, and sociability in addition to decreasing parvalbumin-positive neurons and cortical volume while increasing neuronal apoptosis and stereotypic behaviors (Lim et al. 2012; Neill et al. 2010; Plataki et al. 2021; Table 1).

Although neonatal exposure to NMDA-R antagonists is intended to model the neurodevelopment of schizophrenia, Grayson et al. (2016) state that many outcomes from neonatal PCP exposure do not differ greatly from adult PCP exposure. Consistent with this, other NMDA-R antagonists decrease the number of parvalbumin-positive GABAergic neurons in the prefrontal cortex, alter other neurotransmitter systems, and impair learning and memory regardless of neonatal or adult administration (Lee and Zhou 2019; Ghotbi Ravandi et al. 2019; Lim et al. 2012; Neill et al. 2010; Bubenikova-Valesova et al. 2008; Plataki et al. 2021). Grayson et al. (2016) argue that this lack of separation shows that current neonatal NMDA-R antagonist models may not adequately reproduce neurodevelopmental aspects of schizophrenia, but all models have their limitations and the postnatal administration of NMDA-R antagonists such as PCP to rodents can still successfully recreate some of the behavioral abnormalities linked to the underlying pathologies of schizophrenia.

There are other limitations to consider though when evaluating the validity and translational value of neonatal drug exposure models. Postnatal exposures to high levels of stimulants or NMDA-R antagonists are unlikely to happen in humans and thus these models have limited construct validity. However, infants may be exposed to amphetamines or other drugs prenatally through maternal transmission and this can lead to cognitive impairments in visual motor integration executive function, lower school achievements, and changes in cortical and subcortical brain structures related to cognitive function in exposed children (Chang et al. 2009; Lester and Lagasse 2010; Cernerud et al. 1996; Sanjari Moghaddam et al. 2021; Roos et al. 2015). Importantly, there is, to the best of our knowledge, no link to an increased risk for schizophrenia (yet), though there is a lack of longitudinal outcome data on children exposed to METH or amphetamines in utero (Li et al. 2021). However, given the limitations of human research in this area (due to polydrug use, foster care, lack of longitudinal data, etc.), postnatal drug challenge animal models are an important part of continuing schizophrenia research as they can mimic many aspects of schizophrenia symptoms.

5 Combination Models

Animal laboratory researchers can combine multiple early life stress models to make more complex "two" or even "three" or more hit models (Bilbo et al. 2005; Strzelewicz et al. 2019, 2021). In one classic study, rats displayed memory impairments only if they received both a peripheral challenge with *E. coli* on postnatal day 4 and a "second hit" LPS challenge in adulthood (Bilbo et al. 2005). Other models have utilized different combinations of immunogens (e.g., poly (I:C) and LPS administered during the prenatal and postnatal periods, respectively; Li et al. 2018), postnatal methamphetamine challenges with altered rearing conditions (Brummelte et al. 2007; Lehmann et al. 2009; Vorhees et al. 2008), or even integrated prenatal immunogen exposure with peripubertal stress (Monte et al. 2017; Giovanoli et al. 2014). There is mounting epidemiological and animal model-based evidence demonstrating that multiple hits may better predict neuropsychiatric disease risk than a single environmental insult alone (Giovanoli et al. 2013,

Giovanoli et al. 2014; Mahic et al. 2017; Meyer 2019; Estes and McAllister 2016). Ecologically relevant models such as the *limited bedding model*, which mimics low resource environments by providing rodent dams with reduced nesting and bedding material (Gilles et al. 1996; Ivy et al. 2008), have been combined with diet and other early life stress models to study the developmental impacts of increasing burden on mental health outcomes (Strzelewicz et al. 2019, 2021). Multidimensional models allow investigators to examine the simultaneous contribution and interaction of several risk factors implicated in the development and etiology of diseases such as schizophrenia. This approach provides support for the importance of studying these combination two- and multi-hit models in the animal laboratory (Maynard et al. 2001).

6 Translational Approaches: From Bench to Bedside

6.1 Pharmacological Interventions

Researchers use animal models to study cognitive, behavioral, and physiological impairments relevant to brain diseases to identify their underlying mechanisms. In addition to this, researchers can evaluate the safety and efficacy of potential treatments for these impairments. These animal models are called *preclinical models*. If a preclinical model can significantly mimic prominent features of a disease or disorder, it can help inform the development of clinically relevant treatments that can eventually be translated into patient care.

For example, studies make use of the rat MAM model to induce impairments in cognitive function like those seen in people with schizophrenia. Maternally exposed MAM offspring generally show a reduction in volume in various brain regions including the mediodorsal thalamus, hippocampus, prefrontal cortex, occipital cortex, and parahippocampal cortex (Matricon et al. 2010; Moore et al. 2006), see further details above. In addition, they show motor disturbances like dyskinesia, cognitive inflexibility, and sensorimotor gating deficits (Ratajczak et al. 2015; Ciofalo et al. 1971; Moore et al. 2006). This model has provided scientists a way to develop and test treatment methods aimed at stabilizing cortical function and identify biomarkers implicated in the potential preventative treatment of schizophrenia. As a result, researchers can test the efficacy of various types of drugs on MAM-treated rats to see if they alleviate or minimize symptoms induced by MAM. Studies have tested the safety and efficacy of various nootropic drugs (Mar et al. 2017) and mGlu5 positive allosteric modulators (Gastambide et al. 2012), and have found improvements of cognitive impairments related to schizophrenia. Modafinil is one drug that has shown promise in treating ADHD and narcolepsy (Lanni et al. 2008; Outhoff 2016) and it may ameliorate certain cognitive deficits and impulsivity in people with schizophrenia (Ghahremani et al. 2011). Animal models that have tested the efficacy of modafinil have found mixed results. For example, Mar et al. (2017) found modafinil improved attention and executive function in rats exposed to MAM when testing on a touchscreen-based CPT, although modafinil also improved performance in sham-controlled rats. In humans, modafinil improved attention set shifting in healthy individuals (Turner et al. 2004) and one study showed that modafinil did not improve cognition or reduce negative symptoms in people with schizophrenia when compared with a placebo group (Freudenreich et al. 2009). While this drug has not shown much translational promise for schizophrenia treatment, its prevalent use amongst both healthy and patient populations (Teodorini et al. 2020) warrants continued research on its potential as a cognition enhancing pharmaceutical.

Another drug receiving attention for the treatment of cognitive impairments in schizophrenia is choline. Choline significantly improved cognitive flexibility in combination with working memory training (Waddell et al. 2020) and activates on-time development of cerebral inhibition in children received choline perinatally (Ross et al. 2013). Choline is an essential nutrient and plays significant roles in the development of the brain. Choline is used in the biosynthesis of acetylcholine and is a part of phospholipids and lipoproteins (Zeisel and da Costa 2009). Further, choline is an important methyl donor, and therefore important for the maintenance of epigenetic marks (Zeisel 2017), and abnormalities in methyl or one carbon metabolism have been noted in the study of schizophrenia since the 1960s. In fact, choline is so important that it was designated as an essential nutrient by the Institute of Medicine in the late 1990s.

Sensory gating is also altered in individuals with schizophrenia (Atagun et al. 2020) and can be quantified through P50 response in the dual click paradigm. In this task, two clicks are presented in succession, and the difference in brain response (measured by event-related potential) to the second click is compared against the first click (Adler et al. 1982; Jerger et al. 1992). Generally, people with schizophrenia show less inhibition to the second of the paired stimuli when it is presented compared to healthy patients, indicative of poorer sensory gating (Olincy et al. 2010; Freedman et al. 2021). A randomized, placebo-controlled study with 100 pregnant women found that when mothers received twice the daily recommended dose of choline, via phosphatidylcholine administered during the second trimester of pregnancy through to the third postnatal month, the extra choline-treated children were able to suppress the P50 EEG response (76%) more than the control group children (43%; Ross et al. 2013). Furthermore, researchers also found the presence of a single nucleotide polymorphism (SNP) of the *CHRNA7* gene to lower P50 inhibition among the place-group infants (Ross et al. 2013). Other studies that have implicated SNPs of *CHRNA7*, the gene that codes for the alpha-7 subunit of nicotinic acetylcholine receptor in P50 inhibition in patients with schizophrenia (Stephens et al. 2009; Clementz et al. 1997), and choline has been shown to ameliorate sensory gating deficits presumably through its binding to the alpha-7 subunit of nicotinic acetylcholine receptor (Knott et al. 2015; Choueiry et al. 2019). CNRA7 is also regulated by stress, suggesting it may be a point of interaction between several models of schizophrenia (Hunter 2012). Biomarkers, such as the P50 suppression in infants, can help researchers identify successful interventions that help prevent or reduce the onset of various diseases (Ross et al. 2013). Choline supplementation to dams during neurodevelopment in the above-described models could be tested to determine whether it could normalize deficits described.

6.2 *Environmental Enrichment Interventions*

Researchers have also explored the therapeutic potential of complex environments on rodent models for schizophrenia. *Environmental enrichment (EE)* is a laboratory housing condition that provides more opportunity for stimulation in comparison with standard housing cages, due to increased novelty in alternating toys and increased cage space. As a result, EE promotes more species-typical behaviors in rodents (Kentner et al. 2019b). The link between positive environmental experiences in mitigating neurodevelopmental disruptions is actively being investigated in both humans and animals (Núñez Estevez et al. 2020; Kentner et al. 2019b; Schneider and Przewłocki 2005; Schneider et al. 2006; Woo and Leon 2013; Whittingham et al. 2020; Zhao et al. 2021). In animals, such housing environments have shown improvements in social interaction and general cognitive functioning following MIA. These enrichment mediated improvements were generally associated with an upregulation of genes known to be involved in synaptic plasticity (e.g., excitatory amino acid transporters, brain derived neurotrophic factor, and NMDA receptors) and stress (e.g., corticotropin releasing hormone and oxytocin associated receptors). Each of these genes had been downregulated within the hypothalamus, hippocampus, prefrontal cortex, and amygdala in a sex-specific manner following MIA (Núñez Estevez et al. 2020; Zhao et al. 2021; Zhao et al. 2020; Kentner et al. 2016). These findings are relevant as they may underlie the pathogenesis of various neurodevelopmental disorders like schizophrenia and point to clinical interventions that may target these developmentally induced changes in brain. Moreover, there may be *critical periods* during which environmental manipulations may be effective, and interventions such as EE likely need to be administered early in life for best results (Kentner et al. 2019b).

7 Conclusions

The complex etiology of schizophrenia – consisting of environmental and genetic factors – has made it very difficult to find medications and treatments that are effective among all patients. However, the use of animal models has provided a cost-effective, time-sensitive method to test different hypotheses regarding the underlying mechanisms of schizophrenia. This research is done through the identification of changes in brain structure and genes, and targeted testing of pharmaceutical therapies. Unfortunately, therapeutic interventions identified from animal research often have a high likelihood of not being as effective in humans, partly due to the complex heterogeneity associated with many brain disorders. This complexity has given rise to the National Institute of Mental Health's RDoC initiative. By integrating neurodevelopmental, behavioral, genetic, and environmental perspectives, we hope to obtain a deeper more translational perspective of the spectrum of brain function ranging from "healthy functioning" to disease.

We have discussed several behavioral tasks through this chapter used to assay cognition in animal models of schizophrenia with relevance to such RDoC domains (Table 1). While operant procedures requiring the simultaneous use of many behavioral tasks within a single experiment has been the preferred practice over the last several decades, these methods can be disadvantageous. The repeated handling of animals can promote stress and affect task performance (Horner et al. 2013). More recently, touchscreen technology has become valuable in testing cognitive functioning, such as reversal learning in rodents (Horner et al. 2013). With the introduction of this technology, experimenters can evaluate several cognitive measures with limited animal handling (Horner et al. 2013). The development of touchscreens involves showing animals visual stimuli and training them to make correct response by touching the correct location on a screen, using an appetitive reward as motivation (e.g., a food pellet or liquid milkshake). These automated touchscreen models provide a high level of standardization as they enable limited investigator interference as well as high translational potential given the consistent use of visual stimuli (Kangas and Bergman 2017; Horner et al. 2013). Furthermore, touchscreen testing and operant chambers can be used to test multiple domains within the same group of animals.

In the last decade, there has been a drastic increase in the number of neuroimaging and EEG studies investigating patterns of brain function and connectivity that could be utilized as "biomarkers" of schizophrenia. Machine learning has been particularly useful in extrapolating biomarkers identified by a panoply of imaging and EEG studies across diverse samples (Kim et al. 2020; Park et al. 2021). In addition, new evidence has shown some exciting promise, where the physiological mechanisms of certain RDoC domains are conserved from rodents to humans (Cavanagh et al. 2021). The use of animal models is a cost-effective first step in identifying neural circuits of interest, and when used in tandem with MRI or EEG, will provide more clarity regarding the biochemical pathways and mechanisms seen in neurodevelopmental disorders such as schizophrenia, and aid in the development of more translational pharmacological therapies (Young and Markou 2015; Cavanagh et al. 2021).

Furthermore, there needs to be a better accounting for sex differences in schizophrenia. While the incidence of early onset schizophrenia is higher in males, incidence in later life is higher in females (Pedersen et al. 2014; Häfner 2019). Several animal studies have opted to use only male rodents in their studies (Beery and Zucker 2011) due to a common misconception that males provide more robust data. This myth has been completely discredited (Prendergast et al. 2014) and the exclusion of female animals hinders our ability to fully understand these disorders.

While no single animal model can replicate schizophrenia precisely, they each offer unique opportunities to identify the contributors involved in the etiology and symptomology of this complex disease. By employing these models, we can identify causal risk factors and map out detailed brain circuits involved in the disease process. Although treatments for schizophrenia are still being investigated, the RDoC approach may help accelerate this process, especially if the future rendition of this framework adopts sensory processing and developmental perspectives (Hirjak et al. 2021; Harrison et al. 2019; McLaughlin and Gabard-Durnam 2021).

Acknowledgments This project was funded by NIMH under Award Number R15MH114035 (to ACK) and a Summer Undergraduate Research Fellowship (to S.K). The content is solely the responsibility of the authors and does not necessarily represent the official views of any of the financial supporters. Figures were created with BioRender.com.

References

Acevedo SF, De Esch IJ, Raber J (2007) Sex- and histamine-dependent long-term cognitive effects of methamphetamine exposure. Neuropsychopharmacology 32:665–672

Adler LE, Pachtman E, Franks RD, Pecevich M, Waldo MC, Freedman R (1982) Neurophysiological evidence for a defect in neuronal mechanisms involved in sensory gating in schizophrenia. Biol Psychiatry

Al-Harbi AN, Khan KM, Rahman A (2017) Developmental vitamin D deficiency affects spatial learning in Wistar rats. J Nutr 147(9):1795–1805. https://doi.org/10.3945/jn.117.249953

American Psychiatric Association (2013) Diagnostic and statistical manual of mental disorders, 5th edn. https://doi.org/10.1176/appi.books.9780890425596

Antonelli MC, Pallarés ME, Ceccatelli S, Spulber S (2017) Long-term consequences of prenatal l stress and neurotoxicants exposure on neurodevelopment. Prog Neurobiol 155:21–35

Arnold SJ, Ivleva EI, Gopal TA, Reddy AP, Jeon-Slaughter H, Sacco CB et al (2015) Hippocampal volume is reduced in schizophrenia and schizoaffective disorder but not in psychotic bipolar I disorder demonstrated by both manual tracing and automated parcellation. Schizophr Bull 41(1):233–249

Arsenault D, St-Amour I, Cisbani G, Rousseau LS, Cicchetti F (2014) The different effects of LPS and poly I: C prenatal immune challenges on the behavior, development and inflammatory responses in pregnant mice and their offspring. Brain Behav Immun 38:77–90

Atagun MI, Drukker M, Hall MH, Altun IK, Tatli SZ, Guloksuz S et al (2020) Meta-analysis of auditory P50 sensory gating in schizophrenia and bipolar disorder. Psychiatr Res Neuroimaging 300:111078

Aultman JM, Moghaddam B (2001) Distinct contributions of glutamate and dopamine receptors to temporal aspects of rodent working memory using a clinically relevant task. Psychopharmacology (Berl) 153(3):353–364

Bagorda F, Teuchert-Noodt G, Lehmann K (2006) Isolation rearing or methamphetamine traumatisation induce a "dysconnection" of prefrontal efferents in gerbils: implications for schizophrenia. J Neural Transm (Vienna) 113:365–379

Barcelo F, Suwazono S, Knight RT (2000) Prefrontal modulation of visual processing in humans. Nat Neurosci 3(4):399–403

Basta-Kaim A, Szczęsny E, Leśkiewicz M, Głombik K, Ślusarczyk J, Budziszewska B et al (2012) Maternal immune activation leads to age-related behavioral and immunological changes in male rat offspring-the effect of antipsychotic drugs. Pharmacol Rep 64(6):1400–1410. https://doi.org/10.1016/S1734-1140(12)70937-4

Basu A, Ray A (2016) Nicotine dependence and schizophrenia. https://doi.org/10.1016/B978-0-12-800213-1.00025-0

Becker A, Eyles DW, McGrath JJ, Grecksch G (2005) Transient prenatal vitamin D deficiency is associated with subtle alterations in learning and memory functions in adult rats. Behav Brain Res 161(2):306–312. https://doi.org/10.1016/j.bbr.2005.02.015

Beery AK, Zucker I (2011) Sex bias in neuroscience and biomedical research. Neurosci Biobehav Rev 35(3):565–572

Bennouna-Greene M, Bennouna-Greene V, Berna F, Defranoux L (2011) History of abuse and neglect in patients with schizophrenia who have a history of violence. Child Abuse Negl 35(5): 329–332

Bhakta SG, Young JW (2017) The 5 choice continuous performance test (5C-CPT): a novel tool to assess cognitive control across species. J Neurosci Methods 292:53–60. https://doi.org/10.1016/j.jneumeth.2017.07.011

Bikovsky L, Hadar R, Soto-Montenegro ML, Klein J, Weiner I, Desco M, Pascau J, Winter C, Hamani C (2016) Deep brain stimulation improves behavior and modulates neural circuits in a rodent model of schizophrenia. Exp Neurol 113:142–150. https://doi.org/10.1016/j.expneurol.2016.06.012

Bilbo SD, Levkoff LH, Mahoney JH, Watkins LR, Rudy JW, Maier SF (2005) Neonatal infection induces memory impairments following an immune challenge in adulthood. Behav Neurosci 119(1):293–301. https://doi.org/10.1037/0735-7044.119.1.293

Birrell JM, Brown VJ (2000) Medial frontal cortex mediates perceptual attentional set shifting in the rat. J Neurosci 20(11):4320–4324

Bitanihirwe BK, Peleg-Raibstein D, Mouttet F, Feldon J, Meyer U (2010) Late prenatal immune activation in mice leads to behavioral and neurochemical abnormalities relevant to the negative symptoms of schizophrenia. Neuropsychopharmacology 35(12):2462–2478. https://doi.org/10.1038/npp.2010.129

Blum BP, Mann JJ (2002) The GABAergic system in schizophrenia. Int J Neuropsychopharmacol 5:159–179

Bordeleau M, Fernández de Cossío L, Chakravarty MM, Tremblay MÈ (2021) From maternal diet to neurodevelopmental disorders: a story of neuroinflammation. Front Cell Neurosci 14:612705. https://doi.org/10.3389/fncel.2020.612705

Borovcanin MM, Jovanovic I, Radosavljevic G, Pantic J, Minic Janicijevic S, Arsenijevic N, Lukic ML (2017) Interleukin-6 in schizophrenia – is there a therapeutic relevance? Front Psych 8:221. https://doi.org/10.3389/fpsyt.2017.00221

Brady AM (2016) The neonatal ventral hippocampal lesion (NVHL) rodent model of schizophrenia. Curr Protoc Neurosci 77:9.55.1–9.55.17. https://doi.org/10.1002/cpns.15

Brady AM, Saul RD, Wiest MK (2010) Selective deficits in spatial working memory in the neonatal ventral hippocampal lesion rat model of schizophrenia. Neuropharmacology 59(7-8):605–611. https://doi.org/10.1016/j.neuropharm.2010.08.012

Braff DL, Geyer MA, Light GA, Sprock J, Perry W, Cadenhead KS, Swerdlow NR (2001) Impact of prepulse characteristics on the detection of sensorimotor gating deficits in schizophrenia. Schizophr Res 49(1-2):171–178

Brisch R, Saniotis A, Wolf R, Bielau H, Bernstein HG, Steiner J, Bogerts B, Braun K, Jankowski Z, Kumaratilake J, Henneberg M, Gos T (2014) The role of dopamine in schizophrenia from a neurobiological and evolutionary perspective: old fashioned, but still in vogue. Front Psych 5:47

Brito GN, Davis BJ, Stopp LC, Stanton ME (1983) Memory and the septo-hippocampal cholinergic system in the rat. Psychopharmacology (Berl) 81(4):315–320

Bromley-Brits K, Deng Y, Song W (2011) Morris water maze test for learning and memory deficits in Alzheimer's disease model mice. J Vis Exp 53:2920. https://doi.org/10.3791/2920

Brown MF, Giumetti GW (2006) Spatial pattern learning in the radial arm maze. Learn Behav 34(1):102–108. https://doi.org/10.3758/bf03192875

Brown AS, Meyer U (2018) Maternal immune activation and neuropsychiatric illness: a translational research perspective. Am J Psychiatry 175(11):1073–1083. https://doi.org/10.1176/appi.ajp.2018.17121311

Brown AS, Vinogradov S, Kremen WS, Poole JH, Deicken RF, Penner JD, McKeague IW, Kochetkova A, Kern D, Schaefer CA (2009) Prenatal exposure to maternal infection and executive dysfunction in adult schizophrenia. Am J Psychiatry 166(6):683–690. https://doi.org/10.1176/appi.ajp.2008.08010089

Brummelte S, Teuchert-Noodt G (2006) Postnatal development of dopamine innervation in the amygdala and the entorhinal cortex of the gerbil (Meriones unguiculatus). Brain Res 1125:9–16

Brummelte S, Neddens J, Teuchert-Noodt G (2007) Alteration in the GABAergic network of the prefrontal cortex in a potential animal model of psychosis. J Neural Transm (Vienna) 114:539–547. https://doi.org/10.1007/s00702-006-0613-4

Brummelte S, Grund T, Moll GH, Teuchert-Noodt G, Dawirs RR (2008) Environmental enrichment has no effect on the development of dopaminergic and GABAergic fibers during methylphenidate treatment of early traumatized gerbils. J Negat Results Biomed 7:2

Bubenikova-Valesova V, Horacek J, Vrajova M, Hoschl C (2008) Models of schizophrenia in humans and animals based on inhibition of NMDA receptors. Neurosci Biobehav Rev 32:1014–1023

Burne TH, Alexander S, Turner KM, Eyles DW, McGrath JJ (2014) Developmentally vitamin D-deficient rats show enhanced prepulse inhibition after acute Δ9-tetrahydrocannabinol. Behav Pharmacol 25(3):236–244. https://doi.org/10.1097/FBP.0000000000000041

Burton C, Lovic V, Fleming AS (2006) Early adversity alters attention and locomotion in adult Sprague-Dawley rats. Behav Neurosci 120(3):665–675. https://doi.org/10.1037/0735-7044.120.3.665

Busche A, Bagorda A, Lehmann K, Neddens J, Teuchert-Noodt G (2006) The maturation of the acetylcholine system in the dentate gyrus of gerbils (Meriones unguiculatus) is affected by epigenetic factors. J Neural Transm (Vienna) 113:113–124

Cadenhead KS, Swerdlow NR, Shafer KM, Diaz M, Braff DL (2000) Modulation of the startle response and startle laterality in relatives of schizophrenic patients and in subjects with schizotypal personality disorder: evidence of inhibitory deficits. Am J Psychiatry 157(10):1660–1668. https://doi.org/10.1176/appi.ajp.157.10.1660

Cadet JL, Brannock C (1998) Free radicals and the pathobiology of brain dopamine systems. Neurochem Int 32:117–131

Carcone D, Ruocco AC (2017) Six years of research on the national institute of mental health's research domain criteria (RDoC) initiative: a systematic review. Front Cell Neurosci 11:46. https://doi.org/10.3389/fncel.2017.00046. eCollection 2017. PMID: 28316565

Cariaga-Martinez A, Saiz-Ruiz J, Alelú-Paz R (2016) From linkage studies to epigenetics: what we know and what we need to know in the neurobiology of schizophrenia. Front Neurosci 10:202

Carli M, Robbins TW, Evenden JL, Everitt BJ (1983) Effects of lesions to ascending noradrenergic neurones on performance of a 5-choice serial reaction task in rats; implications for theories of dorsal noradrenergic bundle function based on selective attention and arousal. Behav Brain Res 9(3):361–380. https://doi.org/10.1016/0166-4328(83)90138-9

Castagné, V., Porsolt, R. D., and Moser, P. (2009). Use of latency to immobility improves detection of antidepressant-like activity in the behavioral despair test in the mouse. Eur J Pharmacol, 616 (1-3), 128-133.

Cavanagh JF, Gregg D, Light GA, Olguin SL, Sharp RF, Bismark AW, Bhakta SG, Swerdlow NR, Brigman JL, Young JW (2021) Electrophysiological biomarkers of behavioral dimensions from cross-species paradigms. Transl Psychiatry 11(482)

Cernerud L, Eriksson M, Jonsson B, Steneroth G, Zetterström R (1996) Amphetamine addiction during pregnancy: 14-year follow-up of growth and school performance. Acta Paediatr 85:204–208

Cerveri G, Gesi C, Mencacci C (2019) Pharmacological treatment of negative symptoms in schizophrenia: update and proposal of a clinical algorithm. Neuropsychiatr Dis Treat 15: 1525–1535. https://doi.org/10.2147/NDT.S201726

Chalkiadaki K, Velli A, Kyriazidis E, Stavroulaki V, Vouvoutsis V, Chatzaki E, Aivaliotis M, Sidiropoulou K (2019) Development of the MAM model of schizophrenia in mice: sex similarities and differences of hippocampal and prefrontal cortical function. Neuropharmacology 144:193–207. https://doi.org/10.1016/j.neuropharm.2018.10.026

Chambers RA, Sentir AM (2019) Integrated effects of neonatal ventral hippocampal lesions and impoverished social-environmental rearing on endophenotypes of mental illness and addiction vulnerability. Dev Neurosci 41(5–6):263–273

Chang L, Cloak C, Jiang CS, Farnham S, Tokeshi B, Buchthal S, Hedemark B, Smith LM, Ernst T (2009) Altered neurometabolites and motor integration in children exposed to methamphetamine in utero. Neuroimage 48:391–397

Choueiry J, Blais CM, Shah D, Smith D, Fisher D, Labelle A, Knott V (2019) Combining CDP-choline and galantamine, an optimized α7 nicotinic strategy, to ameliorate sensory gating to speech stimuli in schizophrenia. Int J Psychophysiol 145:70–82

Chow KH, Yan Z, Wu WL (2016) Induction of maternal immune activation in mice at mid-gestation stage with viral mimic poly(I:C). J Vis Exp 109:e53643. https://doi.org/10.3791/53643

Ciofalo VB, Latranyi M, Taber RI (1971) Effect of prenatal treatment of methylazoxymethanol acetate on motor performance, exploratory activity, and maze learning in rats. Commun Behav Biol 6(3–4, Pt. A):223–226

Clementz BA, Geyer MA, Braff DL (1997) P50 suppression among schizophrenia and normal comparison subjects: a methodological analysis. Biol Psychiatry 41(10):1035–1044

Connors EJ, Shaik AN, Migliore MM, Kentner AC (2014) Environmental enrichment mitigates the sex-specific effects of gestational inflammation on social engagement and the hypothalamic pituitary adrenal axis-feedback system. Brain Behav Immun 42:178–190. https://doi.org/10.1016/j.bbi.2014.06.020

Cope ZA, Powell SB, Young JW (2016) Modeling neurodevelopmental cognitive deficits in tasks with cross-species translational validity. Genes Brain Behav 15(1):27–44. https://doi.org/10.1111/gbb.12268

Couch AC, Berger T, Hanger B, Matuleviciute R, Srivastava DP, Thuret S, Vernon AC (2021) Maternal immune activation primes deficiencies in adult hippocampal neurogenesis. Brain Behav Immun

Coyle JT, Basu A, Benneyworth M, Balu D, Konopaske G (2012) Glutamatergic synaptic dysregulation in schizophrenia: therapeutic implications. Handb Exp Pharmacol:267–295

Csatlosova K, Bogi E, Durisova B, Grinchii D, Paliokha R, Moravcikova L et al (2021) Maternal immune activation in rats attenuates the excitability of monoamine-secreting neurons in adult offspring in a sex-specific way. Eur Neuropsychopharmacol 43:82–91. https://doi.org/10.1016/j.euroneuro.2020.12.002

Cui X, Gooch H, Groves NJ, Sah P, Burne TH, Eyles DW, McGrath JJ (2015) Vitamin D and the brain: key questions for future research. J Steroid Biochem Mol Biol 148:305–309. https://doi.org/10.1016/j.jsbmb.2014.11.004

Cui X, McGrath JJ, Burne TH, Eyles D (2021) Vitamin D and schizophrenia: 20 years on. Mol Psychiatry 1–13. https://doi.org/10.1038/s41380-021-01025-0

Curtis EM, Moon RJ, Dennison EM, Harvey NC (2014) Prenatal calcium and vitamin D intake, and bone mass in later life. Curr Osteoporos Rep 12(2):194–204. https://doi.org/10.1007/s11914-014-0210-7

Cuthbert BN, Insel TR (2013) Toward the future of psychiatric diagnosis: the seven pillars of RDoC. BMC Med 11(1):1–8

Cuthbert BN, Morris SE (2021) Evolving concepts of the schizophrenia spectrum: a research domain criteria perspective. Front Psych 12:641319. https://doi.org/10.3389/fpsyt.2021.641319

Dawirs RR, Teuchert-Noodt G, Czaniera R (1993) Maturation of the dopamine innervation during postnatal development of the prefrontal cortex in gerbils (Meriones unguiculatus). A quantitative immunocytochemical study. J Hirnforsch 34:281–290

Dawirs RR, Teuchert-Noodt G, Czaniera R (1996) Ontogeny of PFC-related behaviours is sensitive to a single non invasive dose of methamphetamine in neonatal gerbils (Meriones unguiculatus). J Neural Transm (Vienna) 103:1235–1245

Del Re EC, Konishi J, Bouix S, Blokland GA, Mesholam-Gately RI, Goldstein J, Kubicki M, Wojcik J, Pasternak O, Seidman LJ, Petryshen T, Hirayasu Y, Niznikiewicz M, Shenton ME, McCarley RW (2016) Enlarged lateral ventricles inversely correlate with reduced corpus callosum central volume in first episode schizophrenia: association with functional measures. Brain Imaging Behav 10(4):1264–1273. https://doi.org/10.1007/s11682-015-9493-2

Denninger JK, Smith BM, Kirby ED (2018) Novel object recognition and object location behavioral testing in mice on a budget. J Vis Exp (141)

Di Fausto V, Fiore M, Aloe L (2007) Exposure in fetus of methylazoxymethanol in the rat Alters brain neurotrophins' levels and brain cells' proliferation. Neurotoxicol Teratol 29(2):273–281

Disease and Injury Incidence and Prevalence Collaborators (2016) Global, regional, and national incidence, prevalence, and years lived with disability for 310 diseases and injuries, 1990–2015: a systematic analysis for the global burden of disease study 2015. Lancet 388(10053):1545–1602. https://doi.org/10.1016/S0140-6736(16)31678-6

Ellenbroek BA, Riva MA (2003) Early maternal deprivation as an animal model for schizophrenia. Clin Neurosci Res 3(4-5):297–302

Enthoven L, de Kloet ER, Oitzl MS (2008) Effects of maternal deprivation of CD1 mice on performance in the water maze and swim stress. Behav Brain Res 187(1):195–199. https://doi.org/10.1016/j.bbr.2007.08.037

Ershova ES, Jestkova EM, Chestkov IV, Porokhovnik LN, Izevskaya VL, Kutsev SI et al (2017) Quantification of cell-free DNA in blood plasma and DNA damage degree in lymphocytes to evaluate dysregulation of apoptosis in schizophrenia patients. J Psychiatr Res 87:15–22

Estes ML, McAllister AK (2016) Maternal immune activation: implications for neuropsychiatric disorders. Science 353(6301):772–777. https://doi.org/10.1126/science.aag3194

Everett J, Lavoie K, Gagnon JF, Gosselin N (2001) Performance of patients with schizophrenia on the Wisconsin Card Sorting Test (WCST). J Psychiatry Neurosci 26(2):123–130

Eyles D, Brown J, Mackay-Sim A, McGrath J, Feron F (2003) Vitamin D3 and brain development. Neuroscience 118(3):641–653. https://doi.org/10.1016/s0306-4522(03)00040-x

Fachim HA, Corsi-Zuelli F, Loureiro CM, Iamjan SA, Shuhama R, Joca S et al (2021) Early-life stress effects on BDNF DNA methylation in first-episode psychosis and in rats reared in isolation. Prog Neuro-Psychopharmacol Biol Psychiatr 108:110188

Fajnerová I, Rodriguez M, Levčík D, Konrádová L, Mikoláš P, Brom C, Stuchlík A, Vlček K, Horáček J (2014) A virtual reality task based on animal research – spatial learning and memory in patients after the first episode of schizophrenia. Frontiers in Behavioral Neuroscience 8:157. https://doi.org/10.3389/fnbeh.2014.00157

Featherstone RE, Kapur S, Fletcher PJ (2007a) The amphetamine-induced sensitized state as a model of schizophrenia. Prog Neuropsychopharmacol Biol Psychiatry 31:1556–1571

Featherstone R, Rizos Z, Nobrega J, Kapur S, Fletcher P (2007b) Gestational methylazoxymethanol acetate treatment impairs select cognitive functions: parallels to schizophrenia. Neuropsychopharmacology 32:483–492. https://doi.org/10.1038/sj.npp.1301223

Fillman SG, Cloonan N, Catts VS, Miller LC, Wong J, McCrossin T, Cairns M, Weickert CS (2013) Increased inflammatory markers identified in the dorsolateral prefrontal cortex of individuals with schizophrenia. Mol Psychiatry 18(2):206–214. https://doi.org/10.1038/mp.2012.110

Flagstad P, Mørk A, Glenthøj BY, van Beek J, Michael-Titus AT, Didriksen M (2004) Disruption of neurogenesis on gestational day 17 in the rat causes behavioral changes relevant to positive and negative schizophrenia symptoms and alters amphetamine-induced dopamine release in nucleus accumbens. Neuropsychopharmacology 29(11):2052–2064. https://doi.org/10.1038/sj.npp.1300516

Franklin JC, Jamieson JP, Glenn CR, Nock MK (2015) How developmental psychopathology theory and research can inform the research domain criteria (RDoC) project. J Clin Child Adolesc Psychol 44(2):280–290

Freedman R, Hunter SK, Law AJ, Clark AM, Roberts A, Hoffman MC (2021) Choline, folic acid, vitamin D, and fetal brain development in the psychosis spectrum. Schizophr Res., S0920-9964 (21)00128-6. Advance online publication. https://doi.org/10.1016/j.schres.2021.03.008

Freudenreich O, Henderson DC, Macklin EA, Evins AE, Fan X, Cather C, Walsh JP, Goff DC (2009) Modafinil for clozapine-treated schizophrenia patients: a double-blind, placebo-controlled pilot trial. J Clin Psychiatry 70(12):1674–1680. https://doi.org/10.4088/JCP.08m04683

Garner B, Wood SJ, Pantelis C, van den Buuse M (2007) Early maternal deprivation reduces prepulse inhibition and impairs spatial learning ability in adulthood: no further effect of post-pubertal chronic corticosterone treatment. Behav Brain Res 176(2):323–332. https://doi.org/10.1016/j.bbr.2006.10.020

Gaser C, Nenadic I, Volz HP, Büchel C, Sauer H (2004) Neuroanatomy of 'hearing voices': a frontotemporal brain structural abnormality associated with auditory hallucinations in schizophrenia. Cereb Cortex 14(1):91–96

Gastambide F, Cotel MC, Gilmour G, O'Neill MJ, Robbins TW, Tricklebank MD (2012) Selective remediation of reversal learning deficits in the neurodevelopmental MAM model of schizophrenia by a novel mGlu5 positive allosteric modulator. Neuropsychopharmacology 37(4): 1057–1066. https://doi.org/10.1038/npp.2011.298

Ghahremani DG, Tabibnia G, Monterosso J, Hellemann G, Poldrack RA, London ED (2011) Effect of modafinil on learning and task-related brain activity in methamphetamine-dependent and healthy individuals. Neuropsychopharmacology 36(5):950–959. https://doi.org/10.1038/npp.2010.233

Ghotbi Ravandi S, Shabani M, Bashiri H, Saeedi Goraghani M, Khodamoradi M, Nozari M (2019) Ameliorating effects of berberine on MK-801-induced cognitive and motor impairments in a neonatal rat model of schizophrenia. Neurosci Lett 706:151–157

Gilles EE, Schultz L, Baram TZ (1996) Abnormal corticosterone regulation in an immature rat model of continuous chronic stress. Pediatr Neurol 15(2):114–119. https://doi.org/10.1016/0887-8994(96)00153-1

Gilmour G, Dix S, Fellini L, Gastambide F, Plath N, Steckler T, Talpos J, Tricklebank M (2012) NMDA receptors, cognition and schizophrenia – testing the validity of the NMDA receptor hypofunction hypothesis. Neuropharmacology 62:1401–1412

Giovanoli S, Engler H, Engler A, Richetto J, Voget M, Willi R et al (2013) Stress in puberty unmasks latent neuropathological consequences of prenatal immune activation in mice. Science 339(6123):1095–1099

Giovanoli S, Weber L, Meyer U (2014) Single and combined effects of prenatal immune activation and peripubertal stress on parvalbumin and reelin expression in the hippocampal formation. Brain Behav Immun 40:48–54. https://doi.org/10.1016/j.bbi.2014.04.005

Gogtay N, Vyas NS, Testa R, Wood SJ, Pantelis C (2011) Age of onset of schizophrenia: perspectives from structural neuroimaging studies. Schizophr Bull 37(3):504–513. https://doi.org/10.1093/schbul/sbr030

Goodwin JS, Larson GA, Swant J, Sen N, Javitch JA, Zahniser NR, De Felice LJ, Khoshbouei H (2009) Amphetamine and methamphetamine differentially affect dopamine transporters in vitro and in vivo. J Biol Chem 284:2978–2989

Gourevitch R, Rocher C, Le Pen G, Krebs MO, Jay TM (2004) Working memory deficits in adult rats after prenatal disruption of neurogenesis. Behav Pharmacol 15(4):287–292. https://doi.org/10.1097/01.fbp.0000135703.48799.71

Grace CE, Schaefer TL, Graham DL, Skelton MR, Williams MT, Vorhees CV (2010) Effects of inhibiting neonatal methamphetamine-induced corticosterone release in rats by adrenal autotransplantation on later learning, memory, and plasma corticosterone levels. Int J Dev Neurosci 28:331–342

Grant KM, Levan TD, Wells SM, Li M, Stoltenberg SF, Gendelman HE, Carlo G, Bevins RA (2012) Methamphetamine-associated psychosis. J Neuroimmune Pharmacol 7:113–139

Grayson B, Barnes SA, Markou A, Piercy C, Podda G, Neill JC (2016) Postnatal phencyclidine (PCP) as a neurodevelopmental animal model of schizophrenia pathophysiology and symptomatology: a review. Curr Top Behav Neurosci 29:403–428

Grund T, Teuchert-Noodt G, Busche A, Neddens J, Brummelte S, Moll GH, Dawirs RR (2007) Administration of oral methylphenidate during adolescence prevents suppressive development of dopamine projections into prefrontal cortex and amygdala after an early pharmacological challenge in gerbils. Brain Res 1176:124–132

Haddad FL, Patel SV, Schmid S (2020) Maternal immune activation by Poly I: C as a preclinical model for neurodevelopmental disorders: a focus on autism and schizophrenia. Neurosci Biobehav Rev 113:546–567

Häfner H (2019) From onset and prodromal stage to a life-long course of schizophrenia and its symptom dimensions: how sex, age, and other risk factors influence incidence and course of illness. Psychiatry J 2019

Haijma SV, Van Haren N, Cahn W, Koolschijn PC, Hulshoff Pol HE, Kahn RS (2013) Brain volumes in schizophrenia: a meta-analysis in over 18 000 subjects. Schizophr Bull 39(5): 1129–1138. https://doi.org/10.1093/schbul/sbs118

Harms LR, Cowin G, Eyles DW, Kurniawan ND, McGrath JJ, Burne TH (2012a) Neuroanatomy and psychomimetic-induced locomotion in C57BL/6J and 129/X1SvJ mice exposed to developmental vitamin D deficiency. Behav Brain Res 230(1):125–131. https://doi.org/10.1016/j.bbr.2012.02.007

Harms LR, Turner KM, Eyles DW, Young JW, McGrath JJ, Burne TH (2012b) Attentional processing in C57BL/6J mice exposed to developmental vitamin D deficiency. PLoS One 7(4):e35896. https://doi.org/10.1371/journal.pone.0035896

Harrison LA, Kats A, Williams ME, Aziz-Zadeh L (2019) The importance of sensory processing in mental health: a proposed addition to the research domain criteria (RDoC) and suggestions for RDoC 2.0. Front Psychol 10:103

Hawley WR, Grissom EM, Barratt HE, Conrad TS, Dohanich GP (2012) The effects of biological sex and gonadal hormones on learning strategy in adult rats. Physiol Behav 105(4):1014–1020. https://doi.org/10.1016/j.physbeh.2011.11.021

Hazane F, Krebs MO, Jay TM, Le Pen G (2009) Behavioral perturbations after prenatal neurogenesis disturbance in female rat. Neurotox Res 15(4):311–320. https://doi.org/10.1007/s12640-009-9035-z

Hedberg M, Imbeault S, Erhardt S, Schwieler L (2021) Disrupted sensorimotor gating in first-episode psychosis patients is not affected by short-term antipsychotic treatment. Schizophr Res 228:118–123. https://doi.org/10.1016/j.schres.2020.12.009

Heisler JM, Morales J, Donegan JJ, Jett JD, Redus L, O'Connor JC (2015) The attentional set shifting task: a measure of cognitive flexibility in mice. J Vis Exp 96:51944. https://doi.org/10.3791/51944

Hirjak D, Meyer-Lindenberg A, Sambataro F, Fritze S, Kukovic J, Kubera KM, Wolf RC (2021) Progress in sensorimotor neuroscience of schizophrenia spectrum disorders: lessons learned and future directions. Prog Neuropsychopharmacol Biol Psychiatry 111:110370. https://doi.org/10.1016/j.pnpbp.2021.110370

Horner AE, Heath CJ, Hvoslef-Eide M, Kent BA, Kim CH, Nilsson SR, Alsiö J, Oomen CA, Holmes A, Saksida LM, Bussey TJ (2013) The touchscreen operant platform for testing learning and memory in rats and mice. Nat Protoc 8(10):1961–1984. https://doi.org/10.1038/nprot.2013.122

Howes O, McCutcheon R, Stone J (2015) Glutamate and dopamine in schizophrenia: an update for the 21st century. J Psychopharmacol 29(2):97–115. https://doi.org/10.1177/0269881114563634

Hrubá L, Schutová B, Pometlová M, Rokyta R, Slamberová R (2010) Effect of methamphetamine exposure and cross-fostering on cognitive function in adult male rats. Behav Brain Res 208:63–71

Hunter RG (2012) Stress and the α7 nicotinic acytlcholine receptor. Curr Drug Targets 13:607–612. https://doi.org/10.2174/138945012800398982

Hyppönen E, Läärä E, Reunanen A, Järvelin MR, Virtanen SM (2001) Intake of vitamin D and risk of type 1 diabetes: a birth-cohort study. Lancet (London, England) 358(9292):1500–1503. https://doi.org/10.1016/S0140-6736(01)06580-1

Ivy AS, Brunson KL, Sandman C, Baram TZ (2008) Dysfunctional nurturing behavior in rat dams with limited access to nesting material: a clinically relevant model for early-life stress. Neuroscience 154(3):1132–1142. https://doi.org/10.1016/j.neuroscience.2008.04.019

Jablonski SA, Williams MT, Vorhees CV (2019) Learning and memory effects of neonatal methamphetamine exposure in Sprague-Dawley rats: test of the role of dopamine receptors D1 in mediating the long-term effects. Dev Neurosci 41:44–55

Jahangir M, Zhou JS, Lang B, Wang XP (2021) GABAergic system dysfunction and challenges in schizophrenia research. Front Cell Dev Biol 9:663854

Jerger K, Biggins C, Fein G (1992) P50 suppression is not affected by attentional manipulations. Biol Psychiatry 31(4):365–377

Jones CA, Watson DJ, Fone KC (2011) Animal models of schizophrenia. Br J Pharmacol 164: 1162–1194

Kalinichev M, Easterling KW, Plotsky PM, Holtzman SG (2002) Long-lasting changes in stress-induced corticosterone response and anxiety-like behaviors as a consequence of neonatal maternal separation in Long-Evans rats. Pharmacol Biochem Behav 73(1):131–140. https://doi.org/10.1016/s0091-3057(02)00781-5

Kangas BD, Bergman J (2017) Touchscreen technology in the study of cognition-related behavior. Behav Pharmacol 28(8):623

Kapadia M, Desai M, Parikh R (2020) Fractures in the framework: limitations of classification systems in psychiatry. Dialogues Clin Neurosci 22(1):17

Kentner AC, Khoury A, Lima Queiroz E, MacRae M (2016) Environmental enrichment rescues the effects of early life inflammation on markers of synaptic transmission and plasticity. Brain Behav Immun 57:151–160. https://doi.org/10.1016/j.bbi.2016.03.013

Kentner AC, Bilbo SD, Brown AS, Hsiao EY, McAllister AK, Meyer U, Pearce BD, Pletnikov MV, Yolken RH, Bauman MD (2019a) Maternal immune activation: reporting guidelines to improve the rigor, reproducibility, and transparency of the model. Neuropsychopharmacology 44(2): 245–258. https://doi.org/10.1038/s41386-018-0185-7

Kentner AC, Cryan JF, Brummelte S (2019b) Resilience priming: translational models for understanding resiliency and adaptation to early life adversity. Dev Psychobiol 61(3):350–375. https://doi.org/10.1002/dev.21775

Kesby JP, Burne TH, McGrath JJ, Eyles DW (2006) Developmental vitamin D deficiency alters MK 801-induced hyperlocomotion in the adult rat: An animal model of schizophrenia. Biol Psychiatry 60(6):591–596. https://doi.org/10.1016/j.biopsych.2006.02.033

Kesby JP, Cui X, O'Loan J, McGrath JJ, Burne TH, Eyles DW (2010) Developmental vitamin D deficiency alters dopamine-mediated behaviors and dopamine transporter function in adult female rats. Psychopharmacology (Berl) 208(1):159–168. https://doi.org/10.1007/s00213-009-1717-y

Kesby JP, Turner KM, Alexander S, Eyles DW, McGrath JJ, Burne TH (2017) Developmental vitamin D deficiency alters multiple neurotransmitter systems in the neonatal rat brain. Int J Dev Neurosci 62:1–7

Khashan AS, Abel KM, McNamee R, Pedersen MG, Webb RT, Baker PN, Kenny LC, Mortensen PB (2008) Higher risk of offspring schizophrenia following antenatal maternal exposure to severe adverse life events. Arch Gen Psychiatry 65(2):146–152. https://doi.org/10.1001/archgenpsychiatry.2007.20

Kim SM, Frank LM (2009) Hippocampal lesions impair rapid learning of a continuous spatial alternation task. PLoS One 4(5):e5494

Kim HK, Blumberger DM, Dasakalis ZJ (2020) Neurophysiological biomarkers in schizophrenia-P50, mismatch negativitym and TMS-EMG and TMS-EEG. Front Psych 11(795)

Kinnunen AK, Koenig JI, Bilbe G (2003) Repeated variable prenatal stress alters pre- and postsynaptic gene expression in the rat frontal pole. J Neurochem 86(3):736–748. https://doi.org/10.1046/j.1471-4159.2003.01873.x

Kirby ED, Jensen K, Goosens KA, Kaufer D (2012) Stereotaxic surgery for excitotoxic lesion of specific brain areas in the adult rat. J Vis Exp 65:e4079. https://doi.org/10.3791/4079

Kita T, Wagner GC, Nakashima T (2003) Current research on methamphetamine-induced neurotoxicity: animal models of monoamine disruption. J Pharmacol Sci 92:178–195

Knott V, de la Salle S, Choueiry J, Impey D, Smith D, Smith M et al (2015) Neurocognitive effects of acute choline supplementation in low, medium and high performer healthy volunteers. Pharmacol Biochem Behav 131:119–129

Knuesel I, Chicha L, Britschgi M, Schobel SA, Bodmer M, Hellings JA, Toovey S, Prinssen EP (2014) Maternal immune activation and abnormal brain development across CNS disorders. Nat Rev Neurol 10(11):643–660. https://doi.org/10.1038/nrneurol.2014.187

Koenig JI, Elmer GI, Shepard PD, Lee PR, Mayo C, Joy B, Hercher E, Brady DL (2005) Prenatal exposure to a repeated variable stress paradigm elicits behavioral and neuroendocrinological changes in the adult offspring: potential relevance to schizophrenia. Behav Brain Res 156(2): 251–261. https://doi.org/10.1016/j.bbr.2004.05.030

Konrath L, Beckius D, Tran US (2016) Season of birth and population schizotypy: results from a large sample of the adult general population. Psychiatry Res 242:245–250. https://doi.org/10.1016/j.psychres.2016.05.059

Kraan T, Velthorst E, Smit F, de Haan L, van der Gaag M (2015) Trauma and recent life events in individuals at ultra high risk for psychosis: review and meta-analysis. Schizophr Res 161(2-3): 143–149

Kumari V, Sharma T (2002) Effects of typical and atypical antipsychotics on prepulse inhibition in schizophrenia: a critical evaluation of current evidence and directions for future research. Psychopharmacology (Berl) 162(2):97–101. https://doi.org/10.1007/s00213-002-1099-x

Lanni C, Lenzken SC, Pascale A, Del Vecchio I, Racchi M, Pistoia F, Govoni S (2008) Cognition enhancers between treating and doping the mind. Pharmacol Res 57(3):196–213

Laplante DP, Brunet A, Schmitz N, Ciampi A, King S (2008) Project Ice Storm: prenatal maternal stress affects cognitive and linguistic functioning in 5 1/2-year-old children. J Am Acad Child Adolesc Psychiatry 47(9):1063–1072. https://doi.org/10.1097/CHI.0b013e31817eec80

Lavin A, Moore HM, Grace AA (2005) Prenatal disruption of neocortical development alters prefrontal cortical neuron responses to dopamine in adult rats. Neuropsychopharmacology 30(8):1426–1435. https://doi.org/10.1038/sj.npp.1300696

LeDoux J (2003) The emotional brain, fear, and the amygdala. Cell Mol Neurobiol 23(4–5): 727–738. https://doi.org/10.1023/a:1025048802629

Lee G, Zhou Y (2019) NMDAR hypofunction animal models of schizophrenia. Front Mol Neurosci 12:185

Leggio GM, Torrisi SA, Papaleo F (2020) The discrete paired-trial variable-delay T-maze task to assess working memory in mice. Bio-protocol 10(13):e3664

Lehmann K, Lesting J, Polascheck D, Teuchert-Noodt G (2003) Serotonin fibre densities in subcortical areas: differential effects of isolated rearing and methamphetamine. Brain Res Dev Brain Res 147:143–152

Lehmann K, Hundsdorfer B, Hartmann T, Teuchert-Noodt G (2004) The acetylcholine fiber density of the neocortex is altered by isolated rearing and early methamphetamine intoxication in rodents. Exp Neurol 189:131–140

Lehmann K, Garea Rodriguez E, Kratz O, Moll GH, Daeirs RR, Teuchert-Noodt G (2009) Early preweaning methamphetamine and postweaning rearing conditions interfere with the development of peripheral stress parameters and neural growth factors in gerbils. Int J Neurosci 117: 1621–1638. https://doi.org/10.1080/00207450600934937

Lemaire V, Koehl M, Le Moal M, Abrous DN (2000) Prenatal stress produces learning deficits associated with an inhibition of neurogenesis in the hippocampus. Proc Natl Acad Sci U S A 97(20):11032–11037. https://doi.org/10.1073/pnas.97.20.11032

Leng A, Jongen-Rêlo AL, Pothuizen HH, Feldon J (2005) Effects of prenatal methylazoxymethanol acetate (MAM) treatment in rats on water maze performance. Behav Brain Res 161(2):291–298. https://doi.org/10.1016/j.bbr.2005.02.016

Leonard JA (1959) Medical Research Council, Applied psychology unit reports. In: Five-choice serial reaction apparatus. Cambridge. Vol. Report 326

Lester BM, Lagasse LL (2010) Children of addicted women. J Addict Dis 29:259–276

Li Q, Cheung C, Wei R, Hui ES, Feldon J, Meyer U, Chung S, Chua SE, Sham PC, Wu EX, McAlonan GM (2009) Prenatal immune challenge is an environmental risk factor for brain and behavior change relevant to schizophrenia: evidence from MRI in a mouse model. PLoS One 4: e6354. https://doi.org/10.1371/journal.pone.0006354

Li R, Ma X, Wang G, Yang J, Wang C (2016) Why sex differences in schizophrenia? Transl Neurosci (Beijing) 2016. PMID: 29152382

Li Y, Missig G, Finger BC, Landino SM, Alexander AJ, Mokler EL, Robbins JO, Manasian Y, Kim W, Kim KS, McDougle CJ, Carlezon WA Jr, Bolshakov VY (2018) Maternal and early postnatal immune activation produce dissociable effects on neurotransmission in mPFC-Amygdala circuits. J Neurosci 38(13):3358–3372. https://doi.org/10.1523/JNEUROSCI.3642-17.2018

Li J-H, Liu J-L, Zhang K-K, Chen L-J, Xu J-T, Xie X-L (2021) The adverse effects of prenatal METH exposure on the offspring: a review. Front Pharmacol 12

Lim AL, Taylor DA, Malone DT (2012) Consequences of early life MK-801 administration: long-term behavioural effects and relevance to schizophrenia research. Behav Brain Res 227:276–286

Lipska BK, Weinberger DR (2000) To model a psychiatric disorder in animals: schizophrenia as a reality test. Neuropsychopharmacology 23(3):223–239. https://doi.org/10.1016/S0893-133X(00)00137-8

Lipska BK, Aultman JM, Verma A, Weinberger DR, Moghaddam B (2002) Neonatal damage of the ventral hippocampus impairs working memory in the rat. Neuropsychopharmacology 27(1): 47–54. https://doi.org/10.1016/S0893-133X(02)00282-8

Liu NQ, Kaplan AT, Lagishetty V, Ouyang YB, Ouyang Y, Simmons CF, Equils O, Hewison M (2011) Vitamin D and the regulation of placental inflammation. J Immunol 186(10):5968–5974. https://doi.org/10.4049/jimmunol.1003332

Liu F, Guo X, Wu R, Ou J, Zheng Y, Zhang B, Xie L, Zhang L, Yang L, Yang S, Yang J, Ruan Y, Zeng Y, Xu X, Zhao J (2014) Minocycline supplementation for treatment of negative symptoms in early-phase schizophrenia: a double blind, randomized, controlled trial. Schizophr Res 153(1-3):169–176. https://doi.org/10.1016/j.schres.2014.01.011

Liu J, Wu R, Johnson B, Vu J, Bass C, Li JX (2019) The claustrum-prefrontal cortex pathway regulates impulsive-like behavior. J Neurosci 39(50):10071–10080

Lubow RE (2005) Construct validity of the animal latent inhibition model of selective attention deficits in schizophrenia. Schizophr Bull 31(1):139–153

Lubow RE, Moore AU (1959) Latent inhibition: the effect of nonreinforced pre-exposure to the conditional stimulus. J Comp Physiol Psychol 52(4):415

Mahic M, Mjaaland S, Bøvelstad HM, Gunnes N, Susser E, Bresnahan M et al (2017) Maternal immunoreactivity to herpes simplex virus 2 and risk of autism spectrum disorder in male offspring. MSphere 2(1):e00016–e00017

Malaspina D, Corcoran C, Kleinhaus KR, Perrin MC, Fennig S, Nahon D, Friedlander Y, Harlap S (2008) Acute maternal stress in pregnancy and schizophrenia in offspring: a cohort prospective study. BMC Psychiatry 8:71. https://doi.org/10.1186/1471-244X-8-71

Mar AC, Nilsson S, Gamallo-Lana B, Lei M, Dourado T, Alsiö J, Saksida LM, Bussey TJ, Robbins TW (2017) MAM-E17 rat model impairments on a novel continuous performance task: effects of potential cognitive enhancing drugs. Psychopharmacology (Berl) 234(19):2837–2857. https://doi.org/10.1007/s00213-017-4679-5

Markham JA, Taylor AR, Taylor SB, Bell DB, Koenig JI (2010) Characterization of the cognitive impairments induced by prenatal exposure to stress in the rat. Frontiers in Behavioral Neuroscience 4:173. https://doi.org/10.3389/fnbeh.2010.00173

Maruki K, Izaki Y, Hori K, Nomura M, Yamauchi T (2001) Effects of rat ventral and dorsal hippocampus temporal inactivation on delayed alternation task. Brain Res 895(1-2):273–276. https://doi.org/10.1016/s0006-8993(01)02084-4

Mathalon DH, Sohal VS (2015) Neural Oscillations and Synchrony in Brain Dysfunction and Neuropsychiatric Disorders: It's About Time. JAMA Psychiat 72:840–844

Matheson SL, Shepherd AM, Pinchbeck RM, Laurens KR, Carr VJ (2013) Childhood adversity in schizophrenia: a systematic meta-analysis. Psychol Med 43(2):225–238

Matricon J, Bellon A, Frieling H, Kebir O, Le Pen G, Beuvon F et al (2010) Neuropathological and Reelin deficiencies in the hippocampal formation of rats exposed to MAM: differences and similarities with schizophrenia. PLoS One 5(4):e10291

Maynard TM, Sikich L, Lieberman JA, LaMantia AS (2001) Neural development, cell-cell signaling, and the “two-hit” hypothesis of schizophrenia. Schizophr Bull 27(3):457–476. https://doi.org/10.1093/oxfordjournals.schbul.a006887

McGrath JJ, Burne TH, Féron F, Mackay-Sim A, Eyles DW (2010) Developmental vitamin D deficiency and risk of schizophrenia: a 10-year update. Schizophr Bull 36(6):1073–1078. https://doi.org/10.1093/schbul/sbq101

McGrath J, Brown A, St Clair D (2011) Prevention and schizophrenia – the role of dietary factors. Schizophr Bull 37(2):272–283. https://doi.org/10.1093/schbul/sbq121

McKenna BS, Young JW, Dawes SE, Asgaard GL, Eyler LT (2013) Bridging the bench to bedside gap: validation of a reverse-translated rodent continuous performance test using functional magnetic resonance imaging. Psychiatry Res 212(3):183–191. https://doi.org/10.1016/j.pscychresns.2013.01.005

McLaughlin KA, Gabard-Durnam LJ (2021) Experience-driven plasticity and the emergence of psychopathology: a mechanistic framework integrating development and the environment into the Research Domain Criteria (RDoC) model. https://doi.org/10.31234/osf.io/nue3d

Mednick SA, Machon RA, Huttunen MO, Bonett D (1988) Adult schizophrenia following prenatal exposure to an influenza epidemic. Arch Gen Psychiatry 45(2):189–192. https://doi.org/10.1001/archpsyc.1988.01800260109013

Meehan C, Harms L, Frost JD, Barreto R, Todd J, Schall U, Shannon-Weickert C, Zavitsanou K, Michie PT, Hodgson DM (2017) Effects of immune activation during early or late gestation on schizophrenia-related behaviour in adult rat offspring. Brain Behav Immun 63:8–20. https://doi.org/10.1016/j.bbi.2016.07.144

Meyer U, FEldon J, Schedlowski M, Yee BK (2005) Towards an immno-precipitated neurodevelopmental animal model of schizophrenia. Neurosci Biobehav Rev 29:913–947. https://pubmed.ncbi.nlm.nih.gov/15964075/

Meyer U, Engler A, Weber L, Schedlowski M, Feldon J (2008) Preliminary evidence for a modulation of fetal dopaminergic development by maternal immune activation during pregnancy. Neuroscience 154(2):701–709. https://doi.org/10.1016/j.neuroscience.2008.04.031

Meyer U (2019) Neurodevelopmental resilience and susceptibility to maternal immune activation. Trends Neurosci 42(11):793–806. https://doi.org/10.1016/j.tins.2019.08.001. Epub 2019 Sep 4. PMID: 31493924

Meyer-Lindenberg A, Miletich RS, Kohn PD, Esposito G, Carson RE, Quarantelli M, Weinberger DR, Berman KF (2002) Reduced prefrontal activity predicts exaggerated striatal dopaminergic function in schizophrenia. Nat Neurosci 5(3):267+. https://link.gale.com/apps/doc/A185561768/AONE?u=mcp_mainandsid=bookmark-AONEandxid=62a46842

Mirzaei F, Michels KB, Munger K, O'Reilly E, Chitnis T, Forman MR, Giovannucci E, Rosner B, Ascherio A (2011) Gestational vitamin D and the risk of multiple sclerosis in offspring. Ann Neurol 70(1):30–40. https://doi.org/10.1002/ana.22456

Modinos G, Allen P, Grace AA, McGuire P (2015a) Translating the MAM model of psychosis to humans. Trends Neurosci 38(3):129–138. https://doi.org/10.1016/j.tins.2014.12.005

Modinos G, Allen P, Grace AA, McGuire P (2015b) Translating the MAM model of psychosis to humans. Trends Neurosci 38(3):129–138. https://doi.org/10.1016/j.tins.2014.12.005

Monte AS, Mello B, Borella V, da Silva Araujo T, da Silva F, Sousa F, de Oliveira A, Gama CS, Seeman MV, Vasconcelos S, Lucena DF, Macêdo D (2017) Two-hit model of schizophrenia induced by neonatal immune activation and peripubertal stress in rats: study of sex differences and brain oxidative alterations. Behav Brain Res 331:30–37. https://doi.org/10.1016/j.bbr.2017.04.057

Mooney-Leber SM, Brummelte S (2020) Neonatal pain and reduced maternal care alter adult behavior and hypothalamic-pituitary-adrenal axis reactivity in a sex-specific manner. Sev Psychobiol 62:631–643. https://doi.org/10.1002/dev.21941

Moore H, Jentsch JD, Ghajarnia M, Geyer MA, Grace AA (2006) A neurobehavioral systems analysis of adult rats exposed to methylazoxymethanol acetate on E17: implications for the neuropathology of schizophrenia. Biol Psychiatry 60(3):253–264. https://doi.org/10.1016/j.biopsych.2006.01.003

Mouri A, Nagai T, Ibi D, Yamada K (2013) Animal models of schizophrenia for molecular and pharmacological intervention and potential candidate molecules. Neurobiol Dis 53:61–74

Mueller FS, Richetto J, Hayes LN, Zambon A, Pollak DD, Sawa A et al (2019) Influence of poly (I:C) variability on thermoregulation, immune responses and pregnancy outcomes in mouse models of maternal immune activation. Brain Behav Immun 80:406–418

Murray RM, Paparelli A, Morrison PD, Marconi A, Di Forti M (2013) What can we learn about schizophrenia from studying the human model, drug-induced psychosis? Am J Med Genet B Neuropsychiatr Genet 162B:661–670

Murthy S, Gould E (2018) Early life stress in rodents: animal models of illness or resilience? Front Behav Neurosci 12:157. https://doi.org/10.3389/fnbeh.2018.00157

Nahar L, Delacroix BM, Nam HW (2021) The role of parvalbumin interneurons in neurotransmitter balance and neurological disease. Front Psych 12:679960

Nakazawa K, Jeevakumar V, Nakao K (2017) Spatial and temporal boundaries of NMDA receptor hypofunction leading to schizophrenia. NPJ Schizophr 3:7. https://doi.org/10.1038/s41537-016-0003-3

National Institutes of Health (n.d.) About RDoC. National Institute of Mental Health. https://www.nimh.nih.gov/research/research-funded-by-nimh/rdoc/about-rdoc

Neill JC, Barnes S, Cook S, Grayson B, Idris NF, Mclean SL, Snigdha S, Rajagopal L, Harte MK (2010) Animal models of cognitive dysfunction and negative symptoms of schizophrenia: focus on NMDA receptor antagonism. Pharmacol Ther 128:419–432

Nelson MD, Saykin AJ, Flashman LA, Riordan HJ (1998) Hippocampal volume reduction in schizophrenia as assessed by magnetic resonance imaging: a meta-analytic study. Arch Gen Psychiatry 55(5):433–440. https://doi.org/10.1001/archpsyc.55.5.433

Nieto R, Kukuljan M, Silva H (2013) BDNF and schizophrenia: from neurodevelopment to neuronal plasticity, learning, and memory. Front Psych 4:45. https://doi.org/10.3389/fpsyt.2013.00045

Nieuwenstein MR, Aleman A, De Haan EH (2001) Relationship between symptom dimensions and neurocognitive functioning in schizophrenia: a meta-analysis of WCST and CPT studies. J Psychiatr Res 35(2):119–125

Ning H, Cao D, Wang H, Kang B, Xie S, Meng Y (2017) Effects of haloperidol, olanzapine, ziprasidone, and PHA-543613 on spatial learning and memory in the Morris water maze test in naïve and MK-801-treated mice. Brain Behav 7(8):e00764

Niu Y, Wang T, Liang S, Li W, Hu X, Wu X, Jin F (2020) Sex-dependent aberrant PFC development in the adolescent offspring rats exposed to variable prenatal stress. Int J Dev Neurosci 80(6):464–476

Nossoll M, Teuchert-Noodt G, Dawirs RR (1997) A single dose of methamphetamine in neonatal gerbils affects adult prefrontal gamma-aminobutyric acid innervation. Eur J Pharmacol 340:R3–R5

Núñez Estevez KJ, Rondón-Ortiz AN, Nguyen J, Kentner AC (2020) Environmental influences on placental programming and offspring outcomes following maternal immune activation. Brain Behav Immun 83:44–55. https://doi.org/10.1016/j.bbi.2019.08.192
Ohtani T, Levitt JJ, Nestor PG, Kawashima T, Asami T, Shenton ME, Niznikiewicz M, McCarley RW (2014) Prefrontal cortex volume deficit in schizophrenia: a new look using 3T MRI with manual parcellation. Schizophr Res 152(1):184–190. https://doi.org/10.1016/j.schres.2013.10.026
Olabi B, Ellison-Wright I, McIntosh AM, Wood SJ, Bullmore E, Lawrie SM (2011) Are there progressive brain changes in schizophrenia? A meta-analysis of structural magnetic resonance imaging studies. Biol Psychiatry 70(1):88–96. https://doi.org/10.1016/j.biopsych.2011.01.032
Olincy A, Braff DL, Adler LE, Cadenhead KS, Calkins ME, Dobie DJ, Green MF, Greenwood TA, Gur RE, Gur RC, Light GA, Mintz J, Nuechterlein KH, Radant AD, Schork NJ, Seidman LJ, Siever LJ, Silverman JM, Stone WS, Swerdlow NR et al (2010) Inhibition of the P50 cerebral evoked response to repeated auditory stimuli: results from the Consortium on Genetics of Schizophrenia. Schizophr Res 119(1–3):175–182. https://doi.org/10.1016/j.schres.2010.03.004
Orikabe L, Yamasue H, Inoue H, Takayanagi Y, Mozue Y, Sudo Y et al (2011) Reduced amygdala and hippocampal volumes in patients with methamphetamine psychosis. Schizophr Res 132(2-3):183–189. https://doi.org/10.1016/j.schres.2011.07.006
Outhoff K (2016) Cognitive enhancement: a brief overview. S Afr Fam Pract 58(1):16–18
Overeem K, Alexander S, Burne THJ, Ko P, Eyles DW (2019) Developmental vitamin D deficiency in the rat impairs recognition memory, but has no effect on social approach or hedonia. Nutrients 11(11):2713. https://doi.org/10.3390/nu11112713
Papaleo F, Crawley JN, Song J, Lipska BK, Pickel J, Weinberger DR, Chen J (2008) Genetic dissection of the role of catechol-O-methyltransferase in cognition and stress reactivity in mice. J Neurosci 28(35):8709–8723
Park K, Chung C (2020) Differential alterations in cortico-amygdala circuitry in mice with impaired fear extinction. Mol Neurobiol 57(2):710–721
Park SM, Jeong B, Oh DY, Choi CH, Jung HY, Lee JY, Lee D, Choi JS (2021) Identification of major psychiatric disorders from resting-state electroencephalography using a machine learning approach. Front Psych 12(707581)
Patel KR, Cherian J, Gohil K, Atkinson D (2014) Schizophrenia: overview and treatment options. P and T 39(9):638–645
Pedersen CB, Mors O, Bertelsen A, Waltoft BL, Agerbo E, McGrath JJ et al (2014) A comprehensive nationwide study of the incidence rate and lifetime risk for treated mental disorders. JAMA Psychiat 71(5):573–581
Pezze MA, Dalley JW, Robbins TW (2007) Differential roles of dopamine D1 and D2 receptors in the nucleus accumbens in attentional performance on the five-choice serial reaction time task. Neuropsychopharmacology 32(2):273–283
Pierri JN, Chaudry AS, Woo TU, Lewis DA (1999) Alterations in chandelier neuron axon terminals in the prefrontal cortex of schizophrenic subjects. Am J Psychiatry 156:1709–1719
Pineles SL, Blumenthal TD, Curreri AJ, Nillni YI, Putnam KM, Resick PA, Rasmusson AM, Orr SP (2016) Prepulse inhibition deficits in women with PTSD. Psychophysiology 53(9):1377–1385. https://doi.org/10.1111/psyp.12679
Placek K, Dippel WC, Jones S, Brady AM (2013) Impairments in set-shifting but not reversal learning in the neonatal ventral hippocampal lesion model of schizophrenia: further evidence for medial prefrontal deficits. Behav Brain Res 256:405–413. https://doi.org/10.1016/j.bbr.2013.08.034
Plataki ME, Diskos K, Sougklakos C, Velissariou M, Georgilis A, Stavroulaki V, Sidiropoulou K (2021) Effect of neonatal treatment with the NMDA receptor antagonist, MK-801, during different temporal windows of postnatal period in adult prefrontal cortical and hippocampal function. Front Behav Neurosci 15:689193

Potkin SG, Kane JM, Correll CU, Lindenmayer JP, Agid O, Marder SR et al (2020) The neurobiology of treatment-resistant schizophrenia: paths to antipsychotic resistance and a roadmap for future research. NPJ Schizophr 6(1):1–10

Powell SB, Weber M, Geyer MA (2012) Genetic models of sensorimotor gating: relevance to neuropsychiatric disorders. Curr Top Behav Neurosci 12:251–318. https://doi.org/10.1007/7854_2011_195

Prendergast BJ, Onishi KG, Zucker I (2014) Female mice liberated for inclusion in neuroscience and biomedical research. Neurosci Biobehav Rev 40:1–5

Purves-Tyson TD, Weber-Stadlbauer U, Richetto J, Rothmond DA, Labouesse MA, Polesel M, Robinson K, Shannon Weickert C, Meyer U (2021) Increased levels of midbrain immune-related transcripts in schizophrenia and in murine offspring after maternal immune activation. Mol Psychiatry 26(3):849–863. https://doi.org/10.1038/s41380-019-0434-0

Rajarethinam R, Upadhyaya A, Tsou P, Upadhyaya M, Keshavan MS (2007) Caudate volume in offspring of patients with schizophrenia. Br J Psychiatry 191(3):258–259

Ratajczak P, Kus K, Murawiecka P, Slodzinska I, Giermaziak W, Nowakowska E (2015) Biochemical and cognitive impairments observed in animal models of schizophrenia induced by prenatal stress paradigm or methylazoxymethanol acetate administration. Acta Neurobiol Exp 75(3):314–325

Récamier-Carballo S, Estrada-Camarena E, López-Rubalcava C (2017) Maternal separation induces long-term effects on monoamines and brain-derived neurotrophic factor levels on the frontal cortex, amygdala, and hippocampus: differential effects after a stress challenge. Behav Pharmacol 28(7):545–557

Reisinger S, Khan D, Kong E, Berger A, Pollak A, Pollak DD (2015) The poly(I:C)-induced maternal immune activation model in preclinical neuropsychiatric drug discovery. Pharmacol Ther 149:213–226. https://doi.org/10.1016/j.pharmthera.2015.01.001

Ricaurte GA, Guillery RW, Seiden LS, Schuster CR, Moore RY (1982) Dopamine nerve terminal degeneration produced by high doses of methylamphetamine in the rat brain. Brain Res 235:93–103

Robbins TW (2002) The 5-choice serial reaction time task: behavioural pharmacology and functional neurochemistry. Psychopharmacology (Berl) 163(3-4):362–380. https://doi.org/10.1007/s00213-002-1154-7

Robinson TE, Becker JB (1986) Enduring changes in brain and behavior produced by chronic amphetamine administration: a review and evaluation of animal models of amphetamine psychosis. Brain Res 396:157–198

Roceri M, Cirulli F, Pessina C, Peretto P, Racagni G, Riva MA (2004) Postnatal repeated maternal deprivation produces age-dependent changes of brain-derived neurotrophic factor expression in selected rat brain regions. Biol Psychiatry 55(7):708–714

Roderick RC, Kentner AC (2019) Building a framework to optimize animal models of maternal immune activation: like your ongoing home improvements, it's a work in progress. Brain Behav Immun 75:6–7. https://doi.org/10.1016/j.bbi.2018.10.011

Roffman JL, Lipska BK, Bertolino A, Van Gelderen P, Olson AW, Khaing ZZ, Weinberger DR (2000) Local and downstream effects of excitotoxic lesions in the rat medial prefrontal cortex on in vivo 1H-MRS signals. Neuropsychopharmacology 22(4):430–439. https://doi.org/10.1016/S0893-133X(99)00143-8

Rokita KI, Holleran L, Dauvermann MR, Mothersill D, Holland J, Costello L et al (2020) Childhood trauma, brain structure and emotion recognition in patients with schizophrenia and healthy participants. Soc Cogn Affect Neurosci 15(12):1325–1339

Romeo RD, Mueller A, Sisti HM, Ogawa S, McEwen BS, Brake WG (2003) Anxiety and fear behaviors in adult male and female C57BL/6 mice are modulated by maternal separation. Horm Behav 43(5):561–567. https://doi.org/10.1016/s0018-506x(03)00063-1

Roos A, Kwiatkowski MA, Fouche JP, Narr KL, Thomas KG, Stein DJ, Donald KA (2015) White matter integrity and cognitive performance in children with prenatal methamphetamine exposure. Behav Brain Res 279:62–67

Ross RG, Hunter SK, McCarthy L, Beuler J, Hutchison AK, Wagner BD, Leonard S, Stevens KE, Freedman R (2013) Perinatal choline effects on neonatal pathophysiology related to later schizophrenia risk. Am J Psychiatry 170(3):290–298. https://doi.org/10.1176/appi.ajp.2012.12070940

Sanjari Moghaddam H, Mobarak Abadi M, Dolatshahi M, Bayani Ershadi S, Abbasi-Feijani F, Rezaei S, Cattarinussi G, Aarabi MH (2021) Effects of prenatal methamphetamine exposure on the developing human brain: a systematic review of neuroimaging studies. ACS Chem Nerosci 12:2729–2748

Scarborough J, Mueller F, Arban R, Dorner-Ciossek C, Weber-Stadlbauer U, Rosenbrock H, Meyer U, Richetto J (2020) Preclinical validation of the micropipette-guided drug administration (MDA) method in the maternal immune activation model of neurodevelopmental disorders. Brain Behav Immun 88:461–470. https://doi.org/10.1016/j.bbi.2020.04.015

Schneider T, Przewłocki R (2005) Behavioral alterations in rats prenatally exposed to valproic acid: animal model of autism. Neuropsychopharmacology 30(1):80–89. https://doi.org/10.1038/sj.npp.1300518

Schneider T, Turczak J, Przewłocki R (2006) Environmental enrichment reverses behavioral alterations in rats prenatally exposed to valproic acid: issues for a therapeutic approach in autism. Neuropsychopharmacology 31(1):36–46. https://doi.org/10.1038/sj.npp.1300767

Schroeder H, Grecksch G, Becker A, Bogerts B, Hoellt V (1999) Alterations of the dopaminergic and glutamatergic neurotransmission in adult rats with postnatal ibotenic acid hippocampal lesion. Psychopharmacology (Berl) 145(1):61–66. https://doi.org/10.1007/s002130051032

Shi L, Fatemi SH, Sidwell RW, Patterson PH (2003) Maternal influenza infection causes marked behavioral and pharmacological changes in the offspring. J Neurosci 23(1):297–302. https://doi.org/10.1523/JNEUROSCI.23-01-00297.2003

Shin S, Kim K, Pak K, Nam H-Y, Kim SJ, Kim I (2019) Effects of maturation on striatal dopamine transporter availability in rats. Nuklearmedizin 58:395–400. https://doi.org/10.1055/a-0981-5709

Siegel JA, Park BS, Raber J (2011) Long-term effects of neonatal methamphetamine exposure on cognitive function in adolescent mice. Behav Brain Res 219:159–164

Siemerkus J, Irle E, Schmidt-Samoa C, Dechent P, Weniger G (2012) Egocentric spatial learning in schizophrenia investigated with functional magnetic resonance imaging. Neuroimage Clin 1:153–163

Simeone JC, Ward AJ, Rotella P et al (2015) An evaluation of variation in published estimates of schizophrenia prevalence from 1990—2013: a systematic literature review. BMC Psychiatry 15:193. https://doi.org/10.1186/s12888-015-0578-7

Singh S, Aich TK, Bhattarai R (2017) Wisconsin card sorting test performance impairment in schizophrenia: an Indian study report. Indian J Psychiatry 59(1):88–93. https://doi.org/10.4103/0019-5545.204440

Skelton MR, Williams MT, Schaefer TL, Vorhees CV (2007) Neonatal (+)-methamphetamine increases brain derived neurotrophic factor, but not nerve growth factor, during treatment and results in long-term spatial learning deficits. Psychoneuroendocrinology 32:734–745

Smith SM, Vale WW (2006) The role of the hypothalamic-pituitary-adrenal axis in neuroendocrine responses to stress. Dialogues Clin Neurosci 8(4):383–395. https://doi.org/10.31887/DCNS.2006.8.4/ssmith

Snyder SH (1973) Amphetamine psychosis: a "model" schizophrenia mediated by catecholamines. Am J Psychiatry 130:61–67

Solas M, Aisa B, Mugueta MC, Del Río J, Tordera RM, Ramírez MJ (2010) Interactions between age, stress and insulin on cognition: implications for Alzheimer's disease. Neuropsychopharmacology 35(8):1664–1673. https://doi.org/10.1038/npp.2010.13

Spencer KM, Nestor PG, Perlmutter R, Niznikiewicz MA, Klump MC, Frumin M, Shenton ME, Mccarley RW (2004) Neural synchrony indexes disordered perception and cognition in schizophrenia. Proc Natl Acad Sci U S A 101:17288–17293

Stephens SH, Logel J, Barton A, Franks A, Schultz J, Short M et al (2009) Association of the 5′-upstream regulatory region of the α7 nicotinic acetylcholine receptor subunit gene (CHRNA7) with schizophrenia. Schizophr Res 109(1-3):102–112

Strzelewicz AR, Ordoñes Sanchez E, Rondón-Ortiz AN, Raneri A, Famularo ST, Bangasser DA, Kentner AC (2019) Access to a high resource environment protects against accelerated maturation following early life stress: a translational animal model of high, medium and low security settings. Horm Behav 111:46–59. https://doi.org/10.1016/j.yhbeh.2019.01.003

Strzelewicz AR, Vecchiarelli HA, Rondón-Ortiz AN, Raneri A, Hill MN, Kentner AC (2021) Interactive effects of compounding multidimensional stressors on maternal and male and female rat offspring outcomes. Horm Behav 134:105013. https://doi.org/10.1016/j.yhbeh.2021.105013

Substance Abuse and Mental Health Services Administration (2016) Impact of the DSM-IV to DSM-5 Changes on the National Survey on Drug Use and Health [Internet]. Substance Abuse and Mental Health Services Administration (US), Rockville. Table 3.22, DSM-IV to DSM-5 schizophrenia comparison. Available from: https://www.ncbi.nlm.nih.gov/books/NBK519704/table/ch3.t22/

Szuran TF, Pliska V, Pokorny J, Welzl H (2000) Prenatal stress in rats: effects on plasma corticosterone, hippocampal glucocorticoid receptors, and maze performance. Physiol Behav 71(3-4):353–362. https://doi.org/10.1016/s0031-9384(00)00351-6

Tan T, Wang W, Williams J, Ma K, Cao Q, Yan Z (2019) Stress exposure in dopamine D4 receptor knockout mice induces schizophrenia-like behaviors via disruption of GABAergic transmission. Schizophr Bull 45(5):1012–1023

Tandon R, Gaebel W, Barch DM, Bustillo J, Gur RE, Heckers S et al (2013) Definition and description of schizophrenia in the DSM-5. Schizophr Res 150(1):3–10

Tarazi FI, Baldessarini RJ (2000) Comparative postnatal development of dopamine D1, D2 and D4 receptors in rat forebrain. Int J Dev Neurosci 18:29–37

Teodorini RD, Rycroft N, Smith-Spark JH (2020) The off-prescription use of modafinil: an online survey of perceived risks and benefits. PLoS One 15(2):e0227818. https://doi.org/10.1371/journal.pone.0227818

Tian H, Ding N, Guo M, Wang S, Wang Z, Liu H et al (2019) Analysis of learning and memory ability in an Alzheimer's disease mouse model using the Morris water maze. J Vis Exp 152:e60055

Tseng KY, Chambers RA, Lipska BK (2009) The neonatal ventral hippocampal lesion as a heuristic neurodevelopmental model of schizophrenia. Behav Brain Res 204(2):295–305. https://doi.org/10.1016/j.bbr.2008.11.039

Turner DC, Clark L, Pomarol-Clotet E, McKenna P, Robbins TW, Sahakian BJ (2004) Modafinil improves cognition and attentional set shifting in patients with chronic schizophrenia. Neuropsychopharmacology 29:1363–1373. https://doi.org/10.1038/sj.npp.1300457

Turner KM, Young JW, McGrath JJ, Eyles DW, Burne TH (2013) Cognitive performance and response inhibition in developmentally vitamin D (DVD)-deficient rats. Behav Brain Res 242:47–53. https://doi.org/10.1016/j.bbr.2012.12.029

Uhlhaas PJ, Singer W (2006) Neural synchrony in brain disorders: relevance for cognitive dysfunctions and pathophysiology. Neuron 52:155–168

Umbricht D, Alberati D, Martin-Facklam M, Borroni E, Youssef EA, Ostland M, Wallace TL, Knoflach F, Dorflinger E, Wettstein JG, Bausch A, Garibaldi G, Santarelli L (2014) Effect of bitopertin, a glycine reuptake inhibitor, on negative symptoms of schizophrenia: a randomized, double-blind, proof-of-concept study. JAMA Psychiat 71(6):637–646. https://doi.org/10.1001/jamapsychiatry.2014.163

Veijola J, Guo JY, Moilanen JS, Jääskeläinen E, Miettunen J, Kyllönen M, Haapea M, Huhtaniska S, Alaräisänen A, Mäki P, Kiviniemi V, Nikkinen J, Starck T, Remes JJ, Tanskanen P, Tervonen O, Wink AM, Kehagia A, Suckling J, Kobayashi H et al (2014) Longitudinal changes in total brain volume in schizophrenia: relation to symptom severity, cognition and antipsychotic medication. PLoS One 9(7):e101689. https://doi.org/10.1371/journal.pone.0101689

Vengeliene V, Bespalov A, Roßmanith M, Horschitz S, Berger S, Relo AL, Noori HR, Schneider P, Enkel T, Bartsch D, Schneider M, Behl B, Hansson AC, Schloss P, Spanagel R (2017) Towards trans-diagnostic mechanisms in psychiatry: neurobehavioral profile of rats with a loss-of-function point mutation in the dopamine transporter gene. Dis Model Mech 10(4):451–461. https://doi.org/10.1242/dmm.027623

Vojinovic J (2014) Vitamin D receptor agonists' anti-inflammatory properties. Ann N Y Acad Sci 1317(1):47–56

Vorhees CV, Williams MT (2006) Morris water maze: procedures for assessing spatial and related forms of learning and memory. Nat Protoc 1(2):848–858. https://doi.org/10.1038/nprot.2006.116

Vorhees CV, Williams MT (2016) Cincinnati water maze: a review of the development, methods, and evidence as a test of egocentric learning and memory. Neurotoxicol Teratol 57:1–19

Vorhees CV, Herring NR, Schaefer TL, Grace CE, Skelton MR, Johnson HL, Williams MT (2008) Effects of neonatal (+)-methamphetamine on path integration and spatial learning in rats: effects of dose and rearing conditions. Int J Dev Neurosci 26:599–610

Vorhees CV, Skelton MR, Grace CE, Schaefer TL, Graham DL, Braun AA, Williams MT (2009) Effects of (+)-methamphetamine on path integration and spatial learning, but not locomotor activity or acoustic startle, align with the stress hyporesponsive period in rats. Int J Dev Neurosci 27:289–298

Vorhees CV, He E, Skelton MR, Graham DL, Schaefer TL, Grace CE, Braun AA, Amos-Kroohs R, Williams MT (2011) Comparison of (+)-methamphetamine, +/--methylenedioxymethamphetamine, (+)-amphetamine and +/--fenfluramine in rats on egocentric learning in the Cincinnati water maze. Synapse 65:368–378

Waddell J, Hill E, Tang S, Jiang L, Xu S, Mooney SM (2020) Choline plus working memory training improves prenatal alcohol-induced deficits in cognitive flexibility and functional connectivity in adulthood in rats. Nutrients 12(11):3513. https://doi.org/10.3390/nu12113513

Walder DJ, Walker EF, Lewine RJ (2000) Cognitive functioning, cortisol release, and symptom severity in patients with schizophrenia. Biol Psychiatry 48(12):1121–1132. https://doi.org/10.1016/s0006-3223(00)01052-0

Wang C, Zhang Y (2017) Season of birth and schizophrenia: evidence from China. Psychiatry Res 253:189–196. https://doi.org/10.1016/j.psychres.2017.03.030

Watson JB, Mednick SA, Huttunen M, Wang X (1999) Prenatal teratogens and the development of adult mental illness. Dev Psychopathol 11(3):457–466. https://doi.org/10.1017/s0954579499002151

Weiner B (1985) An attributional theory of achievement motivation and emotion. Psychol Rev 92(4):548

Whittingham K, McGlade A, Kulasinghe K, Mitchell AE, Heussler H, Boys RN (2020) ENACT (Environmental enrichment for infants; parenting with Acceptance and Commitment Therapy): a randomised controlled trial of an innovative intervention for infants at risk of autism spectrum disorder. BMJ Open 10:e034315. https://doi.org/10.1136/bmjopen-2019-034315

Winter C, Djodari-Irani A, Sohr R, Morgenstern R, Feldon J, Juckel G, Meyer U (2009) Prenatal immune activation leads to multiple changes in basal neurotransmitter levels in the adult brain: implications for brain disorders of neurodevelopmental origin such as schizophrenia. Int J Neuropsychopharmacol 12(4):513–524. https://doi.org/10.1017/S1461145708009206

Woo CC, Leon M (2013) Environmental enrichment as an effective treatment for autism: a randomized controlled trial. Behav Neurosci 127(4):487–497. https://doi.org/10.1037/a0033010

Woo TU, Whitehead RE, Melchitzky DS, Lewis DA (1998) A subclass of prefrontal gamma-aminobutyric acid axon terminals are selectively altered in schizophrenia. Proc Natl Acad Sci U S A 95:5341–5346

Xue X, Shao S, Wang W, Shao F (2013) Maternal separation induces alterations in reversal learning and brain-derived neurotrophic factor expression in adult rats. Neuropsychobiology 68(4): 243–249. https://doi.org/10.1159/000356188

Xue J, Schoenrock S, Valdar W, Tarantino L, Ideraabdullah F (2016) Maternal vitamin D depletion alters DNA methylation at imprinted loci in multiple generations. Clin Epigenetics 8. https://doi.org/10.1186/s13148-016-0276-4

Young JW, Markou A (2015) Translational rodent paradigms to investigate neuromechanisms underlying behaviors relevant to amotivation and altered reward processing in schizophrenia. Schizophr Bull 41(5):1024–1032

Young SE, Friedman NP, Miyake A, Willcutt EG, Corley RP, Haberstick BC, Hewitt JK (2009) Behavioral disinhibition: liability for externalizing spectrum disorders and its genetic and environmental relation to response inhibition across adolescence. J Abnorm Psychol 118(1):117

Young JW, Powell SB, Geyer MA (2012) Mouse pharmacological models of cognitive disruption relevant to schizophrenia. Neuropharmacology 62(3):1381–1390

Young JW, Geyer MA, Rissling AJ, Sharp RF, Eyler LT, Asgaard GL, Light G (2013) Reverse translation of the rodent 5C-CPT reveals that the impaired attention of people with schizophrenia is similar to scopolamine-induced deficits in mice. Transl Psychiatry 3(11):e324–e324

Young JW, Winstanley CA, Brady AM, Hall FS (2017) Research domain criteria versus DSM V: how does this debate affect attempts to model corticostriatal dysfunction in animals? Neurosci Biobehav Rev 76(Pt B):301–316. https://doi.org/10.1016/j.neubiorev.2016.10.029

Young JW, Geyer MA, Halberstadt AL, van Enkhuizen J, Minassian A, Khan A, Perry W, Eyler LT (2020) Convergent neural substrates of inattention in bipolar disorder patients and dopamine transporter-deficient mice using the 5-choice CPT. Bipolar Disord 22(1):46–58. https://doi.org/10.1111/bdi.12786

Zeisel S (2017) Choline, other methyl-donors and epigenetics. Nutrients 9:445. https://doi.org/10.3390/nu9050445

Zeisel SH, da Costa KA (2009) Choline: an essential nutrient for public health. Nutr Rev 67(11): 615–623. https://doi.org/10.1111/j.1753-4887.2009.00246.x

Zhao X, Rondòn-Ortiz L, Puracchio M, Roderick RC, Kentner AC (2020) Therapeutic efficacy of environmental enrichment on behavioral, endocrine, and synaptic alterations in an animal model of maternal immune activation. Brain Behav Immun Health 3:100043

Zhao X, Mohammed R, Tran H, Erickson M, Kentner AC (2021) Poly (I:C)-induced maternal immune activation modifies ventral hippocampal regulation of stress reactivity: prevention by environmental enrichment. Brain Behav Immun 95:203–215

Zhu X, Li T, Peng S, Ma X, Chen X, Zhang X (2010) Maternal deprivation-caused behavioral abnormalities in adult rats relate to a non-methylation-regulated D2 receptor levels in the nucleus accumbens. Behav Brain Res 209(2):281–288. https://doi.org/10.1016/j.bbr.2010.02.005

Genetic Influences on Cognitive Dysfunction in Schizophrenia

Tiffany A. Greenwood

Contents

Abstract Schizophrenia is a severe and debilitating psychotic disorder that is highly heritable and relatively common in the population. The clinical heterogeneity associated with schizophrenia is substantial, with patients exhibiting a broad range of deficits and symptom severity. Large-scale genomic studies employing a case–control design have begun to provide some biological insight. However, this strategy combines individuals with clinically diverse symptoms and ignores the genetic risk that is carried by many clinically unaffected individuals. Consequently, the majority of the genetic architecture underlying schizophrenia remains unexplained, and the pathways by which the implicated variants contribute to the clinically observable signs and symptoms are still largely unknown. Parsing the complex, clinical phenotype of schizophrenia into biologically relevant components may have utility in research aimed at understanding the genetic basis of liability. Cognitive dysfunction is a hallmark symptom of schizophrenia that is associated with impaired quality of life and poor functional outcome. Here, we examine the value of quantitative measures of cognitive dysfunction to objectively target the underlying neurobiological pathways and identify genetic variants and gene networks contributing to schizophrenia risk. For a complex disorder, quantitative measures are also more efficient than diagnosis, allowing for the identification of associated genetic variants with fewer subjects. Such a strategy supplements traditional analyses of schizophrenia diagnosis, providing the necessary biological insight to help translate genetic

T. A. Greenwood (✉)
Department of Psychiatry, University of California San Diego, La Jolla, CA, USA
e-mail: tgreenwood@ucsd.edu

Curr Topics Behav Neurosci (2023) 63: 291–314
https://doi.org/10.1007/7854_2022_388
Published Online: 28 August 2022

findings into actionable treatment targets. Understanding the genetic basis of cognitive dysfunction in schizophrenia may thus facilitate the development of novel pharmacological and procognitive interventions to improve real-world functioning.

Keywords Cognition · Endophenotype · Genetics · Schizophrenia

1 Schizophrenia: A Clinically and Genetically Heterogenous Disorder

Schizophrenia (SZ) is a severe and persistent psychotic disorder that is characterized by significant cognitive impairments and psychosocial disability (Green et al. 2000). Patients with SZ exhibit a broad range of deficits and symptom severity that vary over the course of illness and with treatment. Psychosis is defined by symptoms that affect an individual's thoughts, feelings, and behaviors, ranging from positive symptoms of hallucinations, delusions, disorganized speech and/or behavior to negative symptoms of diminished emotional expression, poverty of speech, lack of motivation, an inability to experience pleasure, and social withdrawal. Given the extreme diversity of individual symptom profiles, it is perhaps most accurately described as the "Group of Schizophrenias" (Bleuler 1911).

Treatment of SZ primarily involves antipsychotic medications that were serendipitously discovered and treat the positive symptoms of psychosis. However, antipsychotics are only partially effective, do not improve negative or cognitive symptoms, and have troublesome side effects that, when combined with the lack of insight that is characteristic of SZ, often result in treatment non-compliance (Bitter et al. 2015; Tessier et al. 2017). Indeed, a large-scale investigation of the effectiveness of five commonly used antipsychotic medications found that about 50% of patients discontinue their medications by 6 months and 74% discontinue their medications by 18 months (Lieberman et al. 2005). It is thus imperative that we further our understanding of the underlying causes of SZ to facilitate the development of novel pharmacological agents that can effectively target the debilitating symptoms with fewer side effects.

Genetic factors clearly play a substantial role in the etiology of SZ. Family and twin studies dating back to the 1940s have produced a range of heritability estimates for SZ that were summarized via meta-analysis as the widely quoted estimate of 81% (Sullivan et al. 2003). While these family-based estimates take into account the role of both common and rare variants, more recent estimates obtained from population-based studies of common, additive genetic variation have suggested a heritability of 60–70% (Lichtenstein et al. 2009; Wray and Gottesman 2012). Although sporadic, non-familial cases of SZ are often observed, family history remains the strongest and best replicated risk factor (Walder et al. 2014). Relatives of an individual with SZ have a significantly increased risk of developing the disorder, and the more genes shared contributing to higher risk, ranging from 2–4% for second-degree relatives up to 10–15% for first-degree relatives (Schwab and Wildenauer 2013).

Despite strong evidence for the genetic transmission of vulnerability to SZ, the profound clinical heterogeneity and phenotypic complexity has long frustrated research efforts aimed at understanding the genetic basis of liability. Indeed, early efforts at gene mapping through family-based linkage and association studies served to shed light on the genetic complexity of the illness. While these studies implicated many chromosomal regions and suggested plausible candidate genes, narrowing the source of the signal within broad regions and identifying functional variants within the implicated genes have proven difficult (Baron 2001; Lewis et al. 2003; Owen et al. 2004; Gogos and Gerber 2006; Harrison and Weinberger 2005).

The field of psychiatric genetics was revolutionized in 2007 when the introduction of micro-array-based genotyping and the culmination of efforts to map the structure of the human genome gave birth to genome-wide association (GWA) studies. Such studies rely on allele frequency differences observed between large samples of unrelated case and control subjects to identify common single nucleotide polymorphisms (SNPs) associated with diagnosis. Although the early GWA studies of SZ were underpowered, increasingly large-scale studies have begun to produce replicable findings (O'donovan et al. 2008; Shi et al. 2009; Ripke et al. 2013; Schizophrenia Working Group of the Psychiatric Genomics Consortium 2014; Sekar et al. 2016; International Schizophrenia Consortium 2009; Stefansson et al. 2008, 2009). Several of the implicated genes are consistent with leading hypotheses regarding pathophysiology, such as *DRD2*, the target of most effective antipsychotics, and genes involved in glutamate signaling (e.g., *GRM3*, *GRIN2A*, *GRIA1*) (Schizophrenia Working Group of the Psychiatric Genomics Consortium 2014). The identification of the complement component 4 gene (*C4*) within the strongly associated major histocompatibility complex (MHC) region and its relation to synaptic pruning is particularly intriguing (Sekar et al. 2016). However, the majority of the genetic risk for SZ still remains unexplained, as genome-wide significant variants account for only a small portion of the overall risk and the effect size of each individual variant is very small (Schizophrenia Working Group of the Psychiatric Genomics Consortium 2014). The pathways by which these common variants impact risk also remain largely unknown. While studies of rare and de novo variation have helped shed light on possible underlying pathways, disruptive copy number variants (CNVs) and single nucleotide variants (SNVs) are only detected in only a small percentage of SZ cases. A considerable proportion of the observed heritability is thus not detectable in these large-scale studies of SZ diagnosis among unrelated individuals (Altshuler et al. 2008; Manolio et al. 2009). There remains the challenge of creating a clear pathway from the standard case–control genomic paradigm to the ultimate goal of precision medicine, which envisions the early identification of risk and timely intervention with personalized treatment strategies targeting the core deficits and dysfunction (Braff 2017).

2 The Value of Endophenotypes in Schizophrenia Research

Recent studies have demonstrated that employing more specific phenotype definitions in genetic studies of complex disorders, including SZ, is even more important than large sample sizes for detecting true genetic associations (Liang and Greenwood 2015; Manchia et al. 2013). The use of endophenotypes as objective, laboratory-based measures of specific neurobiological functions with characteristic impairment in SZ (e.g., memory, attention, working memory, etc.) may be particularly helpful in reducing the heterogeneity associated with the considerably more subjective diagnosis, facilitating the detection of risk variants and aberrant molecular pathways (Gottesman and Gould 2003; Braff et al. 2007; Insel and Cuthbert 2009; Greenwood et al. 2019a). Endophenotypes are state-independent traits that are associated with illness and observed at a higher rate in unaffected family members than in the general population (Gottesman and Shields 1972). To be useful in genetic studies, an endophenotype must also be significantly heritable, reliably measured, and stable over time (Braff and Freedman 2002; Braff et al. 2008). As shown in Fig. 1, endophenotypes fall within the genotype-to-phenotype pathway of the disease process, linking genetic risk variants and aberrant neurobiological processes to the clinically observable symptoms of illness (Cannon and Keller 2006; Thaker 2007). The endophenotype strategy thus complements large-scale genomic investigations of diagnosis and provides important neurobiological context for the identified risk variants. As many endophenotypes are also amenable to cross-species investigations, which are important for the development of novel therapeutic interventions, the endophenotype strategy has been advocated by the National Institute of Mental Health (NIMH) as a part of the Research Domain Criteria (RDoC) framework (Cuthbert and Insel 2010; Insel et al. 2010).

In addition to providing increased phenotypic specificity and genetic resolution, the quantitative nature of endophenotypes confers significantly greater power compared to the analysis of diagnosis (Blangero et al. 2003; Lee and Wray 2013). As shown in Fig. 2, polygenic disorders like SZ are best conceptualized as arising from an unobserved continuum of risk according to a liability threshold model (Greenwood et al. 2019a; Gottesman and Shields 1967; Plomin et al. 2009; Falconer 1960). Individuals above the threshold are considered affected cases, while those below are considered unaffected controls. The threshold's position determines both the prevalence of the disorder and the power of case–control studies. While a positive diagnosis of SZ is highly informative with respect to genetic liability, the absence of a diagnosis reveals nothing about where individuals fall on the liability curve, and the inclusion of unaffected individuals with mild-to-moderate liability dilutes the genetic signal in a traditional case–control study. For a disorder like SZ with a 1% prevalence and 80% heritability, the analysis of a quantitative endophenotype that measures the underlying genetic liability is expected to be 100-fold more efficient than the case–control analysis, which translates to a 10-fold increase in power (Blangero et al. 2003). Endophenotype-based studies thus require substantially smaller sample sizes to achieve comparable power to

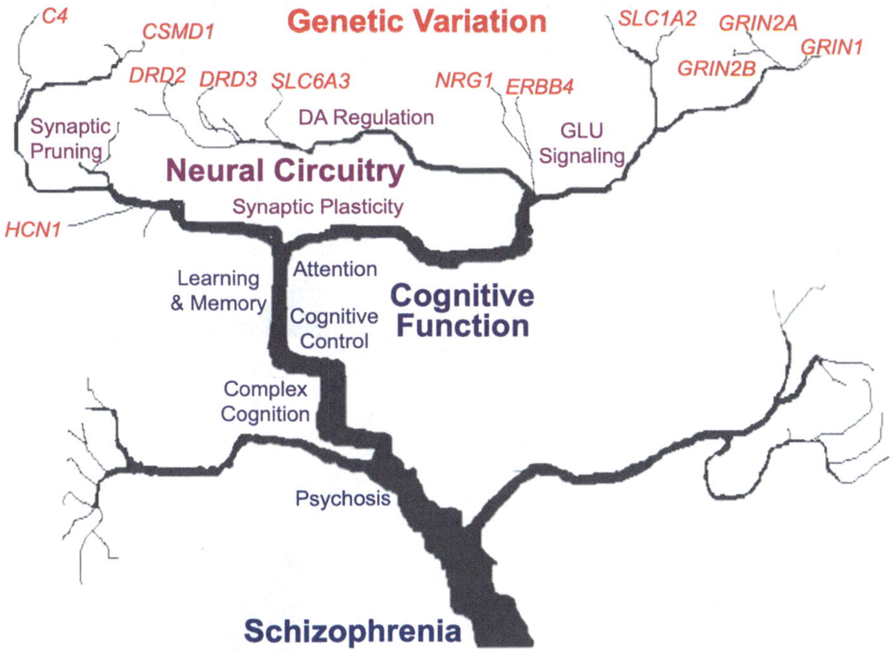

Fig. 1 Watershed model (adapted from Cannon and Keller (2006)) illustrating the heterogeneous nature of schizophrenia and the role of cognitive endophenotypes in linking genetic risk variants and dysregulated neurobiological processes to the clinically observable symptoms of illness. As this model demonstrates, upstream genetic variation affects downstream processes of neural circuit regulation (dopaminergic regulation in the prefrontal cortex, glutamate signaling, synaptic pruning, etc.), disruptions of which lead to broader phenotypes like cognitive dysfunction that can be measured through the use of specific endophenotypes within the RDoC framework. The combination of these and other downstream endophenotypes results in the observed symptoms of schizophrenia (psychosis, etc.). Genetic variants may be of small effect, as in the case of common variants (SNPs), and combine within and across genes in the same pathway to produce an effect on the underlying neural circuitry. Alternatively, a rare mutation of large effect (CNV, SNV) may be sufficient to disrupt the entire pathway

those of SZ diagnosis. Family-based designs provide a further increase in power by enriching for individuals with higher genetic liability to SZ (Abecasis et al. 2001). Additionally, unaffected individuals carrying non-penetrant risk variants do not diminish the genetic signal in the analysis of the endophenotype, as with the analysis of diagnosis. Indeed, affected and unaffected individuals alike provide a range of scores and are thus informative regarding the underlying liability.

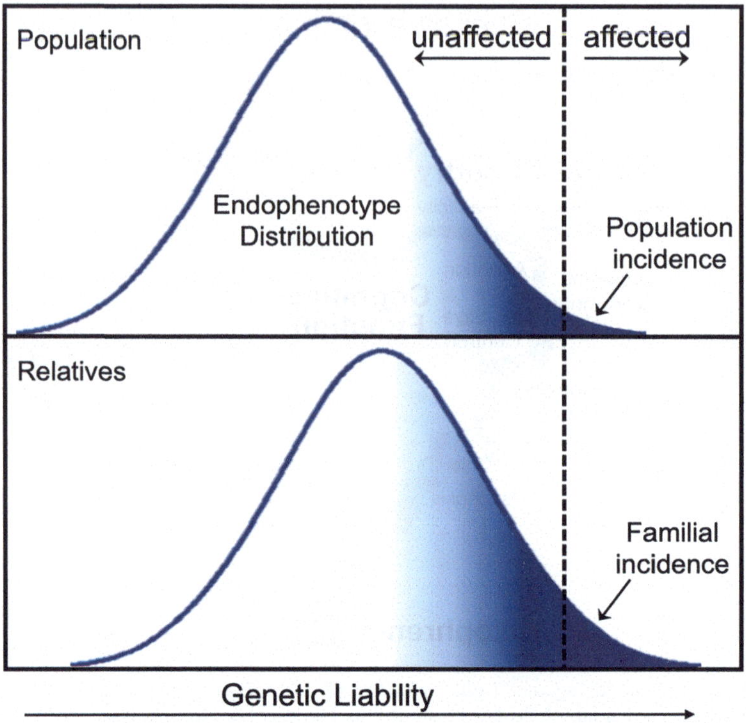

Fig. 2 Liability threshold and the unobserved continuum of genetic liability to schizophrenia that is present in the population. While the use of diagnosis as the phenotype of interest dichotomizes the liability distribution into "affected" and "unaffected" according to a threshold defined by subjective symptom profiles (dashed line), endophenotypes capture the full range of information across "unaffected" and "affected" individuals alike and are thus informative regarding the underlying liability. As shown, "unaffected" individuals reflect a range of genetic liability that is undetectable in standard case–control designs and dilutes the genetic signal. However, by using a quantitative endophenotype to model the genetic liability through a range of endophenotype deficits (attention, learning, memory, social cognition, etc.), such individuals contribute meaningfully to the analysis. By enriching for such individuals with higher genetic liability and stronger expressions of the endophenotype, family-based designs provide greater power for detection of the underlying genetic variation

3 Measures of Cognitive Dysfunction as Endophenotypes for Schizophrenia

Cognitive dysfunction is a hallmark of SZ leading to impaired quality of life and poor functional outcome (Green et al. 2000; Saykin et al. 1991; Elvevag and Goldberg 2000). Examining quantitative measures of cognitive dysfunction may reduce the clinical heterogeneity by targeting specific aspects of the underlying biology, thus providing a complementary approach to unraveling the genetic architecture of SZ (Gottesman and Gould 2003; Braff et al. 2007; Insel and Cuthbert

2009; Glahn et al. 2014). While clinical symptoms vary over the course of illness and treatment, the underlying brain dysfunction forms a more stable trait that cognitive endophenotypes may be able to objectively measure. The study of specific cognitive deficits in SZ can thus inform mechanistic models to help bridge the gap between the identified genes and the clinical phenotype.

Deficits in cognitive performance are not merely an effect of treatment nor a consequence of chronic psychosis. Indeed, cognitive deficits are already prominent at the first clinical presentation of neuroleptic naïve patients; are evident in unaffected individuals at genetic risk for psychosis; have been documented in large-scale prospective studies of children who were asymptomatic when evaluated and received the diagnosis as adults; and are prevalent in youth who report psychosis spectrum symptoms (Cannon et al. 2002, 2006; Saykin et al. 1994; Seidman et al. 2016). Data from the North American Prodrome Longitudinal Study (NAPLS) has further suggested that measures of cognitive functioning may have predictive utility in identifying those clinically high-risk subjects who will eventually convert to psychosis (Seidman et al. 2016; Reichenberg and Mollon 2016). Cognitive deficits are thus as much a defining feature of SZ as the more subjective clinical symptoms used for diagnosis (Gur et al. 2014).

Cognitive deficits play a substantial role in the socio-occupational impairment and disability seen in SZ, suggesting that the study of cognitive endophenotypes has practical benefits in terms of both research and treatment. Indeed, targeted cognitive training has been shown to not only improve verbal memory in SZ patients but also increase their level of real-world functioning (Thomas et al. 2018). Many cognitive endophenotypes are also amenable to neuroimaging studies in humans, as well as translational studies using intrinsic or induced deficits in animal models to mimic those observed in humans, allowing for a direct evaluation of the neural circuit dysfunction (Young et al. 2013; Roalf et al. 2014). As such, the FDA has endorsed cognitive deficits as key targets for the development of novel treatments for SZ (Nuechterlein et al. 2008; Kern et al. 2008).

4 The Genetics of Cognitive Dysfunction in Schizophrenia

The observed overlap between the genetic architectures of cognition and SZ suggests that a portion of the common genetic risk for SZ may be mediated through genetic effects on cognitive functioning. Twin studies of cognitive deficits in SZ have shown that shared genetic effects have a substantial contribution to the phenotypic correlation between cognition and SZ (Toulopoulou et al. 2007, 2010). More recently, large-scale studies of community-based samples confirmed that higher polygenic risk for SZ is associated with lower cognitive functioning (Hubbard et al. 2016; Lencz et al. 2014; Mcintosh et al. 2013; Hagenaars et al. 2016; Trampush et al. 2017). However, to establish a correlation, these studies have relied on global cognitive summaries related to total IQ or estimates of "g" in samples phenotyped using diverse cognitive batteries in conjunction with genomic summaries of SZ risk derived from other samples. Educational attainment has similarly been pursued in large-scale genomic investigations as a proxy for cognitive functioning (Rietveld et al. 2013), yet it represents a long-term life outcome measured across varying educational systems. As such, these large-scale studies of population-representative samples employing crude estimates of cognitive functioning have only captured a small fraction of the shared genetic variance suggested by twin studies and have failed to provide biological insight into the relationship between SZ and specific domains of cognitive functioning.

Several large, multi-site consortia have investigated measures of cognitive dysfunction in SZ as a strategy for dissecting the genetic architecture of the disorder, and these analyses have begun to bear fruit (Gottesman and Gould 2003; Braff et al. 2007). While various cognitive measures have been utilized across these consortia, the Penn Computerized Neuropsychological Battery (CNB) provides a point of convergence from which we can examine some of the initial genetic findings. The CNB provides for a comprehensive evaluation of cognitive functioning in large-scale studies and is featured as part of the Early Psychosis Translational Research Collection of the National Institute of Health's PhenX Toolkit (Gur et al. 2001a, b, 2010, 2012). The CNB is widely used in national and international genomic studies of psychosis, including the Consortium on the Genetics of Schizophrenia (COGS), Multiplex Multigenerational Investigation of Schizophrenia (MGI), Project Among African-Americans to Explore Risks for Schizophrenia (PAARTNERS), North American Prodrome Longitudinal Study (NAPLS), and the Philadelphia Neurodevelopmental Cohort (PNC). As summarized in Table 1, CNB measures have been validated through functional neuroimaging studies and reveal robust prediction accuracy, as well as patterns of brain activation that are domain specific and consistent with the hypothesized neural mechanisms (Roalf et al. 2014; Adler et al. 2001; Jackson and Schacter 2004; Ogg et al. 2008; Crone et al. 2008; Marenco et al. 1993; Specht et al. 2009; Gur et al. 1997, 1982, 2000, 2002; Moser et al. 2007; Derntl et al. 2008). The cognitive domains assessed by the CNB also parallel constructs endorsed as part of the RDoC behavioral classification system (Insel and Cuthbert 2009; Cuthbert and Insel 2010; Insel et al. 2010).

Data across several consortia have demonstrated that all CNB measures shown in Table 1 are significantly heritable and genetically correlated with SZ with deficits observed in unaffected first-degree relatives, thus meeting the key requirements as markers of genetic vulnerability (Greenwood et al. 2007; Calkins et al. 2010; Gur et al. 2007). A comparison of the heritability estimates of these measures across the three SZ family samples is shown in Fig. 3. These estimates range from 15 to 52%, and while individual measures show some degree of variability across the samples, the average heritability across all measures is identical across the samples at 31%. The cognitive deficits identified by CNB measures are also consistent between family-based and case–control studies, which tend to yield SZ patients with different underlying genetic architectures (e.g., polygenic vs. rare) (Gur et al. 2001b). For example, a comparison of SZ probands from the COGS family sample and singleton SZ cases from the COGS case–control sample revealed similar cognitive deficit profiles (Gur et al. 2015). However, despite overall profile similarity, the SZ

Table 1 Relationship of the CNB measures to domains and constructs defined by RDoC, as well as the corresponding brain regions identified through fMRI

RDoC domain	RDoC construct	CNB test	Behavior	Brain region(s)
Cognitive systems	Attention	Attention (ATT)	Attention, vigilance	Frontoparietal network
	Declarative memory	Verbal memory (VMEM)	Learning, recall, recognition	Frontal and bilateral anterior medial temporal lobe
		Face memory (FMEM)		
		Spatial memory (SMEM)		
	Cognitive control	Abstraction and mental flexibility (ABF)	Set-shifting	Prefrontal cortex; temporal, parietal, occipital regions
		Spatial processing (SPA) [a]	Spatial reasoning	Temporoparietal regions
Social processes	Social communication	Emotion processing (EMO)	Emotion identification	Temporolimbic regions
Sensorimotor systems	Motor actions	Sensorimotor processing (SM)	Motor praxis	

[a] Spatial reasoning ability reflects a complex cognitive function, like other aspects of reasoning and problem-solving ability. It involves aspects of several RDoC constructs, including visual perception and working memory

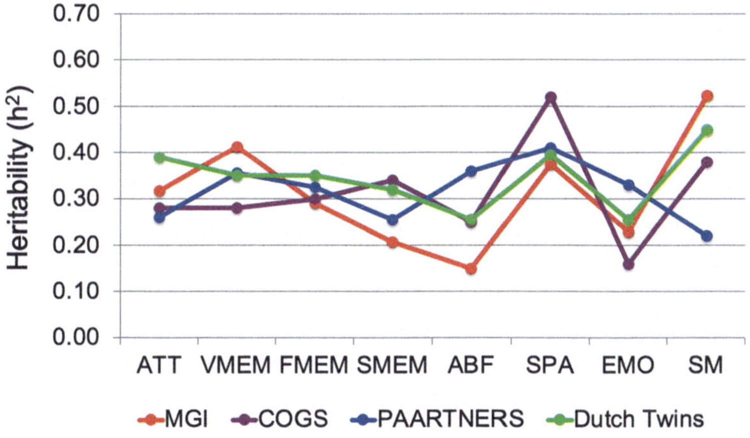

Fig. 3 Heritability estimates of the CNB measures described in Table 1 are consistent across three schizophrenia family-based samples (MGI, COGS, PAARTMNERS) and a population-representative sample (Dutch Twins). For all studies, the heritability of the efficiency of each measure is shown, estimated as the average of accuracy and speed

probands exhibited less cognitive impairment than the singleton cases, which correlated with reduced clinical severity and better real-world functioning (Gur et al. 2015).

The heritability estimates in SZ families produced by COGS, MGI, and PAARTNERS are not only similar to each other but also comparable to population-representative estimates obtained from the Dutch Twin Study of 1,140 participants (age 10–86) from 431 families (see Fig. 3) (Swagerman et al. 2016). A subsample of 246 Dutch participants also received the traditional Wechsler Adult Intelligence Scale (WAIS) for comparison. A latent factor representing the common variance across all CNB measures was found to be 70% heritable and highly correlated ($r = 0.82$) with a measure of total IQ derived from the WAIS (Swagerman et al. 2016). Thus, the CNB can provide an overall cognitive summary that is highly correlated with IQ, yet composed of neurobiologically meaningful parameters that can be further investigated to refine the genetic signal and implicate specific behavioral domains, which have been linked to brain systems through functional neuroimaging studies (see Table 1). Association, linkage, and sequencing studies of the COGS and MGI family samples have also shown that measures of cognitive dysfunction can help resolve the genetic architecture of SZ and offer mechanistic insight into the underlying neurobiological pathways (Greenwood et al. 2011, 2013; Almasy et al. 2008; Yokley et al. 2012; Prasad et al. 2010).

Initial genetic studies of the COGS families involved the investigation of 94 candidate genes for SZ through the use of a custom SNP genotyping array. In a subset of 534 participants from 130 families, the COGS identified 28 genes revealed evidence of association with at least one RDoC construct as captured by cognitive measures derived from the CNB (experiment-wide omnibus p-value <0.001). Examples of single gene associations with specific RDoC constructs included *GRIN3A* with attention, *GABRB2* with cognitive control, and both *GRIN2A* and *DRD3* with social communication. In contrast, 12 genes showed pleiotropic associations across three or more RDoC constructs, including *CTNNA2*, *ERBB4*, *GRID2*, *GRIK3*, *GRIN2B*, *GRM1*, *NOS1AP*, *NRG1*, *RELN*, *SLC1A2*, and *SLC6A3*. Most of these genes were also associated with other cognitive endophenotypes in the COGS sample, as well as in an independently ascertained case–control sample (Greenwood et al. 2011, 2012, 2016). This may be due in part to the observed correlations between many of the CNB measures (Greenwood et al. 2007). Alternatively, pleiotropic effects across multiple constructs may result from the hierarchy of the neurobiological systems involved in cognitive function (see Fig. 1). The perturbation of genes involved in neurodevelopment, for example, would be expected to have multiple downstream effects.

Subsequent linkage analyses of the full sample of 296 COGS families using a genome-wide SNP array identified many regions of at least suggestive evidence for linkage, with several prior candidate genes for SZ located beneath the linkage peaks (Greenwood et al. 2013). These findings generally centered around cognitive endophenotypes related to the RDoC constructs of attention (*ADORA2A*, *GRIK2 GRIN3A*), memory (*CSMD1*, *SLC6A3*, *YWHAE*), or both (*GRIN2B*, *HTR2A*). The linkage results did not show complete convergence with the previous candidate gene association results due to the interaction of a number of factors related to differences in sample composition, the portion of the genome assayed, the density of the coverage of specific genes provided by the different genotyping arrays, and the statistical methodologies that preferentially detect common variants (via association) or larger genomic segments that may be more rare but can be observed to segregate in families (via linkage). However, the linkage results for *GRIN3A*, *SLC6A3*, and *GRIN2B* in particular are in complete agreement with those reported for association. Although not present on the custom candidate gene array due to its large size, the relation of *CSMD1* to the memory construct in the SZ families is intriguing. *CSMD1* is a regulator of complement activation and synaptic pruning which is essential for synaptic plasticity and cognitive development (Stephan et al. 2012; Chung et al. 2015), and recent evidence suggests a role for *CSMD1* and the complement system in risk for SZ (Sekar et al. 2016; Kwon et al. 2013; Koiliari et al. 2014; Schizophrenia Psychiatric Genome-Wide Association Study (GWAS) Consortium 2011).

As summarized in Fig. 4, association and linkage results of the COGS families converge on a functional network dominated by genes involved in neuregulin and glutamate signaling, consistent with prevailing hypotheses regarding the importance of these pathways in the pathophysiology of SZ (Coyle 2006; Sodhi et al. 2008; Buonanno 2010; Silberberg et al. 2006; Stefansson et al. 2002; Hall et al. 2006; Hahn et al. 2006). L-glutamate is the major excitatory neurotransmitter in the mammalian brain and activates ionotropic (GRIDs, GRIKs, GRINs) and metabotropic (GRMs) glutamate receptors. Interestingly, triheteromeric assemblies of GluN1, GluN2A, and GluN2B subunits comprise over half of the N-methyl-D-aspartate (NMDA) receptors in the adult cortex and hippocampus (Rauner and Kohr 2011; Tovar et al. 2013), and the genes encoding these subunits (i.e., *GRIN1, GRIN2A, GRIN2B*) feature prominently in the analyses of cognitive deficits in SZ. *DLG4* is required for synaptic plasticity associated with NMDA receptor signaling, and changes in its expression alter the ratio of excitatory to inhibitory synapses in hippocampal neurons. *SLC1A2* encodes one of the major glutamate transporters, EAAT2 (excitatory amino acid transporter 2), which mediates the rapid reuptake of glutamate from the extracellular space, thereby preventing excitotoxicity and neuronal damage due to excessive activation. *NRG1* encodes a trophic factor that signals through the activation of the ErbB receptor tyrosine kinase encoded by *ERBB4* and plays a crucial role in neurodevelopment and in the modulation of NMDA receptor signaling (Ozaki et al. 1997; Anton et al. 2004). Studies have suggested that alterations in the NRG1-ErbB signaling pathway could account for the observed dysregulation of both glutamate and dopamine signaling in SZ (Li et al. 2007; Roy et al. 2007; Kwon et al. 2008), and this relationship is represented in the gene network as well. *DRD3* encodes the dopamine D3 receptor that is highly expressed in the limbic areas of the brain, which are associated with cognitive and emotional functions, and plays a critical role in cellular and synaptic plasticity throughout neurodevelopment. The D3 receptor is of particular interest as a potential mediator of aberrant dopaminergic neurotransmission and may be involved in the response to antipsychotics (Guma et al. 2019). Another key player in dopamine signaling is *SLC6A3*, the dopamine transporter (DAT), which is expressed most

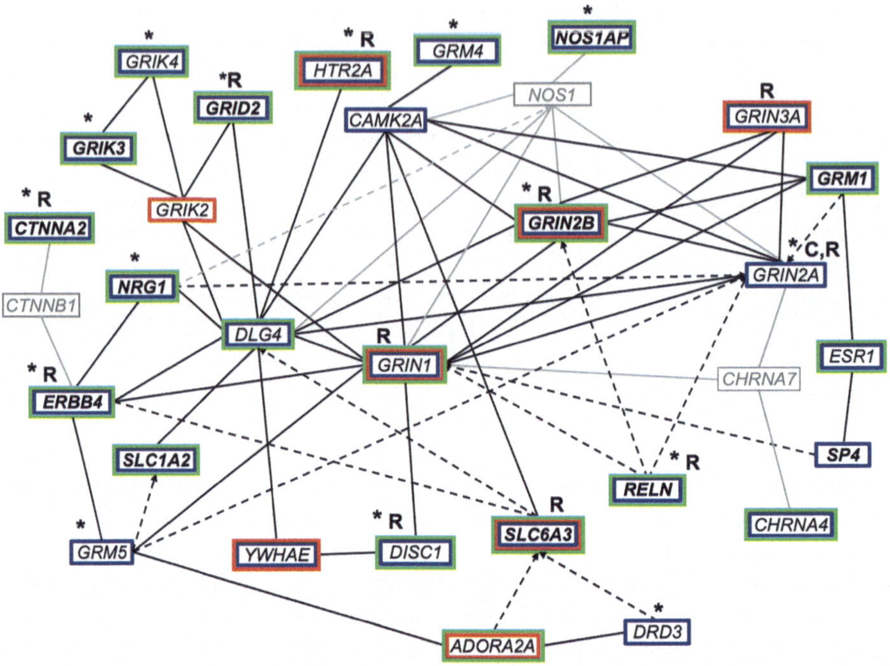

Fig. 4 Network of genes identified by COGS as contributing to cognitive dysfunction in SZ. Genes are represented as nodes with solid lines representing direct protein–protein interactions and dashed arrows representing more indirect effects on expression, activation, or inhibition. A blue box indicates genes associated with at least one RDoC construct in the COGS families, with those associated with three or more RDoC constructs in bold. A red box indicates genes identified through linkage of the COGS families. A green box indicates genes confirmed in the GWA study of the COGS case–control cohort. An asterisk (*) indicates associated with other measures of cognitive function in an independent sample. Genes identified for SZ diagnosis through GWA studies of common variants are indicated with a "C," whereas those identified by studies of rare and de novo variation are indicated with an "R." Note that *GABRB2* was also associated in the COGS sample and links into this network through *AKT1*, which is part of the *DISC1* interactome and has direct and indirect relationships with multiple genes in the network (not shown for simplicity). While *CSMD1* does not directly connect into the defined network, this gene was identified through linkage of the COGS families and is supported by multiple lines of evidence, including association analyses of the COGS case–control cohort and external studies of both common and rare variation in relation to SZ diagnosis

abundantly in the striatum and mediates the rapid clearance of dopamine from the synapse. A final notable aspect of this network is the convergence with the DISC1 Regulome. *DISC1* encodes a scaffolding protein that plays a critical role in cell signaling and neurodevelopment through its multiple interacting partners, which are collectively known as the DISC1 Interactome (Bradshaw and Porteous 2012; Camargo et al. 2007; Millar et al. 2003; Brandon and Sawa 2011). Disruption of the expression of *DISC1*, or its interactors, has been shown to alter the expression of another set of genes, known as the DISC1 Regulome, which is enriched for genes involved in neurodevelopment and synaptogenesis, as well as drug targets for psychiatric and neurological disorders (Hennah and Porteous 2009). Several genes in this network are members of the DISC1 Interactome or Regulome, including *YWHAE, ERBB4*, *NRG1*, *NOS1AP*, *GRIN1*, *GRIN2A*, *GRIN2B*, *SLC1A2,* and *SLC6A3* (Teng et al. 2018; Sialana et al. 2018). Collectively, these data suggest that alterations of the glutaminergic and dopaminergic signaling pathways, perhaps mediated by the DISC Regulome through NRG1-ERBB4 signaling, may be one pathway leading to the cognitive dysfunction observed in SZ, as depicted in Fig. 1.

Genomic studies of the CNB in the MGI sample of large, multiplex families provide points of alignment with the results from the COGS nuclear families. For example, specific variants within *NRG1* revealed associations with CNB measures related to memory (verbal memory in particular), cognitive control (mental flexibility), sensorimotor processing, and especially attention in the MGI families, the same constructs found to be associated in the COGS families (Yokley et al. 2012). Linkage analyses of the MGI families yielded significant evidence of linkage for cognitive control (mental flexibility) on chromosome 5q (LOD $= 3.4$, genome-wide $p = 0.011$), and a joint analysis with diagnosis suggested this region also influences SZ ($p = 0.0024$) (Almasy et al. 2008). Whole exome sequencing was subsequently performed for 134 individuals in the 8 MGI families showing linkage to the 5q region. Of the 407 non-synonymous coding variants identified, associations surviving multiple-test correction were found for two genes, *SYNPO* ($p = 0.0017$) and *WWC1* (i.e., *KIBRA*, $p = 0.0016$), which have known interactions (Kos et al. 2016). *WWC1* also interacts with *YWHAE*, and *SYNPO* is co-expressed with *GRIK5*, which directly interacts with *GRID2* and *GRIK2*. Intriguingly, *SYNPO* and *WWC1* flank the region on 5q containing *GABRB2*, which was found to be uniquely associated with construct of cognitive control in the COGS families. Results derived from the MGI families are thus consistent with those derived from COGS and converge on a common gene network.

Large-scale case–control studies examining common, rare, and de novo variation in SZ offer independent support for many genes implicated through linkage and association studies of cognitive endophenotypes in SZ families. For example, a large GWA study of SZ diagnosis conducted by the Psychiatric Genomics Consortium (PGC) identified associations with *CSMD1*, *GRIN2A*, and *GRIN3A* (Schizophrenia Working Group of the Psychiatric Genomics Consortium 2014). *ERBB4* was among the top GWA findings in the Molecular Genetics of Schizophrenia African-American cohort, supporting overlapping signals across ancestral backgrounds (Shi et al. 2009). Other studies of SZ diagnosis have shown a significant burden of rare variants in *GRIN1*, *GRIN3A*, and *SLC1A2* in SZ patients (Purcell et al. 2014; Fiorentino et al. 2015), as well as a disproportionate disruption of genes in the neuregulin and glutamate pathways (Walsh et al. 2008; Kirov et al. 2012). Studies of de novo variation have implicated *CSMD1*, *CTNNA2*, *DISC1*, *GRID2*, *GRIN2B*, *HTR2A*, *RELN*, and *SLC6A3* in SZ and related disorders (Fromer et al. 2014; Neale et al. 2012; O'roak et al. 2012; Sanders et al. 2012; De Ligt et al. 2012). These findings from large-scale genomic studies of SZ diagnosis thus strengthen the evidence from candidate gene association, linkage, and sequencing analyses of cognitive endophenotypes in SZ family samples implicating glutamatergic neurotransmission and synaptic plasticity pathways in mediating SZ susceptibility. The convergence of genes and pathways arising through these different approaches is key, as genomic studies of cognitive endophenotypes, even in the context of SZ families, may identify variants influencing normal variation in cognitive functioning that do not necessarily increase SZ risk.

Most recently, a GWA study evaluating cognitive endophenotypes in 1,533 participants from the COGS case–control cohort identified six independent regions exceeding the standard genome-wide significance threshold ($p < 5 \times 10^{-8}$) with a mean effect size of 0.70 (Greenwood et al. 2019b). These regions harbor genes that appear to play a role in key cellular and neurodevelopmental processes and have previously shown association with SZ and related disorders. For example, *BASP1* on 5p15 (attention) is involved in neuronal axon growth and guidance and has previously been identified in a GWA study of mood-incongruent psychotic symptoms in bipolar disorder (Goes et al. 2012). *KIF15*on 3p21 (declarative memory, face memory) co-localizes in dendrites and growth cones of axons with microtubules, is differentially expressed in fetal vs. mature astrocytes (Zhang et al. 2016), and is a target of the micro RNA miR-192-5p that is down-regulated in people with SZ (Vachev et al. 2016). *CCNE1* on 19q12 (spatial processing) is another gene in the *DISC1* regulome and has been shown to be upregulated in SZ (Teng et al. 2018; Sun et al. 2015). *C9orf135* on 9q21 (motor actions, sensorimotor processing) has previously been implicated in subsyndromal deficits in cognitive function (Seshadri et al. 2007), as well as cognitive outcome in Parkinson's disease (Chung et al. 2012).

A prime example of the value of cognitive endophenotypes in linking genes to observable symptoms in SZ is provided by the association of cognitive control (mental flexibility) to *NRG3* on chromosome 10q23. Like *NRG1*, which was similarly associated with cognitive control in both the COGS and MGI families, *NRG3* influences neuroblast proliferation, migration, and differentiation by signaling through *ERBB4* and has been associated with SZ in several studies (Kao et al. 2010; Chen et al. 2009; Morar et al. 2011; Benzel et al. 2007). Genetic variants of *NRG3* are also associated with cognitive functioning and psychotic symptom severity, accompanied by increased expression of *NRG3* in the prefrontal cortex (Kao et al. 2010; Tost et al. 2014; Paterson and Law 2014). Furthermore, *NRG3* knockout mice exhibit neurobehavioral alterations that are consistent with aspects of SZ in humans, including novelty-induced hyperactivity, impaired sensorimotor gating, and attenuated fear conditioning, the latter of which may reflect deficiencies in learning and memory (Hayes et al. 2016). These data augment prior reports of association for *NRG1* and *ERBB4*, suggesting that pathogenic variation in the NRG-ErbB pathway may underlie both cognitive functioning and risk for psychosis (Greenwood et al. 2011, 2016; Stefansson et al. 2002; Benzel et al. 2007; Hatzimanolis et al. 2013; Law et al. 2007).

GWA study results of cognitive deficits in SZ have thus identified promising associations for multiple genomic regions and genes involved in critical neurodevelopmental processes. If we apply the enrichment threshold that has been suggested to identify SNPs that regulate gene expression ($p < 10^{-4}$) (Morrow et al.

2018; Wang et al. 2016), we additionally find that most of the genes previously identified through linkage and association analyses of the COGS family cohort (Fig. 4) were at least nominally significant in the COGS GWA of singleton SZ cases and unaffected controls, including nearly all genes that were pleiotropic across three or more RDoC constructs (Greenwood et al. 2011, 2013, 2016). Notably, candidate gene associations observed for specific RDoC constructs in the COGS families were replicated in the COGS case–control cohort, including the associations of both *NRG1* and *ERBB4* with measures of declarative memory, *GRM1* with cognitive control (mental flexibility), and both *NRG1* and *SLC6A3* with motor actions (sensorimotor processing). Additionally, two SNPs in *WWC1,* a gene originally implicated in cognitive control through linkage and sequencing of the MGI sample, were associated with the same construct in the COGS GWA study. Furthermore, 25 of the 108 regions identified by the large-scale PGC study of SZ diagnosis were associated with one or more construct in COGS (Schizophrenia Working Group of the Psychiatric Genomics Consortium 2014; Greenwood et al. 2019b). Such convergence at the pathway level may be more likely to be observed and more meaningful than concordance at the level of an individual gene or SNP in understanding the neurobiological basis of cognitive dysfunction in SZ.

Despite falling just short of genome-wide significance in these initial analyses, the association of declarative memory, specifically spatial memory, with *HCN1* (5p12, $p = 8.3 \times 10^{-8}$) is one of the more intriguing findings that nicely illustrates the potential power of endophenotypes in genomic analyses. *HCN1* is highly expressed in the frontal cortex and regulates neuronal excitability and synaptic plasticity. Large-scale studies of common variation in *HCN1* have revealed associations with SZ diagnosis and educational attainment, whereas rare and de novo variants are associated with a broad phenotypic spectrum that includes neonatal epileptic encephalopathy, generalized seizures, intellectual disability, and autistic spectrum disorders (Schizophrenia Working Group of the Psychiatric Genomics Consortium 2014; Nava et al. 2014; Okbay et al. 2016; Marini et al. 2018). Studies of *HCN1* knockout mice have suggested a role for this gene in spatial learning and memory (Nolan et al. 2004; Thuault et al. 2013), and altered hippocampal expression of *HCN1* in rats is associated with impairments in spatial learning and memory (Zhou et al. 2015). As this example so nicely illustrates, genomic studies of specific cognitive deficits in SZ may provide the necessary biological specificity to enhance the interpretation of large case–control GWA studies and suggest actionable targets for the development of procognitive treatments.

5 Conclusions and Future Directions

SZ is a clinically heterogeneous disorder in which patients exhibit a broad range of deficits and symptom severity, and this profound heterogeneity has complicated efforts to identify genetic risk variants. Traditional case–control studies collapse the substantial phenotypic variation in SZ into a single, categorical diagnosis. However, studies have shown that phenotypic specificity is more important than sample size for detecting true associations in genetic studies of complex diseases (Liang and Greenwood 2015; Manchia et al. 2013). Cognitive endophenotypes can deliver this phenotypic specificity and can help parse the complex etiology of SZ into discreet neurobiological functions, thereby reducing the associated genetic heterogeneity and facilitating the identification of novel genetic risk variants and aberrant molecular pathways (Gottesman and Gould 2003; Braff et al. 2007; Insel and Cuthbert 2009). Furthermore, the RDoC framework may provide a common language for identifying such specific domains so that findings can be readily compared across studies. By capitalizing on the inherent power advantages of such quantitative traits, the analysis of cognitive dysfunction in SZ also requires a substantially smaller sample size to achieve comparable power to an analysis of diagnosis. Although the assessment of cognitive functioning may incur an additional burden at the time of recruitment, the potential payoff suggests that it is well worth the effort.

An endophenotype strategy implemented through the RDoC framework thus complements traditional studies of SZ diagnosis by providing the necessary biological context for interpretation of the observed associations and helping to translate genetic findings into actionable treatment targets, which will ultimately facilitate precision medicine in SZ. Linkage and association analyses of specific cognitive endophenotypes representing several RDoC constructs have implicated a network of genes related to neuregulin and glutamate signaling pathways and synaptic plasticity as underlying liability to SZ (Greenwood et al. 2011, 2013, 2016, 2019b; Almasy et al. 2008; Yokley et al. 2012), consistent with the findings of case–control studies evaluating common, rare, and de novo variation in relation to SZ diagnosis (Schizophrenia Working Group of the Psychiatric Genomics Consortium 2014; Walsh et al. 2008; Kirov et al. 2012). By using polygenic scoring and enrichment methods and leveraging existing large-scale analyses of SZ diagnosis, we can assess how much of the common genetic risk is shared between SZ and a particular construct (International Schizophrenia Consortium 2009; Hart et al. 2014). In addition to estimating the overall genetic correlation, we can also investigate whether individual SNPs that increase the risk for SZ overlap more than we would expect by chance with SNPs that result in deficits in discrete aspects of cognitive functioning. Endophenotypes are also well-suited to multivariate methods, which can be used to identify individual phenotypic profiles and classify subgroups of SZ patients with a similar etiology (Clementz et al. 2016). Methods that can simultaneously incorporate both phenotypic and genomic information may prove particularly useful in this regard (Arnedo et al. 2015). The identified subgroups can then be evaluated in terms of illness severity, clinical course, medication response, and other factors to establish individualized treatment protocols. By investigating the relationship of clinical, genetic, and environmental factors to subgroups defined by RDoC constructs, which reflect the underlying neurobiological dysfunctions, we may gain a better understanding of the "Group of Schizophrenias."

The use of cognitive endophenotypes to go beyond the broad clinical diagnostic category of SZ will undoubtedly facilitate the identification of novel pathways leading from genetic variation to brain dysfunction. While genes associated with cognitive dysfunction may not necessarily increase SZ risk per se, cognitive deficits are debilitating in and of themselves and lead to functional disability. Thus, a better understanding of the genetic underpinnings of cognitive dysfunction, arguably the most salient feature of SZ, will provide a molecular roadmap to guide the development of novel pharmacological interventions aimed at improving real-world functioning, as well as inform precision-based treatment strategies (Green et al. 2000; Green 1996).

References

Abecasis GR, Cookson WO, Cardon LR (2001) The power to detect linkage disequilibrium with quantitative traits in selected samples. Am J Hum Genet 68(6):1463–1474

Adler CM, Sax KW, Holland SK, Schmithorst V, Rosenberg L, Strakowski SM (2001) Changes in neuronal activation with increasing attention demand in healthy volunteers: an fMRI study. Synapse 42(4):266–272

Almasy L, Gur RC, Haack K et al (2008) A genome screen for quantitative trait loci influencing schizophrenia and neurocognitive phenotypes. Am J Psychiatry 165(9):1185–1192

Altshuler D, Daly MJ, Lander ES (2008) Genetic mapping in human disease. Science 322(5903): 881–888

Anton ES, Ghashghaei HT, Weber J et al (2004) Receptor tyrosine kinase Erbb4 modulates neuroblast migration and placement in the adult forebrain. Nat Neurosci 7(12):1319–1328

Arnedo J, Svrakic DM, Del Val C et al (2015) Uncovering the hidden risk architecture of the schizophrenias: confirmation in three independent genome-wide association studies. Am J Psychiatry 172(2):139–153

Baron M (2001) Genetics of schizophrenia and the new millennium: progress and pitfalls. Am J Hum Genet 68(2):299–312

Benzel I, Bansal A, Browning B et al (2007) Interactions among genes in the ErbB-Neuregulin signalling network are associated with increased susceptibility to schizophrenia. Behav Brain Funct 3:31

Bitter I, Feher L, Tenyi T, Czobor P (2015) Treatment adherence and insight in schizophrenia. Psychiatr Hung 30(1):18–26

Blangero J, Williams JT, Almasy L (2003) Novel family-based approaches to genetic risk in thrombosis. J Thromb Haemost 1(7):1391–1397

Bleuler E (1911) Dementia praecox or the group of schizophrenias. In: Zinkin J, Trans. International Universities Press, New York, 1950

Bradshaw NJ, Porteous DJ (2012) Disc1-binding proteins in neural development, signalling and schizophrenia. Neuropharmacology 62(3):1230–1241

Braff D (2017) Nimh neuropsychiatric genomics: crucial foundational accomplishments and the extensive challenges that remain. Mol Psychiatry 22(12):1656–1658

Braff D, Freedman R (2002) The importance of endophenotypes in studies of the genetics of schizophrenia. In: Davis K, Charney D, Coyle JT, Nemeroff C (eds) Neuropsychopharmacology: the fifth generation of progress. Lippincott, Williams and Wilkins, Baltimore, pp 703–716

Braff D, Schork NJ, Gottesman II (2007) Endophenotyping schizophrenia. Am J Psychiatry 164(5): 705–707

Braff D, Greenwood TA, Swerdlow NR, Light GA, Schork NJ (2008) Investigators of the consortium on the genetics of S. advances in endophenotyping schizophrenia. World Psychiatry 7(1):11–18

Brandon NJ, Sawa A (2011) Linking neurodevelopmental and synaptic theories of mental illness through Disc1. Nat Rev Neurosci 12(12):707–722
Buonanno A (2010) The neuregulin signaling pathway and schizophrenia: from genes to synapses and neural circuits. Brain Res Bull 83(3–4):122–131
Calkins ME, Tepper P, Gur RC et al (2010) Project among African-Americans to explore risks for schizophrenia (Paartners): evidence for impairment and heritability of neurocognitive functioning in families of schizophrenia patients. Am J Psychiatry 167(4):459–472
Camargo LM, Collura V, Rain JC et al (2007) Disrupted in schizophrenia 1 Interactome: evidence for the close connectivity of risk genes and a potential synaptic basis for schizophrenia. Mol Psychiatry 12(1):74–86
Cannon TD, Keller MC (2006) Endophenotypes in the genetic analyses of mental disorders. Annu Rev Clin Psychol 2:267–290
Cannon M, Caspi A, Moffitt TE et al (2002) Evidence for early-childhood, pan-developmental impairment specific to schizophreniform disorder: results from a longitudinal birth cohort. Arch Gen Psychiatry 59(5):449–456
Cannon M, Moffitt TE, Caspi A, Murray RM, Harrington H, Poulton R (2006) Neuropsychological performance at the age of 13 years and adult schizophreniform disorder: prospective birth cohort study. Br J Psychiatry 189:463–464
Chen P, Avramopoulos D, Lasseter VK et al (2009) Fine mapping on chromosome 10q22-Q23 implicates Neuregulin 3 in schizophrenia. Am J Hum Genet 84(1):21–34
Chung SJ, Armasu SM, Biernacka JM et al (2012) Genomic determinants of motor and cognitive outcomes in Parkinson's disease. Parkinsonism Relat Disord 18(7):881–886
Chung WS, Welsh CA, Barres BA, Stevens B (2015) Do glia drive synaptic and cognitive impairment in disease? Nat Neurosci 18(11):1539–1545
Clementz BA, Sweeney JA, Hamm JP et al (2016) Identification of distinct psychosis biotypes using brain-based biomarkers. Am J Psychiatry 173(4):373–384
Coyle JT (2006) Glutamate and schizophrenia: beyond the dopamine hypothesis. Cell Mol Neurobiol 26(4–6):365–384
Crone EA, Zanolie K, Van Leijenhorst L, Westenberg PM, Rombouts SA (2008) Neural mechanisms supporting flexible performance adjustment during development. Cogn Affect Behav Neurosci 8(2):165–177
Cuthbert BN, Insel TR (2010) Toward new approaches to psychotic disorders: the Nimh research domain criteria project. Schizophr Bull 36(6):1061–1062
De Ligt J, Willemsen MH, Van Bon BW et al (2012) Diagnostic exome sequencing in persons with severe intellectual disability. N Engl J Med 367(20):1921–1929
Derntl B, Windischberger C, Robinson S et al (2008) Facial emotion recognition and amygdala activation are associated with menstrual cycle phase. Psychoneuroendocrinology 33(8): 1031–1040
Elvevag B, Goldberg TE (2000) Cognitive impairment in schizophrenia is the core of the disorder. Crit Rev Neurobiol 14(1):1–21
Falconer DS (1960) An introduction to quantitative genetics. Ronald Press Co, New York
Fiorentino A, Sharp SI, Mcquillin A (2015) Association of rare variation in the glutamate receptor gene Slc1a2 with susceptibility to bipolar disorder and schizophrenia. Eur J Hum Genet 23(9): 1200–1206
Fromer M, Pocklington AJ, Kavanagh DH et al (2014) De novo mutations in schizophrenia implicate synaptic networks. Nature 506(7487):179–184
Glahn DC, Knowles EE, Mckay DR et al (2014) Arguments for the sake of endophenotypes: examining common misconceptions about the use of endophenotypes in psychiatric genetics. Am J Med Genet B Neuropsychiatr Genet 165b(2):122–130
Goes FS, Hamshere M, Seifuddin F et al (2012) Genome-wide association of mood-incongruent psychotic bipolar disorder. Transl Psychiatry 2:E180
Gogos JA, Gerber DJ (2006) Schizophrenia susceptibility genes: emergence of positional candidates and future directions. Trends Pharmacol Sci 27(4):226–233

Gottesman II, Gould TD (2003) The endophenotype concept in psychiatry: etymology and strategic intentions. Am J Psychiatry 160(4):636–645

Gottesman II, Shields J (1967) A polygenic theory of schizophrenia. Proc Natl Acad Sci U S A 58(1):199–205

Gottesman I, Shields J (1972) Schizophrenia and genetics: a twin study vantage point. Academic Press, New York

Green MF (1996) What are the functional consequences of neurocognitive deficits in schizophrenia? Am J Psychiatry 153(3):321–330

Green MF, Kern RS, Braff D, Mintz J (2000) Neurocognitive deficits and functional outcome in schizophrenia: are we measuring the "Right Stuff"? Schizophr Bull 26(1):119–136

Greenwood TA, Braff D, Light GA et al (2007) Initial heritability analyses of endophenotypic measures for schizophrenia: the consortium on the genetics of schizophrenia. Arch Gen Psychiatry 64(11):1242–1250

Greenwood TA, Lazzeroni LC, Murray SS et al (2011) Analysis of 94 candidate genes and 12 endophenotypes for schizophrenia from the consortium on the genetics of schizophrenia. Am J Psychiatry 168(9):930–946

Greenwood TA, Light GA, Swerdlow NR, Radant AD, Braff D (2012) Association analysis of 94 candidate genes and schizophrenia-related endophenotypes. PLoS One 7(1):E29630

Greenwood TA, Swerdlow NR, Gur RE et al (2013) Genome-wide linkage analyses of 12 endophenotypes for schizophrenia from the consortium on the genetics of schizophrenia. Am J Psychiatry 170(5):521–532

Greenwood TA, Lazzeroni LC, Calkins ME et al (2016) Genetic assessment of additional endophenotypes from the consortium on the genetics of schizophrenia family study. Schizophr Res 170(1):30–40

Greenwood TA, Shutes-David A, Tsuang DW (2019a) Endophenotypes in schizophrenia: digging deeper to identify genetic mechanisms. J Psychiatr Brain Sci 4(2)

Greenwood TA, Lazzeroni LC, Maihofer AX et al (2019b) Genome-wide association of endophenotypes for schizophrenia from the consortium on the genetics of schizophrenia (Cogs). JAMA Psychiat 76(12):1–11

Guma E, Rocchetti J, Devenyi GA et al (2019) Role of D3 dopamine receptors in modulating neuroanatomical changes in response to antipsychotic administration. Sci Rep 9(1):7850

Gur RC, Gur RE, Obrist WD et al (1982) Sex and handedness differences in cerebral blood flow during rest and cognitive activity. Science 217(4560):659–661

Gur RC, Ragland JD, Mozley LH et al (1997) Lateralized changes in regional cerebral blood flow during performance of verbal and facial recognition tasks: correlations with performance and "Effort". Brain Cogn 33(3):388–414

Gur RC, Alsop D, Glahn D et al (2000) An fMRI study of sex differences in regional activation to a verbal and a spatial task. Brain Lang 74(2):157–170

Gur RC, Ragland JD, Moberg PJ et al (2001a) Computerized neurocognitive scanning: I. Methodology and validation in healthy people. Neuropsychopharmacology 25(5):766–776

Gur RC, Ragland JD, Moberg PJ et al (2001b) Computerized neurocognitive scanning: II. The profile of schizophrenia. *Neuropsychopharmacology* 25(5):777–788

Gur RC, Schroeder L, Turner T et al (2002) Brain activation during facial emotion processing. Neuroimage 16(3 Pt 1):651–662

Gur RE, Nimgaonkar V, Almasy L et al (2007) Neurocognitive endophenotypes in a multiplex multigenerational family study of schizophrenia. Am J Psychiatry 164(5):813–819

Gur RC, Richard J, Hughett P et al (2010) A cognitive neuroscience-based computerized battery for efficient measurement of individual differences: standardization and initial construct validation. J Neurosci Methods 187(2):254–262

Gur RC, Richard J, Calkins ME et al (2012) Age group and sex differences in performance on a computerized neurocognitive battery in children age 8-21. Neuropsychology 26(2):251–265

Gur RC, Calkins ME, Satterthwaite TD et al (2014) Neurocognitive growth charting in psychosis spectrum youths. JAMA Psychiat 71(4):366–374

Gur RC, Braff D, Calkins ME et al (2015) Neurocognitive performance in family-based and case-control studies of schizophrenia. Schizophr Res 163(1–3):17–23
Hagenaars SP, Harris SE, Davies G et al (2016) Shared genetic Aetiology between cognitive functions and physical and mental health in UK Biobank (N=112 151) and 24 GWAS consortia. Mol Psychiatry 21(11):1624–1632
Hahn CG, Wang HY, Cho DS et al (2006) Altered neuregulin 1-Erbb4 signaling contributes to Nmda receptor hypofunction in schizophrenia. Nat Med 12(7):824–828
Hall J, Whalley HC, Job DE et al (2006) A neuregulin 1 variant associated with abnormal cortical function and psychotic symptoms. Nat Neurosci 9(12):1477–1478
Harrison PJ, Weinberger DR (2005) Schizophrenia genes, gene expression, and neuropathology: on the matter of their convergence. Mol Psychiatry 10(1):40–68. Image 45
Hart AB, Gamazon ER, Engelhardt BE et al (2014) Genetic variation associated with euphorigenic effects of D-amphetamine is associated with diminished risk for schizophrenia and attention deficit hyperactivity disorder. Proc Natl Acad Sci U S A 111(16):5968–5973
Hatzimanolis A, Mcgrath JA, Wang R et al (2013) Multiple variants aggregate in the Neuregulin signaling pathway in a subset of schizophrenia patients. Transl Psychiatry 3:E264
Hayes LN, Shevelkin A, Zeledon M et al (2016) Neuregulin 3 knockout mice exhibit behaviors consistent with psychotic disorders. *Mol.* Neuropsychiatry 2(2):79–87
Hennah W, Porteous D (2009) The Disc1 pathway modulates expression of neurodevelopmental, synaptogenic and sensory perception genes. PLoS One 4(3):E4906
Hubbard L, Tansey KE, Rai D et al (2016) Evidence of common genetic overlap between schizophrenia and cognition. Schizophr Bull 42(3):832–842
Insel TR, Cuthbert BN (2009) Endophenotypes: bridging genomic complexity and disorder heterogeneity. Biol Psychiatry 66(11):988–989
Insel T, Cuthbert B, Garvey M et al (2010) Research domain criteria (RDoC): toward a new classification framework for research on mental disorders. Am J Psychiatry 167(7):748–751
International Schizophrenia Consortium (2009) Common polygenic variation contributes to risk of schizophrenia and bipolar disorder. Nature 460(7256):748–752
Jackson O, Schacter D (2004) Encoding activity in anterior medial temporal lobe supports subsequent associative recognition. Neuroimage 21(1):456–462
Kao WT, Wang Y, Kleinman JE et al (2010) Common genetic variation in Neuregulin 3 (Nrg3) influences risk for schizophrenia and impacts Nrg3 expression in human brain. Proc Natl Acad Sci U S A 107(35):15619–15624
Kern RS, Nuechterlein KH, Green MF et al (2008) The matrics consensus cognitive battery, part 2: co-norming and standardization. Am J Psychiatry 165(2):214–220
Kirov G, Pocklington AJ, Holmans P et al (2012) De novo CNV analysis implicates specific abnormalities of postsynaptic signalling complexes in the pathogenesis of schizophrenia. Mol Psychiatry 17(2):142–153
Koiliari E, Roussos P, Pasparakis E et al (2014) The Csmd1 genome-wide associated schizophrenia risk variant Rs10503253 affects general cognitive ability and executive function in healthy males. Schizophr Res 154(1–3):42–47
Kos MZ, Carless MA, Peralta J et al (2016) Exome sequence data from multigenerational families implicate Ampa receptor trafficking in neurocognitive impairment and schizophrenia risk. Schizophr Bull 42(2):288–300
Kwon OB, Paredes D, Gonzalez CM et al (2008) Neuregulin-1 regulates Ltp at Ca1 hippocampal synapses through activation of dopamine D4 receptors. Proc Natl Acad Sci U S A 105(40): 15587–15592
Kwon E, Wang W, Tsai LH (2013) Validation of schizophrenia-associated genes Csmd1, C10orf26, Cacna1c and Tcf4 as Mir-137 targets. Mol Psychiatry 18(1):11–12
Law AJ, Kleinman JE, Weinberger DR, Weickert CS (2007) Disease-associated intronic variants in the Erbb4 gene are related to altered Erbb4 splice-variant expression in the brain in schizophrenia. Hum Mol Genet 16(2):129–141

Lee SH, Wray NR (2013) Novel genetic analysis for case-control genome-wide association studies: quantification of power and genomic prediction accuracy. PLoS One 8(8):E71494
Lencz T, Knowles E, Davies G et al (2014) Molecular genetic evidence for overlap between general cognitive ability and risk for schizophrenia: a report from the cognitive genomics consortium (cogent). Mol Psychiatry 19(2):168–174
Lewis CM, Levinson DF, Wise LH et al (2003) Genome scan meta-analysis of schizophrenia and bipolar disorder, part II: schizophrenia. Am J Hum Genet 73(1):34–48
Li B, Woo RS, Mei L, Malinow R (2007) The Neuregulin-1 receptor Erbb4 controls glutamatergic synapse maturation and plasticity. Neuron 54(4):583–597
Liang SG, Greenwood TA (2015) The impact of clinical heterogeneity in schizophrenia on genomic analyses. Schizophr Res 161(2–3):490–495
Lichtenstein P, Yip BH, Bjork C et al (2009) Common genetic determinants of schizophrenia and bipolar disorder in Swedish families: a population-based study. Lancet 373(9659):234–239
Lieberman JA, Stroup TS, Mcevoy JP et al (2005) Effectiveness of antipsychotic drugs in patients with chronic schizophrenia. N Engl J Med 353(12):1209–1223
Manchia M, Cullis J, Turecki G, Rouleau GA, Uher R, Alda M (2013) The impact of phenotypic and genetic heterogeneity on results of genome wide association studies of complex diseases. PLoS One 8(10):E76295
Manolio TA, Collins FS, Cox NJ et al (2009) Finding the missing heritability of complex diseases. Nature 461(7265):747–753
Marenco S, Coppola R, Daniel DG, Zigun JR, Weinberger DR (1993) Regional cerebral blood flow during the Wisconsin card sorting test in Normal subjects studied by Xenon-133 dynamic Spect: comparison of absolute values, percent distribution values, and covariance analysis. Psychiatry Res 50(3):177–192
Marini C, Porro A, Rastetter A et al (2018) Hcn1 mutation spectrum: from neonatal epileptic encephalopathy to benign generalized epilepsy and beyond. Brain 141(11):3160–3178
Mcintosh AM, Gow A, Luciano M et al (2013) Polygenic risk for schizophrenia is associated with cognitive change between childhood and old age. Biol Psychiatry 73(10):938–943
Millar JK, Christie S, Porteous DJ (2003) Yeast two-hybrid screens implicate Disc1 in brain development and function. Biochem Biophys Res Commun 311(4):1019–1025
Morar B, Dragovic M, Waters FA, Chandler D, Kalaydjieva L, Jablensky A (2011) Neuregulin 3 (Nrg3) as a susceptibility gene in a schizophrenia subtype with florid delusions and relatively spared cognition. Mol Psychiatry 16(8):860–866
Morrow JD, Cho MH, Platig J et al (2018) Ensemble genomic analysis in human lung tissue identifies novel genes for chronic obstructive pulmonary disease. Hum Genomics 12(1):1
Moser E, Derntl B, Robinson S, Fink B, Gur RC, Grammer K (2007) Amygdala activation at 3t in response to human and avatar facial expressions of emotions. J Neurosci Methods 161(1): 126–133
Nava C, Dalle C, Rastetter A et al (2014) De novo mutations in Hcn1 cause early infantile epileptic encephalopathy. Nat Genet 46(6):640–645
Neale BM, Kou Y, Liu L et al (2012) Patterns and rates of exonic de novo mutations in autism Spectrum disorders. Nature 485(7397):242–245
Nolan MF, Malleret G, Dudman JT et al (2004) A behavioral role for dendritic integration: Hcn1 channels constrain spatial memory and plasticity at inputs to distal dendrites of Ca1 pyramidal neurons. Cell 119(5):719–732
Nuechterlein KH, Green MF, Kern RS et al (2008) The matrics consensus cognitive battery, part 1: test selection, reliability, and validity. Am J Psychiatry 165(2):203–213
O'donovan MC, Craddock N, Norton N et al (2008) Identification of loci associated with schizophrenia by genome-wide association and follow-up. Nat Genet 40(9):1053–1055
O'roak BJ, Vives L, Girirajan S et al (2012) Sporadic autism exomes reveal a highly interconnected protein network of de novo mutations. Nature 485(7397):246–250
Ogg RJ, Zou P, Allen DN, Hutchins SB, Dutkiewicz RM, Mulhern RK (2008) Neural correlates of a clinical continuous performance test. Magn Reson Imaging 26(4):504–512

Okbay A, Beauchamp JP, Fontana MA et al (2016) Genome-wide association study identifies 74 loci associated with educational attainment. Nature 533(7604):539–542
Owen MJ, Williams NM, O'donovan MC (2004) The molecular genetics of schizophrenia: new findings promise new insights. Mol Psychiatry 9(1):14–27
Ozaki M, Sasner M, Yano R, Lu HS, Buonanno A (1997) Neuregulin-beta induces expression of an Nmda-receptor subunit. Nature 390(6661):691–694
Paterson C, Law AJ (2014) Transient overexposure of Neuregulin 3 during early postnatal development impacts selective behaviors in adulthood. PLoS One 9(8):E104172
Plomin R, Haworth CM, Davis OS (2009) Common disorders are quantitative traits. Nat Rev Genet 10(12):872–878
Prasad KM, Almasy L, Gur RC et al (2010) Rgs4 polymorphisms associated with variability of cognitive performance in a family-based schizophrenia sample. Schizophr Bull 36(5):983–990
Purcell SM, Moran J, Fromer M et al (2014) A polygenic burden of rare disruptive mutations in schizophrenia. Nature 506(7487):185–190
Rauner C, Kohr G (2011) Triheteromeric Nr1/Nr2a/Nr2b receptors constitute the major N-methyl-D-aspartate receptor population in adult hippocampal synapses. J Biol Chem 286(9):7558–7566
Reichenberg A, Mollon J (2016) Challenges and opportunities in studies of cognition in the prodrome to psychosis: no detail is too small. JAMA Psychiat 73(12):1249–1250
Rietveld CA, Medland SE, Derringer J et al (2013) GWAS of 126,559 individuals identifies genetic variants associated with educational attainment. Science 340(6139):1467–1471
Ripke S, O'dushlaine C, Chambert K et al (2013) Genome-wide association analysis identifies 13 new risk loci for schizophrenia. Nat Genet 45(10):1150–1159
Roalf DR, Ruparel K, Gur RE et al (2014) Neuroimaging predictors of cognitive performance across a standardized neurocognitive battery. Neuropsychology 28(2):161–176
Roy K, Murtie JC, El-Khodor BF et al (2007) Loss of erbB signaling in oligodendrocytes alters myelin and dopaminergic function, a potential mechanism for neuropsychiatric disorders. Proc Natl Acad Sci U S A 104(19):8131–8136
Sanders SJ, Murtha MT, Gupta AR et al (2012) De novo mutations revealed by whole-exome sequencing are strongly associated with autism. Nature 485(7397):237–241
Saykin AJ, Gur RC, Gur RE et al (1991) Neuropsychological function in schizophrenia. Selective impairment in memory and learning. Arch Gen Psychiatry 48(7):618–624
Saykin AJ, Shtasel D, Gur RE et al (1994) Neuropsychological deficits in neuroleptic naive patients with first-episode schizophrenia. Arch Gen Psychiatry 51(2):124–131
Schizophrenia Psychiatric Genome-Wide Association Study (GWAS) Consortium (2011) Genome-wide association study identifies five new schizophrenia loci. Nat Genet 43(10):969–976
Schizophrenia Working Group of the Psychiatric Genomics Consortium (2014) Biological insights from 108 schizophrenia-associated genetic loci. Nature 511:421–427
Schwab SG, Wildenauer DB (2013) Genetics of psychiatric disorders in the GWAS era: an update on schizophrenia. Eur Arch Psychiatry Clin Neurosci 263(Suppl 2):S147–S154
Seidman LJ, Shapiro DI, Stone WS et al (2016) Association of neurocognition with transition to psychosis: baseline functioning in the second phase of the north American Prodrome longitudinal study. JAMA Psychiat 73(12):1239–1248
Sekar A, Bialas AR, De Rivera H et al (2016) Schizophrenia risk from complex variation of complement component 4. Nature 530(7589):177–183
Seshadri S, Destefano A, Au R et al (2007) Genetic correlates of brain aging on MRI and cognitive test measures: a genome-wide association and linkage analysis in the Framingham study. BMC Med Genet 8(Suppl 1):S15
Shi J, Levinson DF, Duan J et al (2009) Common variants on chromosome 6p22.1 are associated with schizophrenia. Nature 460(7256):753–757
Sialana FJ, Wang AL, Fazari B et al (2018) Quantitative proteomics of Synaptosomal fractions in a rat overexpressing human Disc1 gene indicates profound synaptic dysregulation in the dorsal striatum. Front Mol Neurosci 11:26

Silberberg G, Darvasi A, Pinkas-Kramarski R, Navon R (2006) The involvement of Erbb4 with schizophrenia: association and expression studies. Am J Med Genet B Neuropsychiatr Genet 141(2):142–148
Sodhi M, Wood KH, Meador-Woodruff J (2008) Role of glutamate in schizophrenia: integrating excitatory avenues of research. Expert Rev Neurother 8(9):1389–1406
Specht K, Lie CH, Shah NJ, Fink GR (2009) Disentangling the prefrontal network for rule selection by means of a non-verbal variant of the Wisconsin card sorting test. Hum Brain Mapp 30(5): 1734–1743
Stefansson H, Sigurdsson E, Steinthorsdottir V et al (2002) Neuregulin 1 and susceptibility to schizophrenia. Am J Hum Genet 71(4):877–892
Stefansson H, Rujescu D, Cichon S et al (2008) Large recurrent microdeletions associated with schizophrenia. Nature 455(7210):232–236
Stefansson H, Ophoff RA, Steinberg S et al (2009) Common variants conferring risk of schizophrenia. Nature 460(7256):744–747
Stephan AH, Barres BA, Stevens B (2012) The complement system: an unexpected role in synaptic pruning during development and disease. Annu Rev Neurosci 35:369–389
Sullivan PF, Kendler KS, Neale MC (2003) Schizophrenia as a complex trait: evidence from a meta-analysis of twin studies. Arch Gen Psychiatry 60(12):1187–1192
Sun L, Cheng Z, Zhang F, Xu Y (2015) Gene expression profiling in peripheral blood mononuclear cells of early-onset schizophrenia. Genom Data 5:169–170
Swagerman SC, De Geus EJ, Kan KJ et al (2016) The computerized neurocognitive battery: validation, aging effects, and heritability across cognitive domains. Neuropsychology 30(1): 53–64
Teng S, Thomson PA, Mccarthy S et al (2018) Rare disruptive variants in the Disc1 Interactome and regulome: association with cognitive ability and schizophrenia. Mol Psychiatry 23(5): 1270–1277
Tessier A, Boyer L, Husky M, Bayle F, Llorca PM, Misdrahi D (2017) Medication adherence in schizophrenia: the role of insight, therapeutic alliance and perceived trauma associated with psychiatric care. Psychiatry Res 257:315–321
Thaker GK (2007) Schizophrenia endophenotypes as treatment targets. Expert Opin Ther Targets 11(9):1189–1206
Thomas M, Bismark AW, Joshi YB et al (2018) Targeted cognitive training improves auditory and verbal outcomes among treatment refractory schizophrenia patients mandated to residential care. Schizophr Res 202:378–384
Thuault SJ, Malleret G, Constantinople CM et al (2013) Prefrontal cortex Hcn1 channels enable intrinsic persistent neural firing and executive memory function. J Neurosci 33(34): 13583–13599
Tost H, Callicott JH, Rasetti R et al (2014) Effects of Neuregulin 3 genotype on human prefrontal cortex physiology. J Neurosci 34(3):1051–1056
Wray NR, Gottesman II (2012) Using summary data from the Danish National Registers to estimate heritabilities for schizophrenia, bipolar disorder, and major depressive disorder. Front Genet 3: 118
Walder DJ, Faraone SV, Glatt SJ, Tsuang MT, Seidman LJ (2014) Genetic liability, prenatal health, stress and family environment: risk factors in the Harvard adolescent family high risk for schizophrenia study. Schizophr Res 157(1–3):142–148
Young JW, Geyer MA, Rissling AJ et al (2013) Reverse translation of the rodent 5c-Cpt reveals that the impaired attention of people with schizophrenia is similar to scopolamine-induced deficits in mice. Transl Psychiatry 3:E324
Toulopoulou T, Picchioni M, Rijsdijk F et al (2007) Substantial genetic overlap between Neurocognition and schizophrenia: genetic modeling in twin samples. Arch Gen Psychiatry 64(12):1348–1355
Toulopoulou T, Goldberg TE, Mesa IR et al (2010) Impaired intellect and memory: a missing link between genetic risk and schizophrenia? Arch Gen Psychiatry 67(9):905–913

Trampush JW, Yang M, Yu J et al (2017) GWAS meta-analysis reveals novel loci and genetic correlates for general cognitive function: a report from the cogent consortium. Mol Psychiatry 22(3):336–345

Yokley J, Prasad KM, Chowdari KV et al (2012) Genetic associations between Neuregulin-1 Snps and neurocognitive function in multigenerational, multiplex schizophrenia families. Psychiatr Genet 22(2):70–81

Tovar KR, Mcginley MJ, Gl W (2013) Triheteromeric NMDA receptors at hippocampal synapses. J Neurosci 33(21):9150–9160

Walsh T, Mcclellan JM, Mccarthy SE et al (2008) Rare structural variants disrupt multiple genes in neurodevelopmental pathways in schizophrenia. Science 320(5875):539–543

Zhang Y, Sloan SA, Clarke LE et al (2016) Purification and characterization of progenitor and mature human astrocytes reveals transcriptional and functional differences with mouse. Neuron 89(1):37–53

Vachev TI, Popov NT, Marchev D, Ivanov H, Stoyanova VK (2016) Characterization of micro Rna signature in peripheral blood of schizophrenia patients using µparaflotm Mirna microarray assay. Int J Curr Microbiol App Sci 5(6):503–512

Wang X, Tucker NR, Rizki G et al (2016) Discovery and validation of sub-threshold genome-wide association study loci using epigenomic signatures. eLife 5

Zhou M, Luo P, Lu Y et al (2015) Imbalance of Hcn1 and Hcn2 expression in hippocampal Ca1 area impairs spatial learning and memory in rats with chronic morphine exposure. Prog Neuropsychopharmacol Biol Psychiatry 56:207–214

Using Nonhuman Primate Models to Reverse-Engineer Prefrontal Circuit Failure Underlying Cognitive Deficits in Schizophrenia

Mathew V. Chafee

Contents

M. V. Chafee (✉)
Department of Neuroscience, University of Minnesota, Minneapolis, MN, USA
e-mail: chafe001@umn.edu

Curr Topics Behav Neurosci (2023) 63: 315–362
https://doi.org/10.1007/7854_2022_407
Published Online: 7 January 2023

Abstract In this chapter, I review studies in nonhuman primates that emulate the circuit failure in prefrontal cortex responsible for working memory and cognitive control deficits in schizophrenia. These studies have characterized how synaptic malfunction, typically induced by blockade of NMDAR, disrupts neural function and computation in prefrontal networks to explain errors in cognitive tasks that are seen in schizophrenia. This work is finding causal relationships between pathogenic events of relevance to schizophrenia at vastly different levels of scale, from synapses, to neurons, local, circuits, distributed networks, computation, and behavior. Pharmacological manipulation, the dominant approach in primate models, has limited construct validity for schizophrenia pathogenesis, as the disease results from a complex interplay between environmental, developmental, and genetic factors. Genetic manipulation replicating schizophrenia risk is more advanced in rodent models. Nonetheless, gene manipulation in nonhuman primates is rapidly advancing, and primate developmental models have been established. Integration of large scale neural recording, genetic manipulation, and computational modeling in nonhuman primates holds considerable potential to provide a crucial schizophrenia model moving forward. Data generated by this approach is likely to fill several crucial gaps in our understanding of the causal sequence leading to schizophrenia in humans. This causal chain presents a vexing problem largely because it requires understanding how events at very different levels of scale relate to one another, from genes to circuits to cognition to social interactions. Nonhuman primate models excel here. They optimally enable discovery of causal relationships across levels of scale in the brain that are relevant to cognitive deficits in schizophrenia. The mechanistic understanding of prefrontal circuit failure they promise to provide may point the way to more effective therapeutic interventions to restore function to prefrontal networks in the disease.

Keywords Cognitive control · Monkey · Neural activity · NMDAR · Prefrontal cortex · Primate · Schizophrenia · Working memory

1 How Does Schizophrenia Alter the Function of Prefrontal Neurons and Synapses, and Can These Changes Be Reversed?

Schizophrenia emerges in late adolescence and early adulthood, when people entering into psychosis undergo a profound shift in their mental experience. Current understanding is that this occurs because neurodevelopmental processes that profoundly remodel cortical neural circuits around this time in human life go awry (Dienel et al. 2022). As a result, physiological dynamics of brain networks are distorted, causing the emergence of hallucinations and delusions. Emotional experience is altered and motivation is reduced. Cognitive function is disrupted. Profound distress and social isolation for people suffering from schizophrenia result. These changes in mental experience must reflect a cataclysmic shift in the physiological dynamics of brain networks. That must mean that the cellular elements making up brain networks (neurons, synapses, and glia) enter into a new operational domain as symptoms emerge. In some sense, the cellular processing elements must themselves become sick, meaning that key physiological parameters within them fall out of the range necessary to support normal function. The change in the functional properties of the cellular processing elements causes a change in the physiological dynamics of brain networks, which is the likely proximal cause of the change in mental life that individuals experience. In spite of intensive research efforts, we have a limited understanding of what the key physiological parameters of neurons and synapses are that schizophrenia alters to produce symptoms. Perhaps as a result, we have achieved only a limited therapeutic ability to effectively reverse changes in brain network function for people with the disease once they occur. Although antipsychotic medications currently in use provide significant benefits for some patients, mostly by helping to manage positive symptoms (such as hallucinations and delusions), they fall short of a cure for millions of people (Potkin et al. 2020). The biological knowledge needed to design dramatically better treatments so far is lacking (Insel 2010). The latest generation of atypical antipsychotics do not appear to be significantly more effective in terms of therapeutic benefits for patients than antipsychotics that were in use six decades ago (Lieberman et al. 2005; Lieberman and Stroup 2011). To better treat people with the disease, what do we need to know about schizophrenia that we do not know already?

This chapter is organized around the thesis that the key piece of information we lack is how schizophrenia alters the functional properties of the cellular processing elements that make up brain networks. The assertion is that we need to know, in particular, how neurons and synapses become physiologically "sick" to cause the disease. Discovering which physiological parameters schizophrenia dysregulates at a cellular scale is likely to enable discovery of better ways to restore function to brain networks, improving mental life for people suffering with the disease. However, as is typical with most theories regarding the origin of the disease, even this simple thesis presents considerable uncertainty. For example, it may not be necessary to discover how schizophrenia alters the function of neurons and synapses because the disease is caused by a change in how brain networks are wired together during development more than how the individual processing elements physiologically operate. Neurons and synapses may be "normal" in a physiological sense (although genetic evidence implies that this is not the case; see below). Similarly, we may discover ways to restore function for people with the disease that exert therapeutic effect at the network level, such as brain stimulation approaches (Brunelin et al. 2022), potentially obviating the necessity to pinpoint functional changes in neurons and synapses that cause the disease. A change in environmental inputs, such as a restructuring of social structures around people with schizophrenia (Insel 2022), or targeted cognitive training regimes (Adcock et al. 2009; Fisher et al. 2013), could prove sufficient to move brain networks into a normative operating regime to reduce suffering of many people with schizophrenia. Or it may prove that fundamental changes in the function of neurons and synapses that cause schizophrenia are irreversible, making their characterization moot. The most effective way to treat schizophrenia may be to prevent it from occurring in the first place, if it is possible to disentangle, and more importantly control, the web of genetic (Timms et al. 2013; Schizophrenia_Working_Group_of_the_Psychiatric_Genomics_Consortium 2014; Sekar et al. 2016), developmental (Dienel et al. 2022), and environmental (van Os et al. 2005) risk factors that precipitate disease well enough to disrupt their interaction. (As daunting as it may prove to fully characterize the full spectrum of risk factors, controlling them is arguably the harder challenge.)

Confronted by numerous unknowns, it seems reasonable for the field to collectively explore many routes at once, to determine which have potential for curative discoveries. One such route leads down levels of scale to determine common failure states in neurons and synapses that can be triggered by diverse risk factors. The level of neurons and synapses (cortical microcircuits) is arguably the level where genetic risk factors exert their deleterious effects on brain network function (Trubetskoy et al. 2022), and it is therefore also the level at which effective therapies must exert countervailing effects to restore brain network function. This line of reasoning encounters an immediate and challenging impasse. Namely, it is not possible to study neurons and synapses in the brain of people suffering from schizophrenia while they are alive to discover how the physiological operation of these processing elements is altered to produce symptoms in the disease state. Therefore, the causal biology most directly responsible for the disease unfolds out of view, beyond the resolving capability of brain imaging technologies such as fMRI or EEG that can be readily utilized in humans. To the extent that the causal biology is immeasurable, it is effectively unknowable. That impasse, as much as any other, is likely responsible for the slow pace of progress in the efficacy of treatments for schizophrenia. Although it is technically feasible to employ invasive neural recording in humans to relate the electrophysiological state of individual neurons to cognitive states (Jamali et al. 2021), single neuron physiological data are not typically obtained in people with schizophrenia because there is no direct clinical benefit of the required experimental procedure (inserting electrodes directly into the functioning brain of awake subjects), a procedure which carries clinical risks. Circumnavigating this impasse will require animal models of brain network failure in schizophrenia that make it possible to establish links between changes in neuron and synaptic function that are likely to cause schizophrenia, on the one hand (using the full array of invasive neurophysiological tools available), and downstream changes in brain network dynamics that are most directly responsible for the symptoms of the disease, on the other hand.

In this chapter, I will focus on the role that nonhuman primate models of brain network failure in schizophrenia have played in the effort to unravel the causal biology of schizophrenia as well as their potential utility going forward.

2 An Emerging Theory of the Failure Cascade Leading to Prefrontal Circuit Collapse in Schizophrenia

The sequence of biological changes in brain circuits that leads to schizophrenia is unknown. However, recent progress supports an emerging theory (Dienel and Lewis 2018; Arnsten et al. 2022; Benoit et al. 2022a; Chafee and Averbeck 2022; Girdhar et al. 2022; Hanson et al. 2022; Howes and Shatalina 2022; Johnson and Hyman 2022; Sheridan et al. 2022; Vinogradov et al. 2022) that constrains where and how nonhuman primate models might fit in future research efforts to establish, and potentially reverse, the causal biological sequence leading to disease. The model is fundamentally neurodevelopmental in nature. In this model, in utero changes in brain development, potentially caused by genomic (Hall and Bray 2022) and epigenomic (Girdhar et al. 2022) variation, or maternal immune activation (Choudhury and Lennox 2021; Hanson et al. 2022), negatively impact the development of microcircuits within the prefrontal cortex, consisting of axon collaterals of pyramidal neurons that establish recurrent excitatory synaptic connections between neighboring neurons (Arnsten et al. 2022; Dienel et al. 2022). Resulting deficits in recurrent prefrontal connections impose cognitive deficits that are detectable in the prodromal period (Reichenberg et al. 2010; MacCabe et al. 2013), but otherwise remain functionally latent due to the superabundance of synaptic connections between prefrontal neurons that is established in early life as part of a normal primate brain development. In the human and nonhuman primate cerebral cortex, the density of synaptic connections between cortical neurons increases postnatally, reaching a peak in early childhood, at which time a protracted period of synaptic pruning and maturation of cortical circuits ensues (Huttenlocher 1990; Bourgeois et al. 1994; Petanjek et al. 2011; Kolk and Rakic 2022). The timing of maturation of cortical circuits is staggered, with primary sensory cortices maturing first, and association cortices including the prefrontal cortex maturing later on (Huttenlocher and Dabholkar 1997; Gogtay et al. 2004; Howes and Shatalina 2022).

There is accumulating evidence that a disruption of synaptic pruning and circuit maturation in the prefrontal cortex may be the proximal cause of symptom onset in schizophrenia. For example, microglia are the immune cells that prune synapses by engulfing them, and microglia derived from people with schizophrenia prune synapses more aggressively in tissue culture than do microglia derived from control subjects (Sellgren et al. 2019; Sheridan et al. 2022). Further, which synapses are pruned is influenced by a molecular tagging mechanism that involves synaptic deposition of the immune component signaling molecule C4 (Yilmaz et al. 2021), and mutations that increase expression of this molecule increase synaptic pruning along with the risk of schizophrenia (Sekar et al. 2016). Dendritic spines are the morphological specialization of dendrites where pyramidal neurons receive the bulk of their synaptic input, and there are fewer dendritic spines in the prefrontal cortex of people that experienced schizophrenia in post-mortem analyses (Glantz and Lewis

2000; Kolluri et al. 2005), consistent with excessive synaptic pruning (although this could equally result from insufficient synaptogenesis during development) (Dienel et al. 2022). These lines of evidence suggest that schizophrenia may be a disease of synaptic pruning, malformation, or retraction that leads to the excessive disconnection of prefrontal circuits (Friston 1999; Dienel et al. 2022). Whereas moderate synaptic pruning improves the stability of attractor states in prefrontal microcircuits, excessive pruning degrades the stability of attractor states, leading to a loss of encoded information and worsened performance on working memory tasks (Averbeck 2022). Attractor states in prefrontal microcircuits are stable patterns of activity over neurons that can be triggered by transient external inputs to the network and are sustained by recurrent excitatory synaptic interactions between neurons (Wang 1999; Compte et al. 2000; Brunel and Wang 2001; Murray et al. 2014). Sustained or temporally dynamic patterns of neural activity in the prefrontal cortex can encode abstract cognitive variables (such as behavioral context, numbers, categories, or rules) in working memory to support cognitive control (Freedman et al. 2001; Wallis et al. 2001; Nieder et al. 2002; Goodwin et al. 2012; Blackman et al. 2016), which can be operationally defined as the ability to respond flexibly to environmental inputs on the basis of internal state variables encoded by neural activity in the prefrontal cortex at the time that environmental inputs arrive (Miller and Cohen 2001). Disruption of these attractor states could underlie deficits in working memory and cognitive control that have been repeatedly observed in schizophrenia (Goldman-Rakic 1999; Barch et al. 2003), and other diagnostic categories including bipolar disorder (Smucny et al. 2018), and major depressive disorder (Wagner et al. 2012; Dotson et al. 2020), although typically to a lesser extent (Smucny et al. 2018). In addition to degrading attractor state stability in prefrontal microcircuits, loss of recurrent excitatory drive during synaptic pruning may induce other pathophysiological states characterized by reduced synchronous spiking between prefrontal neurons (Zick et al. 2018, 2021), potentially accelerating circuit disconnection via spike timing-dependent synaptic plasticity (Dan and Poo 2004). The interdependence of activity states and synaptic connectivity in prefrontal networks is governed by complex signaling cascades in dendritic spines that are sensitive to timing relationships between pre- and postsynaptic depolarization (Hall et al. 2015; He et al. 2015; Clifton et al. 2019; Kasai et al. 2021). The number of interacting variables governing that process is large, spanning both environmental states that generate activity patterns in brain networks and the biochemical pathways that regulate how synaptic strength is adjusted to these environmental inputs. That complexity may render the activity-dependent regulation of synaptic strength in recurrent prefrontal circuits vulnerable to a host of insults and prone to failure or dysregulation in a number of disease states, explaining the transdiagnostic nature of deficits in working memory and cognitive control. Cognitive control and working memory deficits of this type that reflect failure of prefrontal recurrent networks may represent a core axis of biological fault in brain function along which a number of different diagnostic categories are distributed in partially overlapping fashion, consistent with the Research Domain Criterion (RDoC) initiative of the NIH (Kozak and Cuthbert 2016).

In schizophrenia, disruption of recurrent circuits during the in utero development of the prefrontal cortex is likely to reflect a first stage of the failure cascade leading to schizophrenia. A second stage likely occurs as prefrontal circuits disconnect as a result of synaptic pruning late in adolescence acting potentially in concert with activity-dependent synaptic plasticity. Frank psychosis marked by the onset of delusions and hallucinations does not emerge until a third stage of pathogenesis is triggered when falling synaptic connectivity and function in prefrontal local circuits start to dysregulate neural activity in large-scale distributed networks that link the prefrontal cortex to other brain structures. This stage is marked by altered function in loop circuits that link the prefrontal cortex to the basal ganglia, extending from the basal ganglia to the thalamus, and from the thalamus back to the prefrontal cortex (Russchen et al. 1987; Zikopoulos and Barbas 2007). Altered function in this circuit has been detected in schizophrenia at two points. First, PET and SPECT studies that measure displacement of dopamine D2 receptor radioligands by endogenous dopamine or uptake of radiolabeled L-DOPA have detected elevated levels of dopamine release and synthesis capacity in the striatum in schizophrenia (Abi-Dargham et al. 2009; Kegeles et al. 2010; Stone et al. 2010; Howes et al. 2011, 2020; Howes and Shatalina 2022). Elevated dopamine release was detected specifically in the dorsal region of the striatum receiving direct excitatory projections from the prefrontal cortex (Choi et al. 2017; McCutcheon et al. 2018). The magnitude of excess dopamine in the striatum correlated with the severity of psychotic symptoms (Jauhar et al. 2017). This may explain the clinical efficacy of available antipsychotic medications, all of which block dopamine D2 receptors that are concentrated in the striatum (Kaar et al. 2020). Second, functional MRI has detected reduced functional connectivity between the thalamus and the dorsolateral prefrontal cortex in schizophrenia, accompanied by elevated functional connectivity between the thalamus and the sensorimotor cortex (Anticevic et al. 2014, 2015; Cheng et al. 2015; Zhang et al. 2021; Benoit et al. 2022a). Both elevated dopamine in the dorsal striatum (Howes et al. 2009; Howes and Shatalina 2022) and reduced functional connectivity between the thalamus and the prefrontal cortex (Anticevic et al. 2015) are present in individuals at clinical high risk of conversion to psychosis. Reduced functional connectivity between the thalamus and the prefrontal cortex predicted conversion to psychosis in these individuals (Anticevic et al. 2015). Thus, the full-blown disease is likely to result from a complex interplay between developmental events that impact the prefrontal cortex directly, by altering the structure and function of prefrontal microcircuits at the synaptic level, and indirectly, by altering the physiological dynamics of prefrontal macrocircuits that link the prefrontal cortex to other brain structures.

3 Schizophrenia: Convergent Causal Trajectories

Although the disconnection of prefrontal cortical networks and its follow-on impacts on other neural systems are prime suspects for the causal biology leading to schizophrenia currently, these are likely to prove highly complex processes driven by an interaction between a very large number of variables. This fits the complexity of genetic, developmental, and environmental factors that increase the risk that any given individual will develop schizophrenia late in adolescence. More than 200 distinct and relatively common genetic variations (single nucleotide polymorphisms) influencing more than 100 genes are currently known to each impose a small increment in risk (Schizophrenia_Working_Group_of_the_Psychiatric_Genomics_Consortium 2014; Trubetskoy et al. 2022). Implicated genes are highly expressed in cortical pyramidal neurons and interneurons, including genes encoding voltage-sensitive Ca^{2+} channels as well as subunits of the NMDA receptor (Trubetskoy et al. 2022), both of which play a role in activity-dependent modulation of intracellular calcium. A smaller number of rare copy number variants, such as the 22q11.2 microdeletion, which involve larger alterations in gene structure increase risk dramatically, approximately 30-fold (Rees et al. 2014; Merico et al. 2015). Approximately one in three persons with these mutations eventually develops symptoms consistent with a diagnosis of schizophrenia. However, of equal importance, two in three people with the same mutation do not. Genetic influences on their own are not strictly causal, in the sense that none of the risk genetic variations identified to date are sufficient by themselves to dictate whether a specific individual will develop schizophrenia in late adolescence or not. Additional sources of disease risk must come to bear, and they are bewildering in terms of the diversity of biological mechanisms they are likely to engage. As noted, maternal infection and subsequent immune activation can increase the risk that a person will develop schizophrenia later in life (Brown and Derkits 2010; Choudhury and Lennox 2021). Environmental stressors such as early trauma, living in an urban environment, and immigrant status all increase the risk that an individual will develop schizophrenia (van Os et al. 2005). Pharmacological agents can increase risk of schizophrenia or mimic its symptoms. Cannabis use is associated with elevated risk of schizophrenia (Hamilton 2017), whereas drugs that block NMDA receptors (such as ketamine or phencyclidine) induce both positive and negative symptoms of schizophrenia in healthy control subjects (Krystal et al. 1994; Javitt et al. 2012), worsen clinical symptoms in people with schizophrenia (Luby et al. 1959), and in some healthy individuals can induce bouts of psychosis that persist in spite of antipsychotic treatment for more than 30 days (Allen and Young 1978).

The question of how all of these factors, genetic and environmental, intertwine is an important and vexing one: important because answering the question promises to ultimately provide better, possibly curative, therapeutic interventions for people with schizophrenia and vexing because of the high number of variables at play, the levels of scale they span (from molecular genetic to societal risk factors), the complexity of their interaction, and the difficulty of measuring many of the most important variables in the living human brain. These considerations highlight the need for good animal models of the human disease that make it possible to measure these variables.

4 Using Nonhuman Primate Models to Test the Causal Theory

The thrust of the failure cascade model supported by recent data outlined above is that schizophrenia is the end result of a sequence of interlocking pathogenic events, including (a) disruptions of cortical development in utero, that (b) establish a latent physiological vulnerability in prefrontal microcircuits, that (c) is unmasked when synaptic pruning excessively reduces synaptic connectivity in prefrontal microcircuits during late adolescence, triggering pathophysiological states that (d) degrade attractor dynamics in prefrontal microcircuits that normally support working memory and cognitive control, which (e) leads to deficits in working memory and cognitive control in schizophrenia, and (f) elevate dopamine release in the dorsal striatum, thereby (g) disrupting communication between the prefrontal cortex, basal ganglia, and thalamus, (h) leading to psychosis. This is a long and complex causal chain reaction of events that is plausible, consistent with known facts, but only a sketch at present, replete with gaps that contain hypothesized causal relations that are untested and unproven. From one perspective, it is essentially an educated guess, a line connecting a number of experimental observations, where many alternatives are possible. For example, one challenge to this theory is the observation that whereas cognitive control deficits are correlated with negative symptoms in schizophrenia, they are not correlated with positive symptoms (Peng et al. 2021; Nieuwenstein et al. 2001), suggesting that cognitive deficits and positive symptoms may represent two independent pathogenic processes that are only weakly coupled, if at all. On the other side of this coin, lower gray matter volume (D'Ambrosio et al. 2021) and lower N-acetylaspartate levels (indicating neuronal dysfunction) (Bertolino 2000) in the dorsolateral prefrontal cortex are correlated with elevated striatal dopamine in schizophrenia. The degree of altered prefrontal activation during cognitive tasks is correlated with the degree of altered striatal dopamine release in schizophrenia also (Fusar-Poli et al. 2011; Howes and Shatalina 2022). Thus, altered prefrontal function and altered striatal dopamine might be mechanistically coupled in the disease at a network level, as suggested by preclinical rodent models (Adrover et al. 2020; Quiroz et al. 2016; Kim et al. 2015; Howes and Shatalina 2022). However, the relationship between these two aspects of schizophrenia pathogenesis is complex, and each may be responsive to different risk factors to the extent that cognitive deficits and positive symptoms vary independently in people with the disease. In spite of these uncertainties, building and testing causal theories of this type may prove useful in that the theories generate questions that may guide future experiments. The answers to those questions, even if unanticipated and against prediction, may help direct inquiry to the true underlying causal biology. In the following sections, I review how nonhuman primate models have been utilized to test several hypotheses presented by the failure cascade model above, as well as how nonhuman primate models might be employed to test additional hypotheses derived from the model in the future.

The inroad to nonhuman primate models starts with the ability to model cognitive functions that are disrupted in humans with schizophrenia accurately, combined with the ability to relate those cognitive functions to the operations of the individual processing elements of prefrontal brain microcircuits and macrocircuits, namely neurons and synapses. Behavior is the starting point. This is the first link between the outward manifestations of schizophrenia and the underlying biological events that generate them. The ability to make this link between behavior and biology at a cellular scale is the key strength of nonhuman primate models.

Schizophrenia presents with distortions of cognition, affect, and perception. Among these symptoms, distortions of cognition have proven to be most tractable to study in nonhuman primates. A first major strength of nonhuman primate models is that monkeys can perform many of the same cognitive tasks that have been used to measure cognitive deficits in humans with schizophrenia, including, importantly, paradigms that measure working memory and executive control (Jacobsen 1935; Goldman-Rakic 1987; Stoet and Snyder 2003; Dias et al. 2006). In addition, a long history of neuronal physiology experiments in nonhuman primates has related the activation patterns of prefrontal neurons to working memory (Funahashi et al. 1989; Chafee and Goldman-Rakic 1998; Goldman-Rakic 1999; Constantinidis et al. 2001) and executive control (Wallis et al. 2001; Goodwin et al. 2012; Skoblenick and Everling 2012; Blackman et al. 2016). This provides a strong foundation of knowledge on which to base correlations between neural activity and cognitive functions that schizophrenia affects, opening a door to relate distortions of neural activity to distortions of cognition that bear relevance to schizophrenia.

A second major strength of nonhuman primate models is that prefrontal networks are similar in anatomical organization and complexity in monkeys and humans (Goldman-Rakic 1987; Selemon and Goldman-Rakic 1988; Cavada and Goldman-Rakic 1989; Tang et al. 2021). Functional imaging evidence points to malfunction of the granular dorsolateral prefrontal cortex in schizophrenia (Callicott et al. 2000; Holmes et al. 2005; MacDonald 3rd et al. 2005; Yoon et al. 2008; Lesh et al. 2013; Tu et al. 2013; Lopez-Garcia et al. 2016). Careful analysis of the internal structure and connectivity of the granular prefrontal cortex in monkeys and humans provides compelling evidence that there is no homolog in rodents (Preuss 1995; Heilbronner et al. 2016; Balsters et al. 2020; Preuss and Wise 2022). The close similarity in neural architecture between monkeys and humans greatly increases the chances that monkey prefrontal networks may be able to replicate pathophysiological states that produce symptoms in the human disease. At a microscopic level, pathophysiological states that produce schizophrenia must alter the spatial and temporal distribution of action and synaptic potentials in prefrontal networks, since the spatial and temporal evolution of these neural signals mediates cognitive processing, which is altered in the human disease. How patterns of electrical activity are distorted at cellular scale is a crucial question to answer in schizophrenia because as noted there is ample evidence that genetic risk factors in the disease specifically target the molecular mechanisms of activity-dependent synaptic plasticity in brain networks (Hall and Bray 2022), including components of NMDA receptors, voltage-gated calcium channels (Fromer et al. 2014; Schizophrenia_Working_Group_of_the_Psychiatric_Genomics_Consortium 2014; Li et al. 2018; Zhu et al. 2019; Trubetskoy et al. 2022), and other components of postsynaptic density that are likely to influence synaptic function, stability, and plasticity (Kirov et al. 2012; Fromer et al. 2014; Trubetskoy et al. 2022). Both NMDAR and voltage-gated Ca^{2+} channels modulate Ca^{2+} concentrations in dendritic spines which powerfully modulate spine actin dynamics and synaptic plasticity (Kasai et al. 2021). The change in the timing or distribution of action and synaptic potentials in prefrontal networks that emerges when prefrontal networks are pruned may feed back into altered synaptic plasticity mechanisms to accelerate activity-dependent disconnection of prefrontal recurrent networks. Namely, as prefrontal circuits are pruned, loss of synchronous spiking activity in these networks may cause further disconnection via spike timing-dependent mechanisms (Dan and Poo 2004; Zick et al. 2018, 2021). The potential to capture subtle distortions of activity states in prefrontal networks that are relevant to schizophrenia is a strength of nonhuman primate models.

5 Limitations of Nonhuman Primate Models in Schizophrenia Research

By the same token, nonhuman primate models pose several serious limitations in the effort to understand the causal biology of schizophrenia. Chief among these is the difficulty of replicating risk factors of schizophrenia in nonhuman primates, particularly genetic risk factors. The ability to genetically engineer mutations into mice including copy number variants that are known to increase the risk of schizophrenia in humans (Forsingdal et al. 2019; Hiroi and Yamauchi 2019; Hyman 2021) has been productive in elucidating their downstream consequences on neural activity, attractor dynamics, and network synchrony (Sigurdsson et al. 2010; Tamura et al. 2016; Hamm et al. 2017, 2020; Kupferschmidt and Gordon 2018; Zick et al. 2021), cortical structure and neuronal morphology (Meechan et al. 2015; Fernandez et al. 2019), synaptic function and plasticity (Drew et al. 2011; Fénelon et al. 2011, 2013; Earls et al. 2012; Devaraju et al. 2017), and behavior (Ouchi et al. 2013; Meechan et al. 2015; Tamura et al. 2016). Genetic engineering technologies are developing rapidly with successful application in nonhuman primates including cynomolgus monkeys (Aida and Feng 2020) and marmosets (Sasaki et al. 2009; Park et al. 2016; Drummer et al. 2021). Important foundational work on the behavioral (Axelsson et al. 2021; Duan et al. 2021; Ash et al. 2022; Samandra et al. 2022; Stawicka et al. 2022) neuroanatomical (Ash et al. 2022; Garin et al. 2022), and neurophysiological (Miller et al. 2015; Schaeffer et al. 2019, 2020; Feizpour et al. 2021; Jovanovic et al. 2022; Wong et al. 2022) characteristics of marmosets is ongoing. Combining cellular neurophysiology with genetic manipulation in marmosets is technically feasible and holds great promise for unraveling the causal biology of schizophrenia in terms of how risk factors alter neural, synaptic, and network function. However, at present, application of this approach to genetic variation of specific relevance to schizophrenia is marmosets in its infancy in comparison to rodent species.

Similarly, transgenic and optogenetic technologies provide unprecedented ability to manipulate genes and neural circuits and application of these techniques to neural circuit questions of relevance to schizophrenia is considerably more advanced in rodent models (Sohal et al. 2009; Kim et al. 2015; McNally et al. 2021; Benoit et al. 2022b, c), than nonhuman primates, although progress in the application of these technologies to nonhuman primates is ongoing (Okano and Kishi 2018; El-Shamayleh and Horwitz 2019).

The bulk of work in nonhuman primates has used NMDAR antagonists to mimic neural and cognitive malfunction in schizophrenia (Skoblenick and Everling 2012; Blackman et al. 2013; Wang et al. 2013; Kummerfeld et al. 2020). Blocking NMDAR is an artificial means to disrupt prefrontal networks that does not faithfully replicate risk factors in schizophrenia. However, it may capture key features of pathophysiological states that schizophrenia produces (Javitt et al. 2012). A cluster of genetic mutations that increase schizophrenia risk implicate NMDAR malfunction (Timms et al. 2013; Fromer et al. 2014; Schizophrenia_Working_Group_of_the_Psychiatric_Genomics_Consortium 2014; Trubetskoy et al. 2022), and anti-NMDA encephalitis, a condition where the body produces autoimmune antibodies against NMDA receptors, can present clinically with positive symptoms like those seen in schizophrenia, including delusions and auditory hallucinations (Wang et al. 2019b).

Recurrent connections between prefrontal neurons in prefrontal microcircuits are particularly dependent on NMDAR synaptic mechanisms (Wang et al. 2013; Arnsten et al. 2022). Therefore, manipulating NMDAR synaptic mechanisms in prefrontal networks may replicate key features of how these networks fail leading to cognitive deficits in schizophrenia.

6 Neural Basis of Cognitive Functions Disrupted in Schizophrenia: Macaque Prefrontal Delay Neurons and Working Memory

Perhaps, one of the first and to date most successful efforts to uncover the cellular basis of cognitive deficits that occur in schizophrenia has involved the cellular characterization of the neural mechanisms of working memory in the prefrontal cortex of macaques by Goldman-Rakic and her colleagues (Funahashi et al. 1989, 1993a, b; Sawaguchi and Goldman-Rakic 1991; Goldman-Rakic 1999; Constantinidis et al. 2001). Translation of the oculomotor delayed response (ODR) working memory task developed in these experiments for use in nonhuman primates to people with schizophrenia produced one of the first well-controlled and thoroughly documented demonstrations of working memory deficits in people with the disease (Park and Holzman 1992; Smucny et al. 2022) as well as their first-degree relatives (Park et al. 1995). This was an impactful collaboration. A search using the terms "schizophrenia working memory" on PubMed returns more than 4000 publications since the original report in 1992. (The search returned 85 publications before that time.) A recent review provides an authoritative synthesis of the literature linking working memory deficits to prefrontal cortical dysfunction in schizophrenia (Smucny et al. 2022). Robust working memory deficits have now been repeatedly demonstrated in schizophrenia (Gold et al. 1997; Aleman et al. 1999; Forbes et al. 2009), which are present before or at the first psychotic episode (Mesholam-Gately et al. 2009; Bora and Murray 2014), are found to a lesser degree in first-degree relatives (Park et al. 1995; Horan et al. 2008), and are associated with reduced activation of the dorsolateral prefrontal cortex (Glahn et al. 2005) in functional neuroimaging studies.

In the ODR task, initially developed by Hikosaka and Wurtz (1983), and adapted by Goldman-Rakic and her colleagues to the study of working memory in the prefrontal cortex (Funahashi et al. 1989), monkeys were trained to direct their gaze to a central fixation target while a peripheral visual cue was flashed briefly at a randomized location in the visual periphery. After a 3 s delay period, monkeys demonstrated successful spatial working memory by directing a saccadic eye movement to the location where the peripheral cue had been earlier in the trial. The key feature of the task from a behavioral perspective was that there was no informative stimulus in the external environment at the time of the saccade that was available to direct the movement. Rather, the direction of the saccade depended on an internal representation (Goldman-Rakic 1987), an engram of its prior spatial location, sustained in the brain after the cue disappeared and available at the end of the trial to direct the response internally. Goldman-Rakic argued (Goldman-Rakic 1987), elegantly, that this was the functional essence of the prefrontal cortex. She posited that the prefrontal cortex comprised a neural circuit capable of directing behavior on the basis of internally represented information, either when reflexive responses to external stimuli were inappropriate or when the triggering stimuli themselves were not present at the time the response was made. Such a capability would contribute to the autonomous, self-directed, and self-initiated aspects of human behavior. Neural recording in the prefrontal cortex of monkeys performing the ODR task led to the discovery that the memory engram supporting the internal control of behavior in this context was provided by prefrontal neurons that increased their firing rate when the cue appeared and maintained their elevated level of activity throughout the delay period after the cue disappeared until the saccadic eye movement to the remembered location was made (Funahashi et al. 1989). This persistent activity scaled with the length of the delay period imposed between cue and response and faltered on trials where errors were made (Funahashi et al. 1989). “Delay neurons” as cells with this type of activity came to be known were in many cases spatially tuned to the location of the remembered cue, and as a population, they provided an accurate representation of where the cue had appeared in the visual periphery (Takeda and Funahashi 2004). Moreover, temporal evolution of this population code during the delay period was found to reflect cognitive manipulation of the spatial information encoded by prefrontal cortical neurons (Takeda and Funahashi 2004), much like the rotation of the neural population vector previously observed in the primary motor cortex of monkeys performing a mental rotation task (Georgopoulos et al. 1989). Thus, the activity of prefrontal neurons bore a relationship to spatial working memory in terms of the duration over which it operated (the delay period), the information it contained (the spatial location of the remembered cue), and the cognitive manipulation of the encoded information. Watching online displays of spike trains of single prefrontal neurons of monkeys while they performed the ODR task (Funahashi et al. 1993b; Chafee and Goldman-Rakic 1998, 2000) afforded a rare opportunity to directly perceive the potential unity of biological and mental events in the lab. As monkeys formed working memories, prefrontal neurons were activated. The biological process and the inferred mental one unfolded together in time; they mirrored one another. There is no way to demonstrate what, if any, subjective experience monkeys had of the information their delay neurons encoded. (Although see Kiani and Shadlen (2009) for evidence that monkeys can behaviorally report varying degrees of confidence in the information encoded by their own persistent neural activity.) As challenging as it is to link biological and mental events, such links are fundamental to the search for the biological causes of schizophrenia, since functional alterations in neurons, synapses, and networks lead to distortions of conscious experience in the disease.

In the original ODR task, the spatial location of the cue and the direction of the planned saccadic response were overlapping, making it impossible to determine whether the persistent activity of prefrontal delay neurons encoded a sensory memory (the past) or a motor plan (the future). However, subsequent work confirmed that many prefrontal neurons encoded the location of the remembered cue independently of the direction of forthcoming response (Niki and Watanabe 1976; Quintana and Fuster 1992; Funahashi et al. 1993b; Constantinidis et al. 2001), although some delay neurons do predict the direction of the motor response (Niki and Watanabe 1976; Quintana and Fuster 1992; Funahashi et al. 1993b). Prefrontal delay neurons reflect the saccadic choices of animals when they are free to autonomously select among multiple saccade targets (Mochizuki and Funahashi 2016), linking delay neurons to the autonomous control of behavior. Delay neurons are intermingled in the prefrontal cortex with visual neurons transiently activated by the visual cue (Funahashi et al. 1990), and response neurons transiently activated at the time the saccade is made (Funahashi et al. 1991). Since cognition ultimately derives from sensorimotor experience, it is of interest whether and how cognitive signals (such as delay neurons) are derived from sensorimotor signals (such as cue and response neurons) within prefrontal circuits.

7 Spatial Working Memory Deficits Following Manipulation of Prefrontal Cortex

Permanent lesions (Funahashi et al. 1993a), focal injection of compounds blocking D1 receptors (Sawaguchi and Goldman-Rakic 1991), and transient inactivation of the prefrontal cortex by cooling (Chafee and Goldman-Rakic 2000) all induce impairments in spatial working memory in the ODR task that are characterized by deficits in memory-guided saccades. Spatial working memory deficits are greatest for visual cues presented contralateral to the functionally impaired prefrontal hemisphere (Sawaguchi and Goldman-Rakic 1991; Funahashi et al. 1993a; Chafee and Goldman-Rakic 2000). Memory-guided saccade deficits can be dramatic in the sense that at the end of the delay, monkeys may direct their eyes into the incorrect visual quadrant of hemifield on some trials, suggesting a specific failure of spatial working memory, more than a disruption of saccade control circuits. That is further supported by the observation that lesions or functional disruption of the prefrontal cortex does not interfere with saccades so long as saccade targets remain visible during the delay period to provide visual guidance to the eye movement (Sawaguchi and Goldman-Rakic 1991; Funahashi et al. 1993a; Chafee and Goldman-Rakic 2000). This is consistent with the thesis of Goldman-Rakic that the preeminent function of the prefrontal cortex is to guide behavior specifically when informative external stimuli are not available. Such prefrontal manipulations and their behavioral consequences provide models of working memory impairments in schizophrenia.

8 Distributed Network Basis of Spatial Working Memory

The fact that delay neurons and working memory deficits colocalize to the prefrontal cortex would seem to imply that working memory function is localized to the prefrontal cortex also. At least at the level of single neurons, that is not the case. Parietal delay neurons during the ODR task are as robustly activated and spatially selective as their prefrontal counterparts (Chafee and Goldman-Rakic 1998). Likewise cue and response neurons in the prefrontal and parietal cortex bear striking resemblance to one another during the ODR task (Chafee and Goldman-Rakic 1998). The regions of the prefrontal and parietal cortex where these neural populations were seen to undergo parallel modulations in firing rate during behavior share direct reciprocal corticocortical projections (Cavada and Goldman-Rakic 1989). This suggests that the physiological impact of reciprocal projections in cortical networks is to entrain populations of neurons in connected cortical areas to the same patterns of firing rate modulation during behavior. If neural populations in two interconnected cortical areas modulate their firing rate up and down in unison, then the neural populations encode the same information about behavior, whether in relation to externally observable events (such as stimuli and movements) or internal cognitive events (such as working memories). Neural representations, even of a single sensory or cognitive event, appear to be intrinsically network-level phenomena, entraining neurons in multiple cortical areas to the same distributed pattern of firing rate modulation. Computations that generate network representations of this type appear to involve an exchange of information between cortical areas, rather than being restricted to any one cortical area in isolation of the others. Consistent with this view, reversibly inactivating the prefrontal and posterior parietal cortex were equally effective in reducing delay period activity at the network level (Chafee and

Goldman-Rakic 2000). This suggests that persistent activity associated with working memory may be generated by the activation of recurrent excitatory circuits that extend between cortical areas. The exchange of information implied by this physiological dynamic, wired into hierarchical and distributed cortical networks (Felleman and Van Essen 1991), complicates the effort to localize function to individual cortical areas based on the behaviorally defined patterns of single neuron activity they contain. The distribution of single neuron activity patterns between the prefrontal and parietal cortex is not unique to the ODR task, as it has been repeatedly observed in a variety of other task and cognitive contexts (Nieder and Miller 2004a; Qi et al. 2010; Goodwin et al. 2012; Swaminathan and Freedman 2012). Rather, the recruitment of neurons in multiple communicating cortical areas to the same distributed patterns of activity appears to be a general principle of cortical organization,

Although delay neurons are present in the prefrontal and parietal cortex, functional differences between delay neurons in the two areas have been observed. Neural responses exhibit less variability over trials in the prefrontal than the parietal cortex (Qi and Constantinidis 2015). Effective connectivity between neurons as measured by cross-correlation of spike trains is stronger in the parietal than the prefrontal cortex (Katsuki et al. 2014). Delay neurons in the prefrontal cortex are more robust to distractors than delay neurons in the parietal cortex (Qi et al. 2010). Such differences in neural dynamics and neural interactions are likely to reflect differences in the internal architecture of local circuits in the two areas. Moreover, delay activity in the two areas may not play the same role in controlling behavior, as inactivation of the prefrontal cortex produced profound deficits in memory-guided saccades, whereas inactivation of the posterior parietal cortex was without this effect (Chafee and Goldman-Rakic 2000). That may reflect differences in how outputs from the prefrontal and parietal cortex engage downstream saccade control networks. Although differences in activity between prefrontal and parietal neurons are present, they tend to be subtle, related to neural dynamics or how neurons respond differentially across task conditions, and at any given moment as behavior unfolds, coactivation of prefrontal and parietal neurons is the rule rather than the exception (Goodwin et al. 2012; Chafee and Goldman-Rakic 1998). That could explain the common observation that the prefrontal and parietal cortices are coactivated during cognitive control tasks in human functional neuroimaging studies (Lesh et al. 2013; Woolgar et al. 2015; Lopez-Garcia et al. 2016; Sheu and Courtney 2016; Lerman-Sinkoff et al. 2017; A Breukelaar et al. 2018; Smucny et al. 2020b).

9 Plasticity of Prefrontal Working Memory Activity

Typically, neural activity is recorded in the prefrontal cortex after monkeys have undergone many months of training to perform a given cognitive task. This raises the question whether neural activity patterns that are observed reflect the native computational properties of prefrontal networks, or alternatively, how prefrontal networks have adapted to the task demands based on the reinforcement contingencies imposed. Reinforcement signals strongly influence learning in prefrontal circuits (Pasupathy and Miller 2005; Histed et al. 2009), and how prefrontal circuits adapt to reinforcement may be the origin of their computational power during normal behavior as the brain encounters a changing and often unpredictable world. However, determining the extent to which prefrontal neural activity patterns reflect training on a single task over many months requires recording before and after training has taken place. Working memory, as reflected by the persistent activation of prefrontal neurons following presentation of a visual stimulus, appears to be a native capability of prefrontal cortical circuits because this form of activity is present in prefrontal neurons of naive monkeys that have never been trained to perform working memory tasks (Meyer et al. 2007). Persistent activity in task-naive animals can be selective either for the spatial location or visual features of the stimuli (Meyer et al. 2007). Other task-evoked modulations in prefrontal neurons are strongly influenced by training (Meyers et al. 2012; Qi and Constantinidis 2013; Tang et al. 2019, 2022). Behavioral improvements in working memory performance over training have been associated with the recruitment of a larger number of task-responsive neurons in the prefrontal cortex (Tang et al. 2019, 2022) that exhibit a more consistent, less variable time course of activation throughout the trial (Qi and Constantinidis 2012; Tang et al. 2019), reduced noise correlation (Tang et al. 2022), and improvements in stimulus encoding (Tang et al. 2019, 2022) that can depend on the task context in which stimuli are presented (Tang et al. 2022), as well as with alterations in the frequency composition of oscillatory neural activity (Singh et al. 2022; Tang et al. 2022). Generally, learning-dependent changes in the strength of prefrontal neural responses to visual stimuli are modest in comparison to learning-dependent changes in the strength of neural signals that reflect the cognitive rules of the task. For example, in tasks where monkeys view two stimuli and report whether the second matched the first, either in relation to spatial location or visual features, prefrontal neurons acquire signals that reflect the match/nonmatch status of the stimulus abstracted from its location or features as a function of training, and this is the strongest learning effect (Meyers et al. 2012; Tang et al. 2022). These data suggest that visually evoked signals from posterior sensory association cortices passively flow through prefrontal circuits, recruiting both transient stimulus-evoked signals and stimulus-specific persistent activity, on an ongoing basis, regardless of the task significance of stimuli. Reinforcement learning, in contrast, appears to powerfully drive the emergence of cognitive signals in prefrontal neurons that capture rules mapping stimuli to responses (such as the match/nonmatch status of a stimulus) without directly encoding the stimuli or responses themselves. In essence, this suggests that prefrontal circuits utilize reinforcement to learn how to abstract task rules out of sensorimotor experience. How such learning occurs at a neural and synaptic level is likely to provide new insights into the neural basis of intelligent behavior. It may also inform targeted cognitive training strategies that are able to drive improvements in cognitive function in schizophrenia by improving sensory processing ability (Adcock et al. 2009; Fisher et al. 2013; Biagianti et al. 2016; Dale et al. 2016), as these training paradigms may harness the plasticity mechanisms that govern conversion of sensory into cognitive signals in prefrontal neurons.

Schizophrenia disrupts reinforcement learning, although not all forms equally. For example, procedural, "actor-critic" learning is spared (Gold 2012; Geana et al. 2021). This is a form of learning in which reward prediction errors update the value of environmental states (the critic), typically signaled by visual stimuli, which then provide the basis for action selection (the actor) according to state-dependent action weights. Actor-critic models make decisions without explicitly predicting outcomes that selected actions will produce. The fact that this form of learning is intact in schizophrenia suggests that mechanisms of dopamine-mediated synaptic plasticity in the basal ganglia are intact as they pertain to updating state value (critic) or response weight (actor) signals. In other words, learning mechanisms are normal with respect to acquisition of sensorimotor habits. In contrast, schizophrenia impairs a form of learning ("Q-learning") in which the brain learns to make explicit predictions about the outcomes a given action will produce. Because Q-learning models make explicit predictions about outcomes, they distinguish between actions that obtain rewards and actions that avoid losses, even though the two can yield the same reward prediction error, and are indistinguishable in actor-critic models. In line with a deficit in this form of learning, people with schizophrenia are selectively impaired in learning from positive outcomes, and have difficulty discerning actions that gain outcomes from those that avoid losses (Gold 2012; Geana et al. 2021). The fact that this form of learning is disrupted in schizophrenia suggests that mechanisms of dopamine-mediated synaptic plasticity are impaired as they pertain to updating neural representations in the prefrontal cortex that make predictions about future outcomes. That is, forms of reinforcement learning are selectively disrupted that modify cognition more than sensorimotor habit. Discovering whether and how excessive release of dopamine in the striatum (Howes and Shatalina 2022) disrupts cognitive learning in the prefrontal cortex may help unravel the pathogenesis of cognitive deficits in schizophrenia.

10 Changes in Persistent Working Memory Activity Between Adolescence and Adulthood

How the computational properties of prefrontal neurons change from adolescence to adulthood is a question of particular importance to schizophrenia, as this is when symptoms typically emerge. Peripubertal monkeys are more distractable in working memory tasks, but prefrontal neurons exhibit robust persistent activity at this age (Zhou et al. 2013). As monkeys pass through puberty and enter adulthood, the strength of spatially selective persistent activity in prefrontal neurons increases along with improving working memory performance (Zhou et al. 2016). Conversely, sensory responses of prefrontal neurons did not change between puberty and adulthood (Zhou et al. 2016). Gamma frequency oscillations in prefrontal local field potentials in contrast weaken between puberty and adulthood, although correlations between spiking activity and gamma oscillations increase in the adult (Wang et al. 2022). These data suggest that as local prefrontal circuits mature, persistent firing increases, as does coupling between firing and gamma oscillations (although gamma oscillations weaken overall). This echoes the improvement in the performance of simulated prefrontal networks that undergo moderate pruning of weak synapses (Averbeck 2022).

11 "Silent" Mechanisms of Working Memory

Although there is consensus that neural activity during the delay period contributes to working memory, there is less consensus about whether this activity takes the form of persistently elevated firing rates in single neurons (Constantinidis et al. 2018; Lundqvist et al. 2018). In the now classical view of working memory, individual working memories are sustained by step-like changes in the firing rate of individual neurons, with firing rate held steady at elevated levels so long as specific working memories were sustained. However, on any individual trial, spike trains of individual prefrontal neurons are often sporadic and irregular, with brief bouts of elevated firing rate interspersed by periods of inactivity. Given the variable nature of when these increases and decreases in firing rate occur on any given trial, persistent activity is most evident in trial-averaged neural data. Fine-grained analysis of prefrontal neuron spike patterns and local field potentials revealed structure in this apparent noise. At some recording sites, oscillatory dynamics in the local field potential exhibited sporadic bouts of elevated gamma power ("gamma bubbles") that were brief, narrow band, and occurred at variable times in the trial, such that these events were only evident in single-trial data (Lundqvist et al. 2016). The prefrontal neurons that encoded information about remembered stimuli were restricted to sites at which the gamma burst rate was modulated by stimulus presentations throughout the trial. Moreover, the strength of stimulus information encoded by single neuron spike rate closely followed modulation in the local field potential gamma burst rate in the trial, suggesting that information coding by spikes at the single neuron level was coupled to brief, sporadic oscillatory dynamics at the network level (Lundqvist et al. 2016). One implication of this dynamic is that information must be encoded by some mechanism other than elevated neural firing rate in between bouts of oscillatory activity. One candidate is that information is stored by short-term changes in synaptic strength (short-term synaptic plasticity) rather than changes in neuronal firing rate (Stokes 2015). Such models can explain how persistent activity in delay neurons that is interrupted by a distractor or competing task demand (Watanabe and Funahashi 2014) can "reawaken" after a period of silence when information needs to be recalled from working memory. In fact, neural network simulations are able to store working memories solely in the form of short-term changes in synaptic strength, in the absence of overt changes in spike rate (Mongillo et al. 2008; Masse et al. 2019). From that perspective, it is of interest that analysis of synaptic physiology via hippocampal slice recordings in the 22q11.2 microdeletion mouse schizophrenia model has documented altered short-term synaptic plasticity in the mutant (Earls et al. 2010; Devaraju et al. 2017). The degree to which silent (synaptic) and spiking mechanisms of working memory contribute to the storage of information by prefrontal recurrent networks remains to be determined. But these mechanisms are not likely to prove to be mutually exclusive. For example, increasing background inputs to a network simulation of the prefrontal cortex can shift the network from a regime in which information is encoded silently by synaptic changes to a regime in which information is encoded by persistent spiking in the constituent neurons (Mongillo et al. 2008).

12 Dendritic Spines, and Synaptic Mechanisms of Persistent Working Memory Activity in Recurrent Prefrontal Circuits

Dopaminergic and glutamatergic theories of schizophrenia (Stephan et al. 2009; Javitt et al. 2012; Howes and Shatalina 2022) converge on dendritic spines of pyramidal neurons in the prefrontal cortex (Goldman-Rakic et al. 1989), where both synaptic mechanisms modulate the persistent activity of prefrontal neurons in support of working memory (Wang et al. 2013, 2019a). Dendritic spines are increasingly becoming "ground zero" in schizophrenia pathogenesis, the locus where causal biological processes are likely to unfold (Kolluri et al. 2005; Glausier and Lewis 2013; Dienel and Lewis 2018; Kasai et al. 2021; Arnsten et al. 2022). Dynamical processes within spines that are disrupted in schizophrenia may constitute the tipping point past which prefrontal networks structurally disconnect and computationally fail during neural development late in adolescence, as spines are pruned to refine prefrontal circuits, and pathophysiological states in prefrontal microcircuits emerge. A high value goal for the field presently is to better understand how these crucial structures function and malfunction in disease throughout this pruning process, and how disruption of spine function could distort the dynamics of prefrontal recurrent circuits leading to cognitive deficits in schizophrenia.

The axons of pyramidal neurons in the superficial layers of the monkey prefrontal cortex give rise to a dense plexus of axon collaterals that target neighboring neurons (Kritzer and Goldman-Rakic 1995; González-Burgos et al. 2000; Melchitzky et al. 2001). These intrinsic, horizontal projections derive primarily from neurons in the superficial cortical layers (layers II/III) and terminate in a patchy pattern that can extend up to several millimeters along the tangential dimension of the prefrontal cortex (Kritzer and Goldman-Rakic 1995). Near to their point of origin, horizontal projections target both dendritic spines of pyramidal neurons and dendritic shafts of local GABAergic interneurons with equal frequency, but at longer distances, horizontal projections synapse almost exclusively onto the dendritic spines of neighboring pyramidal neurons (Melchitzky et al. 2001). These projections link pyramidal neurons into horizontal, recurrent excitatory networks within the prefrontal cortex.

To unravel the synaptic mechanisms at play in these recurrent prefrontal circuits, and discover their impact on persistent activity and working memory, Arnsten and colleagues have undertaken a series of pharmacological studies employing iontophoresis to introduce minute amounts of drug directly into the local vicinity of individual prefrontal neurons in monkeys performing the ODR task (Vijayraghavan et al. 2007; Paspalas et al. 2013; Wang et al. 2013, 2019a; Yang et al. 2013; Jin et al. 2017; Galvin et al. 2020; Arnsten et al. 2022). Focal application of the nonspecific NMDAR antagonist MK-801 or the NR2B-subtype selective NMDAR antagonist Ro25-6981 powerfully suppressed spatially selective persistent firing in prefrontal neurons of monkeys during task performance in a dose-dependent and reversible manner (Wang et al. 2013). AMPA receptor antagonists CNQX or NBQX also suppressed persistent firing but to a lesser extent (Wang et al. 2013), suggesting that persistent activity in recurrent prefrontal networks is more dependent upon NMDAR than AMPA synaptic currents for its maintenance. This is consistent with predictions from artificial network simulations using recurrent architectures and realistic synaptic conductances which have shown that persistent activity is dependent on NMDAR synaptic actions in the recurrent connections (Wang 1999; Compte et al. 2000; Brunel and Wang 2001; Wang et al. 2013). Iontophoretic application of an α7-nAChR-selective antagonist also powerfully suppressed persistent firing of prefrontal neurons during the ODR task in a dose-dependent manner (Yang et al. 2013), suggesting that nicotinic AChR localized to the dendritic spines of prefrontal pyramidal neurons provide a larger fraction of the fast excitatory synaptic current needed to overcome the Mg^{2+} blockade of NMDAR than do AMPAR (Arnsten et al. 2022). Iontophoresis of α7-nAChR-selective agonist conversely enhanced persistent activity of prefrontal neurons in a dose-dependent manner (Yang et al. 2013). This could explain why deep brain stimulation of the nucleus basalis of Meynert (the primary source of cholinergic afferents to the forebrain) in monkeys enhances persistent activity of prefrontal neurons as well as working memory performance (Qi et al. 2021).

Persistent activity of prefrontal neurons is also powerfully modulated by dopamine, consistent with the fact that dopaminergic afferents synapse onto dendritic spines of prefrontal pyramidal neurons (Goldman-Rakic et al. 1989; Smiley and Goldman-Rakic 1993), often in close proximity to excitatory, presumably glutamatergic, synapses onto the same spine, in a structure termed a "synaptic triad" (Goldman-Rakic et al. 1989). Application of the selective D1R antagonists SCH31966 enhanced persistent firing in prefrontal neurons selectively at the neuron's preferred stimulus location when administered at low doses (Williams and Goldman-Rakic 1995). At higher doses, SCH31966 powerfully suppressed prefrontal activity in all task periods and cue locations (Williams and Goldman-Rakic 1995), indicating an inverted U-shaped dose–response curve, and consistent with working memory impairments on the ODR task produced by microinjection of D1 antagonists into the prefrontal cortex (Sawaguchi and Goldman-Rakic 1991).

Iontophoretic application of the high-affinity D1R agonist SKF81297 also demonstrated an "inverted U"-shaped relationship between D1R activation and persistent activity (Vijayraghavan et al. 2007). At intermediate iontophoretic doses of D1R agonist, the spatial selectivity of delay period activity was strongly enhanced, predominantly by suppressing activity at nonpreferred spatial locations and sharpening the spatial tuning curves of these neurons (Vijayraghavan et al. 2007). At higher doses of D1R agonist, persistent activity at the preferred cue location of each neuron was suppressed, with the effect that the spatial selectivity of delay period activity was reduced overall (Vijayraghavan et al. 2007). The low potency D1R agonist PF-3628, perhaps more closely mimicking the binding properties of endogenous dopamine, enhanced persistent activity in prefrontal neurons at each neuron's preferred cue location (Wang et al. 2019a).

13 Neural Basis of Cognitive Functions Disrupted in Schizophrenia: Prefrontal Activity and Cognitive Control

In addition to deficits in working memory, schizophrenia induces deficits in cognitive control (Smucny et al. 2020a) that are not attributable to antipsychotic medication (Moran et al. 2020) and are present at first episode (MacDonald et al. 2005) and in first-degree relatives (Snitz et al. 2006). Cognitive control and working memory are related constructs (Smucny et al. 2022), in the sense that both involve the ability to govern behavioral responses on the basis of internal neural representations of state. In the case of working memory, internal state variables reflect events in the recent past. In the case of cognitive control, internal state variables include goals, rules, or contextual variables that alter behavioral outputs to environmental stimuli (Miller and Cohen 2001). As such, cognitive control is more directly related to behavioral flexibility, the ability to change how we respond to external stimuli according to what our current behavioral objectives are, or what environmental rules we believe to be in force. The hallmark of cognitive control is the ability to produce different, context-dependent responses to the same sensory input, as a function of internal state variables coded by neural activity in the prefrontal cortex and prefrontal distributed networks (Miller and Cohen 2001). Cognitive control demand is greatest when behavioral responses governed by internal state variables (such as goals or rules) must compete with habitual responses to stimuli. This is generally believed to reflect competition between two behavioral control or decision-making systems in the brain—one deliberative system governed by the prefrontal cortex and explicit models of goals, rules, actions, and predicted outcomes (such as are acquired by "Q-learning" algorithms) and one habitual system governed by reflexive stimulus response associations (such as are acquired by "actor-critic" algorithms) acquired by reinforcement learning encoded into basal ganglia circuits (Sweis et al. 2018). The conflict between these systems has particular relevance for the nature of prefrontal network failure in schizophrenia, because it is precisely when context-dependent or rule-based actions conflict with habitual responses to stimuli that the cognitive deficits of people with schizophrenia become most apparent.

The effort to relate cognitive control to the activity of individual neurons in the nonhuman primate prefrontal cortex was greatly advanced by the work of Miller, Freedman, Nieder, Wallis, and their colleagues (Freedman et al. 2001, 2003; Wallis et al. 2001; Nieder et al. 2002; Nieder and Miller 2003, 2004a, b; Wallis and Miller 2003; Muhammad et al. 2006; McKee et al. 2014). These were pioneering experiments that pushed the boundaries of the complexity of cognitive processes that could be related to the activity of individual neurons in the brain. The ODR task proved a highly effective tool with which to parse the cellular, synaptic, and computational properties of prefrontal networks. But in the end, it is a relatively simple task, in terms of the type of information cortical networks are required to generate and retain to obtain reward (namely, the location of a peripheral visual stimulus, information initially present in the pattern of activity in the retina). Intelligence, whatever it proves to be, will involve more complex processes, for example the capacity for abstraction. The human brain can derive general principles from specific experiences that allow it to predict how the world will behave in novel circumstances. Miller and colleagues tapped into this ability by training monkeys to match visual displays on the basis of abstract characteristics, such as the abstract category to which a stimulus belonged (Freedman et al. 2001, 2003; Meyers et al. 2008; McKee et al. 2014), or the number of items it contained (Nieder et al. 2002; Nieder and Miller 2003, 2004a, b), irrespective of the visual features of the specific stimuli displayed or the parameters of the motor response required. In parallel experiments, they trained monkeys to employ different abstract rules to govern responses to the same set of picture stimuli (Wallis et al. 2001; Wallis and Miller 2003; Muhammad et al. 2006). The key discovery was that individual neurons in the prefrontal cortex were found in which firing rate varied systematically as a function of which specific category (Freedman et al. 2001), number (Nieder et al. 2002), or rule (Wallis et al. 2001) was relevant to the current trial. It was not easy to ascribe this activity to more concrete behavioral correlates, such as stimuli or movements in the task. The information the neurons encoded was abstract. Prefrontal neurons were found to encode an item of information that (a) was decorrelated from features of stimuli or parameters of movement (and therefore outside the domain of sensorimotor processing) and (b) provided a basis for effective mapping of responses to stimuli in novel circumstances based on an underlying, generalized principle. The finding that patterns of activity in individual neurons and neural populations could encode this type of information was a significant step forward in our understanding of the neural basis of cognitive control, in particular, and intelligence, more generally. The utility of neural representations of this type was that they could implement cognitive flexibility in cortical networks. Namely, by establishing different patterns of activity over prefrontal neurons, to encode alternative abstract constructs (such as a category, number, or rule), and thereby changing the initial state of the network, it was possible to alter how the network would respond to subsequent environmental inputs by virtue of this change in the initial physiological state of the network (Miller and Cohen 2001). This would make it possible for the brain to produce different responses to the same stimuli as a function of context, the essence of cognitive control.

We undertook a series of follow-on experiments to investigate how cognitive control and behavioral flexibility were implemented in the prefrontal–parietal network in which we trained monkeys to apply different rules to categorize the same circular array of visual stimuli (Goodwin et al. 2012; Crowe et al. 2013). A peripheral dot stimulus and then a line representing a spatial category boundary were presented in sequence (requiring working memory). Animals were required to report whether the dot fell to the left versus right of the line if the line appeared in a vertical orientation, or above versus below the line if horizontal. Thus, a visual stimulus at a fixed retinal position (a dot in the circular array) could be assigned to the abstract spatial category "up" or "left" depending on the categorization rule imposed later in the trial. We found that prefrontal and also parietal neurons generated a neural representation of the abstract spatial category to which the stimulus belonged (Goodwin et al. 2012). The spatial category was an abstraction, decorrelated from individual stimuli and responses in the task. At the neural population level, differences in the timing and strength of the neural signal were observed between the prefrontal and parietal cortex that suggested specialization of function. Rule signals were earlier and stronger in the parietal cortex (the rule was signaled by a visual stimulus), whereas category signals (derived by an internal computation) were earlier and stronger in the prefrontal cortex (Goodwin et al. 2012). To capture communication between the prefrontal and parietal cortex, we utilized pattern classification to generate single-trial time series measuring temporal variation in the amount of category information encoded by patterns of activity in small groups of prefrontal and parietal neurons that were recorded simultaneously (Crowe et al. 2013). We then evaluated whether the information time series in one cortical area could predict the information time series in the other cortical area at a lag, allowing us to determine whether category signals in prefrontal neurons drove category signals in parietal neurons, or vice versa. We found evidence of top-down transmission of category information from prefrontal to parietal neurons, but not the converse (Crowe et al. 2013). Communication between cortical areas detected by this analysis was abolished by comparing time series in the two areas after trial shuffling to break the simultaneity of the neural activity between the prefrontal and parietal cortex. This was evidence that the analysis detected transmission of task information between cortical areas in real time.

14 Blocking NMDAR in Monkeys to Replicate Cognitive Control Deficits in Schizophrenia

NMDAR antagonists replicate positive, negative, and cognitive deficits of schizophrenia when administered to healthy control subjects (Krystal et al. 1994). NMDAR antagonists also worsen positive symptoms when administered to people with schizophrenia (Malhotra et al. 1997; Lahti et al. 2001), increasing the severity of both auditory hallucinations and paranoia (Malhotra et al. 1997). Early experiments by Roth and colleagues demonstrated that monkeys chronically exposed to NMDAR antagonists exhibit lasting changes both in cognitive function and in dopamine utilization in the prefrontal cortex (Jentsch et al. 1997, 1999). Behavioral deficits outlasted cessation of drug exposure for up to 4 weeks (Jentsch et al. 1997). These data suggest that transient perturbation of NMDAR synaptic function can produce persistent changes in cortical network function.

To optimize the translational relevance of neural recording in nonhuman primates to schizophrenia, several groups have administered NMDAR antagonists to monkeys performing the same behavioral paradigms that detect cognitive control deficits in people with the disease. This makes it possible to relate changes in behavior like those seen in schizophrenia to underlying changes in the function of prefrontal neurons and networks. Everling and colleagues used this approach in monkeys performing an antisaccade task measuring cognitive control deficits in schizophrenia (McDowell et al. 2002). In the task, monkeys have to use cognitive control to produce either a prosaccade toward a peripheral cue or an antisaccade in the opposite direction depending on the color of the central gaze fixation target. This requires switching between two different response rules on a trial-by-trial basis. Administration of the NMDAR antagonist ketamine to monkeys selectively increased the error rate on antisaccade trials that require overriding the prepotent habit of directing a saccade toward the target (Skoblenick and Everling 2012, 2014). Neural recording in the prefrontal cortex demonstrated that ketamine weakened rule signals in prefrontal neurons, by attenuating the difference in firing rate on pro- versus antisaccade trials (Skoblenick and Everling 2012), and reducing the signal-to-noise ratio in rule-selective neural activity at both the single neuron and neural ensemble levels (Ma et al. 2015). These effects were not present on correct trials and were only evident when correct and error trials were pooled in the analysis (Ma et al. 2015). That suggests that NMDAR antagonists alter the dynamics of prefrontal networks in such a way that causes them to fail in a stochastic fashion over trials. The signal-to-noise ratio of neural activity was in the normal range and not affected by ketamine on trials when responses were correct, but it was degraded on the apparently random subset of trials on which errors were committed. Blocking NMDAR additionally weakened neural activity encoding trial outcome (success versus failure) in the prefrontal cortex (Skoblenick and Everling 2014). Such signals could be used to update explicit predictions of action outcomes employed by Q-learning algorithms. Finally, blocking NMDAR attenuated oscillations in prefrontal local field potentials that encoded information about both the rule and trial outcome (Skoblenick et al. 2016; Ma et al. 2018). These data provide cell and network-level descriptions of how prefrontal cortical circuits might fail causing cognitive control deficits in schizophrenia, namely by degrading neural signals that reflect internal state variables (such as rules) and trial outcomes that could serve to update how the rules are applied to control behavior.

One challenge in comparing neurophysiological signals between nonhuman primates and people with schizophrenia is the difference in the nature of the neural signals that are typically measured in the two species (single neuron recording in monkeys; EEG, MEG, or fMRI signals in humans). Albright and colleagues circumvented this problem by recording the same neural signal (EEG) in monkeys and humans performing an auditory oddball paradigm in which pure tones were presented at either high or low sound intensity in random order (Gil-da-Costa et al. 2013). Infrequent "oddball" stimuli evoke a stereotypic sequence of event-related brain potentials in humans performing this task that consists of an early mismatch negativity followed by a later P3a-positive going potential (Gil-da-Costa et al. 2013). Oddball-evoked brain potentials are attenuated both in people with schizophrenia (van der Stelt and Belger 2007; Wynn et al. 2010) and in monkeys given ketamine (Gil-da-Costa et al. 2013), providing a close parallel in neurophysiological phenomena between monkeys and humans that captures changes in brain activity that are seen in schizophrenia.

15 Combining NMDAR Antagonists and the AX-CPT to Translate Cognitive Control Deficits in Schizophrenia to Monkeys

The AX continuous performance task (AX-CPT) is one of the most thoroughly characterized tasks used to measure specific deficits in cognitive control in schizophrenia (Barch et al. 2003; Snitz et al. 2006; MacDonald 3rd 2008; Jones et al. 2010; Carter et al. 2012) as well as the changes in brain activity associated with these deficits using functional neuroimaging (Perlstein et al. 2003; MacDonald et al. 2005; Yoon et al. 2008; Lesh et al. 2013; Niendam et al. 2018; Smucny et al. 2018, 2020b). This task requires that subjects store a contextual cue in working memory to modify their response to a subsequent probe stimulus. One cue stimulus is designated the A-cue, and 5 alternative stimuli are collectively designated B-cues. Similarly, one probe stimulus is designated the X-probe, and 5 alternative stimuli are collectively designated Y-probes. AX cue-probe sequences require a target response (typically a leftward joystick movement or button press). Any other cue-probe sequence requires a nontarget response (rightward joystick movement or button press). The majority of trials (typically 70%) present the AX sequence establishing a prepotent habit to produce the leftward target response whenever the X-probe is presented. The relatively rare BX trials require overriding this habit to produce the rightward, nontarget response to the X-probe instead. As such, BX trials require the greatest cognitive control because they put a response instructed by a contextual cue stored in working memory (the B-cue) in conflict with a reflexive response to a visible stimulus (the X-probe). People with schizophrenia exhibit selectively elevated error rates on BX trials in comparison to the other cue-probe sequences (Barch et al. 2003; MacDonald 3rd 2008; Jones et al. 2010; Henderson et al. 2012), as do their first-degree relatives (MacDonald 3rd et al. 2003; Snitz et al. 2006). The specificity of that error pattern and the underlying computational deficit facilitate search for the specific neural circuit wherein pathophysiological states drive errors in performance. This makes the AX-CPT a high value target for translation to nonhuman primates.

Dias, Javitt, and colleagues directly compared brain activity between a monkey and humans performing the AX-CPT based on EEG recordings in humans and local field potential (LFP) recordings in monkey (Dias et al. 2006). Source localization of EEG recording during task performance in humans identified dipoles in the dorsolateral prefrontal and anterior cingulate cortex. Laminar recordings of cortical local field potentials were directed to homologous regions of the dorsolateral and anterior cingulate cortex in monkey. This comparative approach identified parallels in brain activation patterns during the cue and probe periods between species. In both humans and monkeys, prefrontal activation was greatest under conditions imposing the largest cognitive control demand. During the cue period, this was made evident by greater prefrontal LFP and EEG activation on B-cue than A-cue trials (Dias et al. 2006). During the probe period, this was made evident by greater prefrontal LFP and EEG activation on AY than AX trials (Dias et al. 2006). Both sets of stimulus conditions (presentation of the B-cue during the cue period, and AY cue-probe sequence during the probe period) signal the necessity to override the prepotent target response and are therefore associated with elevated cognitive control demand. Whereas there was close correspondence between LFP and EEG findings in the prefrontal cortex between species, there was weaker correspondence between LFP and EEG findings in the anterior cingulate cortex between species, suggesting that brain networks for cognitive control differ to some degree between them (Dias et al. 2006).

Chafee and colleagues undertook a series of behavioral (Blackman et al. 2013) and single neuron recording studies using multielectrode arrays (Blackman et al. 2016; DeNicola et al. 2020; Kummerfeld et al. 2020) in the prefrontal cortex, posterior parietal cortex, and mediodorsal nucleus of the thalamus in monkeys performing a dot-pattern variant of the AX-CPT, or DPX task (Jones et al. 2010). Administering the NMDAR antagonist ketamine to monkeys produced a transient and dose-dependent cognitive control deficit that manifested as a selective increase in errors on BX trials (Blackman et al. 2013), bearing a striking resemblance to the error pattern in people with schizophrenia performing the same task (Jones et al. 2010). Neural recordings in the prefrontal cortex and thalamus demonstrated a distribution of "switch" neurons between the two structures (DeNicola et al. 2020). Firing rate in these neurons was greatest on B-cue trials during the cue period, and AY trials during the probe period (DeNicola et al. 2020), much like the pattern of LFP modulation observed by Dias and colleagues (Dias et al. 2006). At the single neuron level, this was an interesting signal, because its modulation was better explained by a cognitive variable than a sensorimotor one. Firing rate elevation during the cue period reflects proactive control, the necessity to store contextual cues to override habitual responses to future environmental inputs. Firing rate elevation during the probe period reflects reactive control, the necessity to override a prepotent response when a countermanding stimulus appears. The two forms of cognitive control appeared to be integrated into the activity of single neurons. The strength of switch neuron activity was amplified on prepotent trial sets in which the majority of trials were AX, establishing a strong target response habit, relative to balanced trial sets in which all cue-probe sequences were equiprobable (DeNicola et al. 2020). The distribution of switch neurons between the prefrontal cortex (Blackman et al. 2016), the MD thalamus (DeNicola et al. 2020), and the parietal cortex (unpublished observations) upholds the general principle that neural representations for cognitive control are network-level phenomena rather than properties of any individual brain area. We found differences in the timing and strength of neural signals in the prefrontal cortex and thalamus; however, that suggested differential contributions to their shared activity (DeNicola et al. 2020). Neural signals evoked by the visual cue were earlier in the prefrontal cortex than in the MD thalamus. However, neural signals evoked by the probe or occurring at the time of the manual response were earlier and dramatically stronger in the MD thalamus in comparison to the prefrontal cortex (DeNicola et al. 2020). At the population level, the direction of the motor response (target versus nontarget) could be decoded with significantly greater confidence when based on neural activity patterns in the MD thalamus in comparison to the prefrontal cortex (DeNicola et al. 2020). Both errors in behavioral performance and response times could be better predicted based on neural activity in the MD thalamus than in the prefrontal cortex (DeNicola et al. 2020). Functional communication between the prefrontal cortex and MD thalamus was strongest during the probe period, when information about the cue stored in working memory and the visible probe stimulus had to be integrated to make a decision about which way to move (DeNicola et al. 2020). All of these findings suggest that the prefrontal-MD circuit is preferentially engaged at the time that the decision to execute a specific motor response is made and that MD leads the prefrontal cortex in response-related computations.

Much of the evidence reviewed above provides a compelling argument that schizophrenia is essentially a synaptic disease that interferes with effective communication between neurons in prefrontal circuits, leading to computational failure in these circuits and behavioral errors in cognitive control. To quantify functional interactions between neurons, local circuits, and cortical areas, Kummerfeld and colleagues applied causal discovery analysis to sets of simultaneously recorded single neuron activity and local field potentials in the prefrontal and parietal cortex of monkeys performing the DPX task (Kummerfeld et al. 2020). Causal discovery is a mathematical technique that detects causal relationships between simultaneously observed variables (neurons and local field potentials in this case). The procedure finds the graph of relationships (directed interactions between nodes) that maximizes the probability of the data given the model (Kummerfeld et al. 2020). Each node in this analysis represented a time series capturing fluctuation in the activity of a single prefrontal or parietal neuron, or oscillatory power at a specific frequency in local field potentials recorded at a specific site in the two cortical areas, or behavioral outputs. Functional relationships between neurons and local field potentials detected in this manner provide a proxy for synaptic communication between neurons in networks. Comparison of graphs derived from the prefrontal and parietal cortex under baseline conditions and after administration of NMDAR antagonist in monkeys revealed that loss of NMDAR synaptic actions reduced neuron-to-neuron interactions in the prefrontal cortex but increased neuron-to-neuron interactions in the parietal cortex (Kummerfeld et al. 2020). This indicated that global, systemic administration of an NMDAR antagonist had opposite effects on neural communication in the prefrontal and parietal cortex, likely to reflect different roles of NMDAR synaptic mechanisms in microcircuits within the two cortical regions. These neuron-to-neuron interactions reflected single cell correlates of cognitive control, because they were significantly increased on B-cue trials in relation to A-cue trials, and they predicted BX errors in both cortical areas (Kummerfeld et al. 2020). Blocking NMDAR also disrupted the relationship between spikes in single neurons and local field potentials within and between cortical regions, increasing the strength of bottom-up casual interactions from the parietal to the prefrontal cortex in the drug condition (Kummerfeld et al. 2020). These data relate computations for cognitive control to patterns of functional interaction between neurons and local circuits in prefrontal networks, linking computation to synaptically mediated interactions between cellular processing elements.

16 NMDAR Antagonists and Spiking Timing in Prefrontal Local Circuits

To further explore how loss of NMDAR function as well as genetic risk in schizophrenia might interfere with neuronal communication, Zick and colleagues evaluated spike timing relationships between simultaneously recorded neurons in the monkey prefrontal cortex before and during NMDAR synaptic blockade (Zick et al. 2018). Synaptic interactions between neurons are likely to leave a trace in the form of statistical dependencies between the relative timing structure of their spike trains (Garofalo et al. 2009; Ito et al. 2011). Analysis of spike timing relationships between prefrontal neurons could therefore capture physiological and computational consequences of altered synaptic communication between neurons. This analysis revealed that pairs of prefrontal neurons tended to fire action potentials at precisely the same time (coincident spikes occurring in the same 1 ms time bin) more frequently than predicted by chance based on their firing rates. Moreover, the rate of such synchronous ("0-lag") spike pairs between neurons was strongly modulated by behavior such that 0-lag spiking increased dramatically around the time of the behavioral response and reward in the DPX task (Zick et al. 2018). Administration of NMDAR antagonists strongly suppressed the magnitude of this task-dependent increase in 0-lag spiking without changing overall firing rate. This indicated a disturbance in how spike timing was modulated independently of neural activity during behavior. Synchronous spiking between prefrontal neurons could reflect either common input to the neurons from an extrinsic source or mutual excitation between the neurons in recurrent local circuits (Amit and Brunel 1997; Pipa and Munk 2011; Korndörfer et al. 2017). Unidirectional synaptic interactions between neurons would be reflected instead by lagged changes in spike probability, by which spiking in one neuron would increase (or decrease) the probability that another neuron would spike a short time later. Transfer entropy is a statistical way to measure such lagged interactions that quantifies bits of information transmitted between neurons by measuring conditional probabilities of spiking in a "receiving" neuron as a function of prior spiking in a "transmitting" neuron (Schreiber 2000; Ito et al. 2011; Wibral et al. 2013). Blocking NMDAR reduced the amount of information transmitted between neurons by this measure, both in the acute phase with NMDAR antagonist on board and on subsequent days that saline was injected (Zick et al. 2018). This result suggested that transient and repeated suppression of synchronous spiking in prefrontal microcircuits led to their persistent functional disconnection outlasting the presence of NMDAR antagonist at the receptor. That led to an activity-dependent disconnection hypothesis in which loss of synchronous spiking in recurrent prefrontal networks, perhaps due to excessively aggressive synaptic pruning in adolescence (Sellgren et al. 2019; Sheridan et al. 2022), triggered a feedback cycle by which worsening spike asynchrony and progressive disconnection of prefrontal local circuits amplified each other leading to the synaptic collapse of prefrontal networks (Zick et al. 2018). This dynamic is generally consistent with the principle of spike timing-dependent synaptic plasticity, wherein synapses are strengthened or weakened as a function of precise spike timing relationships in pre- and postsynaptic neurons (Dan and Poo 2004).

17 Convergent Impacts of Genetic Risk and NMDAR Blockade on Prefrontal Circuit Dynamics

It was not clear whether the observed change in the spike synchrony dynamics of prefrontal networks reflected a general failure mode downstream of multiple schizophrenia-relevant risk factors, or an idiosyncratic property of how NMDAR antagonists influenced local circuits in the monkey prefrontal cortex. To answer that question, Zick and colleagues compared 0-lag spike synchrony and transfer entropy profiles in the prefrontal cortex of two different animal models of circuit failure in schizophrenia: in monkeys following administration of NMDAR antagonists, and in mice that bore a genetic mutation increasing the risk of schizophrenia in humans (Zick et al. 2021). The mouse genetic model incorporated selective deletion of *Dgcr8* in neurons. *Dgcr8* is required for the synthesis of microRNA which negatively regulates translation of messenger RNA into protein (Guo and Wang 2019). The *Dgcr8* gene is located within the 22q11.2 microdeletion region comprising one of the strongest identified genetic risk factors for schizophrenia in humans (Merico et al. 2014, 2015; Sellier et al. 2014), and deletion of *Dgcr8* captures many of the phenotypic features of the full 22q11.2 microdeletion in mice (Stark et al. 2008). Zick and colleagues observed convergent impacts of NMDAR blockade in monkeys and *Dgcr8* deletion in mice on the neural dynamics of prefrontal local circuits (Zick et al. 2021). Both manipulations reduced synchronous 0-lag spiking as well as effective communication between neurons as measured by transfer entropy (Zick et al. 2021). The precision of that pathophysiological convergence in prefrontal cortical microcircuits was surprising given the difference in species and manipulations employed. The implication is that synchronous spiking and activity-dependent regulation of synaptic communication in prefrontal local circuits are disrupted in a similar way by different schizophrenia risk factors operating through different molecular and cellular mechanisms. If borne out by subsequent experiments, this implication suggests that treatments that modulate the relationship between spike timing and synaptic plasticity in prefrontal local circuits, perhaps by influencing molecular signaling pathways in dendritic spines that mediate the relationship between electrical activity patterns and synaptic strength in these networks, might restore local circuit connectivity and the computational integrity of the prefrontal cortex in schizophrenia.

18 Developmental NHP Models

Although the studies above provide a starting point in the effort to reverse-engineer prefrontal network failure in schizophrenia, they still suffer from the limitation that in the species with greatest circuit homology to humans (nonhuman primates), the model of the disease state is imposed by administration of a drug, with strong face validity (in terms of behavioral deficits) but restricted construct validity in relation to the causes of schizophrenia in humans. Schizophrenia at its core is a neurodevelopmental disease that is likely to involve a latent physiological vulnerability embedded in prefrontal local circuits that is established during in utero cortical development, and that is functionally unmasked by synaptic pruning as prefrontal circuits are refined in adolescence (Dienel and Lewis 2018; Arnsten et al. 2022; Benoit et al. 2022a; Chafee and Averbeck 2022; Girdhar et al. 2022; Hanson et al. 2022; Howes and Shatalina 2022; Johnson and Hyman 2022; Sheridan et al. 2022; Vinogradov et al. 2022). To investigate the neurodevelopmental origin and cause of these delayed negative impacts on prefrontal cortex structure and function, Bauman and colleagues established a maternal immune activation (MIA) model of altered neural development in nonhuman primates (Hanson et al. 2022). Injection of poly(I:C), a synthetic analog of double-stranded RNA used to simulate viral infections, was administered to pregnant dams in either the first or second trimester of fetal development. Cohorts of offspring in the MIA group exhibited increased repetitive behaviors, decreased affiliative vocalizations, and altered social interactions in comparison to a control cohort (Bauman et al. 2014). Offspring of dams with MIA exposure also exhibit an abnormal pattern of saccades and gaze fixations while viewing pictures of monkey facial expressions (Machado et al. 2015), suggesting a defect in social cognition. Of particular relevance to cognitive control deficits in schizophrenia is that offspring of dams with MIA exposure also commit more false-alarm responses in a continuous performance task (Vlasova et al. 2021). Structural brain changes are also observed in the offspring of dams with MIA exposure, including reduced prefrontal gray matter volume (Vlasova et al. 2021) and changes in the morphology of pyramidal neurons in the dorsolateral prefrontal cortex including a significant reduction in the width and branching pattern of apical dendrites, although spine density was not affected (Weir et al. 2015). Further, PET imaging of a radiolabeled dopamine precursor detected elevated levels of uptake in the dorsal striatum in the offspring of MIA-exposed dams (Bauman et al. 2019). This provided evidence of hyperdopaminergia in the dorsal striatum of the MIA-exposed cohort, a finding that closely parallels molecular imaging results in schizophrenia (Howes et al. 2011; Howes and Shatalina 2022). Thus, the MIA model holds considerable promise as a nonhuman primate model of neurodevelopmental, cognitive, and neural system disruptions in schizophrenia.

Other developmental models have utilized fetal irradiation to disrupt brain development in utero. Offspring exposed to ionizing radiation during development exhibit working memory deficits that emerge in adulthood (Friedman and Selemon 2010), which include an increase in perseverative errors on working memory tasks (Selemon and Friedman 2013). Fetal irradiation early in gestation reduces thalamic volume most prominently in the mediodorsal thalamic nucleus (Selemon et al. 2009). Fetal irradiation also reduces gray matter volume in the prefrontal cortex (Selemon et al. 2013).

Further physiological characterization of these neurodevelopmental models is likely to provide crucial insight into how diverse risk factors in schizophrenia impact neural and synaptic function in prefrontal cortical local circuits and networks, thereby disrupting computations for working memory and cognitive control.

19 Future Potential of Nonhuman Primate Models

The evidence reviewed above documents some of the successes that have been achieved in the effort to translate deficits in working memory and cognitive control from people with schizophrenia to nonhuman primate models, in order to enable characterization of the underlying defects in brain function at a cellular level of scale. This has made it possible to begin to understand how computations mediated by neural interactions in prefrontal microcircuits might be disrupted by synaptic malfunction to produce cognitive deficits in the human disease. These studies also highlight potential pathogenic mechanisms that could cause prefrontal circuits to fail in the first place, including disruption of neural synchrony with follow-on activity-dependent disconnection of prefrontal microcircuits. Theories of this type, if confirmed by subsequent studies, may make it possible to identify the physiological weak points in prefrontal microcircuits that are exploited by multiple schizophrenia risk factors, causing them to fail in fundamentally the same way. That captures a key feature of schizophrenia pathogenesis, namely that a large number of genetic, synaptic, developmental, and social/environmental risk factors impose synergistic risk through mechanistically divergent mechanisms that have functionally convergent impacts on prefrontal cortical circuits. It may be possible to further develop nonhuman primate models to characterize the nature of that functional convergence, by describing the failure state of prefrontal circuits where multiple pathogenic trajectories converge in terms of a fundamental change in how neurons and synapses operate during behavior. That knowledge may guide development of more effective therapeutic interventions, designed and tested to reverse changes in synaptic and neural function that underlie the disease state, therefore normalizing network dynamics and computation in schizophrenia. These advances will require development and enhancement of research tools that can be applied in nonhuman primates, including further refinement of genetic manipulation technologies in nonhuman primates, as well as refinement of optical imaging tools that can measure synaptic and dendritic spine function directly in nonhuman primates. Finally, a new generation of computational models will be required that can capture, predict, and explain how changes in synaptic plasticity and dendritic spine biology implicated in schizophrenia impact spiking patterns and computations in prefrontal recurrent networks. Integration of these approaches will be validated if predictions they provide about how to restore function to prefrontal networks can be demonstrated to work in people with schizophrenia. That last step is, of course, the most challenging, and the most important.

20 Do We Need to Understand Schizophrenia at a Cellular Level to Cure It?

Admittedly, it is an open question whether we need to understand how schizophrenia alters the physiological operation of neurons and synapses to more effectively treat the disease. A recent book by a prior Director of the NIMH (Insel 2022) makes a compelling argument that the problem, at least in the near term, is more of implementing what we know works for people with schizophrenia at scale, rather than finding out more about the neurobiology of the disease. The argument is that basic neuroscience of schizophrenia has yet to translate into significantly better treatments for people dealing with the disease, and the greatest impact for patients now requires modifying the mental health system to increase access to existing treatments that are known to be effective (Insel 2022). This includes increasing access to high-quality in-patient hospital care for acute phases of psychosis, as well as high-quality psychotherapy and community-based interventions that help to alter the course of the disease, in large part by modifying environmental inputs. However, the degree to which interventions that consist of altering environmental inputs can effectively turn the course of the disease for the many millions of individuals suffering from schizophrenia remains to be proven. The underlying change in brain function is unquestionably profound. It may not prove possible to restore function to brain networks completely by altering environmental inputs alone. Rather, the long game in the search for a cure to schizophrenia is likely to strategically require optimizing synergies between environmental and biological interventions, as available evidence indicates this interaction is what sets the disease process in motion at the outset.

References

Abi-Dargham A, van de Giessen E, Slifstein M, Kegeles LS, Laruelle M (2009) Baseline and amphetamine-stimulated dopamine activity are related in drug-naïve schizophrenic subjects. Biol Psychiatry 65:1091–1093

Adcock RA, Dale C, Fisher M, Aldebot S, Genevsky A, Simpson GV, Nagarajan S, Vinogradov S (2009) When top-down meets bottom-up: auditory training enhances verbal memory in schizophrenia. Schizophr Bull 35:1132–1141

Adrover MF, Shin JH, Quiroz C, Ferré S, Lemos JC, Alvarez VA (2020) Prefrontal cortex-driven dopamine signals in the striatum show unique spatial and pharmacological properties. J Neurosci 40(39):7510–7522. https://doi.org/10.1523/JNEUROSCI.1327-20.2020

Aida T, Feng G (2020) The dawn of non-human primate models for neurodevelopmental disorders. Curr Opin Genet Dev 65:160–168

Aleman A, Hijman R, de Haan EH, Kahn RS (1999) Memory impairment in schizophrenia: a meta-analysis. Am J Psychiatry 156:1358–1366

Allen RM, Young SJ (1978) Phencyclidine-induced psychosis. Am J Psychiatry 135:1081–1084

Amit DJ, Brunel N (1997) Model of global spontaneous activity and local structured activity during delay periods in the cerebral cortex. Cereb Cortex 7:237–252

Anticevic A, Cole MW, Repovs G, Murray JD, Brumbaugh MS, Winkler AM, Savic A, Krystal JH, Pearlson GD, Glahn DC (2014) Characterizing thalamo-cortical disturbances in schizophrenia and bipolar illness. Cereb Cortex 24:3116–3130

Anticevic A et al (2015) Association of thalamic dysconnectivity and conversion to psychosis in youth and young adults at elevated clinical risk. JAMA Psychiatry 72:882–891

Arnsten AFT, Woo E, Yang S, Wang M, Datta D (2022) Unusual molecular regulation of dorsolateral prefrontal cortex layer III synapses increases vulnerability to genetic and environmental insults in Schizophrenia. Biol Psychiatry 92:480–490

Ash H, Chang A, Ortiz RJ, Kulkarni P, Rauch B, Colman R, Ferris CF, Ziegler TE (2022) Structural and functional variations in the prefrontal cortex are associated with learning in pre-adolescent common marmosets (Callithrix jacchus). Behav Brain Res 430:113920

Averbeck BB (2022) Pruning recurrent neural networks replicates adolescent changes in working memory and reinforcement learning. Proc Natl Acad Sci U S A 119:e2121331119

Axelsson SFA, Horst NK, Horiguchi N, Roberts AC, Robbins TW (2021) Flexible versus fixed spatial self-ordered response sequencing: effects of inactivation and neurochemical modulation of ventrolateral prefrontal cortex. J Neurosci 41:7246–7258

Balsters JH, Zerbi V, Sallet J, Wenderoth N, Mars RB (2020) Primate homologs of mouse cortico-striatal circuits. eLife 9 Available at: https://doi.org/10.7554/eLife.53680.

Barch DM, Carter CS, MacDonald AW III, Braver TS, Cohen JD (2003) Context-processing deficits in schizophrenia: Diagnostic specificity, 4-week course, and relationships to clinical symptoms. J Abnorm Psychol 112:132–143

Bauman MD, Iosif A-M, Smith SEP, Bregere C, Amaral DG, Patterson PH (2014) Activation of the maternal immune system during pregnancy alters behavioral development of rhesus monkey offspring. Biol Psychiatry 75:332–341

Bauman MD, Lesh TA, Rowland DJ, Schumann CM, Smucny J, Kukis DL, Cherry SR, McAllister AK, Carter CS (2019) Preliminary evidence of increased striatal dopamine in a nonhuman primate model of maternal immune activation. Transl Psychiatry 9:135

Benoit LJ, Canetta S, Kellendonk C (2022a) Thalamocortical development: a neurodevelopmental framework for Schizophrenia. Biol Psychiatry 92:491–500

Benoit LJ, Canetta S, Kellendonk C (2022b) Thalamocortical development: a neurodevelopmental framework for Schizophrenia. Biol Psychiatry 92:491–500

Benoit LJ, Holt ES, Posani L, Fusi S, Harris AZ, Canetta S, Kellendonk C (2022c) Adolescent thalamic inhibition leads to long-lasting impairments in prefrontal cortex function. Nat Neurosci 25:714–725

Bertolino A (2000) The relationship between dorsolateral prefrontal neuronal N-acetylaspartate and evoked release of striatal dopamine in schizophrenia. Neuropsychopharmacol 22(2):125–132. https://doi.org/10.1016/S0893-133X(99)00096-2

Biagianti B, Fisher M, Neilands TB, Loewy R, Vinogradov S (2016) Engagement with the auditory processing system during targeted auditory cognitive training mediates changes in cognitive outcomes in individuals with schizophrenia. Neuropsychology 30:998–1008

Blackman RK, Macdonald AW 3rd, Chafee MV (2013) Effects of ketamine on context-processing performance in monkeys: a new animal model of cognitive deficits in schizophrenia. Neuropsychopharmacology 38:2090–2100. https://doi.org/10.1038/npp.2013.118. Epub 2013 May 10

Blackman RK, Crowe DA, DeNicola AL, Sakellaridi S, MacDonald AW 3rd, Chafee MV (2016) Monkey prefrontal neurons reflect logical operations for cognitive control in a variant of the AX continuous performance task (AX-CPT). J Neurosci 36:4067–4079

Bora E, Murray RM (2014) Meta-analysis of cognitive deficits in ultra-high risk to psychosis and first-episode psychosis: do the cognitive deficits progress over, or after, the onset of psychosis? Schizophr Bull 40:744–755

Bourgeois JP, Goldman-Rakic PS, Rakic P (1994) Synaptogenesis in the prefrontal cortex of rhesus monkeys. Cereb Cortex 4:78–96

Breukelaar IA, Williams LM, Antees C, Grieve SM, Foster SL, Gomes L, Korgaonkar MS (2018) Cognitive ability is associated with changes in the functional organization of the cognitive control brain network. Hum Brain Mapp 39:5028–5038

Brown AS, Derkits EJ (2010) Prenatal infection and schizophrenia: a review of epidemiologic and translational studies. Am J Psychiatry 167:261–280

Brunel N, Wang XJ (2001) Effects of neuromodulation in a cortical network model of object working memory dominated by recurrent inhibition. J Comput Neurosci 11:63–85

Brunelin J, Adam O, Mondino M (2022) Recent advances in noninvasive brain stimulation for schizophrenia. Curr Opin Psychiatry 35:338–344

Callicott JH, Bertolino A, Mattay VS, Langheim FJ, Duyn J, Coppola R, Goldberg TE, Weinberger DR (2000) Physiological dysfunction of the dorsolateral prefrontal cortex in schizophrenia revisited. Cereb Cortex 10:1078–1092

Carter CS, Minzenberg M, West R, Macdonald A 3rd (2012) CNTRICS imaging biomarker selections: Executive control paradigms. Schizophr Bull 38:34–42

Cavada C, Goldman-Rakic PS (1989) Posterior parietal cortex in rhesus monkey: II. Evidence for segregated corticocortical networks linking sensory and limbic areas with the frontal lobe. J Comp Neurol 287:422–445. https://doi.org/10.1002/cne.902870403

Chafee MV, Averbeck BB (2022) Unmasking Schizophrenia: synaptic pruning in adolescence reveals a latent physiological vulnerability in prefrontal recurrent networks. Biol Psychiatry 92: 436–439

Chafee MV, Goldman-Rakic PS (1998) Matching patterns of activity in primate prefrontal area 8a and parietal area 7ip neurons during a spatial working memory task. J Neurophysiol 79:2919–2940

Chafee MV, Goldman-Rakic PS (2000) Inactivation of parietal and prefrontal cortex reveals interdependence of neural activity during memory-guided saccades. J Neurophysiol 83:1550–1566

Cheng W, Palaniyappan L, Li M, Kendrick KM, Zhang J, Luo Q, Liu Z, Yu R, Deng W, Wang Q, Ma X, Guo W, Francis S, Liddle P, Mayer AR, Schumann G, Li T, Feng J (2015) Voxel-based,

brain-wide association study of aberrant functional connectivity in schizophrenia implicates thalamocortical circuitry. NPJ Schizophr 1:15016
Choi EY, Tanimura Y, Vage PR, Yates EH, Haber SN (2017) Convergence of prefrontal and parietal anatomical projections in a connectional hub in the striatum. Neuroimage 146:821–832
Choudhury Z, Lennox B (2021) Maternal immune activation and Schizophrenia-evidence for an immune priming disorder. Front Psychiatry 12:585742
Clifton NE, Trent S, Thomas KL, Hall J (2019) Regulation and function of activity-dependent homer in synaptic plasticity. Mol Neuropsychiatry 5:147–161
Compte A, Brunel N, Goldman-Rakic PS, Wang XJ (2000) Synaptic mechanisms and network dynamics underlying spatial working memory in a cortical network model. Cereb Cortex 10: 910–923
Constantinidis C, Franowicz MN, Goldman-Rakic PS (2001) The sensory nature of mnemonic representation in the primate prefrontal cortex. Nat Neurosci 4:311–316
Constantinidis C, Funahashi S, Lee D, Murray JD, Qi X-L, Wang M, Arnsten AFT (2018) Persistent spiking activity underlies working memory. J Neurosci 38:7020–7028
Crowe DA, Goodwin SJ, Blackman RK, Sakellaridi S, Sponheim SR, MacDonald AW 3rd, Chafee MV (2013) Prefrontal neurons transmit signals to parietal neurons that reflect executive control of cognition. Nat Neurosci 16:1484–1491. https://doi.org/10.1038/nn.3509. Epub 2013 Sep 1
D'Ambrosio E, Jauhar S, Kim S, Veronese M, Rogdaki M, Pepper F, Bonoldi I, Kotoula V, Kempton MJ, Turkheimer F, Kwon JS, Kim E, Howes OD (2021) The relationship between grey matter volume and striatal dopamine function in psychosis: a multimodal 18F-DOPA PET and voxel-based morphometry study. Mol Psychiatry 26(4):1332–1345. https://doi.org/10.1038/s41380-019-0570-6
Dale CL, Brown EG, Fisher M, Herman AB, Dowling AF, Hinkley LB, Subramaniam K, Nagarajan SS, Vinogradov S (2016) Auditory cortical plasticity drives training-induced cognitive changes in Schizophrenia. Schizophr Bull 42:220–228. https://doi.org/10.1093/schbul/sbv087. Epub 2015 Jul 6
Dan Y, Poo MM (2004) Spike timing-dependent plasticity of neural circuits. Neuron 44:23–30
DeNicola AL, Park M-Y, Crowe DA, MacDonald AW 3rd, Chafee MV (2020) Differential roles of mediodorsal nucleus of the thalamus and prefrontal cortex in decision-making and state representation in a cognitive control task measuring deficits in Schizophrenia. J Neurosci 40: 1650–1667
Devaraju P, Yu J, Eddins D, Mellado-Lagarde MM, Earls LR, Westmoreland JJ, Quarato G, Green DR, Zakharenko SS (2017) Haploinsufficiency of the 22q11.2 microdeletion gene Mrpl40 disrupts short-term synaptic plasticity and working memory through dysregulation of mitochondrial calcium. Mol Psychiatry 22:1313–1326
Dias EC, McGinnis T, Smiley JF, Foxe JJ, Schroeder CE, Javitt DC (2006) Changing plans: neural correlates of executive control in monkey and human frontal cortex. Exp Brain Res 174:279–291
Dienel SJ, Lewis DA (2018) Alterations in cortical interneurons and cognitive function in schizophrenia. Neurobiol Dis. https://doi.org/10.1016/j.nbd.2018.06.020
Dienel SJ, Schoonover KE, Lewis DA (2022) Cognitive dysfunction and prefrontal cortical circuit alterations in Schizophrenia: developmental trajectories. Biol Psychiatry 92:450–459
Drew LJ, Stark KL, Fénelon K, Karayiorgou M, Macdermott AB, Gogos JA (2011) Evidence for altered hippocampal function in a mouse model of the human 22q11.2 microdeletion. Mol Cell Neurosci 47:293–305
Drummer C, Vogt E-J, Heistermann M, Roshani B, Becker T, Mätz-Rensing K, Kues WA, Kügler S, Behr R (2021) Generation and breeding of EGFP-transgenic marmoset monkeys: cell chimerism and implications for disease modeling. Cells 10. Available at: https://doi.org/10.3390/cells10030505
Dotson VM, McClintock SM, Verhaeghen P, Kim JU, Draheim AA, Syzmkowicz SM, Gradone AM, Bogoian HR, De Wit L (2020) Depression and cognitive control across the lifespan: a

systematic review and meta-analysis. Neuropsychol Rev 30(4):461–476. https://doi.org/10.1007/s11065-020-09436-6
Duan LY, Horst NK, Cranmore SAW, Horiguchi N, Cardinal RN, Roberts AC, Robbins TW (2021) Controlling one's world: identification of sub-regions of primate PFC underlying goal-directed behavior. Neuron 109:2485–2498.e5
Earls LR, Bayazitov IT, Fricke RG, Berry RB, Illingworth E, Mittleman G, Zakharenko SS (2010) Dysregulation of presynaptic calcium and synaptic plasticity in a mouse model of 22q11 deletion syndrome. J Neurosci 30:15843–15855
Earls LR, Fricke RG, Yu J, Berry RB, Baldwin LT, Zakharenko SS (2012) Age-dependent microRNA control of synaptic plasticity in 22q11 deletion syndrome and schizophrenia. J Neurosci 32:14132–14144
El-Shamayleh Y, Horwitz GD (2019) Primate optogenetics: progress and prognosis. Proc Natl Acad Sci U S A. https://doi.org/10.1073/pnas.1902284116
Feizpour A, Majka P, Chaplin TA, Rowley D, Yu H-H, Zavitz E, Price NSC, Rosa MGP, Hagan MA (2021) Visual responses in the dorsolateral frontal cortex of marmoset monkeys. J Neurophysiol 125:296–304
Felleman DJ, Van Essen DC (1991) Distributed hierarchical processing in the primate cerebral cortex. Cereb Cortex 1:1–47
Fénelon K, Mukai J, Xu B, Hsu P-K, Drew LJ, Karayiorgou M, Fischbach GD, Macdermott AB, Gogos JA (2011) Deficiency of Dgcr8, a gene disrupted by the 22q11.2 microdeletion, results in altered short-term plasticity in the prefrontal cortex. Proc Natl Acad Sci U S A 108:4447–4452
Fénelon K, Xu B, Lai CS, Mukai J, Markx S, Stark KL, Hsu P-K, Gan W-B, Fischbach GD, MacDermott AB, Karayiorgou M, Gogos JA (2013) The pattern of cortical dysfunction in a mouse model of a schizophrenia-related microdeletion. J Neurosci 33:14825–14839
Fernandez A, Meechan DW, Karpinski BA, Paronett EM, Bryan CA, Rutz HL, Radin EA, Lubin N, Bonner ER, Popratiloff A, Rothblat LA, Maynard TM, LaMantia A-S (2019) Mitochondrial dysfunction leads to cortical under-connectivity and cognitive impairment. Neuron. https://doi.org/10.1016/j.neuron.2019.04.013
Fisher M, Loewy R, Hardy K, Schlosser D, Vinogradov S (2013) Cognitive interventions targeting brain plasticity in the prodromal and early phases of schizophrenia. Annu Rev Clin Psychol 9: 435–463
Forbes NF, Carrick LA, McIntosh AM, Lawrie SM (2009) Working memory in schizophrenia: a meta-analysis. Psychol Med 39:889–905
Forsingdal A, Jørgensen TN, Olsen L, Werge T, Didriksen M, Nielsen J (2019) Can animal models of copy number variants that predispose to Schizophrenia elucidate underlying biology? Biol Psychiatry 85:13–24
Freedman DJ, Riesenhuber M, Poggio T, Miller EK (2001) Categorical representation of visual stimuli in the primate prefrontal cortex. Science 291:312–316. https://doi.org/10.1126/science.291.5502.312
Freedman DJ, Riesenhuber M, Poggio T, Miller EK (2003) A comparison of primate prefrontal and inferior temporal cortices during visual categorization. J Neurosci 23:5235–5246
Friedman HR, Selemon LD (2010) Fetal irradiation interferes with adult cognition in the nonhuman primate. Biol Psychiatry 68:108–111
Friston KJ (1999) Schizophrenia and the disconnection hypothesis. Acta Psychiatr Scand Suppl 395:68–79
Fromer M et al (2014) De novo mutations in schizophrenia implicate synaptic networks. Nature 506:179–184. https://doi.org/10.1038/nature12929. Epub 2014 Jan 22
Funahashi S, Bruce CJ, Goldman-Rakic PS (1989) Mnemonic coding of visual space in the monkey's dorsolateral prefrontal cortex. J Neurophysiol 61:331–349
Funahashi S, Bruce CJ, Goldman-Rakic PS (1990) Visuospatial coding in primate prefrontal neurons revealed by oculomotor paradigms. J Neurophysiol 63:814–831
Funahashi S, Bruce CJ, Goldman-Rakic PS (1991) Neuronal activity related to saccadic eye movements in the monkey's dorsolateral prefrontal cortex. J Neurophysiol 65:1464–1483

Funahashi S, Bruce CJ, Goldman-Rakic PS (1993a) Dorsolateral prefrontal lesions and oculomotor delayed-response performance: evidence for mnemonic "scotomas.". J Neurosci 13:1479–1497
Funahashi S, Chafee MV, Goldman-Rakic PS (1993b) Prefrontal neuronal activity in rhesus monkeys performing a delayed anti-saccade task. Nature 365:753–756
Fusar-Poli P, Howes OD, Allen P, Broome M, Valli I, Asselin M-C, Montgomery AJ, Grasby PM, McGuire P (2011) Abnormal prefrontal activation directly related to pre-synaptic striatal dopamine dysfunction in people at clinical high risk for psychosis. Mol Psychiatry 16(1):67–75. https://doi.org/10.1038/mp.2009.108
Galvin VC, Yang ST, Paspalas CD, Yang Y, Jin LE, Datta D, Morozov YM, Lightbourne TC, Lowet AS, Rakic P, Arnsten AFT, Wang M (2020) Muscarinic M1 receptors modulate working memory performance and activity via KCNQ potassium channels in the primate prefrontal cortex. Neuron 106:649–661.e4
Garin CM, Hori Y, Everling S, Whitlow CT, Calabro FJ, Luna B, Froesel M, Gacoin M, Ben Hamed S, Dhenain M, Constantinidis C (2022) An evolutionary gap in primate default mode network organization. Cell Rep 39:110669
Garofalo M, Nieus T, Massobrio P, Martinoia S (2009) Evaluation of the performance of information theory-based methods and cross-correlation to estimate the functional connectivity in cortical networks. PLoS One 4:e6482
Geana A, Barch DM, Gold JM, Carter CS, MacDonald AW III, Ragland JD, Silverstein SM, Frank MJ (2021) Using computational modeling to capture schizophrenia-specific reinforcement learning differences and their implications on patient classification. Biol Psychiatry Cogn Neurosci Neuroimaging. https://doi.org/10.1016/j.bpsc.2021.03.017
Georgopoulos AP, Lurito JT, Petrides M, Schwartz AB, Massey JT (1989) Mental rotation of the neuronal population vector. Science 243:234–236
Gil-da-Costa R, Stoner GR, Fung R, Albright TD (2013) Nonhuman primate model of schizophrenia using a noninvasive EEG method. Proc Natl Acad Sci U S A 110:15425–15430
Girdhar K, Rahman S, Dong P, Fullard JF, Roussos P (2022) The neuroepigenome: implications of chemical and physical modifications of genomic DNA in schizophrenia. Biol Psychiatry 92: 443–449
Glahn DC, Ragland JD, Abramoff A, Barrett J, Laird AR, Bearden CE, Velligan DI (2005) Beyond hypofrontality: a quantitative meta-analysis of functional neuroimaging studies of working memory in schizophrenia. Hum Brain Mapp 25:60–69
Glantz LA, Lewis DA (2000) Decreased dendritic spine density on prefrontal cortical pyramidal neurons in schizophrenia. Arch Gen Psychiatry 57:65–73
Glausier JR, Lewis DA (2013) Dendritic spine pathology in schizophrenia. Neuroscience 251:90–107. https://doi.org/10.1016/j.neuroscience.2012.04.044. Epub 2012 Apr 27
Gogtay N, Giedd JN, Lusk L, Hayashi KM, Greenstein D, Vaituzis AC, Nugent TF 3rd, Herman DH, Clasen LS, Toga AW, Rapoport JL, Thompson PM (2004) Dynamic mapping of human cortical development during childhood through early adulthood. Proc Natl Acad Sci U S A 101: 8174–8179
Gold JM (2012) Negative symptoms and the failure to represent the expected reward value of actions. Arch Gen Psychiatry 69(2):129. https://doi.org/10.1001/archgenpsychiatry.2011.1269
Gold JM, Carpenter C, Randolph C, Goldberg TE, Weinberger DR (1997) Auditory working memory and Wisconsin card sorting test performance in schizophrenia. Arch Gen Psychiatry 54:159–165
Goldman-Rakic PS (1987) Circuitry of primate prefrontal cortex and regulation of behavior by representational memory. Compr Physiol:373–417 Available at: https://onlinelibrary.wiley.com/doi/10.1002/cphy.cp010509
Goldman-Rakic PS (1999) The physiological approach: functional architecture of working memory and disordered cognition in schizophrenia. Biol Psychiatry 46:650–661
Goldman-Rakic PS, Leranth C, Williams SM, Mons N, Geffard M (1989) Dopamine synaptic complex with pyramidal neurons in primate cerebral cortex. Proc Natl Acad Sci U S A 86:9015–9019

González-Burgos G, Barrionuevo G, Lewis DA (2000) Horizontal synaptic connections in monkey prefrontal cortex: an in vitro electrophysiological study. Cereb Cortex 10:82–92
Goodwin SJ, Blackman RK, Sakellaridi S, Chafee MV (2012) Executive control over cognition: stronger and earlier rule-based modulation of spatial category signals in prefrontal cortex relative to parietal cortex. J Neurosci 32:3499–3515
Guo W-T, Wang Y (2019) Dgcr8 knockout approaches to understand microRNA functions in vitro and in vivo. Cell Mol Life Sci 76:1697–1711
Hall J, Bray NJ (2022) Schizophrenia genomics: convergence on synaptic development, adult synaptic plasticity, or both? Biol Psychiatry 91:709–717
Hall J, Trent S, Thomas KL, O'Donovan MC, Owen MJ (2015) Genetic risk for schizophrenia: convergence on synaptic pathways involved in plasticity. Biol Psychiatry 77:52–58
Hamilton I (2017) Cannabis, psychosis and schizophrenia: unravelling a complex interaction. Addiction 112:1653–1657
Hamm JP, Peterka DS, Gogos JA, Yuste R (2017) Altered cortical ensembles in mouse models of Schizophrenia. Neuron 94:153–167.e8
Hamm JP, Shymkiv Y, Mukai J, Gogos JA, Yuste R (2020) Aberrant cortical ensembles and Schizophrenia-like sensory phenotypes in Setd1a+/- Mice. Biol Psychiatry 88:215–223
Hanson KL, Grant SE, Funk LH, Schumann CM, Bauman MD (2022) Impact of maternal immune activation on nonhuman primate prefrontal cortex development: insights for Schizophrenia. Biol Psychiatry 92:460–469
He K, Huertas M, Hong SZ, Tie X, Hell JW, Shouval H, Kirkwood A (2015) Distinct eligibility traces for LTP and LTD in cortical synapses. Neuron 88:528–538
Heilbronner SR, Rodriguez-Romaguera J, Quirk GJ, Groenewegen HJ, Haber SN (2016) Circuit-based corticostriatal homologies between rat and primate. Biol Psychiatry 80:509–521
Henderson D, Poppe AB, Barch DM, Carter CS, Gold JM, Ragland JD, Silverstein SM, Strauss ME, MacDonald AW 3rd (2012) Optimization of a goal maintenance task for use in clinical applications. Schizophr Bull 38:104–113
Hikosaka O, Wurtz RH (1983) Visual and oculomotor functions of monkey substantia nigra pars reticulata. III. Memory-contingent visual and saccade responses. J Neurophysiol 49:1268–1284
Hiroi N, Yamauchi T (2019) Modeling and predicting developmental trajectories of neuropsychiatric dimensions associated with copy number variations. Int J Neuropsychopharmacol. https://doi.org/10.1093/ijnp/pyz026
Histed MH, Pasupathy A, Miller EK (2009) Learning substrates in the primate prefrontal cortex and striatum: sustained activity related to successful actions. Neuron 63:244–253. https://doi.org/10.1016/j.neuron.2009.06.019
Holmes AJ, MacDonald A 3rd, Carter CS, Barch DM, Andrew Stenger V, Cohen JD (2005) Prefrontal functioning during context processing in schizophrenia and major depression: an event-related fMRI study. Schizophr Res 76:199–206
Horan WP et al (2008) Verbal working memory impairments in individuals with schizophrenia and their first-degree relatives: findings from the consortium on the genetics of Schizophrenia. Schizophr Res 103:218–228
Howes O, Bose S, Turkheimer F, Valli I, Egerton A, Stahl D, Valmaggia L, Allen P, Murray R, McGuire P (2011) Progressive increase in striatal dopamine synthesis capacity as patients develop psychosis: a PET study. Mol Psychiatry 16:885–886
Howes OD, Shatalina E (2022) Integrating the neurodevelopmental and dopamine hypotheses of Schizophrenia and the role of cortical excitation-inhibition balance. Biol Psychiatry 92:501–513
Howes OD, Montgomery AJ, Asselin M-C, Murray RM, Valli I, Tabraham P, Bramon-Bosch E, Valmaggia L, Johns L, Broome M, McGuire PK, Grasby PM (2009) Elevated striatal dopamine function linked to prodromal signs of schizophrenia. Arch Gen Psychiatry 66:13–20
Howes OD, Hird EJ, Adams RA, Corlett PR, McGuire P (2020) Aberrant salience, information processing, and dopaminergic signaling in people at clinical high risk for psychosis. Biol Psychiatry 88:304–314

Huttenlocher PR (1990) Morphometric study of human cerebral cortex development. Neuropsychologia 28:517–527

Huttenlocher PR, Dabholkar AS (1997) Regional differences in synaptogenesis in human cerebral cortex. J Comp Neurol 387:167–178

Hyman SE (2021) Use of mouse models to investigate the contributions of CNVs associated with schizophrenia and autism to disease mechanisms. Curr Opin Genet Dev 68:99–105

Insel T (2022) Healing: our path from mental illness to mental health. Penguin Press

Insel TR (2010) Rethinking schizophrenia. Nature 468:187–193. https://doi.org/10.1038/nature09552

Ito S, Hansen ME, Heiland R, Lumsdaine A, Litke AM, Beggs JM (2011) Extending transfer entropy improves identification of effective connectivity in a spiking cortical network model. PLoS One 6:e27431. https://doi.org/10.1371/journal.pone.0027431. Epub 2011 Nov 15

Jacobsen CF (1935) Functions of frontal association area in primates. Arch NeurPsych 33:558–569

Jamali M, Grannan BL, Fedorenko E, Saxe R, Báez-Mendoza R, Williams ZM (2021) Single-neuronal predictions of others' beliefs in humans. Nature 591:610–614

Jauhar S, Nour MM, Veronese M, Rogdaki M, Bonoldi I, Azis M, Turkheimer F, McGuire P, Young AH, Howes OD (2017) A test of the transdiagnostic dopamine hypothesis of psychosis using positron emission tomographic imaging in bipolar affective disorder and Schizophrenia. JAMA Psychiatry 74:1206–1213

Javitt DC, Zukin SR, Heresco-Levy U, Umbricht D (2012) Has an angel shown the way? Etiological and therapeutic implications of the PCP/NMDA model of schizophrenia. Schizophr Bull 38: 958–966

Jentsch JD, Redmond DE Jr, Elsworth JD, Taylor JR, Youngren KD, Roth RH (1997) Enduring cognitive deficits and cortical dopamine dysfunction in monkeys after long-term administration of phencyclidine. Science 277:953–955

Jentsch JD, Taylor JR, Elsworth JD, Redmond DE Jr, Roth RH (1999) Altered frontal cortical dopaminergic transmission in monkeys after subchronic phencyclidine exposure: involvement in frontostriatal cognitive deficits. Neuroscience 90:823–832

Jin LE, Wang M, Yang S-T, Yang Y, Galvin VC, Lightbourne TC, Ottenheimer D, Zhong Q, Stein J, Raja A, Paspalas CD, Arnsten AFT (2017) mGluR2/3 mechanisms in primate dorsolateral prefrontal cortex: evidence for both presynaptic and postsynaptic actions. Mol Psychiatry 22:1615–1625

Johnson MB, Hyman SE (2022) A critical perspective on the synaptic pruning hypothesis of Schizophrenia pathogenesis. Biol Psychiatry 92:440–442

Jones JA, Sponheim SR, MacDonald AW 3rd (2010) The dot pattern expectancy task: reliability and replication of deficits in schizophrenia. Psychol Assess 22:131–141. https://doi.org/10.1037/a0017828

Jovanovic V, Fishbein AR, de la Mothe L, Lee K-F, Miller CT (2022) Behavioral context affects social signal representations within single primate prefrontal cortex neurons. Neuron 110:1318–1326.e4

Kaar SJ, Natesan S, McCutcheon R, Howes OD (2020) Antipsychotics: mechanisms underlying clinical response and side-effects and novel treatment approaches based on pathophysiology. Neuropharmacology 172:107704

Kasai H, Ziv NE, Okazaki H, Yagishita S, Toyoizumi T (2021) Spine dynamics in the brain, mental disorders and artificial neural networks. Nat Rev Neurosci 22:407–422

Katsuki F, Qi X-L, Meyer T, Kostelic PM, Salinas E, Constantinidis C (2014) Differences in intrinsic functional organization between dorsolateral prefrontal and posterior parietal cortex. Cereb Cortex 24:2334–2349

Kegeles LS, Abi-Dargham A, Frankle WG, Gil R, Cooper TB, Slifstein M, Hwang D-R, Huang Y, Haber SN, Laruelle M (2010) Increased synaptic dopamine function in associative regions of the striatum in schizophrenia. Arch Gen Psychiatry 67:231–239

Kiani R, Shadlen MN (2009) Representation of confidence associated with a decision by neurons in the parietal cortex. Science 324:759–764

Kim T, Thankachan S, McKenna JT, McNally JM, Yang C, Choi JH, Chen L, Kocsis B, Deisseroth K, Strecker RE, Basheer R, Brown RE, McCarley RW (2015) Cortically projecting basal forebrain parvalbumin neurons regulate cortical gamma band oscillations. Proc Natl Acad Sci U S A 112:3535–3540

Kirov G et al (2012) De novo CNV analysis implicates specific abnormalities of postsynaptic signalling complexes in the pathogenesis of schizophrenia. Mol Psychiatry 17:142–153. https://doi.org/10.1038/mp.2011.154. Epub 2011 Nov 15

Kolk SM, Rakic P (2022) Development of prefrontal cortex. Neuropsychopharmacology 47:41–57

Kolluri N, Sun Z, Sampson AR, Lewis DA (2005) Lamina-specific reductions in dendritic spine density in the prefrontal cortex of subjects with schizophrenia. Am J Psychiatry 162:1200–1202

Korndörfer C, Ullner E, García-Ojalvo J, Pipa G (2017) Cortical spike synchrony as a measure of input familiarity. Neural Comput 29:2491–2510

Kozak MJ, Cuthbert BN (2016) The NIMH research domain criteria initiative: background issues and pragmatics. Psychophysiol 53(3):286–297. https://doi.org/10.1111/psyp.12518

Kritzer MF, Goldman-Rakic PS (1995) Intrinsic circuit organization of the major layers and sublayers of the dorsolateral prefrontal cortex in the rhesus monkey. J Comp Neurol 359:131–143

Krystal JH, Karper LP, Seibyl JP, Freeman GK, Delaney R, Bremner JD, Heninger GR, Bowers MB Jr, Charney DS (1994) Subanesthetic effects of the noncompetitive NMDA antagonist, ketamine, in humans. Psychotomimetic, perceptual, cognitive, and neuroendocrine responses. Arch Gen Psychiatry 51:199–214

Kummerfeld E, Ma S, Blackman RK, DeNicola AL, Redish AD, Vinogradov S, Crowe DA, Chafee MV (2020) Cognitive control errors in nonhuman primates resembling those in Schizophrenia reflect opposing effects of NMDA receptor Blockade on causal interactions between cells and circuits in prefrontal and parietal cortices. Biol Psychiatry Cogn Neurosci Neuroimaging 5:705–714

Kupferschmidt DA, Gordon JA (2018) The dynamics of disordered dialogue: prefrontal, hippocampal and thalamic miscommunication underlying working memory deficits in schizophrenia. Brain Neurosci Adv 2 Available at: https://doi.org/10.1177/2398212818771821

Lahti AC, Weiler MA, Tamara Michaelidis BA, Parwani A, Tamminga CA (2001) Effects of ketamine in normal and schizophrenic volunteers. Neuropsychopharmacology 25:455–467

Lerman-Sinkoff DB, Sui J, Rachakonda S, Kandala S, Calhoun VD, Barch DM (2017) Multimodal neural correlates of cognitive control in the human connectome project. Neuroimage 163:41–54

Lesh TA, Westphal AJ, Niendam TA, Yoon JH, Minzenberg MJ, Ragland JD, Solomon M, Carter CS (2013) Proactive and reactive cognitive control and dorsolateral prefrontal cortex dysfunction in first episode schizophrenia. Neuroimage Clin 2:590–599

Li W, Fan CC, Mäki-Marttunen T, Thompson WK, Schork AJ, Bettella F, Schizophrenia Working Group of the Psychiatric Genomics Consortium, Djurovic S, Dale AM, Andreassen OA, Wang Y (2018) A molecule-based genetic association approach implicates a range of voltage-gated calcium channels associated with schizophrenia. Am J Med Genet B Neuropsychiatr Genet 177:454–467

Lieberman JA, Stroup TS (2011) The NIMH-CATIE Schizophrenia study: what did we learn? Am J Psychiatry 168:770–775

Lieberman JA, Stroup TS, McEvoy JP, Swartz MS, Rosenheck RA, Perkins DO, Keefe RSE, Davis SM, Davis CE, Lebowitz BD, Severe J, Hsiao JK, Clinical Antipsychotic Trials of Intervention Effectiveness (CATIE) Investigators (2005) Effectiveness of antipsychotic drugs in patients with chronic schizophrenia. N Engl J Med 353:1209–1223

Lopez-Garcia P, Lesh TA, Salo T, Barch DM, MacDonald AW 3rd, Gold JM, Ragland JD, Strauss M, Silverstein SM, Carter CS (2016) The neural circuitry supporting goal maintenance during cognitive control: a comparison of expectancy AX-CPT and dot probe expectancy paradigms. Cogn Affect Behav Neurosci 16:164–175

Luby ED, Cohen BD, Rosenbaum G, Gottlieb JS, Kelley R (1959) Study of a new schizophrenomimetic drug; sernyl. AMA Arch Neurol Psychiatry 81:363–369

Lundqvist M, Rose J, Herman P, Brincat SL, Buschman TJ, Miller EK (2016) Gamma and beta bursts underlie working memory. Neuron 90:152–164. https://doi.org/10.1016/j.neuron.2016.02.028. Epub 2016 Mar 17

Lundqvist M, Herman P, Miller EK (2018) Working memory: delay activity, Yes! persistent activity? Maybe not. J Neurosci 38:7013–7019

Ma L, Skoblenick K, Seamans JK, Everling S (2015) Ketamine-induced changes in the signal and noise of rule representation in working memory by lateral prefrontal neurons. J Neurosci 35:11612–11622

Ma L, Skoblenick K, Johnston K, Everling S (2018) Ketamine alters lateral prefrontal oscillations in a rule-based working memory task. J Neurosci 38:2482–2494

MacCabe JH, Wicks S, Löfving S, David AS, Berndtsson Å, Gustafsson J-E, Allebeck P, Dalman C (2013) Decline in cognitive performance between ages 13 and 18 years and the risk for psychosis in adulthood: a Swedish longitudinal cohort study in males. JAMA Psychiatry 70:261–270

MacDonald AW 3rd (2008) Building a clinically relevant cognitive task: case study of the AX paradigm. Schizophr Bull 34:619–628

MacDonald AW 3rd, Pogue-Geile MF, Johnson MK, Carter CS (2003) A specific deficit in context processing in the unaffected siblings of patients with schizophrenia. Arch Gen Psychiatry 60:57–65

MacDonald AW 3rd, Carter CS, Kerns JG, Ursu S, Barch DM, Holmes AJ, Stenger VA, Cohen JD (2005) Specificity of prefrontal dysfunction and context processing deficits to schizophrenia in never-medicated patients with first-episode psychosis. Am J Psychiatry 162:475–484

Machado CJ, Whitaker AM, Smith SEP, Patterson PH, Bauman MD (2015) Maternal immune activation in nonhuman primates alters social attention in juvenile offspring. Biol Psychiatry 77:823–832

Malhotra AK, Pinals DA, Adler CM, Elman I, Clifton A, Pickar D, Breier A (1997) Ketamine-induced exacerbation of psychotic symptoms and cognitive impairment in neuroleptic-free schizophrenics. Neuropsychopharmacology 17:141–150

Masse NY, Yang GR, Song HF, Wang X-J, Freedman DJ (2019) Circuit mechanisms for the maintenance and manipulation of information in working memory. Nat Neurosci 22:1159–1167

McCutcheon R, Beck K, Jauhar S, Howes OD (2018) Defining the locus of dopaminergic dysfunction in Schizophrenia: a meta-analysis and test of the mesolimbic hypothesis. Schizophr Bull 44:1301–1311

McDowell JE, Brown GG, Paulus M, Martinez A, Stewart SE, Dubowitz DJ, Braff DL (2002) Neural correlates of refixation saccades and antisaccades in normal and schizophrenia subjects. Biol Psychiatry 51:216–223

McKee JL, Riesenhuber M, Miller EK, Freedman DJ (2014) Task dependence of visual and category representations in prefrontal and inferior temporal cortices. J Neurosci 34:16065–16075. https://doi.org/10.1523/JNEUROSCI.1660-14.2014

McNally JM, Aguilar DD, Katsuki F, Radzik LK, Schiffino FL, Uygun DS, McKenna JT, Strecker RE, Deisseroth K, Spencer KM, Brown RE (2021) Optogenetic manipulation of an ascending arousal system tunes cortical broadband gamma power and reveals functional deficits relevant to schizophrenia. Mol Psychiatry 26:3461–3475

Meechan DW, Rutz HLH, Fralish MS, Maynard TM, Rothblat LA, LaMantia A-S (2015) Cognitive ability is associated with altered medial frontal cortical circuits in the LgDel mouse model of 22q11.2DS. Cereb Cortex 25:1143–1151

Melchitzky DS, González-Burgos G, Barrionuevo G, Lewis DA (2001) Synaptic targets of the intrinsic axon collaterals of supragranular pyramidal neurons in monkey prefrontal cortex. J Comp Neurol 430:209–221

Merico D, Costain G, Butcher NJ, Warnica W, Ogura L, Alfred SE, Brzustowicz LM, Bassett AS (2014) MicroRNA dysregulation, gene networks, and risk for Schizophrenia in 22q11.2 deletion syndrome. Front Neurol 5:238

Merico D, Zarrei M, Costain G, Ogura L, Alipanahi B, Gazzellone MJ, Butcher NJ, Thiruvahindrapuram B, Nalpathamkalam T, Chow EWC, Andrade DM, Frey BJ, Marshall CR, Scherer SW, Bassett AS (2015) Whole-genome sequencing suggests Schizophrenia risk mechanisms in humans with 22q11.2 deletion syndrome. G3 5:2453–2461

Mesholam-Gately RI, Giuliano AJ, Goff KP, Faraone SV, Seidman LJ (2009) Neurocognition in first-episode schizophrenia: a meta-analytic review. Neuropsychology 23:315–336

Meyer T, Qi X-L, Constantinidis C (2007) Persistent discharges in the prefrontal cortex of monkeys naive to working memory tasks. Cereb Cortex 17(Suppl 1):i70–i76

Meyers EM, Freedman DJ, Kreiman G, Miller EK, Poggio T (2008) Dynamic population coding of category information in inferior temporal and prefrontal cortex. J Neurophysiol 100:1407–1419. https://doi.org/10.1152/jn.90248.2008. Epub 2008 June 18

Meyers EM, Qi X-L, Constantinidis C (2012) Incorporation of new information into prefrontal cortical activity after learning working memory tasks. Proc Natl Acad Sci U S A 109:4651–4656

Miller CT, Thomas AW, Nummela SU, de la Mothe LA (2015) Responses of primate frontal cortex neurons during natural vocal communication. J Neurophysiol 114:1158–1171

Miller EK, Cohen JD (2001) An integrative theory of prefrontal cortex function. Annu Rev Neurosci 24:167–202. https://doi.org/10.1146/annurev.neuro.24.1.167

Mochizuki K, Funahashi S (2016) Prefrontal spatial working memory network predicts animal's decision making in a free choice saccade task. J Neurophysiol 115:127–142

Mongillo G, Barak O, Tsodyks M (2008) Synaptic theory of working memory. Science 319:1543–1546

Moran EK, Gold JM, Carter CS, MacDonald AW, Ragland JD, Silverstein SM, Luck SJ, Barch DM (2020) Both unmedicated and medicated individuals with schizophrenia show impairments across a wide array of cognitive and reinforcement learning tasks. Psychol Med:1–11.

Muhammad R, Wallis JD, Miller EK (2006) A comparison of abstract rules in the prefrontal cortex, premotor cortex, inferior temporal cortex, and striatum. J Cogn Neurosci 18:974–989. https://doi.org/10.1162/jocn.2006.18.6.974

Murray JD, Anticevic A, Gancsos M, Ichinose M, Corlett PR, Krystal JH, Wang X-J (2014) Linking microcircuit dysfunction to cognitive impairment: effects of disinhibition associated with schizophrenia in a cortical working memory model. Cereb Cortex 24:859–872

Nieder A, Miller EK (2003) Coding of cognitive magnitude: compressed scaling of numerical information in the primate prefrontal cortex. Neuron 37:149–157

Nieder A, Miller EK (2004a) A parieto-frontal network for visual numerical information in the monkey. Proc Natl Acad Sci U S A 101:7457–7462. https://doi.org/10.1073/pnas.0402239101. Epub 2004 May 3

Nieder A, Miller EK (2004b) Analog numerical representations in rhesus monkeys: evidence for parallel processing. J Cogn Neurosci 16:889–901. https://doi.org/10.1162/089892904970807

Nieder A, Freedman DJ, Miller EK (2002) Representation of the quantity of visual items in the primate prefrontal cortex. Science 297:1708–1711. https://doi.org/10.1126/science.1072493

Niendam TA, Ray KL, Iosif A-M, Lesh TA, Ashby SR, Patel PK, Smucny J, Ferrer E, Solomon M, Ragland JD, Carter CS (2018) Association of age at onset and longitudinal course of prefrontal function in youth with Schizophrenia. JAMA Psychiatry 75:1252–1260

Nieuwenstein MR, Aleman A, de Haan EHF (2001) Relationship between symptom dimensions and neurocognitive functioning in schizophrenia: a meta-analysis of WCST and CPT studies. J Psychiatr Res 35(2):119–125. https://doi.org/10.1016/S0022-3956(01)00014-0

Niki H, Watanabe M (1976) Prefrontal unit activity and delayed response: relation to cue location versus direction of response. Brain Res 105:79–88

Okano H, Kishi N (2018) Investigation of brain science and neurological/psychiatric disorders using genetically modified non-human primates. Curr Opin Neurobiol 50:1–6

Ouchi Y, Banno Y, Shimizu Y, Ando S, Hasegawa H, Adachi K, Iwamoto T (2013) Reduced adult hippocampal neurogenesis and working memory deficits in the Dgcr8-deficient mouse model of 22q11.2 deletion-associated schizophrenia can be rescued by IGF2. J Neurosci 33:9408–9419

Park JE, Zhang XF, Choi S-H, Okahara J, Sasaki E, Silva AC (2016) Generation of transgenic marmosets expressing genetically encoded calcium indicators. Sci Rep 6:34931
Park S, Holzman PS (1992) Schizophrenics show spatial working memory deficits. Arch Gen Psychiatry 49:975–982
Park S, Holzman PS, Goldman-Rakic PS (1995) Spatial working memory deficits in the relatives of schizophrenic patients. Arch Gen Psychiatry 52:821–828
Paspalas CD, Wang M, Arnsten AFT (2013) Constellation of HCN channels and cAMP regulating proteins in dendritic spines of the primate prefrontal cortex: potential substrate for working memory deficits in schizophrenia. Cereb Cortex 23:1643–1654
Pasupathy A, Miller EK (2005) Different time courses of learning-related activity in the prefrontal cortex and striatum. Nature 433:873–876. https://doi.org/10.1038/nature03287
Peng X-J, Hei G-R, Yang Y, Liu C-C, Xiao J-M, Long Y-J, Huang J, Zhao J-P, Ren-Rong W (2021) The association between cognitive deficits and clinical characteristic in first-episode drug naïve patients with schizophrenia. Front Psychiatry 12:638773. https://doi.org/10.3389/fpsyt.2021.638773
Perlstein WM, Dixit NK, Carter CS, Noll DC, Cohen JD (2003) Prefrontal cortex dysfunction mediates deficits in working memory and prepotent responding in schizophrenia. Biol Psychiatry 53:25–38
Petanjek Z, Judaš M, Šimic G, Rasin MR, Uylings HBM, Rakic P, Kostovic I (2011) Extraordinary neoteny of synaptic spines in the human prefrontal cortex. Proc Natl Acad Sci U S A 108:13281–13286
Pipa G, Munk MH (2011) Higher order spike synchrony in prefrontal cortex during visual memory. Front Comput Neurosci 5:23. https://doi.org/10.3389/fncom.2011.00023. eCollection 2011
Potkin SG, Kane JM, Correll CU, Lindenmayer J-P, Agid O, Marder SR, Olfson M, Howes OD (2020) The neurobiology of treatment-resistant schizophrenia: paths to antipsychotic resistance and a roadmap for future research. NPJ Schizophr 6:1
Preuss TM (1995) Do rats have prefrontal cortex? The Rose-Woolsey-Akert program reconsidered. J Cogn Neurosci 7:1–24
Preuss TM, Wise SP (2022) Evolution of prefrontal cortex. Neuropsychopharmacology 47:3–19
Qi X-L, Constantinidis C (2012) Variability of prefrontal neuronal discharges before and after training in a working memory task. PLoS One 7:e41053
Qi X-L, Constantinidis C (2013) Neural changes after training to perform cognitive tasks. Behav Brain Res 241:235–243
Qi X-L, Constantinidis C (2015) Lower neuronal variability in the monkey dorsolateral prefrontal than posterior parietal cortex. J Neurophysiol 114:2194–2203
Qi X-L, Katsuki F, Meyer T, Rawley JB, Zhou X, Douglas KL, Constantinidis C (2010) Comparison of neural activity related to working memory in primate dorsolateral prefrontal and posterior parietal cortex. Front Syst Neurosci 4:12
Qi X-L, Liu R, Singh B, Bestue D, Compte A, Vazdarjanova AI, Blake DT, Constantinidis C (2021) Nucleus basalis stimulation enhances working memory by stabilizing stimulus representations in primate prefrontal cortical activity. Cell Rep 36:109469
Quintana J, Fuster JM (1992) Mnemonic and predictive functions of cortical neurons in a memory task. Neuroreport 3:721–724
Quiroz C, Orrú M, Rea W, Ciudad-Roberts A, Yepes G, Britt JP, Ferré S (2016) Local control of extracellular dopamine levels in the medial nucleus accumbens by a glutamatergic projection from the infralimbic cortex. J Neurosci 36(3):851–859. https://doi.org/10.1523/JNEUROSCI.2850-15.2016
Rees E, Walters JT, Georgieva L, Isles AR, Chambert KD, Richards AL, Mahoney-Davies G, Legge SE, Moran JL, McCarroll SA, O'Donovan MC, Owen MJ, Kirov G (2014) Analysis of copy number variations at 15 schizophrenia-associated loci. Br J Psychiatry 204:108–114. https://doi.org/10.1192/bjp.bp.113.131052. Epub 2013 Dec 5

Reichenberg A, Caspi A, Harrington H, Houts R, Keefe RSE, Murray RM, Poulton R, Moffitt TE (2010) Static and dynamic cognitive deficits in childhood preceding adult schizophrenia: a 30-year study. Am J Psychiatry 167:160–169

Russchen FT, Amaral DG, Price JL (1987) The afferent input to the magnocellular division of the mediodorsal thalamic nucleus in the monkey, Macaca fascicularis. J Comp Neurol 256:175–210

Samandra R, Haque ZZ, Rosa MGP, Mansouri FA (2022) The marmoset as a model for investigating the neural basis of social cognition in health and disease. Neurosci Biobehav Rev 138: 104692

Sasaki E et al (2009) Generation of transgenic non-human primates with germline transmission. Nature 459:523–527

Sawaguchi T, Goldman-Rakic PS (1991) D1 dopamine receptors in prefrontal cortex: involvement in working memory. Science 251:947–950

Schaeffer DJ, Gilbert KM, Gati JS, Menon RS, Everling S (2019) Intrinsic functional boundaries of lateral frontal cortex in the common marmoset monkey. J Neurosci 39:1020–1029

Schaeffer DJ, Selvanayagam J, Johnston KD, Menon RS, Freiwald WA, Everling S (2020) Face selective patches in marmoset frontal cortex. Nat Commun 11:4856

Schizophrenia_Working_Group_of_the_Psychiatric_Genomics_Consortium (2014) Biological insights from 108 schizophrenia-associated genetic loci. Nature 511:421–427. https://doi.org/10.1038/nature13595. Epub 2014 July 22

Schreiber T (2000) Measuring information transfer. Phys Rev Lett 85:461–464

Sekar A, Bialas AR, de Rivera H, Davis A, Hammond TR, Kamitaki N, Tooley K, Presumey J, Baum M, Van Doren V, Genovese G, Rose SA, Handsaker RE, Daly MJ, Carroll MC, Stevens B, McCarroll SA (2016) Schizophrenia risk from complex variation of complement component 4. Nature 530:177–183. https://doi.org/10.1038/nature16549. Epub 2016 Jan 27

Selemon LD, Friedman HR (2013) Motor stereotypies and cognitive perseveration in non-human primates exposed to early gestational irradiation. Neuroscience 248:213–224

Selemon LD, Goldman-Rakic PS (1988) Common cortical and subcortical targets of the dorsolateral prefrontal and posterior parietal cortices in the rhesus monkey: evidence for a distributed neural network subserving spatially guided behavior. J Neurosci 8:4049–4068

Selemon LD, Begović A, Rakic P (2009) Selective reduction of neuron number and volume of the mediodorsal nucleus of the thalamus in macaques following irradiation at early gestational ages. J Comp Neurol 515:454–464

Selemon LD, Ceritoglu C, Ratnanather JT, Wang L, Harms MP, Aldridge K, Begović A, Csernansky JG, Miller MI, Rakic P (2013) Distinct abnormalities of the primate prefrontal cortex caused by ionizing radiation in early or midgestation. J Comp Neurol 521:1040–1053

Sellgren CM, Gracias J, Watmuff B, Biag JD, Thanos JM, Whittredge PB, Fu T, Worringer K, Brown HE, Wang J, Kaykas A, Karmacharya R, Goold CP, Sheridan SD, Perlis RH (2019) Increased synapse elimination by microglia in schizophrenia patient-derived models of synaptic pruning. Nat Neurosci 22:374–385

Sellier C, Hwang VJ, Dandekar R, Durbin-Johnson B, Charlet-Berguerand N, Ander BP, Sharp FR, Angkustsiri K, Simon TJ, Tassone F (2014) Decreased DGCR8 expression and miRNA dysregulation in individuals with 22q11.2 deletion syndrome. PLoS One 9:e103884

Sheridan SD, Horng JE, Perlis RH (2022) Patient-derived in vitro models of microglial function and synaptic engulfment in Schizophrenia. Biol Psychiatry Available at: https://doi.org/10.1016/j.biopsych.2022.01.004.

Sheu Y-S, Courtney SM (2016) A neural mechanism of cognitive control for resolving conflict between abstract task rules. Cortex 85:13–24

Sigurdsson T, Stark KL, Karayiorgou M, Gogos JA, Gordon JA (2010) Impaired hippocampal-prefrontal synchrony in a genetic mouse model of schizophrenia. Nature 464:763–767

Singh B, Wang Z, Qi X-L, Constantinidis C (2022) Plasticity after cognitive training reflected in prefrontal local field potentials. iScience 25:104929

Skoblenick K, Everling S (2012) NMDA antagonist ketamine reduces task selectivity in macaque dorsolateral prefrontal neurons and impairs performance of randomly interleaved prosaccades and antisaccades. J Neurosci 32:12018–12027
Skoblenick K, Everling S (2014) N-methyl-d-aspartate receptor antagonist ketamine impairs action-monitoring activity in the prefrontal cortex. J Cogn Neurosci 26:577–592. https://doi.org/10.1162/jocn_a_00519. Epub 2013 Nov 4
Skoblenick KJ, Womelsdorf T, Everling S (2016) Ketamine alters outcome-related local field potentials in monkey prefrontal cortex. Cereb Cortex 26:2743–2752
Smiley JF, Goldman-Rakic PS (1993) Heterogeneous targets of dopamine synapses in monkey prefrontal cortex demonstrated by serial section electron microscopy: a laminar analysis using the silver-enhanced diaminobenzidine sulfide (SEDS) immunolabeling technique. Cereb Cortex 3:223–238
Smucny J, Lesh TA, Newton K, Niendam TA, Ragland JD, Carter CS (2018) Levels of cognitive control: a functional magnetic resonance imaging-based test of an RDoC domain across bipolar disorder and Schizophrenia. Neuropsychopharmacology 43:598–606
Smucny J, Iosif A-M, Eaton NR, Lesh TA, Ragland JD, Barch DM, Gold JM, Strauss ME, MacDonald AW, Silverstein SM, Carter CS (2020a) Latent profiles of cognitive control, episodic memory, and visual perception across psychiatric disorders reveal a dimensional structure. Schizophr Bull 46:154–162
Smucny J, Lesh TA, Zarubin VC, Niendam TA, Ragland JD, Tully LM, Carter CS (2020b) One-year stability of frontoparietal cognitive control network connectivity in recent onset Schizophrenia: a task-related 3T fMRI study. Schizophr Bull. https://doi.org/10.1093/schbul/sbz122
Smucny J, Dienel SJ, Lewis DA, Carter CS (2022) Mechanisms underlying dorsolateral prefrontal cortex contributions to cognitive dysfunction in schizophrenia. Neuropsychopharmacology 47:292–308
Snitz BE, Macdonald AW 3rd, Carter CS (2006) Cognitive deficits in unaffected first-degree relatives of schizophrenia patients: a meta-analytic review of putative endophenotypes. Schizophr Bull 32:179–194. Epub 2005 Sep 15
Sohal VS, Zhang F, Yizhar O, Deisseroth K (2009) Parvalbumin neurons and gamma rhythms enhance cortical circuit performance. Nature 459:698–702
Stark KL, Xu B, Bagchi A, Lai W-S, Liu H, Hsu R, Wan X, Pavlidis P, Mills AA, Karayiorgou M, Gogos JA (2008) Altered brain microRNA biogenesis contributes to phenotypic deficits in a 22q11-deletion mouse model. Nat Genet 40:751–760
Stawicka ZM, Massoudi R, Oikonomidis L, McIver L, Mulvihill K, Quah SKL, Cockcroft GJ, Clarke HF, Horst NK, Wood CM, Roberts AC (2022) Differential effects of the inactivation of anterior and posterior orbitofrontal cortex on affective responses to proximal and distal threat, and reward anticipation in the common marmoset. Cereb Cortex 32:1319–1336
Stephan KE, Friston KJ, Frith CD (2009) Dysconnection in schizophrenia: from abnormal synaptic plasticity to failures of self-monitoring. Schizophr Bull 35:509–527
Stoet G, Snyder LH (2003) Executive control and task-switching in monkeys. Neuropsychologia 41:1357–1364
Stokes MG (2015) "Activity-silent" working memory in prefrontal cortex: a dynamic coding framework. Trends Cogn Sci 19:394–405
Stone JM, Howes OD, Egerton A, Kambeitz J, Allen P, Lythgoe DJ, O'Gorman RL, McLean MA, Barker GJ, McGuire P (2010) Altered relationship between hippocampal glutamate levels and striatal dopamine function in subjects at ultra high risk of psychosis. Biol Psychiatry 68:599–602
Swaminathan SK, Freedman DJ (2012) Preferential encoding of visual categories in parietal cortex compared with prefrontal cortex. Nat Neurosci 15:315–320. https://doi.org/10.1038/nn.3016
Sweis BM, Thomas MJ, Redish AD (2018) Beyond simple tests of value: measuring addiction as a heterogeneous disease of computation-specific valuation processes. Learn Mem 25:501–512

Takeda K, Funahashi S (2004) Population vector analysis of primate prefrontal activity during spatial working memory. Cereb Cortex 14:1328–1339

Tamura M, Mukai J, Gordon JA, Gogos JA (2016) Developmental inhibition of Gsk3 rescues behavioral and neurophysiological deficits in a mouse model of Schizophrenia predisposition. Neuron 89:1100–1109

Tang H, Qi X-L, Riley MR, Constantinidis C (2019) Working memory capacity is enhanced by distributed prefrontal activation and invariant temporal dynamics. Proc Natl Acad Sci U S A 116:7095–7100

Tang H, Riley MR, Singh B, Qi X-L, Blake DT, Constantinidis C (2022) Prefrontal cortical plasticity during learning of cognitive tasks. Nat Commun 13:90

Tang W, Choi EY, Heilbronner SR, Haber SN (2021) Nonhuman primate meso-circuitry data: a translational tool to understand brain networks across species. Brain Struct Funct 226:1–11

Timms AE, Dorschner MO, Wechsler J, Choi KY, Kirkwood R, Girirajan S, Baker C, Eichler EE, Korvatska O, Roche KW, Horwitz MS, Tsuang DW (2013) Support for the N-methyl-D-aspartate receptor hypofunction hypothesis of schizophrenia from exome sequencing in multiplex families. JAMA Psychiatry 70:582–590

Trubetskoy V et al (2022) Mapping genomic loci implicates genes and synaptic biology in schizophrenia. Nature 604:502–508

Tu P-C, Lee Y-C, Chen Y-S, Li C-T, Su T-P (2013) Schizophrenia and the brain's control network: aberrant within- and between-network connectivity of the frontoparietal network in schizophrenia. Schizophr Res 147:339–347

van der Stelt O, Belger A (2007) Application of electroencephalography to the study of cognitive and brain functions in schizophrenia. Schizophr Bull 33:955–970

van Os J, Krabbendam L, Myin-Germeys I, Delespaul P (2005) The schizophrenia envirome. Curr Opin Psychiatry 18:141–145

Vijayraghavan S, Wang M, Birnbaum SG, Williams GV, Arnsten AFT (2007) Inverted-U dopamine D1 receptor actions on prefrontal neurons engaged in working memory. Nat Neurosci 10: 376–384

Vinogradov S, Hamid AA, Redish AD (2022) Etiopathogenic models of psychosis spectrum illnesses must resolve four key features. Biol Psychiatry 92:514–522

Vlasova RM et al (2021) Maternal immune activation during pregnancy alters postnatal brain growth and cognitive development in nonhuman primate offspring. J Neurosci 41:9971–9987

Wallis JD, Miller EK (2003) From rule to response: neuronal processes in the premotor and prefrontal cortex. J Neurophysiol 90:1790–1806. https://doi.org/10.1152/jn.00086.2003. Epub 2003 May 7

Wallis JD, Anderson KC, Miller EK (2001) Single neurons in prefrontal cortex encode abstract rules. Nature 411:953–956. https://doi.org/10.1038/35082081

Wang M, Yang Y, Wang C-J, Gamo NJ, Jin LE, Mazer JA, Morrison JH, Wang X-J, Arnsten AFT (2013) NMDA receptors subserve persistent neuronal firing during working memory in dorsolateral prefrontal cortex. Neuron 77:736–749

Wang M, Datta D, Enwright J, Galvin V, Yang S-T, Paspalas C, Kozak R, Gray DL, Lewis DA, Arnsten AFT (2019a) A novel dopamine D1 receptor agonist excites delay-dependent working memory-related neuronal firing in primate dorsolateral prefrontal cortex. Neuropharmacology 150:46–58

Wang W, Zhang L, Chi X-S, He L, Zhou D, Li J-M (2019b) Psychiatric symptoms of patients with anti-NMDA receptor encephalitis. Front Neurol 10:1330

Wang XJ (1999) Synaptic basis of cortical persistent activity: the importance of NMDA receptors to working memory. J Neurosci 19:9587–9603

Wang Z, Singh B, Zhou X, Constantinidis C (2022) Strong gamma frequency oscillations in the adolescent prefrontal cortex. J Neurosci 42:2917–2929

Wagner S, Doering B, Helmreich I, Lieb K, Tadić A (2012) A meta-analysis of executive dysfunctions in unipolar major depressive disorder without psychotic symptoms and their

changes during antidepressant treatment. Acta Psychiatr Scand 125(4):281–292. https://doi.org/10.1111/j.1600-0447.2011.01762.x
Watanabe K, Funahashi S (2014) Neural mechanisms of dual-task interference and cognitive capacity limitation in the prefrontal cortex. Nat Neurosci 17:601–611
Weir RK, Forghany R, Smith SEP, Patterson PH, McAllister AK, Schumann CM, Bauman MD (2015) Preliminary evidence of neuropathology in nonhuman primates prenatally exposed to maternal immune activation. Brain Behav Immun 48:139–146
Wibral M, Pampu N, Priesemann V, Siebenhuhner F, Seiwert H, Lindner M, Lizier JT, Vicente R (2013) Measuring information-transfer delays. PLoS One 8:e55809. https://doi.org/10.1371/journal.pone.0055809. Epub 2013 Feb 28
Williams GV, Goldman-Rakic PS (1995) Modulation of memory fields by dopamine D1 receptors in prefrontal cortex. Nature 376:572–575
Wong RK, Selvanayagam J, Johnston KD, Everling S (2022) Delay-related activity in marmoset prefrontal cortex. Cereb Cortex. https://doi.org/10.1093/cercor/bhac289
Woolgar A, Afshar S, Williams MA, Rich AN (2015) Flexible coding of task rules in frontoparietal cortex: an adaptive system for flexible cognitive control. J Cogn Neurosci 27:1895–1911. https://doi.org/10.1162/jocn_a_00827. Epub 2015 May 26
Wynn JK, Sugar C, Horan WP, Kern R, Green MF (2010) Mismatch negativity, social cognition, and functioning in schizophrenia patients. Biol Psychiatry 67:940–947
Yang Y, Paspalas CD, Jin LE, Picciotto MR, Arnsten AFT, Wang M (2013) Nicotinic α7 receptors enhance NMDA cognitive circuits in dorsolateral prefrontal cortex. Proc Natl Acad Sci USA 110:12078–12083
Yilmaz M, Yalcin E, Presumey J, Aw E, Ma M, Whelan CW, Stevens B, McCarroll SA, Carroll MC (2021) Overexpression of schizophrenia susceptibility factor human complement C4A promotes excessive synaptic loss and behavioral changes in mice. Nat Neurosci 24:214–224
Yoon JH, Minzenberg MJ, Ursu S, Ryan Walter BS, Wendelken C, Ragland JD, Carter CS (2008) Association of dorsolateral prefrontal cortex dysfunction with disrupted coordinated brain activity in schizophrenia: relationship with impaired cognition, behavioral disorganization, and global function. Am J Psychiatry 165:1006–1014
Zhang M, Palaniyappan L, Deng M, Zhang W, Pan Y, Fan Z, Tan W, Wu G, Liu Z, Pu W (2021) Abnormal thalamocortical circuit in adolescents with early-onset Schizophrenia. J Am Acad Child Adolesc Psychiatry 60:479–489
Zhou X, Zhu D, Qi X-L, Lees CJ, Bennett AJ, Salinas E, Stanford TR, Constantinidis C (2013) Working memory performance and neural activity in prefrontal cortex of peripubertal monkeys. J Neurophysiol 110:2648–2660
Zhou X, Zhu D, Qi X-L, Li S, King SG, Salinas E, Stanford TR, Constantinidis C (2016) Neural correlates of working memory development in adolescent primates. Nat Commun 7:13423
Zhu D, Yin J, Liang C, Luo X, Lv D, Dai Z, Xiong S, Fu J, Li Y, Lin J, Lin Z, Wang Y, Ma G (2019) CACNA1C (rs1006737) may be a susceptibility gene for schizophrenia: An updated meta-analysis. Brain Behav 9:e01292
Zick JL, Blackman RK, Crowe DA, Amirikian B, DeNicola AL, Netoff TI, Chafee MV (2018) Blocking NMDAR disrupts spike timing and decouples monkey prefrontal circuits: implications for activity-dependent disconnection in Schizophrenia. Neuron 98:1243–1255.e5
Zick JL, Crowe DA, Blackman RK, Schultz K, Bergstrand DW, DeNicola AL, Carter RE, Ebner TJ, Lanier LM, Netoff TI, Chafee MV (2021) Disparate insults relevant to schizophrenia converge on impaired spike synchrony and weaker synaptic interactions in prefrontal local circuits. Curr Biol. https://doi.org/10.1016/j.cub.2021.10.009
Zikopoulos B, Barbas H (2007) Parallel driving and modulatory pathways link the prefrontal cortex and thalamus. PLoS One 2:e848

Olfactory Dysfunction in Schizophrenia: Evaluating Olfactory Abilities Across Species

Taitum O. Cothren, Christopher J. Evonko, and David A. MacQueen

Contents

Abstract Though understudied relative to perturbations in the auditory and visual domains, olfactory dysfunction is a common symptom of schizophrenia. Over the past two decades, the availability of standardized assessments to quantify human olfactory abilities, and enhance understanding of the neurophysiology supporting olfaction, has increased, enabling a more thorough characterization of these deficits. In contrast to other psychiatric conditions for which olfactory dysfunction has been observed (e.g., major depressive disorder, bipolar disorder, Alzheimer's disease), the impairments observed in schizophrenia are particularly global and profound. At this level, such deficits in olfactory abilities likely impact the enjoyment of food, detection of environmental hazards, and influence social relationships. More broadly, the study of olfactory phenotypes in schizophrenia presents new avenues for detection of those at-risk for the condition, identification of therapeutic targets for treatment development, and for the characterization of novel animal models relevant to schizophrenia and psychosis. This review will consider the olfactory performance of individuals with schizophrenia in domains for which standardized assessments are available (odor sensitivity, discrimination, identification, and memory). Paradigms available for assessing these abilities in rodents will also be discussed with the aim of facilitating translation. Thus, future studies will be able to include cross-species

T. O. Cothren, C. J. Evonko, and D. A. MacQueen (✉)
Department of Psychology, University of North Carolina at Wilmington, Wilmington, NC, USA
e-mail: macqueend@uncw.edu

Curr Topics Behav Neurosci (2023) 63: 363–392
https://doi.org/10.1007/7854_2022_390
Published Online: 5 September 2022

translation of mechanisms relevant to olfactory function and cognition, what has gone awry in the disease state, and test potential therapeutics.

Keywords Odor discrimination · Odor identification · Odor memory · Odor sensitivity · Odor threshold · Olfaction · Schizophrenia

1 Olfactory Dysfunction in Schizophrenia: Evaluating Olfactory Abilities Across Species

The presentation of schizophrenia varies substantially across individuals, but the clinical diagnosis outlined in the Diagnostic and Statistical Manual (DSM-I through DSM-5) has long required that delusions, hallucinations, or both, are present. Accordingly, a great deal of work has been conducted to characterize these cognitive and perceptual disturbances that are characteristic of the disorder. For many reasons, such work has primarily focused on, or relied upon, the visual and auditory senses. This focus might be expected given that language-based assessments (e.g., list learning) will naturally make use of visual and/or auditory modalities. It is also fitting that studies of perception have focused on audition and vision given that associated hallucinatory experiences are most frequently reported to be of an auditory and/or visual nature. Such focus on the auditory domain has been fruitful; leading to perceptual testing paradigms, such as the pre-pulse inhibition (PPI) assay that has contributed greatly to the development of therapeutics for schizophrenia (Geyer et al. 2001). Until fairly recently however, there has been a paucity of perceptual and cognitive studies inspecting the sense of olfaction as it relates to schizophrenia. This gap has stemmed in part from an underdeveloped understanding of the olfactory apparatus relative to the human auditory and visual systems. The study of olfaction has also long been hampered by the difficulty of controlling the presentation of odorous stimuli in a consistent, reliable, and reproducible manner. Yet, much has been learned about odor perception over the past 20 years, as reflected in the Nobel prize awarded to Richard Axel and Linda Buck for outlining the organization of the olfactory system (Miller 2004). Standardized methods for assessing olfactory abilities in both the human and non-human species are now widely available. As such, olfactory assessment is providing new windows into the clinical presentation and neurobiological substrates of schizophrenia.

It has long been recognized that individuals with schizophrenia commonly experience olfactory dysfunction. An early twentieth century report from psychiatrists at Bellevue Hospital (New York) outlines no less than 20 cases of patients with schizophrenia reporting olfactory experiences considered to be hallucinations (Bromberg and Schilder 1934). In the report, the authors lament that "the paucity of olfactory studies from a psychologic or sensational point of view is in marked contrast to the enormous literature concerned with optic and tactual sensation," and that "textbooks practically neglect the subject." Nearly three decades later, Rubert et al. (1961) documented that olfactory hallucinations are frequently reported by patients with schizophrenia but, only when providers intentionally inquired about such experiences. Similar to the sentiments expressed by Bromberg and Schilder (1934), the authors noted "The belief that olfactory hallucinations are uncommon and portend a poor prognosis is widely held among psychiatrists. It has been handed down by word of mouth and in print...".

In one sense, it is easy to understand why research focus has been targeted primarily at evaluating auditory, visual, and language-based deficits. One can readily imagine how impairments in a domain such as verbal list learning could substantially impact quality of life. Yet, olfactory dysfunction has a consequential impact on quality of life as well. The sense of smell is important to the enjoyment of food and beverage, aids in the detection of spoiled foods, and alerts one to hazards in the environment such as smoke or hazardous chemicals (Croy et al. 2014). Olfaction also plays an important role in social relations. For example, individuals with impaired or absent olfaction (hyposmia or anosmia, respectively) often report concerns that they may be expressing offensive bodily odors of which they are unaware. In a study of 278 patients with olfactory dysfunction, 41% of participants reported this concern (Temmel et al. 2002). Notably, in the cases of schizophrenia-related olfactory hallucinations reported by Bromberg and Schilder (1934), 12 out of 20 patients reported a foul odor emanating from themselves, or another's body, and at least three patients explicitly expressed concern about how others perceived them due to bodily smells. An ensuing report documented three cases of patients with schizophrenia who sought care as a result of "the uncontrollable escape of flatus, which they imagined was constantly present and detected by everybody about them". In each case, proctologic examination failed to uncover physical abnormalities accounting for the symptoms, which were presumed to reflect olfactory hallucinations (Forte 1952). Thus, either deficits in olfactory abilities or the presence of olfactory hallucinations can impact social relations in a manner disruptive to quality of life.

While it is important to study the presence of olfactory hallucinations and/or olfactory impairments in schizophrenia given the potential impacts on quality of life, the use of olfactory assessment might also provide other advantages for characterizing schizophrenia-associated neuropathology. Measures of olfactory perception and cognition may be particularly useful for investigating the role of schizophrenia-associated biomarkers given the significant overlap and interplay between structures supporting olfaction and those supporting cognitive and affective functions which are disrupted in schizophrenia. In short, odorants activate olfactory receptor neurons in the nasal epithelium, and signals generated from such activation are transmitted to glomeruli in the olfactory bulb. Projections from the olfactory bulb then project to areas including the piriform cortex, entorhinal cortex, and portions of the amygdala (see Fig. 1). It is believed that such close connection with the hippocampal formation and amygdala underlies the powerful associations of smell with memory and affect. In contrast with the visual and auditory senses, signals derived from the olfactory sensory apparatus are not transmitted through the thalamus before being relayed to cortical areas. As a result, the relative simplicity of olfactory circuits may facilitate

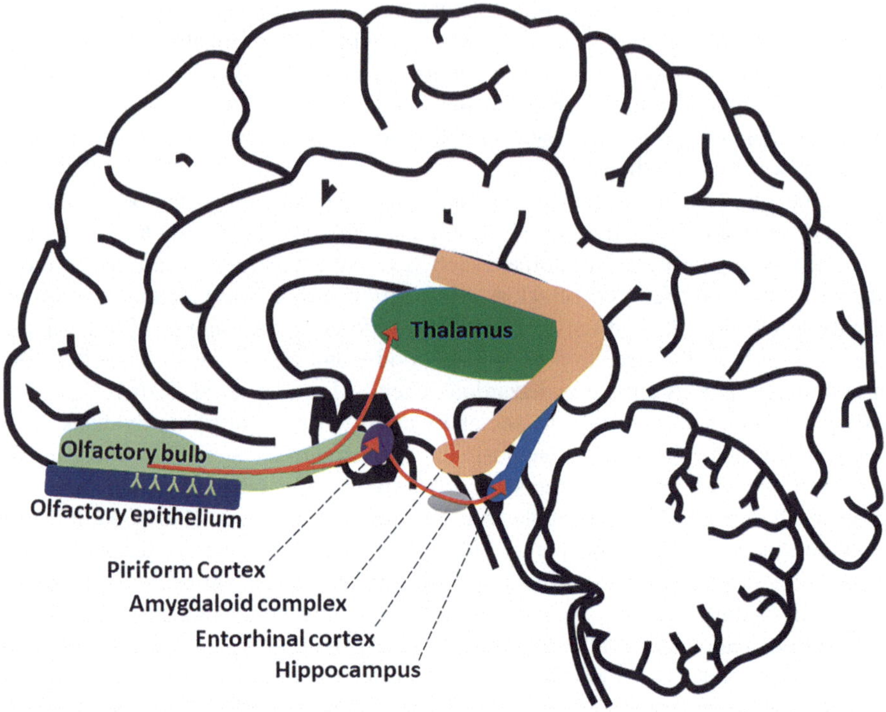

Fig. 1 A schematic of olfactory input to the central nervous system

evaluation of the association between neurophysiological function and behavioral performance. Further, the configuration of olfactory system is reasonably well conserved across mammalian species (Su et al. 2009), facilitating translational research that will be necessary for mapping neurobiological substrates of olfactory performance, testing disease-relevant manipulations, and for evaluating novel therapeutics targeting mechanisms perturbed in schizophrenia.

As mentioned previously, a limiting factor to the study of olfaction in psychiatric patients in the twentieth century stemmed from the lack of standardized tools for evaluating olfactory performance. In the present day, there are now a variety of standardized olfactory measures for which normative data, stratified by variables such as age and gender, are readily available. Such measures include the University of Pennsylvania Smell Identification Test (UPSIT), the odor discrimination/memory test (ODMT), and the Sniffin' Sticks test battery, which provide individual tests of olfactory sensitivity, discrimination, and identification. In addition to these standardized measures, olfactometers, which allow for computer-controlled, time-locked presentation of odorants are now commercially available for testing with human participants and with model species, such as rodents. Furthermore, as a result of their keen sense of olfaction, mice and rats can often be trained on operant tasks rapidly when odorants serve as relevant stimuli, and the automated nature of olfactometer-based tasks can support high-throughput testing (Kraemer and Apfelbach 2004). Coupled with a modern understanding of the neural substrates of olfaction, olfactory testing paradigms may be ideal for translational research aimed at identifying individuals at risk of developing schizophrenia, screening potential therapeutics for the condition, and identifying the causal mechanisms involved in effective treatments.

The present review is intended to provide a background on perceptual and cognitive olfactory testing paradigms and their use in research on schizophrenia. The review will focus on domains for which reliable and valid assessments of olfactory performance are readily available, including odor sensitivity, discrimination, identification, and memory.

1.1 Odor Sensitivity

Olfactory sensitivity refers to the concentration of an odorant necessary to stimulate subjective awareness. Tests of olfactory sensitivity seek to establish the concentration *threshold* at which an odor can be detected. As such, these paradigms are interchangeably referred to as tests of olfactory sensitivity, threshold, or detection. With this terminology, it is important to recognize that results revealing a *low* olfactory threshold are demonstrating a *high* degree of olfactory sensitivity. The detection of an odor represents the most basic process involved in using olfactory information to guide behavior. Odorant detection is most principally influenced by processes occurring in the peripheral olfactory system (e.g., olfactory epithelium and olfactory bulb). Thus, olfactory sensitivity paradigms allow for the study of human behavior as influenced by relatively limited circuitry.

Olfactory sensitivity tests typically proceed by probing an examinee's ability to detect an odor across serial dilutions of an odorant. These procedures can be conducted in a great variety of manners and with any odorant chosen by the experimenter. Several standardized assessments of olfactory sensitivity are presently available, allowing for consistent study across laboratories. These include the Burghart Sniffin' Sticks tests (SS; (Kobal et al. 1996)) and the Sensonics Smell Threshold Test (STT; (Doty et al. 1986)). The SS is composed of a battery of olfactory tests including sensitivity, discrimination, and identification. The SS sensitivity test presents stimuli through a collection of felt-tip "markers" that have been soaked in serial dilutions of the odorant, or water. In the STT, the examinee sniff from a series of bottles containing the requisite dilutions. Both the SS and STT are available with phenyl ethyl alcohol (PEA) used as the odorant. PEA is frequently selected because it is colorless, has a pleasant, floral scent and does not cause activation of the trigeminal nerve (also present in the nasal sinuses). Alternatively, the SS sensitivity test is also available with n-butanol, an odorant that produces some stimulation of the trigeminal nerve in addition to olfactory receptor neurons.

In a typical threshold test, an examinee is asked to sample two or more comparisons (e.g., odor pens) and identify the only comparison that contained the odorant.

These tests are forced choice, meaning that the individual must choose one and cannot "pass" if unsure. A staircase method is then used to determine the individual's odor threshold. This method means that testing concentration decreases across trials until the examinee begins to make errors, at which point the testing concentration will increase until the examinee is reliably correct. The procedure of ascending and descending concentrations is usually repeated multiple times until the concentration that can reliably be detected (threshold) is established. An individual scoring a low threshold would have high olfactory sensitivity.

A meta-analysis by Cohen et al. (2012) including 14 studies which evaluated sensitivity in individuals with schizophrenia demonstrated a significant small to moderate sized deficit ($d = -0.45$), relative to controls. Notably, every study included in this analysis yielded a negative effect size, demonstrating reliably poorer performance amongst those with the condition. Yet, from these studies it is not possible to establish whether olfactory sensitivity deficits emerge in tandem with psychosis, or whether impaired sensitivity is a dispositional aspect associated with individuals at risk for developing schizophrenia. As such, Cohen et al. (2012) also provide an analysis of sensitivity from studies evaluating individuals with traits of schizotypy compared with healthy controls. This approach included ultra-high-risk individuals (individuals with a family history of psychosis and functional decline), individuals with a biological family member who has schizophrenia, and those presenting with high but subclinical levels of Schizotypal traits. The analysis yielded a similar effect size ($d = -0.38$) and again, the effect size was negative for all studies included. This suggests that olfactory sensitivity deficits do not simply emerge as part of the initial psychotic episode but rather, are detectable in individuals who are at risk of and may yet experience a psychotic episode.

A more recent meta-analysis of olfactory function reached a similar conclusion from studies of patients with schizophrenia, at-risk youth, family members of individuals with schizophrenia, and those expressing schizotypal features (Moberg et al. 2014). In the evaluation of olfactory sensitivity, a review of 40 separate comparisons yielded an effect size of $d = -0.51$, consistent with the earlier analysis by Cohen et al. (2012). Again, the vast majority of comparisons (all but 4) included means reflecting better sensitivity amongst healthy controls. Despite the general reliability of olfactory threshold deficits amongst individuals with schizophrenia, those at-risk, and familial relationships, meta-analysis has been necessary to fully establish the relationship (see Fig. 2). Given the challenges of recruiting such samples, most patient/control studies reporting on olfactory threshold have included 40 patients or less. With an estimated effect size in the small to moderate range it is thus not unexpected that quite a few investigations have not reported significant olfactory detection deficits in these groups (Kayser et al. 2013; Kohler et al. 2001; Malaspina et al. 2012, 2016; Moberg et al. 2006; Takahashi et al. 2018; Woolley et al. 2015). It is plausible that the deficits in olfactory sensitivity amongst patients with schizophrenia (and those at risk) reported in these meta-analyses result from publication bias favoring studies which detected significant differences between groups. Indeed, Moberg et al. (2014) did report significant evidence of possible publication bias. Yet, this analysis also revealed that there would need to be an

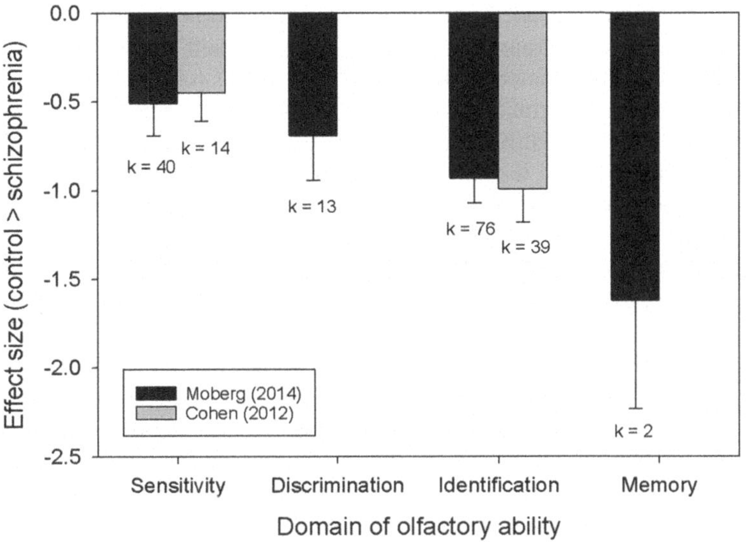

Fig. 2 The effect size of olfactory deficits amongst individuals with schizophrenia relative to healthy controls by olfactory domain as derived from meta-analysis. Data reproduced from Moberg et al. (2014) and Cohen et al. (2012)

exceptionally large number of studies finding null effects (7,103 studies) to reverse the general conclusions of the meta-analysis.

In considering olfactory sensitivity deficits amongst individuals with schizophrenia it is important to recognize that tobacco smoking rates amongst this population are exceptionally high relative to the general population (NIH State of the Science Panel 2006). Cigarette smoking is a known cause of olfactory dysfunction. Otherwise healthy smokers self-report hyposmia, a reduced ability to smell, at greatly elevated rates when compared with never smokers (Duffy et al. 2019; Glennon et al. 2019). Well-controlled laboratory studies have also demonstrated a decreased sensitivity to odors amongst smokers relative to non-smokers (Hayes and Jinks 2012; Ozmen et al. 2016; Rosenblatt et al. 1998). The olfactory dysfunction produced by smoking can be long lasting but is, typically, not permanent. A study of change in olfactory performance amongst smokers following smoking cessation demonstrated significant improvements in olfactory discrimination and identification, but not sensitivity, within 45 days (Dinc et al. 2020). Recovery of these olfactory abilities was related to smoking history such that the greatest improvement was observed amongst those with shortest duration of smoking. Though it is important to consider the role of smoking in the olfactory sensitivity deficits observed in schizophrenia it is notable that such deficits have been observed even in studies in which smoking variables were reasonably balanced between groups and/or used as covariates in statistical analyses (e.g., (Rupp et al. 2005)).

An advantage of evaluating olfactory dysfunction as a phenotype of schizophrenia is that olfactory function can be assessed relatively easily in rodents, which serve as the primary animal model for pharmacology (rats and mice) and genetic manipulation (mice) in schizophrenia-related research. As a result of their strong olfactory acuity and ethological reliance on this sense (Doty 1986), rodents can be trained and tested on olfactory paradigms with relative ease. Multiple paradigms exist for testing olfactory detection, or sensitivity with rodents. For a simple evaluation of olfactory detection, the buried food test can be completed in a single session and does not require behavioral training (Yang and Crawley 2009). The test is conducted by recording the latency of a rodent to uncover a familiar piece of food hidden underneath a layer of bedding. This time can then be compared to the latency of the animal in approaching a visible piece of the same food in the same environment recorded during a separate trial. Disrupted olfactory detection is inferred when latencies for retrieval of the buried food exceed latencies for approach to visible food or differ substantially between groups. This manner of testing relies on the propensity in rodents to use olfaction for foraging. While prior operant training is not required to conduct the test, familiarization with the food item and some degree of pre-test food deprivation (e.g., 18–24 h) is recommended for ideal testing conditions. Though the buried food test is adequate for identifying gross disruptions in olfactory detection, such testing does not allow for a precise evaluation of olfactory sensitivity and can be impacted by manipulations that alter food motivation or sensorimotor abilities (e.g., ambulation).

The olfactory habituation/dishabituation testing paradigm is a procedure that can be used both to evaluate olfactory detection and discrimination (For detailed protocols, see (Yang and Crawley 2009)). It relies on the propensity of rodents to approach and investigate novelty. The task proceeds through a series of trials in which the animal is presented with odorous and non-odorous stimulus. For example, on an initial trial an odor is introduced into the animal's cage. This can be accomplished by coating a cotton tipped applicator in the odorous material and entering the tip into the cage through a hole in the lid. The animal is assessed over the next few minutes, scoring the number of approaches to the stimulus and the time spent inspecting the stimulus. This test is repeated for three separate trials using the same odorant. Typically, the animal will progressively reduce the time they spend inspecting the stimulus, demonstrating habituation to the stimulus. Following the habituation trials, the odorant can be replaced with a novel odorant and the trials repeated. If the animal is able to detect the novel odorant the experimenter can inspect to see if measures of stimulus approach/inspection increased relative to the last trial of the initial odorant, illustrating dishabituation. When the animal demonstrates dishabituation, it can be presumed that the animal can both detect the odorant and distinguish it as novel (odor discrimination). This format of testing can be used to compare behavior elicited by odorous and non-odorous stimuli (e.g., water), or compare social odors (e.g., bedding from conspecifics) with non-social odors. Standard applications of this procedure can be used to confirm detection and, in some arrangements, discrimination of odorants but, does not provide a quantification of sensitivity/threshold. However, threshold can be measured with this arrangement through a series of trials intended to determine the concentration of a novel odorant necessary to produce dishabituation.

The buried food and the habituation tests are advantageous in that they provide a simple paradigm for assessing odor detection that utilizes readily available materials. Yet, the most sensitive means of evaluating olfactory sensitivity in rodents utilize an olfactometer; a computer directed apparatus designed for the controlled delivery of odors. Olfactometers built for rodent testing are now available from multiple vendors or can be constructed from component parts. In a typical arrangement, rodents are trained to place their nose into a tube or port through which odorous air is directed. There is also typically a response element (e.g., a lever or a lick sensor) that the animal can act on to respond to programmed stimulus–response contingencies. Olfactometer setups vary most prominently with regard to the number and form of response elements and the number of odor "channels" available, which determines the number of odors that can be used in training or testing. Various formats can be used with this equipment to test odor sensitivity. For example, a paradigm could consist of training the animal to respond on a lick sensor when an odor is delivered but, inhibit licking when the odor is absent. After demonstrating reliably accurate performance with this discrimination, the subject can then be tested with trials presenting varied concentrations of the odorant to determine what concentration yields responding (odor threshold).

All the strategies described above have been used to evaluate odor detection in schizophrenia-relevant rodent models. For example, the buried food test has been conducted in transgenic mice engineered to express a dominant-negative form of the Disrupted-in-Schizophrenia-1 gene (DN-DISC1). When tested, DN-DISC1 mice took significantly longer to locate buried food relative to wild-type control subjects, suggesting dysfunction in odor detection (Hikida et al. 2007). It is important to note however, that other phenotypes were also disrupted in DN-DISC1 animals (e.g., locomotor activity, immobility) that could have potentially impacted performance on the buried food task. A separate study evaluating mice engineered to express humanized DISC1 (hDISC1) exclusively in forebrain region did not find disrupted performance of the buried food task despite confirmation of hDISC1 expression in the olfactory bulb. Mutations in genes coding for neurexins, a family of cell adhesion proteins associated with schizophrenia, have also been explored in mouse models. A study of mice lacking a form of neurexin (Nrxn1α KO) exhibited schizophrenia-relevant phenotypes of altered social approach and investigation but, did not exhibit deficits in retrieving buried food (Intact olfaction; (Grayton et al. 2013)).

Deficient expression and/or function of the NMDA subtype glutamate receptor has been implicated in the development of schizophrenia, and the relationship of NMDAr blockade and olfactory function has been assessed in rodent models. Acute doses of the NMDAr antagonist phencyclidine (PCP) produced deficits in the buried food task. Further, postnatal administration of PCP resulted in similar deficits expressed in adulthood (Shan et al. 2018). Such deficits were accompanied by alterations in field potentials derived from the olfactory bulb and were reversed by co-administration of the antipsychotic medication olanzapine. While these data suggest decreased olfactory sensitivity, it is unlikely that moderate NMDAr antagonism fully abolishes odor detection, as many studies have demonstrated intact odor discrimination in rats administered moderate to moderate-high doses of NMDAr antagonists (MacQueen et al. 2011, 2016). High doses of NMDAr antagonists, such as PCP, produce gross multi-sensory deficits (Kesner et al. 1981). A variety of mechanisms by which NMDAr expression or function may impact olfactory function have been explored using mouse models. Yet, deficits in the buried food task have not been reported for glutamate aspartate transporter deficient mice (Karlsson et al. 2009), SynGAP deficient mice (Guo et al. 2009), mice with reduced NMDA receptor glycine affinity (Grin1-d481n) (Labrie et al. 2008, 2010), mice deficient in the growth factor neuregulin 1 (Nrg1+/−) (Moy et al. 2009; O'Tuathaigh et al. 2007), or serine racemase deficient mice (Labrie et al. 2009). Conditional deletion of the neuregulin receptor Erbb4 did yield deficits on the buried food test (Moy et al. 2009). It is conceivable that such manipulations may in fact impact olfactory sensitivity but, not to a degree that disturbs finding an odorous and highly attractive food located in the proximal vicinity.

As mentioned previously, a limitation to the buried food test is that performance can be impacted by non-olfactory factors such as food motivation. The olfactory habituation/dishabituation paradigm offers an advantage in this regard as the behaviors assessed by the task are not inherently food motivated. Like the buried food test, the olfactory habituation/dishabituation test has been used to evaluate the effects of NMDAr antagonists. Yet, a study of male rats receiving sub chronic dosing with PCP performed as well as control animals (receiving vehicle) on this task in response to both social and non-social odors (Tarland and Brosda 2018). Olfactometer-based tasks have also been used to assess the role of the NMDAr in odor detection. Staubli and colleagues (1989) used an olfactometer to train mice to acquire a two-choice odor discrimination before implanting minipumps providing intracerebroventricular infusion of the competitive NMDAr antagonist AP5 over 14 days. During this period, animals receiving AP5 were significantly slower at acquiring a novel odor discrimination relative to control animals when diluted odorants (weak intensity) were used in training. Though this would appear to suggest an odor sensitivity deficit, the interpretation was complicated in that weak intensity odors only yielded deficits when long (10 min), but not short (2 min), intertrial intervals were employed. Moreover, NMDAr antagonism produces a limited effect on olfactory sensitivity at doses that disrupt other aspects of olfactory or cognitive performance. For example, several NMDAr antagonist drugs including MK-801, CPP, and ketamine impair performance of the olfactory span task, an odor-based memory task, while sparing the accuracy of well-learned olfactory discriminations (MacQueen et al. 2011, 2016; Galizio et al. 2016). Thus, while NMDAr antagonists may profoundly disrupt olfactory sensitivity at high doses (Kesner et al. 1981), doses typically used to model schizophrenia-relevant phenotypes appear to have modest deleterious effect on odor sensitivity. This point is particularly salient when using tests that require olfactory discrimination to guide cognition, such as the attentional set-shifting task (Birrell and Brown 2000).

Dopaminergic mechanisms have also been evaluated with regard to their impact on olfactory sensitivity. In a study of knockout mice engineered to lack either the dopamine transporter (DAT −/−) or the D2 dopamine receptor (D2 −/−), Tillerson and colleagues utilized both the habituation/dishabituation paradigm, and a series of concentration-based discriminations, to evaluate olfactory function. Both the DAT −/− and D2 −/− animals demonstrated initial odor habituation consistent with controls however, when a novel odor was then introduced, both knockout groups failed to exhibit dishabituation (in contrast to control animals). When subjects were tested on discriminations of various concentrations of paprika, both mutant and wild-type groups performed similarly, successfully completing discrimination trials at the 100 ng/ml concentration but, not at the 10 ng/ml concentration. This combination of findings suggests that mice lacking DAT exhibit a deficit in odor discrimination but, not sensitivity. Pharmacological studies have also been informative for evaluating the relationship between dopaminergic tone and olfactory sensitivity. Doty and Ferguson-Segall (1987) evaluated the dose–response curve of amphetamine in rats on an olfactometer-based task requiring go/no-go discrimination of an odorant at varying concentrations. Low doses of amphetamine improved odor detection at the lowest concentrations of the odorant (weakest intensity), while high doses of amphetamine impaired odor detection even at the highest concentrations of the odorant (highest intensity). A follow-up study evaluated the effects of the D2 agonist quinpirole on the same olfactometer-based task and observed dose-dependent impairments in odor detection that were rescued by co-administration of the D2 antagonist spiperone (Doty and Risser 1989).

There is a wealth of evidence implicating hyperdopaminergia and glutamatergic dysregulation in the pathophysiology of schizophrenia. Thus, it is unsurprising that mechanisms related to these biomarkers have been a focus of investigation in preclinical studies assessing odor detection. It is also not unexpected that manipulations of glutamatergic and dopaminergic processes impact odor sensitivity given the physiology of the peripheral olfactory system. Olfactory receptor neurons signal to mitral and tufted cells within the olfactory bulb using glutamate, and this transmission is regulated by presynaptic D1 and GABAb receptors (Doty and Kamath 2014), as well as D2 receptors (Koster et al. 1999). Given the alignment between the known pathophysiology of schizophrenia and the signaling processes of the peripheral olfactory system, odor detection/olfactory sensitivity tasks represent a useful endophenotype for characterizing model animals. In this regard, the peripheral olfactory system provides the benefit of being a relatively limited circuit. While the buried food task and habituation/dishabituation models can be useful in screening for odor detection deficits, olfactometer-based paradigms are typically most useful for precision in evaluating olfactory sensitivity.

Meta-analyses have confirmed odor sensitivity deficits amongst individuals with schizophrenia and those at risk for the condition. Though such deficits appear relatively reliable, the magnitude of the effect is rather modest. Thus, preclinical research seeking to model schizophrenia phenotypes will need to employ sensitive paradigms to demonstrate consistency with the human condition. Given the high rates of smoking amongst patients with schizophrenia, there are remaining questions regarding the extent that tobacco use is responsible for the observed deficits in odor sensitivity. As with the study of other endophenotypes in schizophrenia, ambiguity regarding medication effects further complicates interpretation of patient studies. Yet importantly, observations from studies utilizing at-risk populations (rather than patients) suggest that sensitivity deficits are not entirely attributable to tobacco or medication effects.

1.2 Odor Discrimination

Odor discrimination is the ability to distinguish one odor from another. To evaluate olfactory discrimination, several standardized assessments are available. The most common test of olfactory discrimination for human participants is the odor discrimination component of the Sniffin' Sticks Battery. The assessment proceeds through 16 trials in which the participant samples three odor pens on each trial. The examinee is blind folded, asked to smell each pen sequentially in a random order, and is then asked to report which pen smelled different from the other pens presented. The examinees score is the sum of each item they answered correctly. The score from the discrimination test can be assessed alone or it can be summed with the other assessments in the Sniffin' Sticks battery (odor threshold and odor identification) for a total TDI (threshold, discrimination, and identification) score (Kobal et al. 1996). This manner of olfactory discrimination testing can also be conducted with a modified version of the University of Pennsylvania Smell Identification Test (UPSIT). The test is comprised of one booklet with 16 items, with each item containing three scratch and sniff microcapsule panels. The panels contain two identical odors, and one odor that is different. After smelling each triad, the examinee is asked to report which odor was different from the others (Doty et al. 1994; Smith et al. 1993). Another option is the Munich Olfaction Test (MOT) that can be administered to assess discrimination as well as several other domains of olfaction. The discrimination portion of the assessment consists of eight trials in which triplets of bottles are presented in random order with two bottles containing the same odor and one bottle containing a different odor. Once again, subjects are asked to distinguish the different odor from the other two presented (Rupp et al. 2005).

Moberg et al. (1999) conducted a quantitative review of the literature on olfaction in schizophrenia, with gender, medication, and smoking history as moderator variables. Findings indicated that substantial olfactory deficits were observed in patients with schizophrenia across all domains of olfaction with no differential deficits observed across domains of olfactory (identification, threshold, sensitivity, discrimination, and memory). Influence of gender, medication, and smoking did not show significant effect sizes across the studies reviewed (Moberg et al. 1999). However, that it is important to note that only two studies were included in this review that assessed olfactory discrimination, both using a match-to-sample testing format to evaluate discrimination. Over the past two decades, olfactory research in patients with schizophrenia has grown substantially allowing for a meta-analysis of domain-specific reports. In a meta-analysis including 13 studies which assessed odor discrimination, Moberg et al. (2014) reported significant odor discrimination impairments amongst patients with schizophrenia, first-degree family members, and youths at risk for psychosis. This deficit ($k = 13$, $d = -0.69$) was on par with the impairment observed for measures of odor detection/sensitivity ($k = 40, d = -0.51$). Deficits also appeared to be relatively reliable with 11 of 13 studies reporting means that favored the performance of healthy controls. As with odor detection deficits, there remains the question of whether discrimination impairments are dispositional (present from an early age) or emerge with the positive symptoms of the condition in late adolescence/early adulthood. The Moberg et al. (2014) analysis reported that across olfaction measures, youth at-risk for schizophrenia were significantly more impaired than either first-degree family members or schizotypy groups. While this analysis suggests that olfactory deficits are likely present early in the progression of the condition, this assessment was not specific to odor discrimination.

Given the reliable deficits in odor sensitivity observed in patients with schizophrenia, it is conceivable that odor discrimination impairment may directly result from an inability to adequately detect the odorant. Yet, this seems unlikely given that standardized assessments of olfaction, such as the Sniffin' Sticks battery, utilize suprathreshold odorants that should remain detectable even with the modest levels of odor sensitivity impairment observed in patients with schizophrenia. It remains possible however, that long-standing deficits in odor sensitivity may limit opportunities for learning that give rise to more sophisticated odor discrimination. As with odor sensitivity, there is also the question of the degree to which odor discrimination impairments in schizophrenia is driven or exacerbated by high rates of smoking, or the effects of antipsychotic treatment. Cigarette smoking is associated with odor discrimination deficits and amongst smokers and odor discrimination ability is predicted by pack-years smoking (Katotomichelakis et al. 2007). Smoking related dysfunction in odor discrimination can be reversed by smoking cessation and rebounds relatively quickly (within 45 days of cessation) however, there is some evidence that reversal may be more limited for individuals with more intensive smoking histories (Dinc et al. 2020).

The effects of smoking in schizophrenia-relevant olfactory dysfunction have been evaluated in a meta-analysis, and while smoking status did not moderate effect sizes, pack-year history of smoking did moderate effect sizes amongst the patient group (Moberg et al. 2014). This association was negative however, indicating that smaller olfactory deficits were observed amongst patients with more intensive smoking histories. As a whole, it does not appear that the odor discrimination deficits observed in schizophrenia are primarily attributable to tobacco use. To evaluate the potential that olfactory deficits observed in schizophrenia are caused or exacerbated by antipsychotic medications, Chen et al. (2018) evaluated olfactory performance amongst medication naïve patients during the initial episode of psychosis. Olfactory discrimination was impaired in patients relative to age and sex matched controls, demonstrating that schizophrenia-associated discrimination deficits are not solely the product of antipsychotic treatments. Further, odor discrimination scores were inversely related to negative symptom scores derived from the Positive and Negative Syndrome Scale (PANSS) suggesting that odor discrimination deficits may be related to processes involved in producing the negative symptoms of the condition.

The association between odor discrimination and cognitive performance has also been evaluated in schizophrenia patients during the first episode of psychosis. Odor discrimination performance (derived from the Sniffin' Sticks battery) was inversely related to perseverative errors on the Wisconsin Card Sorting Task amongst patients ($r = -0.46$) but not amongst controls ($r = -0.04$) (Kamath et al. 2019). Further, it was possible to establish reasonable identification of schizophrenia cases (78.6% accurate classification) based upon a combination of test scores that included measures of speeded manual dexterity, verbal fluency, and odor discrimination. Thus, if odor discrimination deficits are indeed present prior to the first episode of psychosis, it is conceivable that odor discrimination performance may have utility in identifying those at risk for schizophrenia. Associations between odor discrimination and sensorimotor performance have also been observed in patients with schizophrenia. For example, odor discrimination deficits have been found to be highly associated with smooth pursuit eye movement dysfunction amongst patients (Malaspina et al. 1994). Experimentation in model species is likely necessary to determine whether the associations between odor discrimination, sensorimotor behavior, and cognitive task performance are driven by shared dependency on circuits outside of the peripheral olfactory system that are disturbed in schizophrenia or rather, that the pathophysiology of schizophrenia produces similar deleterious effects on discrete circuits which independently subserve these abilities.

Odor discrimination can be evaluated in rodents in a variety of ways. As previously described, the odor habituation/dishabituation paradigm can be employed to evaluate both odor detection and odor discrimination. In this task, elevated levels of approach/inspection of a novel odorant, along with subsequent habituation to the odorant across trials, can be inferred to reflect adequate odor detection. Following trials with the initial odorant, subsequent testing with a novel odorant should yield dishabituation (a return to higher levels of approach/inspection), signifying intact capacity to discriminate the novel odorant from the odorant the animal habituated to in earlier trials. Again, an advantage of the habituation/dishabituation paradigm is that it can be completed in a single session with readily available materials and does not require training. Yet, rodents can be trained to high levels of accuracy in odor discrimination relatively easily. A simple method of training olfactory discrimination in rodents involves presenting odor stimuli to the animal in an open field. For example, odorants, such as household spices, can be mixed with sand and presented to the animal in small cups. Through a shaping process, rodents can be trained to dig in these "odor cups" to retrieve buried food rewards. By selectively baiting one of the two odor cups, rodents can be subsequently trained to selectively respond (dig) to a single odorant across a series of trials. Highly accurate responding emerges within a few sessions of training and remains consistent with maintenance training (MacQueen et al. 2011). This form of olfactory discrimination training can also be accomplished with an olfactometer in both mice and rats, allowing for automated training and testing (Kraemer and Apfelbach 2004; Bodyak and Slotnick 1999).

Whether trained in an olfactometer or by manual administration, simple discrimination training/testing is among the most popular procedures for assessing odor discrimination in rodents. This testing can be conducted in a go/no-go format with a single odor presented in each trial, or in a simultaneous discrimination format in which multiple comparisons are available on each trial. The most common form of odor discrimination testing in humans, the Sniffin' Sticks odor discrimination task, uses a simultaneous discrimination format; that is, three pens are presented on each trial and only one odor is different (correct). There is a great variability between rodent studies of odor discrimination regarding the choice of odorants. Such variability in human odor discrimination studies has been reduced by the availability of standardized tests for olfactory function. Additionally, odor discrimination testing with rodents has demonstrated that strains of rats and mice can detect certain odorants below human thresholds (Blount and Coppola 2020). For example, rats have even trained to discriminate the smell of mineral oils obtained from different sources even though the mineral oils themselves were purported to be "odorless" (Gamble and Smith 2009). The ease of training rodents to perform olfactory discriminations (Bodyak and Slotnick 1999) make odor discrimination-based tasks an attractive method for modeling human cognitive processes.

As previously described, NMDAr antagonist drugs have been tested extensively in studies which included well-trained simple discrimination of suprathreshold odors. Both competitive and non-competitive antagonists have been tested in rats and in all cases, odor discrimination performance is spared at doses that impact short-term odor memory as assessed by the odor span task (MacQueen et al. 2011, 2016; Galizio et al. 2013, 2019; Mathews et al. 2018). In these studies, odor discrimination was only impaired at high doses, which caused deficits in multiple domains and produced readily observable sensorimotor disruption. Thus, while there is evidence of NMDAr involvement in the development of odor conditioning (Mukherjee and Yuan 2016), the NMDAr has not demonstrated appreciable involvement in the discrimination of suprathreshold (easily detectable), well-known odors. There are indications that moderate doses of NMDAr antagonists impair formation of short-term odor memory and/or disrupt acquisition of operant procedures to quantify odor discrimination however (MacQueen et al. 2011).

Several studies have also investigated the effects of dopaminergic manipulations on olfactory discrimination in rodents. In an olfactometer-based odor discrimination paradigm, Doty and Risser (1989) tested the effects of selective dopamine D2 agents in rats. The D2 agonist quinpirole dose-dependently impaired odor discrimination performance and this effect was reversed with co-administration of the D2 antagonist spiperone. Importantly, subjects were well-trained on the odor discrimination prior to the administration of drug. As such, the deleterious effect of quinpirole on performance cannot be attributed to deficits in acquisition of the testing procedure. The disruptive effect of quinpirole in rats has been further replicated with a manually delivered odor discrimination task in a study that also demonstrated enhanced discrimination with the antipsychotic spiperone (Wei et al. 2006). By evaluating the effects of these drugs across concentrations of the odorant, Wei et al. (2006) showed that the enhancing effects of this D2 antagonist resembled performance with increased odor concentrations, while the deleterious effect of the D2 agonist resembled performance with decreased odor concentrations. As such, the impact of D2 targeted drugs on odor discrimination paradigms has been interpreted to reflect dose-dependent alterations of odor sensitivity rather than discrimination. Yet, these findings are somewhat at odds with the findings of Tillerson et al. (2006) who evaluated odor discrimination abilities in mice lacking either the dopamine transporter (DAT) or the D2 receptor. These mice were equivalent to wild-type controls with regard to their detection threshold for paprika but, failed to show dishabituation in the presence of a novel odor in the habituation/dishabituation paradigm; a pattern of results that would suggest intact odor sensitivity with impaired odor discrimination. A separate investigation of D2 receptor-deficient mice found that relative to wild-type controls, mutant animals took longer to acquire a 2-odor discrimination and failed to adjust responding during a reversal of contingencies. Of course, knockout studies cannot guarantee non-specific developmental changes, just as pharmacology studies cannot offer receptor specificity. In sum, odor discrimination performance appears to be highly modulated by dopaminergic signaling and activity at the D2 receptor in particular. It remains unclear however, the extent to which discrimination performance is driven by reduced odor sensitivity or the cumulative effects of reduced sensitivity across time. As a result, given D2-selectivity for current antipsychotic treatments, their role should be carefully considered in studies evaluating odor discrimination performance in individuals with schizophrenia.

1.3 Odor Identification

If one is able to both perceive an odor and tell the difference between odors, then they may also be able to identify the odor; that is, report back an object or material that is understood to emit the odor. In addition to processes assessed by odor threshold and odor discrimination tasks, odor identification tasks evaluate the degree to which an odor percept is linked with semantic memory (Cain et al. 1998). As part of a battery which also includes odor threshold and odor discrimination tests, odor identification is frequently evaluated with the Sniffin' Sticks. To conduct the test, a series of 16 trials are performed in which the examinee is presented with a single odor pen. Prior to each odor exposure, the examinee is given a selection key of four words representing objects that might emit the smell the examinee will be asked to sample. Subsequently, an odor pen is presented below the subject's nose for approximately 3 s. The subject is then asked to pick the response that corresponds with the odor emitted from the pen. Each pen presents a different odor and comes with a unique response key. The subject receives a score representing the number of items answered correctly (0–16). The identification test score can be summed with the threshold and discrimination scores of the Sniffin' Stick battery to yield the Threshold Discrimination and Identification (TDI) score (Kobal et al. 1996).

A separate stand-alone test of odor identification, the University of Pennsylvania Smell Identification Test (UPSIT), is the most widely used measure of odor identification and has greatly accelerated interest in this domain of olfactory abilities. The UPSIT consists of four booklets with each containing 10 test pages. Each page contains a unique odorant embedded in scratch and sniff panel, along with four words describing objects that might emit the odor. The examinee is instructed to scratch and sniff the odor strip, then choose the word that best corresponds with the odor. The subject is asked to choose a response even if the subject cannot perceive the odor. The final score is determined by summing the number of correct responses across all 40 items (Doty et al. 1984). Both the Sniffin' Sticks Identification test and the UPSIT provide normative data stratified by gender and age (Hummel et al. 2007; Kamrava et al. 2020). An advantage of the UPSIT is that it can be completed by an examinee in a self-guided manner, whereas the Sniffin' Sticks odor identification test is administered by an examiner. In general, odor identification abilities appear to improve across childhood and adolescence, as individuals accumulate olfactory experience and develop semantic memory, reaching stability in adulthood (Lehrner et al. 1999). Beyond the age of 50, odor identification performance begins to deteriorate (Doty and Kamath 2014; Zhang and Wang 2017), with more rapid and profound deterioration observed amongst individuals with neurodegenerative diseases including Alzheimer's and Parkinson's disease (Woodward et al. 2017).

Of the domains of olfaction investigated in reference to schizophrenia, olfactory identification is the most frequently studied (see Fig. 2). In a meta-analysis of studies reporting on odor identification performance in individuals with schizophrenia or schizotypy, Cohen et al. (2012; Woodward et al. 2017) identified 40 studies providing odor identification measures in the relevant groups. The analysis estimated an odor identification deficit amongst individuals with schizophrenia nearing a full standard deviation in magnitude ($d = -0.99$). The vast majority of the included studies evaluated odor identification using the UPSIT measure, though a few studies utilized the Sniffin' Sticks test, or an abbreviated version of the UPSIT (the Brief Smell Identification Test; BSIT). As described previously, Cohen and colleagues (2012) reported similar deficits in odor sensitivity amongst schizophrenia and schizotypy cohorts ($d = -0.45$ and -0.38, respectively). In contrast, individuals with schizophrenia displayed a much more profound deficit in odor identification relative to schizotypy groups ($d = -0.99$ and -0.25, respectively). Notably, studies utilizing samples at high-risk of developing schizophrenia yielded deficits approaching the levels of deficit observed in schizophrenia ($d = -0.67$). While too few studies on odor identification in high-risk groups were identified in order to arrive at firm conclusions, the analysis suggests that in contrast to odor sensitivity, odor identification deficits may be exacerbated in those predisposed to schizophrenia who go on to manifest the illness.

A separate meta-analysis of olfactory function in individuals with schizophrenia identified 76 studies reporting odor identification performance (Moberg et al. 2014). Again, significant deficits were observed relative to control groups and the magnitude of the impairment ($d = -0.93$) was consistent with that observed in the earlier Cohen and colleagues (2012) analysis. Odor identification performance was also assessed for studies including related participant groups (i.e., those at clinical risk, family members of individuals with schizophrenia, and those expressing schizotypy) and again, youth at clinical risk of developing schizophrenia displayed a deficit of intermediate severity ($d = -0.71$). The observed impairment in at-risk youth was significantly elevated relative to first-degree family members ($d = -0.36$), and those displaying schizotypy ($d = -0.19$), but was not significantly different from the impairment in those for who had developed schizophrenia. Consistent with the conclusion of earlier studies Moberg et al. (1997, 2006, 2014); Ugur et al. (2005) reported a negative relationship between the duration of illness and the severity of odor identification deficits.

Though the level of risk for developing schizophrenia appears to be associated with the magnitude of odor identification deficits, the developmental trajectory by which odor identification deficits become pronounced has yet to be fully described. A study of odor identification in 7-year-old children at familial high risk of schizophrenia or bipolar disorder did not detect a significant difference in these groups (Loren et al. 2020). Yet, children at risk of schizophrenia produced the lowest scores, followed by the bipolar group, and then controls. When the recommended cutoff for impaired ability (microsmia) was applied, significantly more boys in the schizophrenia risk group were deemed microsmic (27.6%) relative to population-based controls (10.8%). These data provide some modest support for the notion that the odor identification deficits associated with schizophrenia emerge at a relatively early age within the prodromal period. Given that odor identification abilities develop across adolescence as semantic knowledge and odor experiences accumulate (Lehrner et al. 1999), it may be the case that individuals with schizophrenia fail to make these developmental gains. Such a pattern might be expected, in part, as a result of the impact of reduced olfactory sensitivity on the acquisition of odor-associated semantic memory across time. A comparison of olfactory abilities amongst monozygotic twins discordant for schizophrenia has suggested that relative to odor sensitivity and discrimination, odor identification is less impacted by genetic influences (Ugur et al. 2005), and thus, more susceptible to environmental factors. Thus, odor identification deficits may be specific to schizophrenia and manifest in the prodrome stage, driven in part by environmental interactions.

Odor identification deficits occur in other psychiatric conditions as well. For example, such deficits are amongst the first symptoms observed in Alzheimer's disease. As a result, standardized assessments of odor identification have promising utility for early detection of that condition (Devanand et al. 2008). Such deficits are also seen amongst patients with bipolar disorder and major depressive disorder though, with smaller magnitude impairments when compared with schizophrenia (Kamath et al. 2018; Li et al. 2021). In a study of 183 hospitalized patients carrying diagnoses of either schizophrenia, depression, or an eating disorder, Kopala et al. (1994) reported that only patients with schizophrenia displayed pronounced odor identification deficits. Despite the fact that multiple psychiatric conditions have been associated with odor identification deficits, measures of odor identification have utility as a marker of schizophrenia vulnerability to the extent that schizophrenia-associated deficits can be distinguished from other conditions. In this regard, Alzheimer's disease and other neurodegenerative disorders pose less of an issue as the olfactory identification deficits typically emerge with advanced age. Mood disorders may present with similar deficits in odor identification but, of a lesser magnitude. Also, it remains unclear whether odor identification deficits are present in the premorbid phase of these conditions, or extend to domains of odor sensitivity and discrimination, as appears to be the case with schizophrenia. Notably, odor identification deficits in schizophrenia are not the direct result of antipsychotic medication treatment, as these deficits have been observed in non-medicated patients during the first episode of psychosis (Chen et al. 2018; Brewer et al. 2001).

Odor identification deficits offer promise as a vulnerability marker of schizophrenia. Investigations using animal models will likely be necessary to explicate relevant neuropathology contributing to these effects. Yet, evaluating odor identification in non-human species presents a challenge. The standardized odor identification tests for human participants require the participant to match their subjective odor experience with a written word describing an object widely understood to emit that odor. Obviously, this process cannot be faithfully replicated in species lacking human verbal capacity. Avoiding the necessity of verbal labeling, odor identification testing procedures have been introduced in which the participant matches their odor experience against pictures of objects that might emit the particular odor (Aguillon-Hernandez et al. 2015). Whether or not the task requires verbal labeling, both versions of the test require a comparison of objects retrieved from semantic memory (the objects represented in the list of response options), and a determination of which object is most associated with the odor percept. It is not uncommon to observe reports in which performance on odor detection or discrimination paradigms is interpreted as a form of odor identification. It is important to recognize that these tasks lack key features of human odor identification tests. Odor identification relies upon a subject having a history of odor experiences common to the species and culture. The process in which odor associations are consolidated into semantic memory is primarily passive; that is, they are acquired without intentional learning or explicit reward/punishment. Well-conditioned odor discrimination performance does not require retrieval of semantic memory which has been passively acquired. Similarly, in rodent olfactory tasks, performance is likely more heavily influenced by food motivation and odor sensitivity than the ability to retrieve semantic memory of the object associated with the odor. More generally, poor odor identification performance in schizophrenia likely stems from a combination of dispositional and environmental factors impacting peripheral olfaction abilities (e.g., odor sensitivity), dispositional and environmental factors impacting cognitive abilities (e.g., attention, learning, and memory retrieval), and environmental factors such as in an impoverished odor learning history. Given the role of semantic memory retrieval in human odor identification, olfactory tasks developed for rodents that are relevant to odor identification will be explored in the more general consideration of odor memory.

1.4 Odor Memory

Several standardized tests exist for the evaluation of odor memory in human participants. The Odor Memory Test (OMT) is an examiner guided assessment in which odors are presented through the use of scratch and sniff panels (as used in the

UPSIT). The test is conducted through a series of trials which begin with the examiner scratching a panel and presenting it below the examinees nose so that they may sample the odor. The examiner then removes the panel and waits a specified amount of time before presenting four more odors sequentially to the examinee. They are then asked to choose the panel that matched the odor they sampled. During the delay between sample and choice, the examinee is instructed to count backward from 280 by intervals of 3, to avoid the use of verbal labeling as means of enhancing retention of the odor percept. Normative data is available for the OMT stratified by age (10–68 years of age) and gender (Choudhury et al. 2003). As with odor sensitivity, females outperform males on the OMT. Performance on the OMT also declines with age in a manner similar to that observed with odor identification. Interestingly, no differences as a result of the delay period (10, 30, and 60 s) were observed in the normative sample. Thus, OMT instructions describe that longer or shorter intervals may be preferred and encourage researchers to utilize delay intervals that are most relevant to their needs.

If the OMT did not include delay intervals, the procedure would otherwise represent an odor discrimination task. More precisely, the OMT procedure would be considered a match-to-sample (MTS) task, and with the incorporation of delay periods, a delayed match-to-sample (dMTS) task. The format of the OMT has also been adapted for use with Sniffin' Sticks in a procedure described as the odor discrimination memory test (ODMT) (Besser et al. 2019). Both versions use rose, peppermint, and banana as odorants. The ODT utilizes shoe leather as the fourth odor, while the ODMT includes peanut. An advantage of Sniffin' Sticks based procedures is that the odor pens can be reused between participants. Thus, Sniffin' Sticks testing may be more cost-efficient when the test is used to assess many individuals over a short period of time. In contrast, the microencapsulated odor format of the ODT (scratch and sniff panels) has a longer shelf-life (Besser et al. 2019). Thus, this format of testing might be preferred for low-density testing, when tests need to be space out over time. More broadly, the benefit of using OMT/ODMT is that the stimuli and procedures are standardized with age and gender stratified norms readily available. Nonetheless, Sniffin' Sticks odor pens, as well as other means of odor presentation, can and have been used to create a variety of olfactory memory assays. For example, Croy and colleagues (2015) have described a test of olfactory memory using Sniffin' Sticks pens titled the Sniffin' Test of Odor Memory (TOM). The TOM is an odor recognition test in which the participant is instructed to memorize eight unique odor pens sampled sequentially. A recognition test immediately follows sampling. The examinee is presented with 16 odors sequentially and for each odor they are asked to report whether the odor appeared on the sample list (yes/no). Eight odors in the recognition phase were previously presented during the sample phase while the remaining eight odors were not. In this arrangement memory can also be taxed by introducing delays between the sample and choice phases (delayed recognition).

The Moberg and colleagues (2014) meta-analysis of olfactory function in schizophrenia reported a larger effect size for odor memory tests ($d = -1.62$) than other forms of olfactory testing, including threshold, discrimination, identification, and hedonics (see Fig. 2). However, this effect size should be interpreted cautiously given that only two studies using an odor memory test were included. In both cases an MTS format was used to assess odor memory. In the Wu and colleagues (Wu et al. 1993) study, examinees were asked to sample an odor and then subsequently choose the matching odor from three presented comparisons (forced choice). This procedure was repeated through the course of 15 trials in which different odors were utilized. Individuals with schizophrenia performed significantly worse than control participants on the olfactory MTS task, a visual MTS task, and odor identification (UPSIT). Deficits in olfactory MTS were evident even when the sample was restricted to non-medicated patients, demonstrating that the effects were not a result of antipsychotic treatment. Interestingly, while olfactory MTS and UPSIT performance were highly correlated amongst control participants ($r = 0.74$), this correlation was markedly reduced amongst patients with schizophrenia ($r = 0.18$). In fact, deficits in in the olfactory MTS task remained apparent even when variance in UPSIT performance was factored out. This finding suggests that while both odor identification and odor memory tasks demonstrate deficits of a similar magnitude in patients with schizophrenia, the two tasks appear to be differentially sensitive to processes disrupted in the condition.

Odor memory performance, as assessed by tasks such the OMT/ODMT has been understudied in patients with schizophrenia. More commonly, olfactory abilities (sensitivity, discrimination, and identification) are assessed in individuals with schizophrenia and compared with mnemonic performance on cognitive tasks utilizing auditory or visual stimuli; As previously noted however, odor identification tasks require semantic memory retrieval and thus may be considered primarily a mnemonic task. In contrast, there is an abundance of studies examining odor memory in rodents that bear relevance to schizophrenia neuropathology. The odor span task (OST) has received particular attention as a means of evaluating working memory in schizophrenia-associated research with rodents (Dudchenko et al. 2013; Young et al. 2009).

The OST, as developed by Dudchenko et al. (2000) is based on a non-match-to sample principle. In an initial trial an animal is released onto an open field upon which rests a small cup of scented sand, placed in a random location. If the animal digs in this cup, it is rewarded by discovery of bit of attractive food. This is immediately followed by a second trial in which two odor cups are present on the open field, one presenting the odor used on the prior trial, and one presenting a novel odor. In this case, only a response (digging) to the novel odor yields discovery of a food reward. This trial format can be continued for many trials. On each trial, a novel odor is introduced along with all of the odors that served as novel odors on previous trial. Only responses to the novel odor are ever reinforced. Animals are trained across sessions. On each day the same odorants are used, only appearing in a different order within the task. Thus, to respond accurately, the animal must maintain a short-term memory of each odor it has been presented with in the current session, as that list grows progressively larger. Both rats and mice acquire the OST rapidly and reach high levels of accuracy (MacQueen et al. 2011; Young et al. 2007). Rats remain highly accurate (>80% accuracy) when tested with as many as 72 individual odorants (April et al. 2013). Importantly however, the OST provides a mechanism to evaluate the effects of capacity (the number of stimuli to remember) on short-term memory performance. Multiple investigations have demonstrated that accuracy is indeed capacity dependent (declining with increased memory load), even when confounds related to the number of comparisons presented are avoided (MacQueen et al. 2011; Galizio et al. 2019; Dudchenko et al. 2000; April et al. 2013).

Relevant to schizophrenia, rodent performance on the OST appears particularly dependent on adequate function of the NMDAr. This link was demonstrated through the administration of NMDAr antagonists, selectively and dose-dependently impairing OST accuracy, e.g. the competitive antagonists CPP, the non-competitive antagonists ketamine, MK-801 (dizocilpine), phencyclidine (PCP), and methoxetamine in rats (MacQueen et al. 2016; Galizio et al. 2016, 2019; Mathews et al. 2018; Davies et al. 2013; Rushforth et al. 2011). Importantly, most of these studies included a control task in which the animals were tested on a well-learned 2-odor simple discrimination. Each of the NMDAr antagonist drugs substantially impaired OST performance at a dose which spared simple discrimination performance. This control demonstrates that the OST impairments cannot be attributed to effects of the drug on motivation or odor discrimination and shows that mnemonic effects at these doses are selective to short-term memory. Given that the OST deficits produced by these drugs become more pronounced as the memory load increases, it appears that NMDAr blockade limits the quantity of odorants that can be retained in short-term memory (Galizio et al. 2019).

The OST has also been adapted for testing with mice (Young et al. 2007). Interestingly, in a study of transgenic mice engineered to overexpress the GluN2B subunit of the NMDAr, these mice outperformed wild-type controls on the OST. Transgenic animals also demonstrated an enhancement of long-term potentiation (LTP) in the medial prefrontal cortex (mPFC) that was eliminated by administration of a GluN2B subunit NMDAr antagonist (Cui et al. 2011). Relatedly, bilateral infusion of this same NR2B antagonist (Ro 25-6981) into the dorsomedial striatum (dmSTR), or pharmacological decoupling of mPFC and dmSTR, impaired OST of rats (Davies et al. 2017). These findings are particularly relevant in that hypoexpression and/or hypofunction of the NMDAr has been implicated in the pathogenesis of schizophrenia (Snyder and Gao 2013), a condition in which working memory deficits are pronounced (Lett et al. 2014). It has also been suggested that in genetically disposed individuals, a trajectory for developing schizophrenia may arise from events occurring in the prenatal or neonatal period (McGrath et al. 2003). Consistent with this hypothesis, maternal immune activation (mimicking infection during pregnancy) impaired OST during adulthood in impacted rat pups (Murray et al. 2017). Thus, multiple manipulations relevant to hypothesized determinants of schizophrenia have been demonstrated to produce odor memory deficits as assessed by the OST. Additionally, an automated version of OST testing for rats has recently been developed which should enable for high-throughput testing with the task (Wagner et al. 2022).

Another advantage of the OST is that it has been successfully adapted for human testing. In humans, it has been shown that OST performance declines with memory load as observed in rodents (MacQueen and Drobes 2017), and that OST performance is only very modestly impacted in individuals with verified hippocampal lesions (Levy et al. 2003). Intact OST performance is similarly observed in hippocampectomized rats (Dudchenko et al. 2000). Unfortunately, OST performance has yet to be characterized in individuals with schizophrenia. The availability of a great variety of standardized odor pens (Sniffin' Sticks) should allow for the further development of a human OST protocol that can be more easily implemented consistently across research groups. Reliability and precision of a human OST protocol might be further enhanced by olfactometer automation, as has been accomplished in rodents. While it is not clear that the form of short-term odor memory assessed by the OST is analogous to odor memory in the ODT/MDT, the shared features of these tasks suggest recruitment of similar cognitive processing resources. Given the substantial impairments of OMT/ODMT amongst individuals with schizophrenia, it would be advantageous to develop a protocol for testing these abilities in an analogous manner with model species. It is important to note that the OMT/ODMT utilizes a match-to-sample format and that odor match-to-sample is more difficult to establish in rats when compared with a similarly constructed non-match-to-sample procedure (Bruce et al. 2018). Thus, it may be more advantageous to reverse translate odor memory tasks from rodent models for human testing, especially since the literature with animal models is becoming quite robust in this domain.

As described above, odor identification remains the most frequently studied aspect of olfactory-based performance amongst individuals with schizophrenia. Odor identification tasks require sufficient odor sensitivity to detect the odorants used, intact odor discrimination, semantic memory retrieval, and in most cases, verbal ability. Though the use of pictures and/or objects can obviate the dependency on verbal ability, developing an odor-based memory task that demonstrates semantic retrieval remains challenging in rodents. Paradigms have been developed for rodents with the goal of evidencing episodic-like memory in these species. Episodic memory refers to memory for multiple aspects of an event (e.g., place, time, and additional details) that an individual personally experienced (Tulving 1983). Semantic memory is similar in that it requires memory for multiple aspects of an object, concept, or event but, this form of memory is not tied to a single particular event an individual experienced and is often acquired passively through many learning experiences distributed across time. In order to evaluate the ability of rodents to encode and retrieve episodic memory, tasks have been developed which require subjects to respond differentially based upon what stimulus is encountered, when the stimulus has previously been encountered, and where that encounter took place. Thus, subjects are required to demonstrate memory for multiple aspects of a previous encounter with a stimulus. In such "what-where-when" testing, great pains are taken to limit the stimulus exposure history of the animal such that the ultimate test of memory requires episodic memory (Crystal 2010). Yet, for the purposes of evaluating semantic memory, stimulus–context associations need not be acquired in a single learning event. Thus, adaptations of what-where-when paradigms incorporating olfaction may present a useful avenue for modeling human odor identification paradigms in rodents. In such an approach, a greater quantity of odor-context exposures prior to testing would be preferred.

In sum, individuals with schizophrenia have been shown to demonstrate a profound deficit in odor memory as assessed by odor MTS tasks (OMT/ODMT), albeit in limited study. The substantial deficits observed in odor identification tasks amongst individuals with schizophrenia may also suggest impairments in semantic memory retrieval. However, it is important to note that human odor identification tasks may also be impacted by deficits in odor sensitivity and discrimination, a limited history of odor experiences, or disruption of verbal processes. Odor MTS and NMTS tasks have been developed for rodents which allow for evaluation of effects of delay in short-term memory in manner analogous to the OMT/ODMT. Yet, odor identification tasks are more challenging to model in rodents as they require a demonstration that presentation of one aspect of a stimulus (i.e., smell) generates retrieval of an associated characteristic of the stimulus (i.e., verbal label, or visual image). The OST represents a task of short-term odor memory which can be used to evaluate both the effects of capacity (i.e., memory load) and delay. Several manipulations relevant to the neuropathology of schizophrenia (e.g., NMDAr blockade and maternal immune activation) have been evaluated using the OST and result in deficits akin to those observed in human tasks of odor memory amongst individuals with schizophrenia. The extent to which the OST maps onto processes evaluated by human odor memory tasks remains somewhat unclear however, adaptation of the OST for human testing should allow for further clarification of mnemonic abilities in the domain of olfaction that are perturbed in schizophrenia. The OST can serve as a cross-species platform by the which the neurobiological determinants of odor memory performance can be explored and may also serve as useful paradigm for screening the relevance of novel animal models for schizophrenia-relevant phenotypes.

2 Conclusions

It is clear that olfactory dysfunction is a common symptom of schizophrenia. While deficits in at least one aspect of olfactory function have been observed in a variety of psychiatric and neurodegenerative conditions including Alzheimer's disease, major depressive disorder, and bipolar disorder, impairments observed in schizophrenia appear to be more global and profound than in other psychiatric conditions. Such impairments are likely to negatively impact the enjoyment of food, detection of environmental hazards such as fire or the presence of noxious chemicals, and influence social relationships, including an individual's comfort with social situations. Meta-analyses have confirmed that schizophrenia is associated with impairments in each of the domains reviewed (odor sensitivity, discrimination, identification, and memory) with the largest deficits observed in odor identification and odor memory tasks. Odor sensitivity deficits are reliably observed in the condition but, these impairments are relatively modest. Odor threshold deficits may be of value as a vulnerability marker for schizophrenia given that these impairments appear to manifest early in development. Of the domains of olfaction evaluated, odor sensitivity is reported to be the most heritable phenotype. As such, odor threshold measures may be particularly useful for evaluating genetic disposition for the disorder. Given that odor sensitivity is believed to be primarily mediated by processes in the peripheral olfactory system (i.e., olfactory epithelium and olfactory bulb), the limited circuitry involved may facilitate research intended to evaluate the neurophysiological correlates of genetic variation. In this regard, genetic manipulations related to DAT, the D2 dopamine receptor, and the human DISC1 risk variant have all been shown to impact odor detection. Notably, D2 receptor antagonists have been observed to rescue disrupted odor detection abilities and thus, the effects of antipsychotic medications warrant consideration in the design of patient trials in which odor sensitivity is assessed.

Odor discrimination is also impaired in schizophrenia at a level similar to observed deficits in sensitivity. As with odor sensitivity, odor discrimination deficits are also notable in first-degree family members and those expressing schizotypy. Yet, youth deemed at risk of schizophrenia have been observed to have greater deficits than these other two groups, suggesting that odor discrimination may have some predictive utility for the ultimate manifestation of the condition amongst those with a disposition for the disorder. Odor discrimination deficits are likely to stem in part from the observed impairments in odor sensitivity and the long-term impact of poor sensitivity on the acquisition of odor associations. Odor identification is the most often studied domain of olfactory performance in individuals with schizophrenia and at-risk groups. Odor identification depends on adequate sensitivity and discrimination but, also requires higher order processes such as semantic memory retrieval and verbal processing. Odor identification deficits in schizophrenia are of a greater magnitude than is observed with sensitivity and discrimination. This likely results from impairments in basic olfactory processing combined with cognitive dysfunction. It is conceivable that the early emergence of impaired sensitivity and discrimination limits the acquisition of odor associations across childhood and adolescence and contributes to odor identification deficits in adulthood. Large deficits have also been observed amongst individuals with schizophrenia on other tests of odor memory, such as the OMT or ODMT (albeit in limited study). In rodents, the OST has been used extensively to evaluate manipulations relevant to schizophrenia and has also been reverse translated to allow for human testing. Though OST performance has yet to be characterized in individuals with schizophrenia, this cross-species task holds promise for explicating the relationship between the olfactory and cognitive deficits present in the condition.

As they relate to the condition of schizophrenia, olfactory abilities have received considerably less attention when compared with the auditory and visual domains. In tandem with an improved understanding of the olfactory apparatus, the development of standardized assessment of olfactory function has opened new avenues for investigating the dispositional and environmental determinants of schizophrenia, as well as the neuropathology underlying phenotypes disrupted in the condition. Continued research in this area may allow for enhanced detection of those at-risk for the condition, identification of therapeutic targets for treatment development, and for evaluating the relevance of novel animal models related to schizophrenia and psychosis.

References

Aguillon-Hernandez N et al (2015) An odor identification approach based on event-related pupil dilation and gaze focus. Int J Psychophysiol 96(3):201–209

April LB, Bruce K, Galizio M (2013) The magic number 70 (plus or minus 20): variables determining performance in the rodent odor span task. Learn Motiv 44(3):143–158

Besser G et al (2019) The Sniffin' sticks odor discrimination memory test: a rapid, easy-to-use, reusable procedure for testing olfactory memory. Ann Otol Rhinol Laryngol 128(3):227–232

Birrell JM, Brown VJ (2000) Medial frontal cortex mediates perceptual attentional set shifting in the rat. J Neurosci 20(11):4320–4324

Blount A, Coppola DM (2020) The effect of odor enrichment on olfactory acuity: olfactometric testing in mice using two mirror-molecular pairs. PLoS One 15(7):e0233250

Bodyak N, Slotnick B (1999) Performance of mice in an automated olfactometer: odor detection, discrimination and odor memory. Chem Senses 24(6):637–645

Brewer WJ et al (2001) Stability of olfactory identification deficits in neuroleptic-naive patients with first-episode psychosis. Am J Psychiatry 158(1):107–115

Bromberg W, Schilder P (1934) Olfactory imagination and olfactory hallucinations: an experimental and clinical study of the sense of smell in normal and in psychotic persons. Arch Neurol Psychiatry 32(3):467–492

Bruce K et al (2018) Successive odor matching- and non-matching-to-sample in rats: a reversal design. Behav Processes 155:26–32

Chen X et al (2018) Olfactory impairment in first-episode schizophrenia: a case-control study, and sex dimorphism in the relationship between olfactory impairment and psychotic symptoms. BMC Psychiatry 18(1):199

Choudhury ES, Moberg P, Doty RL (2003) Influences of age and sex on a microencapsulated odor memory test. Chem Senses 28(9):799–805

Cohen AS, Brown LA, Auster TL (2012) Olfaction, "olfiction," and the schizophrenia-spectrum: an updated meta-analysis on identification and acuity. Schizophr Res 135(1):152–157

Croy I, Nordin S, Hummel T (2014) Olfactory disorders and quality of life – an updated review. Chem Senses 39(3):185–194

Croy I et al (2015) Test-retest reliability and validity of the Sniffin' TOM odor memory test. Chem Senses 40(3):173–179

Crystal JD (2010) Episodic-like memory in animals. Behav Brain Res 215(2):235–243

Cui Y et al (2011) Forebrain NR2B overexpression facilitating the prefrontal cortex long-term potentiation and enhancing working memory function in mice. PLoS One 6(5):e20312

Davies DA, Greba Q, Howland JG (2013) GluN2B-containing NMDA receptors and AMPA receptors in medial prefrontal cortex are necessary for odor span in rats. Front Behav Neurosci 7:183

Davies DA et al (2017) Interactions between medial prefrontal cortex and dorsomedial striatum are necessary for odor span capacity in rats: role of GluN2B-containing NMDA receptors. Learn Mem 24(10):524–531

Devanand DP et al (2008) Combining early markers strongly predicts conversion from mild cognitive impairment to Alzheimer's disease. Biol Psychiatry 64(10):871–879

Dinc AS et al (2020) Smoking cessation improves olfactory functions. Laryngoscope 130(2):E35–E38

Doty RL (1986) Odor-guided behavior in mammals. Experientia 42(3):257–271

Doty RL, Ferguson-Segall M (1987) Odor detection performance of rats following d-amphetamine treatment: a signal detection analysis. Psychopharmacology (Berl) 93(1):87–93
Doty R, Kamath V (2014) The influences of age on olfaction: a review. Front Psychol 5(20)
Doty RL, Risser JM (1989) Influence of the D-2 dopamine receptor agonist quinpirole on the odor detection performance of rats before and after spiperone administration. Psychopharmacology (Berl) 98(3):310–315
Doty RL et al (1984) University of Pennsylvania smell identification test: a rapid quantitative olfactory function test for the clinic. Laryngoscope 94(2 Pt 1):176–178
Doty RL, Gregor TP, Settle RG (1986) Influence of intertrial interval and sniff-bottle volume on phenyl ethyl alcohol odor detection thresholds. Chem Senses 11(2):259–264
Doty RL et al (1994) Tests of human olfactory function: principal components analysis suggests that most measure a common source of variance. Percept Psychophys 56(6):701–707
Dudchenko PA, Wood ER, Eichenbaum H (2000) Neurotoxic hippocampal lesions have no effect on odor span and little effect on odor recognition memory but produce significant impairments on spatial span, recognition, and alternation. J Neurosci 20(8):2964–2977
Dudchenko PA et al (2013) Animal models of working memory: a review of tasks that might be used in screening drug treatments for the memory impairments found in schizophrenia. Neurosci Biobehav Rev 37(9, Part B):2111–2124
Duffy VB et al (2019) Heightened olfactory dysfunction and oral irritation among chronic smokers and heightened propylthiouracil (PROP) bitterness among menthol smokers. Physiol Behav 201:111–122
Forte FS (1952) Olfactory hallucinations as a proctologic manifestation of early schizophrenia. Am J Surg 84(5):620–622
Galizio M et al (2013) Working memory in the odor span task: effects of chlordiazepoxide, dizocilpine (MK801), morphine, and scopolamine. Psychopharmacology (Berl) 225(2): 397–406
Galizio M et al (2016) Behavioral pharmacology of the odor span task: effects of flunitrazepam, ketamine, methamphetamine and methylphenidate. J Exp Anal Behav 106(3):173–194
Galizio M et al (2019) Effects of NMDA antagonist dizocilpine (MK-801) are modulated by the number of distractor stimuli in the rodent odor span task of working memory. Neurobiol Learn Mem 161:51–56
Gamble KR, Smith DW (2009) Discrimination of "odorless" mineral oils alone and as diluents by behaviorally trained mice. Chem Senses 34(7):559–563
Geyer MA et al (2001) Pharmacological studies of prepulse inhibition models of sensorimotor gating deficits in schizophrenia: a decade in review. Psychopharmacology (Berl) 156(2): 117–154
Glennon SG et al (2019) Chronic cigarette smoking associates directly and indirectly with self-reported olfactory alterations: analysis of the 2011-2014 National Health and Nutrition Examination Survey. Nicotine Tob Res 21(6):818–827
Grayton HM et al (2013) Altered social behaviours in neurexin 1alpha knockout mice resemble core symptoms in neurodevelopmental disorders. PLoS One 8(6):e67114
Guo X et al (2009) Reduced expression of the NMDA receptor-interacting protein SynGAP causes behavioral abnormalities that model symptoms of schizophrenia. Neuropsychopharmacology 34(7):1659–1672
Hayes JE, Jinks AL (2012) Evaluation of smoking on olfactory thresholds of phenyl ethyl alcohol and n-butanol. Physiol Behav 107(2):177–180
Hikida T et al (2007) Dominant-negative DISC1 transgenic mice display schizophrenia-associated phenotypes detected by measures translatable to humans. Proc Natl Acad Sci 104(36):14501
Hummel T et al (2007) Normative data for the "Sniffin' Sticks" including tests of odor identification, odor discrimination, and olfactory thresholds: an upgrade based on a group of more than 3,000 subjects. Eur Arch Otorhinolaryngol 264(3):237–243
Kamath V et al (2018) Olfactory processing in bipolar disorder, major depression, and anxiety. Bipolar Disord 20(6):547–555

Kamath V et al (2019) Contributions of olfactory and neuropsychological assessment to the diagnosis of first-episode schizophrenia. Neuropsychology 33(2):203–211

Kamrava SK et al (2020) Validity and reliability of Persian smell identification test. Iran J Otorhinolaryngol 32(109):65–71

Karlsson R-M et al (2009) Assessment of glutamate transporter GLAST (EAAT1)-deficient mice for phenotypes relevant to the negative and executive/cognitive symptoms of schizophrenia. Neuropsychopharmacology 34(6):1578–1589

Katotomichelakis M et al (2007) The effect of smoking on the olfactory function. Rhinology 45(4): 273–280

Kayser J et al (2013) Olfaction in the psychosis prodrome: electrophysiological and behavioral measures of odor detection. Int J Psychophysiol 90(2):190–206

Kesner RP, Hardy JD, Calder LD (1981) Phencyclidine and behavior: I. sensory-motor function, activity level, taste aversion and water intake. Pharmacol Biochem Behav 15(1):7–13

Kobal G et al (1996) “Sniffin’ sticks”: screening of olfactory performance. Rhinology 34(4): 222–226

Kohler CG et al (2001) Olfactory dysfunction in schizophrenia and temporal lobe epilepsy. Neuropsychiatry Neuropsychol Behav Neurol 14(2):83–88

Kopala LC, Good KP, Honer WG (1994) Olfactory hallucinations and olfactory identification ability in patients with schizophrenia and other psychiatric disorders. Schizophr Res 12(3): 205–211

Koster NL et al (1999) Olfactory receptor neurons express D2 dopamine receptors. J Comp Neurol 411(4):666–673

Kraemer S, Apfelbach R (2004) Olfactory sensitivity, learning and cognition in young adult and aged male Wistar rats. Physiol Behav 81(3):435–442

Labrie V, Lipina T, Roder JC (2008) Mice with reduced NMDA receptor glycine affinity model some of the negative and cognitive symptoms of schizophrenia. Psychopharmacology (Berl) 200(2):217–230

Labrie V et al (2009) Serine racemase is associated with schizophrenia susceptibility in humans and in a mouse model. Hum Mol Genet 18(17):3227–3243

Labrie V et al (2010) Genetic loss of D-amino acid oxidase activity reverses schizophrenia-like phenotypes in mice. Genes Brain Behav 9(1):11–25

Lehrner JP, Glück J, Laska M (1999) Odor identification, consistency of label use, olfactory threshold and their relationships to odor memory over the human lifespan. Chem Senses 24(3):337–346

Lett TA et al (2014) Treating working memory deficits in schizophrenia: a review of the neurobiology. Biol Psychiatry 75(5):361–370

Levy DA et al (2003) Impaired visual and odor recognition memory span in patients with hippocampal lesions. Learn Mem 10(6):531–536

Li SB et al (2021) Odour identification impairment is a trait but not a disease-specific marker for bipolar disorders: comparisons of bipolar disorder with different episodes, major depressive disorder and schizophrenia. Aust N Z J Psychiatry:4867421998774

Loren V, van Themaat AH et al (2020) Odor identification in 7-year-old children at familial high risk of schizophrenia or bipolar disorder – the Danish high risk and resilience study VIA 7. Schizophr Res 216:77–84

MacQueen DA, Drobes DJ (2017) Validation of the human odor span task: effects of nicotine. Psychopharmacology (Berl) 234(19):2871–2882

MacQueen DA, Bullard L, Galizio M (2011) Effects of dizocilpine (MK801) on olfactory span in rats. Neurobiol Learn Mem 95(1):57–63

MacQueen DA et al (2016) Influence of pharmacological manipulations of NMDA and cholinergic receptors on working versus reference memory in a dual component odor span task. Learn Mem 23(6):270–277

Malaspina D et al (1994) Odor discrimination deficits in schizophrenia: association with eye movement dysfunction. J Neuropsychiatry Clin Neurosci 6(3):273–278

Malaspina D et al (2012) Olfaction and cognition in schizophrenia: sex matters. J Neuropsychiatry Clin Neurosci 24(2):165–175
Malaspina D et al (2016) Parental age effects on odor sensitivity in healthy subjects and schizophrenia patients. Am J Med Genet B Neuropsychiatr Genet 171(4):513–520
Mathews MJ, Mead RN, Galizio M (2018) Effects of N-methyl-D-aspartate (NMDA) antagonists ketamine, methoxetamine, and phencyclidine on the odor span test of working memory in rats. Exp Clin Psychopharmacol 26(1):6–17
McGrath JJ et al (2003) The neurodevelopmental hypothesis of schizophrenia: a review of recent developments. Ann Med 35(2):86–93
Miller G (2004) Nobel prizes. Axel, Buck share award for deciphering how the nose knows. Science 306(5694):207
Moberg PJ et al (1997) Olfactory identification deficits in schizophrenia: correlation with duration of illness. Am J Psychiatry 154(7):1016–1018
Moberg PJ et al (1999) Olfactory dysfunction in schizophrenia: a qualitative and quantitative review. Neuropsychopharmacology 21(3):325–340
Moberg PJ et al (2006) Olfactory functioning in schizophrenia: relationship to clinical, neuropsychological, and volumetric MRI measures. J Clin Exp Neuropsychol 28(8):1444–1461
Moberg PJ et al (2014) Meta-analysis of olfactory function in schizophrenia, first-degree family members, and youths at-risk for psychosis. Schizophr Bull 40(1):50–59
Moy SS et al (2009) Deficient NRG1-ERBB signaling alters social approach: relevance to genetic mouse models of schizophrenia. J Neurodev Disord 1(4):302–312
Mukherjee B, Yuan Q (2016) NMDA receptors in mouse anterior piriform cortex initialize early odor preference learning and L-type calcium channels engage for long-term memory. Sci Rep 6: 35256
Murray BG et al (2017) Maternal immune activation during pregnancy in rats impairs working memory capacity of the offspring. Neurobiol Learn Mem 141:150–156
O'Tuathaigh CMP et al (2007) Phenotypic characterization of spatial cognition and social behavior in mice with 'knockout' of the schizophrenia risk gene neuregulin 1. Neuroscience 147(1): 18–27
Ozmen S et al (2016) Olfactory and erectile dysfunction association in smoking and non-smoking men. Physiol Behav 160:1–5
Rosenblatt MR et al (1998) Olfactory thresholds for nicotine and menthol in smokers (abstinent and nonabstinent) and nonsmokers. Physiol Behav 65(3):575–579
Rubert SL, Hollender MH, Mehrhof EG (1961) Olfactory hallucinations. Arch Gen Psychiatry 5: 313–318
Rupp CI et al (2005) Olfactory functions and volumetric measures of orbitofrontal and limbic regions in schizophrenia. Schizophr Res 74(2–3):149–161
Rushforth SL, Steckler T, Shoaib M (2011) Nicotine improves working memory span capacity in rats following sub-chronic ketamine exposure. Neuropsychopharmacology 36(13):2774–2781
Shan L et al (2018) Schizophrenia-like olfactory dysfunction induced by acute and postnatal phencyclidine exposure in rats. Schizophr Res 199:274–280
Smith RS et al (1993) Smell and taste function in the visually impaired. Percept Psychophys 54(5): 649–655
Snyder MA, Gao WJ (2013) NMDA hypofunction as a convergence point for progression and symptoms of schizophrenia. Front Cell Neurosci 7:31
Staubli U et al (1989) Antagonism of NMDA receptors impairs acquisition but not retention of olfactory memory. Behav Neurosci 103(1):54–60
Su C-Y, Menuz K, Carlson JR (2009) Olfactory perception: receptors, cells, and circuits. Cell 139(1):45–59
Takahashi T et al (2018) Olfactory deficits in individuals at risk for psychosis and patients with schizophrenia: relationship with socio-cognitive functions and symptom severity. Eur Arch Psychiatry Clin Neurosci 268(7):689–698

Tarland E, Brosda J (2018) Male rats treated with subchronic PCP show intact olfaction and enhanced interest for a social odour in the olfactory habituation/dishabituation test. Behav Brain Res 345:13–20

Temmel AF et al (2002) Characteristics of olfactory disorders in relation to major causes of olfactory loss. Arch Otolaryngol Head Neck Surg 128(6):635–641

Tillerson JL et al (2006) Olfactory discrimination deficits in mice lacking the dopamine transporter or the D2 dopamine receptor. Behav Brain Res 172(1):97–105

Tulving E (1983) Elements of episodic memory, Oxford psychology series. Oxford University Press, Oxford. xi, 351 p

Ugur T et al (2005) Olfactory impairment in monozygotic twins discordant for schizophrenia. Eur Arch Psychiatry Clin Neurosci 255(2):94–98

Wagner TJ, Bruce K, Galizio M (2022) Incrementing non-matching- but not matching-to-sample is rapidly learned in an automated version of the odor span task. Anim Cogn

Wei CJ, Linster C, Cleland TA (2006) Dopamine D_2 receptor activation modulates perceived odor intensity. Behav Neurosci 120(2):393–400

Woodward MR et al (2017) Validation of olfactory deficit as a biomarker of Alzheimer disease. Neurol Clin Pract 7(1):5–14

Woolley JD et al (2015) Oxytocin administration selectively improves olfactory detection thresholds for lyral in patients with schizophrenia. Psychoneuroendocrinology 53:217–222

Wu J et al (1993) Olfactory memory in unmedicated schizophrenics. Schizophr Res 9(1):41–47

Yang M, Crawley JN (2009) Simple behavioral assessment of mouse olfaction. Curr Protoc Neurosci 48(1):8.24.1–8.24.12

Young JW et al (2007) The odour span task: a novel paradigm for assessing working memory in mice. Neuropharmacology 52(2):634–645

Young JW et al (2009) Using the MATRICS to guide development of a preclinical cognitive test battery for research in schizophrenia. Pharmacol Ther 122(2):150–202

Zhang C, Wang X (2017) Initiation of the age-related decline of odor identification in humans: a meta-analysis. Ageing Res Rev 40:45–50

Cholinergic Functioning, Cognition, and Anticholinergic Medication Burden in Schizophrenia

Yash B. Joshi

Contents

Abstract Acetylcholine (ACh) signaling is critical for central nervous function and is known to be abnormal in schizophrenia (SZ), a chronic neuropsychiatric disorder in which cognitive deficits persist, despite treatment. This review provides a summary of the clinical evidence linking ACh abnormalities to SZ-associated cognitive deficits, an overview of ACh-based pro-cognitive strategies attempted in SZ, and a survey of recent studies that describe the impact of anticholinergic medication burden on cognitive outcomes in SZ. Methodological challenges that currently limit more substantial investigation of ACh in SZ patients and future directions are also discussed.

Keywords Anticholinergic · Cognition · Muscarinic receptor · Nicotinic receptor · Schizophrenia

---

Y. B. Joshi (✉)
Desert Pacific Mental Illness Research Education and Clinical Center, VA San Diego Healthcare System, San Diego, CA, USA

Department of Psychiatry, University of California, San Diego, La Jolla, CA, USA
e-mail: yajoshi@health.ucsd.edu

Curr Topics Behav Neurosci (2023) 63: 393–406
https://doi.org/10.1007/7854_2022_400
Published Online: 29 November 2022

1 Introduction

Schizophrenia (SZ) is one of the most disabling neuropsychiatric conditions known. Despite a prevalence of ~1%, it accounts for over 12 million years lost due to disability or early death annually (He et al. 2020). While multiple factors account for disability, cognitive impairment associated with SZ is thought to be a key factor (Green et al. 2004). Indeed, cognitive impairment seen in people with SZ has been associated with poor educational attainment, limited vocational success, impaired social functioning, driving poor quality of life, and long-term disability (Mohamed et al. 2008). Informed by decades of basic, translational, and clinical science, the mainstay of contemporary pharmacotherapy in SZ through the use of antipsychotics centers on attenuating dopamine-signaling abnormalities, and while this is effective for some symptoms, it does not materially attenuate cognitive deficits seen in this illness. Due to observations that acetylcholine (ACh) is important for a number of cognitive functions, and that many cognitive disorders have abnormalities related to ACh, there has been a longstanding interest in this neurotransmitter for the treatment of SZ. While investigation of ACh in SZ spans multiple levels of analysis, the aim of this chapter is to: (1) provide an overview of cholinergic signaling abnormalities in studies of SZ patients; (2) summarize major cholinergic pro-cognitive treatment strategies in SZ thus far attempted; and (3) characterize the impact of anticholinergic medication burden on cognitive outcomes in SZ.

2 Abnormalities of Central Nervous System Cholinergic Functioning in Schizophrenia

ACh was the first neurotransmitter identified and has multiple roles in the central nervous system (CNS). ACh is synthesized by the enzyme choline acetyltransferase from acetyl-coenzyme and choline in neurons and is metabolized by acetylcholinesterase into choline and acetate extracellularly (Picciotto et al. 2012). In the CNS, ACh is primarily neuromodulatory and binds to one of the two primary classes of ACh receptors: muscarinic ACh (mAChR) and nicotinic ACh (nAChR) receptors. mAChRs are G protein-coupled receptors (GPCRs) which exert cellular effects through second messenger systems. In mammals, five subtypes of muscarinic receptors are widely studied, M1 through M5 (for a review, see Picciotto et al. (2012)). M1, M3, and M5 receptors are G_q-coupled and their activation leads to phospholipase C-mediated increases in intracellular levels of inositol triphosphate and calcium, while M2 and M4 receptors are $G_{i/o}$-coupled and their activation leads to adenylyl cyclase-mediated reduction of cyclic adenosine monophosphate. Muscarinic receptors are both pre- and post-synaptic and can have a variety of excitatory or inhibitory effects depending on the cellular context. By contrast, nAChRs are ligand-gated ion channels which are permeable to cations and are assembled as homeric or heteromeric assemblies of alpha (α) and beta (β) subunits (for a review, see Albuquerque et al. (2009)). nAChR activation leads to subtype-specific actions based on subunit composition. nAChRs are widely distributed across neurons not only at pre- and post-synaptic sites, but across other neuronal regions, including the soma and axon. Cholinergic signaling informs neural signal propagation not only distally but also through local circuits. Major projections include: (1) projections from the basal forebrain (e.g., nucleus basalis) to multiple cortical areas; (2) basal forebrain projections to subcortical areas (e.g., hippocampus, amygdala, etc.); (3) brainstem projections to thalamus, midbrain, and brainstem; and (4) local ACh interneuron inhibitory circuitry (e.g., striatal cholinergic interneurons (Scarr and Dean 2009; Agostinelli et al. 2019)).

The convergence of abnormalities related to ACh in SZ spans several decades and includes dozens of studies, only some of which will be highlighted here. In magnetic resonance spectroscopy studies of antipsychotic-naïve patients with SZ, elevated levels of choline have been observed in multiple brain regions, including caudate nucleus, anterior cingulate, and thalamus, suggesting abnormal ACh metabolism (Bustillo et al. 2002; Theberge et al. 2004). It is interesting to note in this context that choline acetyltransferase activity is elevated in hippocampus and basal ganglia; it has been theorized that these changes could reflect compensatory response due to illness, chronic use of psychotropics or both (McGeer and McGeer 1977). However, some SZ postmortem studies also suggest that cortical choline acetyltransferase activity may not be significantly diminished compared to those without psychosis; nevertheless, lower cortical levels of choline acetyltransferase are correlated with reduced cognitive functioning in SZ (Powchik et al. 1998).

Multiple postmortem and radioligand studies have revealed abnormalities in ACh receptors expression and/or binding in SZ patients. Among many observations, reduction of mAChR expression has been seen in frontal (Mancama et al. 2003; Bennett et al. 1979; Crook et al. 2001), cingulate (Zavitsanou et al. 2004), temporal (Deng and Huang 2005), and occipital (Raedler et al. 2003) cortices, as well as subcortical structures, including hippocampus (Crook et al. 2000), thalamus (Raedler et al. 2003), basal ganglia, and pons (Nagao et al. 1975). These abnormalities are present even in unmedicated patients (Nagao et al. 1975). Synthesizing results from multiple receptor-specific radioligand studies, the M1 receptor abnormalities seem to be of clear importance in SZ (Dean et al. 1996, 2002; Crook et al. 2000, 2001). Similarly, abnormalities in nAChR expression have also been observed, with reduced $\alpha4\beta2$ nAChR binding in cortex, striatum, and hippocampus (Breese et al. 2000; Durany et al. 2000), and $\alpha7$ nAChR alterations in hippocampus and frontal cortex (Freedman et al. 1995). Delineating the origin of these changes remains important however, as it is unclear if they are due to disease state, substance use, or chronic medication treatment (or a combination of these factors).

In parallel, it has been well documented that the prevalence of tobacco use and degree of cigarette smoking are increased in SZ, with some estimating 40–80% of those with SZ regularly smoke, compared to ~15–20% of the general population (de Leon et al. 1995; de Leon and Diaz 2005). In individuals without SZ, tobacco use results in upregulated nAChRs in areas such as the hippocampus and thalamus in a dose-dependent and reversible way (Breese et al. 1997). However, in those with SZ, this response is not observed, and there is a weaker relationship between packs smoked per day and nicotinic radioligand binding in multiple brain regions (hippocampus, thalamus, cortex, caudate (Breese et al. 2000)). Beyond receptor and ACh metabolism abnormalities, other observations support the central role of cholinergic signaling in SZ. For example, in sleep studies, SZ patients show reduced rapid eye movement sleep latency, which is associated with abnormal muscarinic signaling (Tandon et al. 1992). Additionally, SZ patients respond robustly to pyridostigmine, a cholinesterase inhibitor (O'Keane et al. 1994). Thus, despite elevated tobacco use, abnormal central cholinergic functioning seems to be persistent in people with SZ.

3 Attempted Cholinergic-Based Treatment Strategies in SZ

Based on the strength of these observations, attempts have been made to use existing pro-cholinergic medications or develop novel cholinergic-based medications for SZ. There have been several studies which tested the ability of approved medications for Alzheimer's disease in SZ, including the acetylcholinesterase inhibitors galantamine, donepezil, and rivastigmine, among others. In open-label and double-blind placebo-controlled trials, galantamine, a reversible cholinesterase inhibitor that potentiates action of nicotinic receptors, produced variable effects on cognitive outcomes: many studies report little to no effects, though some point to improvements in various domains, albeit inconsistently (Sacco et al. 2008; Schubert et al. 2006; Buchanan et al. 2008; Lee et al. 2007a; Dyer et al. 2008). For example, in a double-blind, placebo-controlled trial which tested the pro-cognitive effects of galantamine on individuals who had been stabilized on biweekly long-acting risperidone for 6 months, the combination of galantamine and risperidone over the following 6 months did not produce cognitive benefit compared to placebo and galantamine (Lindenmayer and Khan 2011). In double-blind, placebo-controlled trials, donepezil (Akhondzadeh et al. 2008; Lee et al. 2007b; Fagerlund et al. 2007; Friedman et al. 2002; Tugal et al. 2004; Mazeh et al. 2006) was not associated with significant improvement in cognitive functioning, though some open-label trials have reported modest improvement (Chung et al. 2009; Buchanan et al. 2003). Similarly, the acetylcholinesterase inhibitor rivastigmine has not produced cognitive gains (Chouinard et al. 2007). Collectively, there appears to be weak evidence for using these cholinergic agents approved for Alzheimer's disease as adjunctive pro-cognitive therapeutics for SZ, though modest improvements in selective cognitive domains or measures have been described (Santos et al. 2018; Choi et al. 2013). For example, there is moderate quality evidence that speed of processing is enhanced, and low quality evidence that attention, working memory, and verbal memory are enhanced by acetylcholinesterase inhibitors in randomized clinical trials (Santos et al. 2018; Choi et al. 2013).

Varenicline, a partial $\alpha4\beta2$ nACh agonist and low affinity $\alpha7$ agonist, used for smoking cessation pharmacotherapy, has also been investigated for pro-cognitive effects. In an 8-week double-blind randomized placebo-controlled trial (Hong et al.

2011), Hong and colleagues observed improved executive functioning in 59 SZ patients treated adjunctively with varenicline. Similarly, in another placebo-controlled study with both smokers and nonsmokers, beneficial effects of varenicline on some cognitive tasks were noted, though results were mixed and dependent on smoking status (Shim et al. 2012). Beneficial effects of varenicline on spatial memory have also been reported (Wing et al. 2013), though not supported or reproduced elsewhere (Roh et al. 2014; Kozak et al. 2018; Smith et al. 2016). Based on these and other observations (Olincy et al. 2006; Tregellas et al. 2010), encenicline, a selective partial α7 nACh agonist was developed to treat cognitive impairment in SZ (Barbier et al. 2015). Encenicline produced encouraging results in a 12-week phase 2, double-blind, randomized, placebo-controlled, multi-center trial where beneficial effects were noted on multiple cognitive assessments, as well as negative symptoms, with good tolerability (Keefe et al. 2015); however, these benefits were not observed in two larger phase 3 studies which enrolled ~1,500 patients at more than 200 sites (Brannan 2019).

More recently, xanomeline, an M1- and M4-muscarinic agonist, has received attention as another promising therapeutic in early phase clinical trials in SZ. In a small ($n = 20$) 4-week double-blind, placebo-controlled study, xanomeline produced reduction in psychotic symptoms, as well as attenuation of verbal learning and short-term memory deficits (Shekhar et al. 2008). Informed by parallel studies in which xanomeline was given to Alzheimer's disease patients, which reported a high degree of discontinuation due to gastrointestinal side effects (Bodick et al. 1997), xanomeline was paired with trospium, a peripheral muscarinic antagonist in a placebo-controlled double-blind, phase 2 study (Brannan et al. 2021). In this 5-week study ($n = 182$ SZ inpatients), the combination of xanomeline and trospium was associated with an improvement in symptoms, though cholinergic side effects were noted; additional trials are ongoing.

In summary, central cholinergic nervous system dysfunction has historically been an attractive target for re-purposing medications developed for other indications and illnesses (Alzheimer's disease, smoking cessation, etc.) and continues to be an active area of study for novel drug development. However, the cognitive benefit seen across studies has been fairly modest when observed and often inconsistent across studies.

4 Clinical Evidence Linking Anticholinergic Medication Burden to Cognitive Outcomes in Schizophrenia

Despite the current lack of success from pro-cognitive cholinergic strategies, there is a substantial literature on the deleterious effects of anticholinergic burden on cognitive outcomes in SZ. Radioligand or immunoassay studies from blood/peripheral biofluids have described the relationship between serum anticholinergic drug or activity and cognitive performance. Tune and colleagues (1982) found an inverse relationship between anticholinergic drug burden and verbal recall in a small cross-sectional SZ patient cohort medicated on first generation antipsychotics; they noted in this early report that even SZ patients stabilized on similar doses of anticholinergic medications had a wide variety of anticholinergic drug burden as measured by radioligand assay. Perlick and colleagues (1986) further reported that serum anticholinergic activity was associated with verbal but not recognition memory. Similarly, differences in cognitive performance were reported when SZ cohorts were separated on the basis of serum anticholinergic activity: verbal learning was worse in the high anticholinergic burden SZ group (Strauss et al. 1990). These studies strongly suggested that reducing anticholinergic medication burden may improve cognitive functioning. Indeed, this premise has been supported to some degree in many studies over the last several decades. In a 4-week double-blind study, withdrawal of benztropine (a strongly anticholinergic medication) was associated with improved performance on memory tasks (Baker et al. 1983). In a separate study, a cohort of SZ patients were randomized to benztropine or amantadine for the treatment of extrapyramidal side effects, with those in the amantadine group reporting improved performance on tasks of memory (McEvoy et al. 1987). These results paralleled similar double-blind crossover studies in healthy adults which tested both benztropine and amantadine: benztropine, but not amantadine, was associated with both objective evidence and subjective report of cognitive impairment (Gelenberg et al. 1989). Aside from verbal memory, Tracy and colleagues (2001) also described associations between poorer performance on attentionally demanding tasks like executive control or effortful memory recall and greater peripheral anticholinergic activity.

Such studies were instructive, but many were carried out prior to the widespread utilization of second-generation/atypical antipsychotics, which often have a lower incidence of extrapyramidal side effects (requiring less anticholinergic medications to treat), but also have a greater likelihood of having strong anticholinergic properties. Several studies offer insight into possible dissociable effects of antipsychotics and anticholinergic burden effects on cognition. In a 14-week, double-blind trial involving 101 SZ patients, the neurocognitive effects of haloperidol (first-generation/typical antipsychotic, minimal anticholinergic medication burden), risperidone (second-generation/atypical antipsychotic, minimal anticholinergic medication burden), olanzapine and clozapine (both second-generation/atypical antipsychotics, high anticholinergic medication burden) were explored (Bilder et al. 2002). Both risperidone and olanzapine showed superiority to haloperidol, but not to clozapine on general neurocognitive outcomes. Interestingly, olanzapine was associated with improvement in processing speed, attention, and executive functioning, while risperidone appeared to show greater effects on declarative verbal learning and memory; blood levels of antipsychotics were not related to changes in cognitive measures. It should be noted that in this study participants were given benztropine based on observed motoric side effects, and few clinical studies have yet to comprehensively disentangle how anticholinergic medication burden impacts cognition independently of antipsychotic dose, motor function (including antipsychotic-associated side effects), and symptom severity.

Studies also provide evidence that even among similar antipsychotics, there can be a wide variety of anticholinergic activity. For example, Chengappa et al. (2000) report that in a variety of patients with SZ, schizoaffective disorder, and bipolar disorder, olanzapine-treated patients had significant, but substantially lower, anticholinergic activity compared to those on clozapine. More recent studies have also attempted to establish a clinically useful standard on which to judge anticholinergic medication effects in SZ. Minzenberg and colleagues (2004) carried out analyses comparing clinical (i.e., expert rated) and pharmacological indices on cognitive outcomes in 106 SZ patients. They found both clinical and pharmacological indices were highly correlated and related to cognitive measures: they observed a negative association between anticholinergic burden and complex attention, and auditory and visual memory, but not simple attention, working memory, executive function, conceptual fluency, or motor speed. Ang and colleagues studied over 700 SZ patients across outpatient and inpatient settings and also found anticholinergic medication burden-associated impairments in executive function, memory, and speed of processing (Ang et al. 2017). More recently, we also reported the impact of anticholinergic medication burden on cognitive outcomes in ~1,000 SZ outpatients (Joshi et al. 2021) as part of the Consortium on the Genetics of Schizophrenia (COGS-2) study. These analyses revealed that all cognitive domains tested had anticholinergic medication burden-associated vulnerability. When compared with those with minimal anticholinergic medication burden, those with the greatest anticholinergic medication burden had substantially worse performance on measures of abstraction, attention, working memory, verbal memory, spatial memory, spatial ability, and emotion processing. Additional analyses in this report also suggested that the effect of anticholinergic medication burden was not anchored by a specific deficit: anticholinergic medication affected all domains relatively equally. In this large-scale analysis, covarying for effects of antipsychotic dose, symptoms, duration of illness, age, and number of past hospitalizations also did not affect the relationship between anticholinergic medication burden and cognitive outcomes. While the above analysis largely described SZ patients that were middle-aged, in older-aged SZ patients higher anticholinergic burden also was associated with a cognitive profile similar to early-stage Alzheimer's disease (Tsoutsoulas et al. 2017). These observations parallel large studies that describe the negative impact of anticholinergic medication burden in healthy individuals, where high anticholinergic burden increases odds of developing dementia (Coupland et al. 2019). Interestingly, when comparing clinically stable patients with SZ, schizoaffective disorder and bipolar disorder with psychotic features, degree of anticholinergic burden was associated with cognitive deficits only in those with SZ, despite a comparable anticholinergic burden across groups, suggesting unique disease-specific vulnerability (Eum et al. 2017).

5 Measuring and Accounting for Anticholinergic Medication Burden: Limitations and Implications for Translational Biomarker Development

While the above studies describe the negative impact of anticholinergic medication burden on cognitive outcomes in SZ, they bring up key methodological barriers in quantifying anticholinergic medication burden. Common methods of quantifying anticholinergic medication in typical clinical and research settings fall into two broad categories: scale-based ratings of individual medications based on expert consensus panels or pharmacological data, which are then summed to generate a total anticholinergic burden score; and blood-based assays of anticholinergic activity.

Many anticholinergic scales have been described: Anticholinergic Activity Scale (Ehrt et al. 2010), Anticholinergic Burden Classification (Ancelin et al. 2006), Anticholinergic Risk Scale (Rudolph et al. 2008), Anticholinergic Loading Scale (Sittironnarit et al. 2011), Anticholinergic Drug Scale (Carnahan et al. 2006), Anticholinergic Cognitive Burden scale (Coupland et al. 2019; Cai et al. 2013; Campbell et al. 2010) are among the most notable. Lozano-Ortega et al. (2020) provide a comprehensive review of these scales and will be paraphrased here. The majority of these scales have been developed from observations in older adults, and most are dose-independent, which means that the lowest dose of a strongly anticholinergic medication is rated higher in terms of anticholinergic medication burden than a very high dose of a minimally or moderately anticholinergic medication (the Anticholinergic Drug Scale and Anticholinergic Risk Scale are exceptions, and include dose). Furthermore, many of these scales are rated on a 0–3 scale with 0 indicating no anticholinergic burden, and 3 indicating a highly anticholinergic drug – it is not clear to what degree there are cognitively-salient ceiling and floor effects of such ratings. Another limitation is that it is often difficult to classify medications that are not included in these lists; Lozano-Ortega and colleagues note that while scales include many medications approved in the USA (range 67–100%), they are variable in scope ($n = 27$–520 medications), and have variably skewed ratings (i.e., some scales are highly populated with medications with no anticholinergic medication burden). There is also inter-scale variability between ratings of individual medications. Despite these barriers, these scales are convenient, easily deployable in clinical settings and allow for cross-sectional and longitudinal database analyses with some inter-scale correlations as high as $r = 0.82$.

In contrast to anticholinergic drug rating scales, blood-based assessments of serum anticholinergic activity typically use radioreceptor assays or in vitro measurements of mAChR (Salahudeen et al. 2016). The quantitative nature of these assays offers a more nuanced way to measure anticholinergic burden. However, the degree to which peripheral anticholinergic activity reflects central nervous system anticholinergic activity (Thomas et al. 2008) and the degree to which peripheral anticholinergic activity predicts cognitive impairment have been called into question (Carnahan et al. 2002). Furthermore, a wide variability in basal anticholinergic activity has been reported, with acute illness or effects of endogenous substances impacting results (Carnahan et al. 2002). Therefore, blood-based assessments of anticholinergic activity are limited in their ability to disentangle which cognitive deficits in SZ are due to acute effects of anticholinergic medications, chronic exposure, or inherent to SZ even in the absence of any treatment (Ribe et al. 2015; Harvey et al. 1996; Solis-Vivanco et al. 2020). Another methodological consideration is that many anticholinergic drugs have other significant receptor activity which inform cognitive performance in complex ways (for example, many anticholinergic medications also have antihistaminic effects), but these have not been adequately characterized. Finally, many SZ studies either are biased to exclude SZ patients with medical issues or are not adequately powered or designed to account for non-psychiatric medical factors, which further obfuscate the impact anticholinergic medication burden on cognition in complex ways (Taipale et al. 2022).

Cholinergic activity has also been assayed from cerebrospinal fluid, enabling more ready quantification of central ACh activity. Unfortunately, this technique is invasive, clinically impractical, and does not offer spatial resolution. On the other hand, radioligand binding studies offer superior spatial resolution, but are similarly not clinically feasible due to costs and logistics required. Neurophysiological measures relevant to cognition, cholinergic functioning, and anticholinergic effects have been increasingly investigated as clinic-ready cross-species biomarkers (see Kumari et al. 2001; Kumari et al. 2000; Light et al. 2015; Naicker et al. 2017). Similarly, dissection of cholinergic signaling in animal models using emerging molecular tools and approaches offers potential to develop future translational measures or tasks for clinical application (Crouse et al. 2020; Papouin et al. 2017). In a complementary way, utilizing specific tests of cognitive function, such as those afforded by the Research Domain Criteria (RDoC), may enable more direct assessment of neuronal function and translational comparability across species (Young et al. 2017). Thus, using the RDoC as a framework, the more direct impact of pro-cholinergic treatments and anticholinergic medication burden can be assessed in patients and compared with direct treatment studies to animals.

6 Summary and Future Directions

Basic, clinical, and epidemiologic studies have established that cholinergic functioning is of critical importance in SZ and is associated with cognitive deficits observed in this chronic neuropsychiatric illness. While there are clear indications that SZ-associated abnormalities are present in the metabolism of ACh and ACh receptor expression across brain regions, pro-cholinergic treatments and reduction of anticholinergic medication burden have produced cognitive benefits that are modest or inconsistent. There are methodological reasons for this discrepancy: both expert consensus panel-based medication rating systems for anticholinergic medication burden and peripheral assessment of central cholinergic functioning that inform these studies have limitations. Future work must produce novel methods of assessing anticholinergic medication burden in SZ and quantifying its impact on SZ-associate cognitive impairment. These future assessments must also account for a variety of factors to contextualize important ACh-cognition relationships in SZ, including – but not limited to – smoking status, myriad direct and indirect effects of both psychotropic and non-psychotropics medications on cognition, and medical illnesses that impact cognition in SZ. Development of objective biomarkers of cholinergic functioning and anticholinergic medication burden, particularly those that allow cross-species investigation, would help bridge the divide between the substantial clinical and epidemiological data identifying ACh as a key target in SZ and the limited efficaciousness of ACh-specific interventions to date.

Acknowledgments The author would like to thank Jared Young, PhD for reviewing the manuscript and discussion. The author has been supported by Department of Veterans Affairs grant IK2 RX003395, NIMH grants R33-MH125114, R33-MH123603, R01-AG059640, and the Brain Behavior Research Foundation (#27428).

References

Agostinelli LJ, Geerling JC, Scammell TE (2019) Basal forebrain subcortical projections. Brain Struct Funct 224(3):1097–1117

Akhondzadeh S et al (2008) A 12-week, double-blind, placebo-controlled trial of donepezil adjunctive treatment to risperidone in chronic and stable schizophrenia. Prog Neuropsychopharmacol Biol Psychiatry 32(8):1810–1815

Albuquerque EX et al (2009) Mammalian nicotinic acetylcholine receptors: from structure to function. Physiol Rev 89(1):73–120

Ancelin ML et al (2006) Non-degenerative mild cognitive impairment in elderly people and use of anticholinergic drugs: longitudinal cohort study. BMJ 332(7539):455–459

Ang MS et al (2017) The impact of medication anticholinergic burden on cognitive performance in people with schizophrenia. J Clin Psychopharmacol 37(6):651–656

Baker LA, Cheng LY, Amara IB (1983) The withdrawal of benztropine mesylate in chronic schizophrenic patients. Br J Psychiatry 143:584–590

Barbier AJ et al (2015) Pharmacodynamics, pharmacokinetics, safety, and tolerability of encenicline, a selective alpha7 nicotinic receptor partial agonist, in single ascending-dose and bioavailability studies. Clin Ther 37(2):311–324

Bennett JP Jr et al (1979) Neurotransmitter receptors in frontal cortex of schizophrenics. Arch Gen Psychiatry 36(9):927–934

Bilder RM et al (2002) Neurocognitive effects of clozapine, olanzapine, risperidone, and haloperidol in patients with chronic schizophrenia or schizoaffective disorder. Am J Psychiatry 159(6): 1018–1028

Bodick NC et al (1997) Effects of xanomeline, a selective muscarinic receptor agonist, on cognitive function and behavioral symptoms in Alzheimer disease. Arch Neurol 54(4):465–473

Brannan S (2019) 32.2 two global phase iii trials of encenicline for cognitive impairment in chronic schizophrenia patients: red flags and lessons learned. Schizophr Bull 45(Supplement_2):S141–S142

Brannan SK et al (2021) Muscarinic cholinergic receptor agonist and peripheral antagonist for schizophrenia. N Engl J Med 384(8):717–726

Breese CR et al (1997) Effect of smoking history on [3H]nicotine binding in human postmortem brain. J Pharmacol Exp Ther 282(1):7–13

Breese CR et al (2000) Abnormal regulation of high affinity nicotinic receptors in subjects with schizophrenia. Neuropsychopharmacology 23(4):351–364
Buchanan RW et al (2003) An open-labeled trial of adjunctive donepezil for cognitive impairments in patients with schizophrenia. Schizophr Res 59(1):29–33
Buchanan RW et al (2008) Galantamine for the treatment of cognitive impairments in people with schizophrenia. Am J Psychiatry 165(1):82–89
Bustillo JR et al (2002) High choline concentrations in the caudate nucleus in antipsychotic-naive patients with schizophrenia. Am J Psychiatry 159(1):130–133
Cai X et al (2013) Long-term anticholinergic use and the aging brain. Alzheimers Dement 9(4): 377–385
Campbell NL et al (2010) Use of anticholinergics and the risk of cognitive impairment in an African American population. Neurology 75(2):152–159
Carnahan RM et al (2002) A critical appraisal of the utility of the serum anticholinergic activity assay in research and clinical practice. Psychopharmacol Bull 36(2):24–39
Carnahan RM et al (2006) The anticholinergic drug scale as a measure of drug-related anticholinergic burden: associations with serum anticholinergic activity. J Clin Pharmacol 46(12): 1481–1486
Chengappa KN, Pollock BG, Parepally H, Levine J, Kirshner MA, Brar JS, Zoretich RA (2000) Anticholinergic differences among patients receiving standard clinical doses of olanzapine or clozapine. J Clin Psychopharmacol 20(3):311–316. https://doi.org/10.1097/00004714-200006000-00004
Choi KH, Wykes T, Kurtz MM (2013) Adjunctive pharmacotherapy for cognitive deficits in schizophrenia: meta-analytical investigation of efficacy. Br J Psychiatry 203(3):172–178
Chouinard S et al (2007) Rivastigmine treatment as an add-on to antipsychotics in patients with schizophrenia and cognitive deficits. Curr Med Res Opin 23(3):575–583
Chung YC et al (2009) Effect of donepezil added to atypical antipsychotics on cognition in patients with schizophrenia: an open-label trial. World J Biol Psychiatry 10(2):156–162
Coupland CAC et al (2019) Anticholinergic drug exposure and the risk of dementia: a nested case-control study. JAMA Intern Med 179(8):1084–1093
Crook JM et al (2000) Decreased muscarinic receptor binding in subjects with schizophrenia: a study of the human hippocampal formation. Biol Psychiatry 48(5):381–388
Crook JM et al (2001) Low muscarinic receptor binding in prefrontal cortex from subjects with schizophrenia: a study of Brodmann's areas 8, 9, 10, and 46 and the effects of neuroleptic drug treatment. Am J Psychiatry 158(6):918–925
Crouse RB et al (2020) Acetylcholine is released in the basolateral amygdala in response to predictors of reward and enhances the learning of cue-reward contingency. eLife 9
de Leon J, Diaz FJ (2005) A meta-analysis of worldwide studies demonstrates an association between schizophrenia and tobacco smoking behaviors. Schizophr Res 76(2–3):135–157
de Leon J et al (1995) Schizophrenia and smoking: an epidemiological survey in a state hospital. Am J Psychiatry 152(3):453–455
Dean B et al (1996) The density of muscarinic M1 receptors is decreased in the caudate-putamen of subjects with schizophrenia. Mol Psychiatry 1(1):54–58
Dean B et al (2002) Decreased muscarinic1 receptors in the dorsolateral prefrontal cortex of subjects with schizophrenia. Mol Psychiatry 7(10):1083–1091
Deng C, Huang XF (2005) Decreased density of muscarinic receptors in the superior temporal gyrusin schizophrenia. J Neurosci Res 81(6):883–890
Durany N et al (2000) Human post-mortem striatal alpha4beta2 nicotinic acetylcholine receptor density in schizophrenia and Parkinson's syndrome. Neurosci Lett 287(2):109–112
Dyer MA et al (2008) High-dose galantamine augmentation inferior to placebo on attention, inhibitory control and working memory performance in nonsmokers with schizophrenia. Schizophr Res 102(1–3):88–95
Ehrt U et al (2010) Use of drugs with anticholinergic effect and impact on cognition in Parkinson's disease: a cohort study. J Neurol Neurosurg Psychiatry 81(2):160–165

Eum S et al (2017) Cognitive burden of anticholinergic medications in psychotic disorders. Schizophr Res 190:129–135
Fagerlund B et al (2007) Effects of donepezil adjunctive treatment to ziprasidone on cognitive deficits in schizophrenia: a double-blind, placebo-controlled study. Clin Neuropharmacol 30(1): 3–12
Freedman R et al (1995) Evidence in postmortem brain tissue for decreased numbers of hippocampal nicotinic receptors in schizophrenia. Biol Psychiatry 38(1):22–33
Friedman JI et al (2002) A double blind placebo controlled trial of donepezil adjunctive treatment to risperidone for the cognitive impairment of schizophrenia. Biol Psychiatry 51(5):349–357
Gelenberg AJ et al (1989) Anticholinergic effects on memory: benztropine versus amantadine. J Clin Psychopharmacol 9(3):180–185
Green MF et al (2004) Approaching a consensus cognitive battery for clinical trials in schizophrenia: the NIMH-MATRICS conference to select cognitive domains and test criteria. Biol Psychiatry 56(5):301–307
Harvey PD et al (1996) Cognitive impairment and negative symptoms in geriatric chronic schizophrenic patients: a follow-up study. Schizophr Res 22(3):223–231
He H et al (2020) Trends in the incidence and DALYs of schizophrenia at the global, regional and national levels: results from the global burden of disease study 2017. Epidemiol Psychiatr Sci 29:e91
Hong LE et al (2011) Effects of moderate-dose treatment with varenicline on neurobiological and cognitive biomarkers in smokers and nonsmokers with schizophrenia or schizoaffective disorder. Arch Gen Psychiatry 68(12):1195–1206
Joshi YB et al (2021) Anticholinergic medication burden-associated cognitive impairment in schizophrenia. Am J Psychiatry 178(9):838–847
Keefe RS et al (2015) Randomized, double-blind, placebo-controlled study of encenicline, an alpha7 nicotinic acetylcholine receptor agonist, as a treatment for cognitive impairment in schizophrenia. Neuropsychopharmacology 40(13):3053–3060
Kozak K et al (2018) Effects of varenicline on cognitive function in non-smokers with schizophrenia. Schizophr Res 197:562–563
Kumari V et al (2000) Prepulse inhibition of the startle response in men with schizophrenia: effects of age of onset of illness, symptoms, and medication. Arch Gen Psychiatry 57(6):609–614
Kumari V et al (2001) Effects of procyclidine on prepulse inhibition of the acoustic startle response in healthy human volunteers. Psychopharmacology (Berl) 154(3):221–229
Lee SW et al (2007a) A 12-week, double-blind, placebo-controlled trial of galantamine adjunctive treatment to conventional antipsychotics for the cognitive impairments in chronic schizophrenia. Int Clin Psychopharmacol 22(2):63–68
Lee BJ, Lee JG, Kim YH (2007b) A 12-week, double-blind, placebo-controlled trial of donepezil as an adjunct to haloperidol for treating cognitive impairments in patients with chronic schizophrenia. J Psychopharmacol 21(4):421–427
Light GA et al (2015) Validation of mismatch negativity and P3a for use in multi-site studies of schizophrenia: characterization of demographic, clinical, cognitive, and functional correlates in COGS-2. Schizophr Res 163(1–3):63–72
Lindenmayer JP, Khan A (2011) Galantamine augmentation of long-acting injectable risperidone for cognitive impairments in chronic schizophrenia. Schizophr Res 125(2–3):267–277
Lozano-Ortega G et al (2020) A review of published anticholinergic scales and measures and their applicability in database analyses. Arch Gerontol Geriatr 87:103885
Mancama D et al (2003) Reduced expression of the muscarinic 1 receptor cortical subtype in schizophrenia. Am J Med Genet B Neuropsychiatr Genet 119B(1):2–6
Mazeh D et al (2006) Donepezil for negative signs in elderly patients with schizophrenia: an add-on, double-blind, crossover, placebo-controlled study. Int Psychogeriatr 18(3):429–436
McEvoy JP, McCue M, Freter S (1987) Replacement of chronically administered anticholinergic drugs by amantadine in outpatient management of chronic schizophrenia. Clin Ther 9(4): 429–433

McGeer PL, McGeer EG (1977) Possible changes in striatal and limbic cholinergic systems in schizophrenia. Arch Gen Psychiatry 34(11):1319–1323

Minzenberg MJ et al (2004) Association of anticholinergic load with impairment of complex attention and memory in schizophrenia. Am J Psychiatry 161(1):116–124

Mohamed S et al (2008) Relationship of cognition and psychopathology to functional impairment in schizophrenia. Am J Psychiatry 165(8):978–987

Nagao T et al (1975) Statistical studies on therapy of leukemia with tumor formation (author's transl). Rinsho Ketsueki 16(1):19–24

Naicker P et al (2017) Medications influencing central cholinergic neurotransmission affect saccadic and smooth pursuit eye movements in healthy young adults. Psychopharmacology (Berl) 234(1):63–71

O'Keane V, Abel K, Murray RM (1994) Growth hormone responses to pyridostigmine in schizophrenia: evidence for cholinergic dysfunction. Biol Psychiatry 36(9):582–588

Olincy A, Harris JG, Johnson LL, Pender V, Kongs S, Allensworth D, Ellis J, Zerbe GO, Leonard S, Stevens KE, Stevens JO, Martin L, Adler LE, Soti F, Kem WR, Freedman R (2006) Proof-of-concept trial of an alpha7 nicotinic agonist in schizophrenia. Arch Gen Psychiatry 63(6): 630–638. https://doi.org/10.1001/archpsyc.63.6.630

Papouin T et al (2017) Septal cholinergic neuromodulation tunes the astrocyte-dependent gating of hippocampal NMDA receptors to wakefulness. Neuron 94(4):840–854.e7

Perlick D et al (1986) Memory deficits and anticholinergic levels in chronic schizophrenia. Am J Psychiatry 143(2):230–232

Picciotto MR, Higley MJ, Mineur YS (2012) Acetylcholine as a neuromodulator: cholinergic signaling shapes nervous system function and behavior. Neuron 76(1):116–129

Powchik P et al (1998) Postmortem studies in schizophrenia. Schizophr Bull 24(3):325–341

Raedler TJ et al (2003) In vivo determination of muscarinic acetylcholine receptor availability in schizophrenia. Am J Psychiatry 160(1):118–127

Ribe AR et al (2015) Long-term risk of dementia in persons with schizophrenia: a Danish population-based cohort study. JAMA Psychiat 72(11):1095–1101

Roh S et al (2014) Acute effects of mecamylamine and varenicline on cognitive performance in non-smokers with and without schizophrenia. Psychopharmacology (Berl) 231(4):765–775

Rudolph JL et al (2008) The anticholinergic risk scale and anticholinergic adverse effects in older persons. Arch Intern Med 168(5):508–513

Sacco KA et al (2008) Effects of galantamine on cognitive deficits in smokers and non-smokers with schizophrenia. Schizophr Res 103(1–3):326–327

Salahudeen MS, Chyou TY, Nishtala PS (2016) Serum anticholinergic activity and cognitive and functional adverse outcomes in older people: a systematic review and meta-analysis of the literature. PLoS One 11(3):e0151084

Santos B et al (2018) Cognitive improvement of acetylcholinesterase inhibitors in schizophrenia. J Psychopharmacol 32(11):1155–1166

Scarr E, Dean B (2009) Role of the cholinergic system in the pathology and treatment of schizophrenia. Expert Rev Neurother 9(1):73–86

Schubert MH, Young KA, Hicks PB (2006) Galantamine improves cognition in schizophrenic patients stabilized on risperidone. Biol Psychiatry 60(6):530–533

Shekhar A et al (2008) Selective muscarinic receptor agonist xanomeline as a novel treatment approach for schizophrenia. Am J Psychiatry 165(8):1033–1039

Shim JC et al (2012) Adjunctive varenicline treatment with antipsychotic medications for cognitive impairments in people with schizophrenia: a randomized double-blind placebo-controlled trial. Neuropsychopharmacology 37(3):660–668

Sittironnarit G et al (2011) Effects of anticholinergic drugs on cognitive function in older Australians: results from the AIBL study. Dement Geriatr Cogn Disord 31(3):173–178

Smith RC et al (2016) Varenicline effects on smoking, cognition, and psychiatric symptoms in schizophrenia: a double-blind randomized trial. PLoS One 11(1):e0143490

Solis-Vivanco R et al (2020) Cognitive impairment in never-medicated individuals on the schizophrenia spectrum. JAMA Psychiat 77(5):543–545

Strauss ME et al (1990) Effects of anticholinergic medication on memory in schizophrenia. Schizophr Res 3(2):127–129

Taipale H et al (2022) Representation and outcomes of individuals with schizophrenia seen in everyday practice who are ineligible for randomized clinical trials. JAMA Psychiat 79(3): 210–218

Tandon R, Shipley JE, Taylor S, Greden JF, Eiser A, DeQuardo J, Goodson J (1992) Electroencephalographic sleep abnormalities in schizophrenia. Relationship to positive/negative symptoms and prior neuroleptic treatment. Arch Gen Psychiatry 49(3):185–194. https://doi.org/10.1001/archpsyc.1992.01820030017003

Theberge J et al (2004) Duration of untreated psychosis vs. N-acetylaspartate and choline in first episode schizophrenia: a 1H magnetic resonance spectroscopy study at 4.0 Tesla. Psychiatry Res 131(2):107–114

Thomas C et al (2008) Serum anticholinergic activity and cerebral cholinergic dysfunction: an EEG study in frail elderly with and without delirium. BMC Neurosci 9:86

Tracy JI et al (2001) Anticholinergicity and cognitive processing in chronic schizophrenia. Biol Psychol 56(1):1–22

Tregellas JR, Olincy A, Johnson L, Tanabe J, Shatti S, Martin LF, Singel D, Du YP, Soti F, Kem WR, Freedman R (2010) Functional magnetic resonance imaging of effects of a nicotinic agonist in schizophrenia. Neuropsychopharmacology 35(4):938–942. https://doi.org/10.1038/npp.2009.196

Tsoutsoulas C et al (2017) Anticholinergic burden and cognition in older patients with schizophrenia. J Clin Psychiatry 78(9):e1284–e1290

Tugal O et al (2004) A double-blind, placebo controlled, cross-over trial of adjunctive donepezil for cognitive impairment in schizophrenia. Int J Neuropsychopharmacol 7(2):117–123

Tune LE et al (1982) Serum levels of anticholinergic drugs and impaired recent memory in chronic schizophrenic patients. Am J Psychiatry 139(11):1460–1462

Wing VC et al (2013) Varenicline modulates spatial working memory deficits in smokers with schizophrenia. Schizophr Res 149(1–3):190–191

Young JW et al (2017) Research domain criteria versus DSM V: how does this debate affect attempts to model corticostriatal dysfunction in animals? Neurosci Biobehav Rev 76 (Pt B):301–316

Zavitsanou K et al (2004) Investigation of m1/m4 muscarinic receptors in the anterior cingulate cortex in schizophrenia, bipolar disorder, and major depression disorder. Neuropsychopharmacology 29(3):619–625

An Update on Treatment of Cognitive Impairment Associated with Schizophrenia

William P. Horan, Lauren T. Catalano, and Michael F. Green

Contents

Abstract Cognitive impairment associated with schizophrenia (CIAS) is widely regarded as a critically important treatment target for schizophrenia. Despite major efforts and a number of promising findings, we do not yet have an approved drug for CIAS. Similarly, promising cognitive remediation approaches are limited in their ability to help patients achieve real-world functional gains on a wide scale. This

W. P. Horan (✉)
WCG VeraSci, Durham, NC, USA

Department of Psychiatry and Biobehavioral Sciences, David Geffen School of Medicine, University of California, Los Angeles, Los Angeles, CA, USA
e-mail: Bill.Horan@verasci.com

L. T. Catalano and M. F. Green
Department of Psychiatry and Biobehavioral Sciences, David Geffen School of Medicine, University of California, Los Angeles, Los Angeles, CA, USA

Veterans Affairs Greater Los Angeles Healthcare System, Los Angeles, CA, USA

Curr Topics Behav Neurosci (2023) 63: 407–436
https://doi.org/10.1007/7854_2022_382
Published Online: 2 August 2022

article provides an update and critical evaluation of recent treatment development activities for CIAS. First, we provide update on pharmacological approaches, which include a glutamatergic drug that is currently in Phase III trials for CIAS, and discuss factors that may have impacted past efforts to identify efficacious drugs. Second, we review positive findings, limitations, and current trends involving cognitive remediation approaches. Third, we consider newer transdiagnostic approaches aimed at looking beyond, or identifying more homogenous subgroups within, the diagnostic category schizophrenia to advance treatment development. Despite its many challenges, treatment development for CIAS remains a major public health issue and research continues to push forward on several encouraging fronts.

Keywords Clinical trials · Cognition · Remediation · Schizophrenia · Treatment

1 Introduction

Cognitive impairment associated with schizophrenia (CIAS) is widely regarded as a critically important treatment target for schizophrenia. Its importance is based on extensive evidence that cognitive impairment is a core feature of schizophrenia and is among the most robust determinants of the poor functional outcome that characterizes this disorder (Green et al. 2019). While typical and atypical antipsychotic medications are generally efficacious treatments for positive symptoms, they do not meaningfully impact the cognitive impairment that is frequently found in schizophrenia, and thus do not help patients' ability to function independently and achieve their personal goals in daily life in the community when significant CIAS is present. The hope, therefore, is that by improving cognition through alternative intervention approaches, we can enable those with schizophrenia to function more productively.

Schizophrenia is associated with broad, substantial compromise of cognitive functioning on the order of 1.0–2.0 standard deviations below the normal mean across multiple cognitive domains (Gold 2004; Heinrichs and Zakzanis 1998). For clinical trials in schizophrenia, cognition is assessed using standard performance-based pencil-and-paper or computerized tasks, most of which were derived from clinical neuropsychology. The most commonly used clinical trial test battery, the MATRICS Consensus Cognitive Battery (MCCB) (Nuechterlein et al. 2008), assesses six consensus-based noncognitive domains of speed of processing, verbal learning and memory, visuospatial learning and memory, working memory, attention/vigilance, and reasoning/problem-solving, as well as social cognition (which is not a focus of this review). These domains can also be assessed using more specialized tasks grounded in cognitive neuroscience (Carter et al. 2008). Cognition in schizophrenia has also been considered from a transdiagnostic RDoC-based perspective (Cuthbert and Morris 2021; Smucny et al. 2019; Tamminga et al. 2017). The RDoC "Cognitive Systems" domain includes the constructs of attention, declarative memory, cognitive control, and working memory, which map onto four of the key domains assessed in CIAS trials.

While the rationale for developing novel treatments for CIAS is clear, the goal has been elusive. Despite major efforts, and a number of promising findings, we do not yet have an approved drug for CIAS. Similarly, despite promising findings for other approaches, such as resource-intensive cognitive remediation, limitations in their ability to help patients, at a scalable level, achieve real-world functional gains persist. Although the challenge is formidable, research on several fronts continues to push forward toward the goal of enhancing cognition and its associated disability in schizophrenia.

In a recent review, our team surveyed of the available evidence through 2018 for pharmacological, psychosocial, and novel approaches to treating cognitive impairment in schizophrenia (Green et al. 2019). Building on that foundation, the current article provides an update and critical evaluation of treatment development activities from 2018 up to the present time. This descriptive review covers three main areas. First, we provide an update on pharmacological approaches to CIAS, including a discussion of factors that may (or may not) have impeded efforts to identify efficacious new drugs. Second, we review the positive findings, limitations, and current trends involving cognitive remediation approaches. Third, we consider forward-looking conceptual, and related regulatory, issues for treatment development such as identifying more homogenous subgroups within schizophrenia or looking beyond schizophrenia to transdiagnostic approaches to cognitive enhancement.

2 Pharmacological Treatments

2.1 Background

In the early 2000s, the NIMH-MATRICS initiative created a pathway through which new drugs could ultimately receive regulatory approval for CIAS (Green et al. 2004; Marder and Fenton 2004). This large, multi-disciplinary initiative brought together representatives from academia, industry, and the FDA to establish consensus-based guidelines on trial methodology and design. It also led to the creation of the MCCB, which is accepted as an endpoint by the FDA. This milestone set of achievements energized drug development through an influx of resources from pharmacological industry sponsors, both big and small. A wide range of candidate neurotransmitter mechanisms was initially considered (Marder 2006). Notably, many of these candidates have also been considered in drug development programs for the negative symptoms of schizophrenia (Davis et al. 2014). A wave of initial trials for CIAS using add-on designs focused on glutamatergic and cholinergic agents and, to a lesser extent, agents targeting serotonin, dopamine, GABA, and noradrenaline.

Unfortunately, achieving functionally meaningful cognitive enhancement proved to be quite challenging. Overall, the initial wave of findings was mixed and inconsistent. This pattern was comprehensively documented in a 2018 meta-analytic review (Sinkeviciute et al. 2018) of all available pharmacological treatment studies ($n = 93$). The review reported a statistically significant, though very small (Hedge's $g = 0.10$), effect for overall cognition with no significant effects for any particular cognitive subdomain.

Regarding particular neurotransmitter systems, only a few agents showed initial benefits and these, unfortunately, did not hold up in subsequent trials. The strongest findings were for agents acting predominantly on the glutamatergic system (overall cognition: $g = 0.19$, $n = 29$; working memory: $g = 0.13$, $n = 20$). Within specific glutamatergic agents, results were strongest (small-to-medium) for AMPA receptor agonists on working memory ($g = 0.28$; $n = 5$) and for memantine/amantadine on overall cognition ($g = 0.34$; $n = 6$). There were a few significant findings for other neurotransmitter systems: cholinesterase inhibitors showed a small yet significant effect on working memory ($g = 0.26$; $n = 6$), and dopaminergic agents showed a non-significant effect on the domain of reasoning ($g = 0.34$; $n = 4$).

One notable drug development program focused on the selective α7 nicotinic agonist encenicline (EVP-6124), the only agent for CIAS that had advanced to Phase III. Positive Phase II results (Keefe et al. 2015) led to the launch of two global Phase III trials (EVP-6124-015/016) aimed at assessing once-daily encenicline (1 mg or 2 mg) as a pro-cognitive treatment in stable patients with schizophrenia. In two identical, global (primarily North America, South America, eastern and western Europe), placebo-controlled 6-month trials involving over 1,500 patients, highly robust within-group improvements were observed in both trials on the MCCB neurocognitive composite score, as well as an index of cognition-relevant daily functioning, across all three trials arms, including both drug doses and placebo. However, no statistically significant differences between encenicline and placebo emerged for either cognition or functioning. Despite some indication of greater improvement on drug in one of the trials, the encenicline development program was terminated.

It is worth noting that the number of trials conducted, and the amount of resources invested, in CIAS has been quite small compared to drug development efforts in other therapeutic areas. For example, in 2018, the number of clinical trials for cancer outnumbered those for CIAS by over 1,000 to 1 (see Keefe (2019)), despite a similar likelihood of successful progression from Phase 1 to ultimate FDA approval for indications in cancer (5.1%) and in psychiatry (6.2%) (Thomas et al. 2016). Similarly, within CNS indications, the number of trials for Alzheimer's Disease is much larger than for CIAS, despite a very high failure rate in Alzheimer's (Cummings et al. 2014, 2020).

2.2 *Why Did These Trials Fail?*

The field struggled through 2018 to find efficacious pharmacological interventions for CIAS as compounds that showed promise in early trials failed as they moved forward into larger RCTs. In attempting to explain the negative findings for drugs that showed early promise but failed to replicate in later stage clinical trials, there has been debate about whether the discouraging findings may be attributable to a number of potentially confounding factors rather than a true lack of efficacy (Keefe et al. 2016; Marder et al. 2017). Aside from scientific considerations related to our incomplete understanding of the pathophysiology of cognitive impairment in the heterogeneous diagnostic category of schizophrenia (to which we return below in Sect. 4), a number of methodological factors in later stage trials have been proposed as potential impediments to breakthroughs. These trials are typically multi-site and often multi-national and are logistically complex and challenging. For example, the encenicline Phase III trials enrolled about 1,500 patients from over 150 sites in over a dozen countries. While negative CIAS trials do not appear to be attributable to any single factor, three general types of factors have been considered: the suitability of cognitive assessment measures, patient characteristics/selection, and clinical trial implementation issues.

The first issue concerns the measurement of cognition in CIAS trials. Later phase trials have typically used the MCCB, which has been accepted as a gold-standard by the FDA. Although positive studies using the MCCB have been reported, most have been negative, including the failed, and highly publicized, Phase III encenicline program. A few early, relatively small studies raised concerns about the psychometric properties of the MCCB, such as reliability, practice effects, ceiling effects, and sensitivity to treatment effects. These concerns have not held up to empirical scrutiny. For example, the MCCB has consistently demonstrated strong test–retest reliability (Georgiades et al. 2017; Green et al. 2014; Keefe et al. 2011).

Concerns that an unusually large practice effect or a ceiling effect on the MCCB has impeded detection of treatment benefit have been allayed by an analysis of pooled data from 12 separate clinical trials that focused on 813 patients who were randomized to receive placebo during double-blind pharmacologic intervention studies (Keefe et al. 2017). Overall, the mean MCCB composite T-score at baseline was 22.8 points below the normative mean (Mean = 50, SD = 10), and the mean total change in the MCCB during receipt of placebo was 1.8 (SD = 0.2) T-score points (95%CI, 1.40–2.18), equivalent to a change of 0.18 SD. Practice effects in the seven studies in which there was a pre-baseline assessment were essentially identical to the post-baseline placebo changes. Given that the patients performed 2.28 SDs below normative standards on average at baseline, a mean placebo-associated improvement of <0.2 SD provides evidence that ceiling effects do not occur in these trials. Regarding sensitivity to treatment effects, it is very unlikely that these minimal changes in the MCCB are responsible for effective active treatments failing to separate from placebo. Furthermore, although pharmacological studies using the MCCB have more often than not been negative, as described below (Sect. 3), studies using cognitive remediation approaches have actually been quite consistent in demonstrating significant treatment benefits on the MCCB.

Another potential measurement-related concern is that nearly all trials have focused on a global composite score from the MCCB rather than a specific cognitive domain. This approach lumps diverse cognitive functions together that may not be uniformly responsive to a particular drug's mechanism of action, which could wash out the effect on a particular cognitive domain. Although there is nothing in the MATRICS consensus guidelines that require a global score endpoint in CIAS trials, efforts to target a specific aspect of cognition have been rare in late phase trials. Translation of specific drug–cognitive domain linkages from preclinical neuroscience into human clinical studies is complex and unpredictable, and has thus far not led to many strong predictions that compounds will show specific cognitive effects in participants with schizophrenia. An exception is the glutamatergic drug, BIIB-104 (Singer et al. 2015), whose impact on the working memory domain score from the MCCB is currently being evaluated (discussed further below).

The second issue concerns whether certain sample characteristics may contribute to negative findings. For example, most trials have used older patients (mean age in the 40s and predominantly male) who are chronically ill. It could be that older patients with entrenched cognitive impairment have limited neuroplasticity to demonstrate improvements as compared to younger, less chronic patients. Although the moderating effect of age has been extensively evaluated in the cognitive remediation treatment outcome literature (see Sect. 3 below), this issue has received little systematic consideration for pharmacological treatments (e.g., (Keefe et al. 2016; Umbricht et al. 2014)). Some trials do focus on early course patients or even at-risk samples (Levkovitz et al. 2010; McClure et al. 2019), though recruiting a sufficient number of these patients is a substantial challenge.

Another factor concerns the level of cognitive impairment among trial participants, which typically varies substantially. Some argue that clinical trials are biased toward recruiting higher functioning patients who are sufficiently motivated to engage in the trial requirements, whereas those most likely to benefit from cognitive enhancing treatments are patients with at least moderate cognitive impairment. At the same time, it could be that those with persistently severe cognitive impairment, which may even be present premorbidly in some patients, are less likely to benefit from cognitive enhancers. Again, while there is considerable data on the moderating effect of baseline cognition for cognitive remediation, there is little direct evidence that level of impairment moderates pharmacological treatment outcome (Cotter et al. 2019; Granger et al. 2018; Keefe 2021). To mitigate potential risks associated with age and baseline cognition, some have proposed conducting cognitive screening and/or incorporating stratification on these factors the statistical analysis plan.

The third issue relates to the real-world implementation of clinical trials. The implementation of a multi-site/multi-national trial is a complex, expensive endeavor that involves multi-faceted regulatory, scientific, and practical challenges and constraints. We consider two of the major implementation challenges: addressing sources of noise in cognitive data collection and trial implementation factors. Cognitive assessments are prone to many sources of noise that can impede signal detection. One involves variability in test administration and scoring (Keefe and Harvey 2008). The background experience and skill of those administering cognitive measures in multi-site, multi-national trials can vary enormously (Keefe and Harvey 2008). Learning to adequately administer cognitive tasks requires considerable up-front training for inexperienced assessors. Regular data quality monitoring throughout a trial is also critically important; for example, among low recruiting sites, raters with limited opportunity to practice can drift from standard administration and scoring practices. During the course of a trial, if the number of sites expands, available resources to provide rigorous training and data quality monitor become stretched. Furthermore, in multi-national studies, it is not uncommon to find regional differences in cognition levels or treatment effects. Aside from the complexities of translating and culturally adapting cognitive tests, maintaining standardization and administration significantly expands logistical challenges and resources required for global trials. For example, even factors such as variability over a trial in the time of day at which assessments are administered can impact findings (Hufford et al. 2014).

Another key factor concerns participant enrollment. CIAS trials never have an abundance of willing and able participants. Rather, recruitment is nearly always a challenge and recruitment problems are a common reason for discontinuing trials. Participation in a clinical trial requires a substantial commitment, sustained effort, and scheduling and organization skills (e.g., transportation to a trial site), which all can be challenging for schizophrenia patients with cognitive difficulties, negative symptoms, and/or financial/social resource limitations. Recruitment challenges, as well as cost-driven recruitment targets, also contribute to the fact that many trials are significantly underpowered (Keefe et al. 2013). Furthermore, poor adherence to treatment and high drop-out rates are common. There are also concerns that both patients and staff may be incentivized to participate for the wrong reasons. For example, some participants may be motivated by financial gain ("professional patients") rather than contributing to research, which can motivate them to report their symptoms/experiences to "fit" inclusion criteria. Sites may be incentivized or pressured to enroll large numbers of patients quickly in accordance with aggressive sponsor timelines, which may impact the suitability of the patients who are enrolled in trials (Marder et al. 2017). Furthermore, as trials experience recruitment challenges, adding sites and relaxing recruitment criteria are common, which can further contribute to noise.

In the context of these real-world implementation challenges, it is interesting to consider post-hoc analyses of the negative Phase III encenicline trial (Brannon 2017). As this program moved forward, recruitment challenges led to the addition of new sites. Protocol changes intended to accelerate enrollment were also made, including a switch from allowing only one background antipsychotic to two. Post-hoc analyses revealed substantial differences in the early stage of the trial, during which the placebo response rate was much lower than later in the trial. Furthermore, drug-related cognitive change (versus placebo) was much larger in those taking one antipsychotic medication (particularly those with low cholinergic effects) than those taking two antipsychotic medications. Other findings included: notable regional variation; high rates of treatment non-compliance that ranged from 5% of subjects (based on showing no plasma encenicline concentration at any time throughout the trial) up to 18% of subjects (depending on how non-compliance was defined); low recruiting sites (< 6 subjects) showed almost no difference between treatment groups; and a sizable number of subjects showed suspiciously large MCCB changes from screening to baseline. In a "clean" study population that excluded subjects who were on two antipsychotics, were non-adherent, or had large pre-baseline MCCB changes, encenicline was significantly better than placebo. While these findings are of course post hoc, they highlight the range of factors than can impact the ultimate outcome of large Phase III efficacy trials.

Before turning to recent trials, a few other developments in the literature are worth noting. First, recent work highlights the known, substantial link between anticholinergic burden, which accompanies many psychotropic and other medications, and cognitive impairment in schizophrenia (Joshi et al. 2021). Thus, one pro-cognitive therapeutic strategy is to minimize the use of medications with significant anticholinergic properties when clinically appropriate. Furthermore, the anticholinergic properties of permissible background antipsychotics are important considerations when designing CIAS trials for add-on drugs. Second, regarding potential moderators of treatment response, a meta-analysis alpha-7 nicotinic acetylcholine receptor agonist trials found no evidence of heterogeneity (based on I^2 values) for any cognitive subdomain, indicating that characteristics such as age, duration of illness, and sex did not moderate the overall absence of treatment-related benefit (Recio-Barbero et al. 2021). Third, there is emerging interest in alternative approaches to cognitive enhancement, such as neurostimulation approaches (Ciullo et al. 2021), targeting the microbiome (e.g., nutraceuticals), gut–brain axis hormones, and neuroinflammation (Bioque et al. 2021; Dickerson et al. 2021; Hong and Bang 2020; Marx et al. 2021), and anti-diabetic agents (Chen et al. 2021), though these will not be covered in this review.

2.3 *Clinical Trials Since 2018*

Despite major efforts by pharmaceutical companies, the overall status of pharmacological treatments has not changed substantially since 2018. There are still no drugs approved for CIAS though, as alluded to above, the number of trials and amount of resources devoted to CIAS remain relatively small in comparison to many other indications. Trials focused on CIAS have generally continued to target the same neural mechanisms and further negative findings have been reported. However, the news has not been entirely bleak and reasons for hope on a few fronts have emerged. In fact, it is possible that one active drug development program could lead to the approval of the first cognition enhancing drug for CIAS within the next few years.

A summary of industry sponsored efficacy trials from 2018 to the present that focused on cognition as the primary endpoint is shown in Table 1. The most substantial progress in the past 4 years involves Boehringer Ingelheim's drug development program for the glycine transporter-1 (glyT1) inhibitor, BI 425809. This compound enhances glutamatergic transmission by increasing synaptic levels of glycine, a co-agonist required for NMDA receptor-mediated signaling. Inhibitors of glycine transporter-1 (GlyT1) are thought to elevate synaptic glycine levels and consequently enhance glutamatergic neurotransmission and downstream

Table 1 Industry sponsored efficacy trials for CIAS from 2018 to present

NCT number	Title	Phase	Sponsor	Drug and mechanism of action	Status/primary endpoint
NCT02832037	Clinical Trial of BI 425809 Effect on Cognition and Functional Capacity in Schizophrenia	Phase 2	Boehringer Ingelheim	BI 425809: glycine transporter-1 (glyT1) inhibitor	Completed: positive – MCCB composite score (Fleischhacker et al. 2021)
NCT04846868	Clinical Trial of BI 425809 Effect on Cognition and Functional Capacity in Schizophrenia (CONNEX-1)	Phase 3	Boehringer Ingelheim	BI 425809: glycine transporter-1 (glyT1) inhibitor	Active: MCCB composite score
NCT04846881	Clinical Trial of BI 425809 Effect on Cognition and Functional Capacity in Schizophrenia (CONNEX-2)	Phase 3	Boehringer Ingelheim	BI 425809: glycine transporter-1 (glyT1) inhibitor	Active: MCCB composite score
NCT04860830	Clinical Trial of BI 425809 Effect on Cognition and Functional Capacity in Schizophrenia (CONNEX-3)	Phase 3	Boehringer Ingelheim	BI 425809: glycine transporter-1 (glyT1) inhibitor	Active: MCCB composite score
NCT03859973	This Study Tests Whether BI 425809 Together With Brain Training Using a Computer Improves Mental Functioning in Patients With Schizophrenia	Phase 2	Boehringer Ingelheim	BI 425809: glycine transporter-1 (glyT1) inhibitor + computerized cognitive training (exercises from HappyNeuron)	Active: MCCB composite score
NCT03745820	A Study to Evaluate the Safety and Efficacy of BIIB104 in	Phase 2	Biogen	BIIB-104 (also known as PF-04958242): Positive allosteric	Active: targets working memory domain of the MCCB

(continued)

Table 1 (continued)

NCT number	Title	Phase	Sponsor	Drug and mechanism of action	Status/primary endpoint
	Participants With Cognitive Impairment Associated With Schizophrenia (CIAS)			modulator (PAM) of the AMPA receptor	
NCT03557931	A Study to Assess the Safety and Efficacy of ASP4345 as Add-on Treatment for Cognitive Impairment in Subjects With Schizophrenia on Stable Doses of Antipsychotic Medication	Phase 2	Astellas Pharma Global Development, Inc.I Astellas Pharma Inc	ASP4345: Positive allosteric modulator (PAM) of the dopamine type 1 (D_1) receptor	Completed: negative for MCCB composite score (results not published)
NCT02953639	A Study to Evaluate the Effects of Basmisanil in Participants With Cognitive Impairment Associated With Schizophrenia (CIAS) Treated With Antipsychotics	Phase 2	Hoffmann-La Roche	Basmisanil: $GABA_A$-α5 selective negative allosteric modulator (NAM)	Completed: negative for MCCB neurocognitive composite score (results not published)
NCT05182476	Study to Evaluate the Efficacy, Safety, and Tolerability of Luvadaxistat in Subjects With Cognitive Impairment Associated With Schizophrenia	Phase 2	Neurocrine	Luvadaxistat	Active: Brief Assessment of Cognition (BAC) composite score

neuroplasticity processes that may improve CIAS (Balu and Coyle 2015; Javitt 2009). Following compelling preclinical proof of mechanism studies and phase I studies demonstrating good tolerability in doses up to 75 mg, a phase II randomized, double-blind, parallel-groups trial evaluated the efficacy of BI 425809 (2, 5, 10, or 25 mg) compared with placebo as add-on to standard of care in stable adult patients (18–50 years old) with schizophrenia (Fleischhacker et al. 2021). This 12-week trial randomized 509 patients recruited from 81 specialist psychiatric centers (including hospitals, research centers, outpatient clinics, and private practices) in 11 countries. For the MCCB composite score primary endpoint, BI 425809 showed a significant benefit over placebo, with the greatest improvement found for 10 mg (standardized effect size = 0.34) and 25 mg (effect size = 0.30). However, on the secondary endpoint, an interview-based measure of cognition-related functioning, there was no significant improvement in functioning compared with placebo in any treatment group. BI 425809 was generally well tolerated.

In the context of potential methodological concerns raised in prior CIAS studies (see Sect. 2.2. above), a few findings and post-hoc analyses from this phase II trial are noteworthy. For example, the sample had comparable baseline levels of cognitive impairment to prior studies (about 2 SD below normative mean) and the results were similar whether the MCCB overall composite or neurocognitive composite was evaluated. Exploratory subgroup analyses indicated no differences for MCCB Composite Score in patients receiving or not receiving anticholinergic medications, in patients receiving only one versus two concurrent antipsychotic, and in patients with or without negative symptoms at baseline. However, separation from placebo in the BI 425809 10 mg group was slightly better in patients aged 38 or less, in females, in those with greater cognitive impairment (MCCB T-score < 40), and in those with a shorter duration of illness, compared with the full analysis dataset. Thus, although some patient characteristics related to small mean score shifts on the MCCB, none substantially impacted the overall pattern of results.

In May of 2021, BI 425809 was granted Breakthrough Therapy Designation by the US Food and Drug Administration (FDA) for CIAS. Boehringer Ingelheim's CONNEX Phase III clinical trial program is currently recruiting participants to assess the safety and efficacy of BI 425809 for improving cognition in adults with schizophrenia. The program is comprised of three clinical trials, all of which are Phase III randomized, double-blind, placebo-controlled parallel group trials to examine the efficacy and safety of BI 425809 once daily over a 26-week treatment period. The program aims to recruit over 1,500 patients from over 25 countries. The primary outcome measure is change from baseline to end of treatment in overall composite T-score of the MCCB. The trials are currently estimated to be completed in mid-2024. Notably, a separate, ongoing Phase II trial (NCT03859973) is exploring the efficacy of BI425809 (10 mg) in patients with schizophrenia who are also receiving computerized cognitive training. In line with the notion that GlyT1 inhibitors may promote activity-dependent neuroplasticity processes, cognitive benefits of BI 425809 might possibly be increased further by adjunctive cognitive training.

The efficacy of another glutamatergic drug, BIIB-104, is currently being evaluated in a phase IIb study by Biogen. Previously known as PF-04958242 (when under development by Pfizer), BIIB-104 is a positive allosteric modulator (PAM) of the AMPA receptor (AMPAR), an ionotropic glutamate receptor. BIIB-104 has also been reported to act as a GlyT1 glycine transporter blocker and, by increasing extracellular levels of glycine, may indirectly activate the glycine receptor and the glycine co-agonist site of the NMDA receptor (Singer et al. 2015). The primary endpoint in this trial of over 200 participants focuses on the working memory domain score from the MCCB and has an anticipated completion date of late 2022.

Regarding other glutamatergic drugs, another interesting development involves luvadaxistat, which had been in development by Neurocrine for treatment of negative symptoms. Luvadaxistat (NBI-1065844; formerly TAK-831) is a highly selective and potent inhibitor of D-amino acid oxidase (DAAO), the major enzyme responsible for the catabolism/degradation of D-serine. Inhibition of DAAO leads to higher D-serine levels and thereby increases NMDA-dependent and glutamate receptor (GluRδ2) glutamatergic signaling, which has been proposed as a treatment strategy for both negative symptoms and cognitive impairment. Although a phase II negative symptoms trial with 256 patients (three dosages vs. placebo) did not meet its primary endpoint (negative symptom factors score on the PANSS), positive results for luvadaxistat 50 mg were reported for cognitive functioning as measured by the composite score on the Brief Assessment of Cognition, as well as cognition-related functioning on the SCoRS (NCT03382639). The findings for cognition supported Neurocrine's decision to further evaluate luvadaxistat in a phase IIb trial, which just recently initiated recruitment.

Over the past 4 years, two additional efficacy trials focused on other neurotransmitter systems, including dopamine and GABA, were both negative. First, Astellas was developing ASP4345, a positive allosteric modulator of the dopamine type 1 (D_1) receptor that selectively binds to, and enhances the activity of, D_1 receptors. Their 12-week phase II trial of over 233 patients from 27 sites in the USA failed to show a significant benefit over placebo for the MCCB neurocognitive composite score. Second, Roche reported negative results for basmisanil, a $GABA_A$-α5 selective negative allosteric modulator (NAM). Their phase II trial of 214 patients from 37 centers in the USA reported no benefit for the MCCB neurocognitive composite score. This drug was also under development for cognitive impairment in Downs Syndrome, but a phase II trial was terminated due to lack of efficacy.

Aside from efficacy studies in which cognition was the primary endpoint, it is noteworthy that several recent trials focused on negative or positive symptoms also include cognitive measures as secondary or exploratory endpoints. Although the methods and patients enrolled in these types of trials differ considerably from CIAS trials (e.g., Kirkpatrick et al. (2006)), they can shed light on the promise of new drugs targeting various mechanisms for cognitive enhancement. For example, one trial from Minerva found that monotherapy with MIN-101, a molecule that combines sigma-2 and 5HT2A antagonism (and low affinity for dopaminergic, cholinergic, and histaminergic receptors), improved both negative symptoms and cognition (Keefe et al. 2018). However, Minerva went forward with Phase III trials for negative symptoms only (the original treatment target for which the trial was designed). Examples of other recently completed or ongoing trials targeting novel mechanisms include: an NMDA receptor positive allosteric modulator (PAM) (NCT04306146); Cannabidiol (NCT04421456); PDE10A inhibitors (EudraCT number: 2020-002316-51; NCT04624243); a lysine specific demethylase 1 (LSD1) inhibitor (EudraCT number 2021-000350-26); RL-007, a cholinergic, glutamatergic, and GABA-B receptor modulator (NCT04822883); and SEP-363856, a trace amine-associated receptor 1 (TAAR1) and 5-hydroxytryptamine type 1A (5-HT_{1A}) receptor agonist (NCT02969382). Thus, a variety of mechanistically novel compounds with potential relevance for cognitive enhancement are in early clinical development.

3 Cognitive Remediation

3.1 Background

Considerable attention has been directed toward the development and implementation of cognitive remediation (CR) – broadly defined as behavioral training interventions designed to improve cognition and generalize improvements to community functioning for people with schizophrenia (Bowie et al. 2020). Training approaches for CR can be divided into compensatory and restorative methods. Compensatory training aims to reduce cognitive burden by providing skills that compensate for, or circumvent, cognitive deficits (Best and Bowie 2017). In contrast, restorative training applies learning principles to enhance or restore cognitive functions (Barlati et al. 2019; Wykes et al. 2011). This approach aims to facilitate neuroplasticity (i.e., changes in cortical organization and interaction between neural systems) and support more efficient information processing (Best and Bowie 2017).

The majority of CR interventions for schizophrenia employ restorative training and that approach will be the focus for this section. These interventions are delivered via computerized or paper-and-pencil exercises of varying length and complexity, and adjust for difficulty level based on individual performance. CR includes a range of treatment modalities and targets (Best and Bowie 2017). Treatment modalities range from self-directed practice with minimal or no therapist involvement (e.g., "drill-and-practice"), to intensive, guided practice (e.g., strategy coaching), often with adjunctive group or individual psychotherapy in rehabilitation settings (Saperstein and Kurtz 2013). Treatment targets range from lower-level sensory, perceptual skills (i.e., "bottom-up"), to higher-level executive processes (i.e., "top-down"). The range of intervention durations vary, with the average length of treatment being approximately 15 weeks (ranging from 3–104 weeks) (Vita et al. 2021).

3.2 Fundamental Elements

Given the wide variety of evidence-based CR interventions, an expert consensus group held a workshop to establish the key ingredients of CR for schizophrenia (Bowie et al. 2020). The group identified four core elements included in most, but not all CR, interventions: (1) an active and trained therapist; (2) repetition of cognitive exercises; (3) development of problem-solving strategies (i.e., strategy-based learning); and (4) development of strategies to transfer cognitive skills into the real world (i.e., bridging strategies). First, CR therapists work collaboratively with patients to identify the cognitive strategies that are most useful to them during training exercises. Therapists then connect these exercises with everyday activities, encourage the patient to use learned strategies while pursuing recovery goals, and address barriers. Second, CR interventions require intensive (e.g., 3–6 months), repetitive exercises that are engaging yet challenging for each participant to build mastery. Third, CR interventions provide opportunities for participants to monitor and modify strategies during training with the support of the therapist. Lastly, CR interventions typically involve discussions for skill application (i.e., in individual or group settings), opportunities for direct practice (i.e., using role-plays, social cognitive training, or homework assignments), and psychiatric rehabilitation.

3.3 Meta-Analyses of Efficacy for Cognitive Remediation

Since 2018, six meta-analyses were published that considered restorative approaches to CR for schizophrenia. The studies and their main findings are summarized in Table 2 and are briefly described in this section.

Prikken and colleagues (Prikken et al. 2019) conducted a meta-analysis examining the efficacy of computerized "drill-and-practice" restorative interventions unaccompanied by concomitant approaches. Computerized "drill-and-practice" interventions emphasize repetition of cognitive exercises with little or no human guidance. These interventions have generated enthusiasm over the past 4 years as a cost-effective option for large-scale dissemination. However, there is debate as to whether this type of training alone will lead to meaningful and sustained functional improvements (Harvey et al. 2018). Results indicated that "drill-and-practice" interventions alone can improve cognitive abilities in specific domains, such as attention and working memory, and some psychiatric symptoms, such as depression and positive symptoms, but they do not significantly improve global cognition or global functioning.

A second meta-analysis by Kambeitz-Ilankovic and colleagues (2019) examined the efficacy of computerized "drill-and-practice" cognitive training, but this meta-analysis included studies with and without supplementary human guidance. Supplementary human guidance refers to any clinician-mediated learning enhancement or transfer strategies provided during cognitive training or concomitant psychosocial

Table 2 Meta-analyses of cognitive remediation for schizophrenia from 2018 to present

Study (first author, year)	Research question	Number of included studies and participants (*N*)	Recruited sample	Cognitive outcomes (effect size, 95% CI); heterogeneity	Functional outcomes (effect size, 95% CI); heterogeneity	Symptom outcomes (effect size, 95% CI); heterogeneity	Moderators/subgroup analyses
(Prikken et al. 2019)	Computerized CR without human guidance vs. non-CR control group	24 studies ($N = 1{,}262$)	Psychosis Schizophrenia Schizoaffective disorder Schizophreniform disorder	*Global cognition*: No significant improvements *Domains*: Attention and working memory showed significant improvements with computerized CR (Hedge's $g > 0.31$; $I^2 < 35.84\%$)	*Global functioning*: No significant improvements	*Global symptoms*: No significant improvements *Domains*: Positive and depressive symptoms showed significant improvements with computerized CR (Hedge's $g > 0.31$; $I^2 < 23.86\%$)	No influence of age Longer illness duration was associated with larger effect sizes for attention Shorter treatment duration (with higher intensity) was associated with larger effect sizes for working memory, visual memory, and verbal memory
(Kambeitz-Ilankovic et al. 2019)	Computerized CR vs. non-CR control group, with versus without human guidance	67 studies ($N = 4{,}067$)	Psychosis Schizophrenia Schizoaffective disorder Schizophreniform disorder	*Global cognition*: Hedge's $g = 0.26$ (95% CI: 0.15–0.36) $I^2 = 19.16\%$ *Domains*: Attention, verbal memory, social	*Global functioning*: No significant improvements Social and vocational outcomes showed significant improvements with computerized CR	*Global symptoms*: No significant improvements *Domains*: Negative and depressive symptoms showed significant improvements with	Younger age, shorter duration of illness, and being female were associated with larger effect sizes for reasoning and problem-solving Verbal memory ($Q = 3.38$, $p = 0.05$) and working memory ($Q = 4.35$, $p = 0.04$) showed significant improvements when computerized CR included human guidance

(continued)

Table 2 (continued)

Study (first author, year)	Research question	Number of included studies and participants (*N*)	Recruited sample	Cognitive outcomes (effect size, 95% CI); heterogeneity	Functional outcomes (effect size, 95% CI); heterogeneity	Symptom outcomes (effect size, 95% CI); heterogeneity	Moderators/subgroup analyses
				cognition, working memory, processing speed, and reasoning showed significant improvements with computerized CR (Hedge's $g > 0.21$; $I^2 < 59.87\%$)	(Hedge's $g > 0.26$; $I^2 < 67.95\%$)	computerized CR (Hedge's $g > 0.13$; $I^2 < 31.92$)	versus computerized CR alone
(van Duin et al. 2019)	Psychiatric rehabilitation plus CR vs. psychiatric rehabilitation alone	23 studies ($N = 1{,}819$)	Serious mental illness	*Global cognition*: SMD = 0.31, (95% CI: 0.17–0.45) $I^2 = 0\%$	*Global functioning*: Not assessed Social and vocational outcomes showed significant improvements with psychiatric rehabilitation plus CR (SMD > 0.24; $I^2 < 89.00\%$	*Global symptoms*: Not assessed	Fewer years of education was associated with larger effect sizes for functional outcomes CR with strategy-based learning, shorter treatment duration (with lower intensity) was associated with larger effect sizes for functional outcomes

(Cella et al. 2020)	CR vs. non-CR control group	20 studies ($N = 1{,}509$)	Inpatients Schizophrenia-spectrum disorders	*Global cognition*: Not assessed *Domains*: Processing speed and working memory showed significant improvements with CR (Hedge's $g > 0.48$); $I^2 < 67\%$	*Global functioning*: No significant improvements in global, vocational, or social functioning	*Global symptoms*: Not assessed	Not assessed
(Vita et al. 2021)	CR vs. non-CR control group	130 studies ($N = 8{,}851$)	Serious mental illness	*Global cognition*: Cohen's $d = 0.29$ (95% CI: 0.24–0.34) $I^2 = 24.00\%$ *Domains*: Processing speed, working memory, verbal memory, visual memory, executive functions, and social cognition showed significant improvements with CR ($d > 0.20$)	*Global functioning*: Cohen's $d = 0.22$ (95% CI: 0.16–0.29); $I^2 = 37.00\%$	*Global symptoms*: Cohen's $d = 0.14$ (95% CI: 0.08–0.20)	No influence of age, gender, or duration of illness Fewer years of education, lower premorbid IQ, and higher baseline symptom severity were associated with larger effect sizes for cognition and functioning Longer treatment duration was associated with larger effect sizes for functioning Integration with all four core CR elements (plus psychiatric rehabilitation) was associated with larger effect sizes for global cognition and functioning

(continued)

Table 2 (continued)

Study (first author, year)	Research question	Number of included studies and participants (*N*)	Recruited sample	Cognitive outcomes (effect size, 95% CI); heterogeneity	Functional outcomes (effect size, 95% CI); heterogeneity	Symptom outcomes (effect size, 95% CI); heterogeneity	Moderators/subgroup analyses
(Lejeune et al. 2021)	CR (non-social only) vs. non-CR control group	73 studies ($N = 4{,}594$)	Schizophrenia Schizoaffective disorder	*Global cognition*: Hedge's $g = 0.29$ (95% CI: 0.12, 0.45) $I^2 = 60.55\%$ *Domains*: Verbal learning, working memory, attention, reasoning and problem-solving, processing speed, and visual learning showed significant improvements with CR ($g > 0.19$)	*Global functioning*: Hedge's $g = 0.21$ (95% CI: 0.08, 0.34) $I^2 = 52.77\%$	*Negative symptoms*: Hedge's $g = 0.16$ (95% CI: 0.04, 0.29) $I^2 = 42.88\%$	No influence of age, gender, symptoms, or adjunctive psychiatric rehabilitation Fewer years of education was associated with larger effect sizes for reasoning, problem-solving, and processing speed Lower IQ was associated with larger effect sizes for visual memory Longer duration of illness was associated with larger effect sizes for global functioning Strategy coaching was associated with larger effect sizes for verbal learning and visual learning Bridging groups were associated with larger effect sizes for global cognition and verbal memory Longer treatment duration was associated with larger effect sizes for attention

Note: *95% CI* 95% confidence interval, *SMD* standardized mean difference. Only significant effect sizes ($p < 0.05$) are reported. I^2 describes the heterogeneity of effect sizes across studies. Larger %'s indicate that effects are due to differences among studies rather than chance intervention. The studies in this meta-analysis yielded small to moderate improvements in global cognition, the subdomains of social and vocational functioning (though not global functioning), negative symptoms, and depression. A subgroup analysis compared treatment outcomes between studies with computerized training alone versus computerized training with supplementary human guidance and it indicated that the addition of human guidance was associated with significantly greater improvements in an index of global cognition and the cognitive domains of verbal memory and working memory.

Psychiatric rehabilitation (e.g., supported employment, social skills training, cognitive behavioral therapy, etc.) is a type of supplementary human guidance that has been previously shown to boost cognitive skill acquisition and functional outcomes (Barlati et al. 2019; Wykes et al. 2011). A meta-analysis by van Duin and colleagues (Van Duin et al. 2019) evaluated the efficacy of CR plus psychiatric rehabilitation versus psychiatric rehabilitation alone. The addition of CR led to a significant favorable outcome for global cognition. Furthermore, there were improvements in vocational outcomes (i.e., increased employment rate, hours worked, job duration, and work/education quality) and social functioning (i.e., social skills).

Two studies examined CR in diverse patient populations (outpatient and inpatient samples). One study by Lejeune et al. focused solely on non-social cognitive training (Lejeune et al. 2021), while the other by Vita et al. included both social and non-social cognitive training (Vita et al. 2021). Both studies found that CR has an overall positive effect on global cognition, and a small but significant effect on functioning. The two types of training improved different aspects of symptoms. Non-social CR interventions showed improvements in negative symptoms, whereas CR interventions with both social and non-social training showed improvements in global psychiatric symptoms. The effect sizes observed in these meta-analyses were smaller than those found in an earlier meta-analysis (Wykes et al. 2011), which may be due to greater heterogeneity of the samples and interventions included.

Lastly, a meta-analysis by Cella and colleagues (Cella et al. 2020) examined the efficacy of CR for patients in an inpatient setting. Findings indicated that CR significantly improved processing speed and working memory. However, CR did not lead to significant improvements in functional outcome beyond the inpatient setting. These findings suggest that, although CR improves specific domains of cognition, inpatients likely need follow-up CR and/or adjunctive rehabilitation after discharge to improve community functioning.

3.4 Variability of Treatment Response

Because of considerable variability in individual response to CR (Barlati et al. 2019; Reser et al. 2019), there is a need to identify moderators of treatment response, with the ultimate goal of personalizing CR interventions to maximize individual gains (Medalia et al. 2018). Only tentative conclusions can be reached at this stage.

3.4.1 Patient-Associated Moderators

Researchers have attempted to identify the those most likely to benefit from CR. One variable of interest is age, which in theory can impact treatment response in one of two ways. On the one hand, young people may benefit more from CR because they have greater neural plasticity potential. On the other hand, older people may benefit more because they have greater deficits due to a longer illness duration. The majority of evidence since 2018 suggests that age does not significantly moderate treatment response when examined as a continuous variable (Allott et al. 2020; Saperstein et al. 2021; Seccomandi et al. 2021a; Van Duin et al. 2019; Vita et al. 2021). However, one study reported that individuals with longer illness durations showed the largest functional gains (Lejeune et al. 2021).

Findings related to clinical status have been mixed. Some studies indicate that CR shows greater benefits for individuals with lower baseline IQ, fewer years of education, and greater symptom severity (Lejeune et al. 2021; Vita et al. 2021). These individuals with particularly poor functioning may show larger improvements because they have more room for growth. In contrast, CR is also shown to benefit higher functioning individuals with greater premorbid intelligence, baseline cognition, and training task progress (Reser et al. 2019). These individuals improve because they have a high capacity to learn. Cognitive decline may also play a role in CR treatment response in that one study found that individuals with preserved IQ had more cognitive gains than deteriorated or compromised IQ groups, and those with deteriorated IQ had more gains than those with compromised IQ (Seccomandi et al. 2021b).

3.4.2 Treatment-Associated Moderators

Researchers have also attempted to identify the optimal aspects of treatment for CR. Treatment format (i.e., individual versus group sessions) and delivery method (i.e., computerized versus paper-and-pencil) do not significantly influence cognitive outcomes (Vita et al. 2021). Rather, cognitive outcomes are enhanced by specific CR techniques, such as strategy coaching, bridging discussions, and the identification of personalized goals (Lejeune et al. 2021; Prikken et al. 2019; Saperstein et al. 2021; Vita et al. 2021). These techniques reinforce skill development and transfer to the real world. Longer-term treatments are associated with improved functioning (Allott et al. 2020; Vita et al. 2021).

Some effort has been made to disentangle the benefits of human guidance from non-specific treatment factors, such as therapeutic engagement and support. One study found that therapeutic support alone did not improve cognition, but human guidance with strategy coaching did (Lejeune et al. 2021). The role of the therapist may be especially important in maintaining negative symptom improvements (Kambeitz-Ilankovic et al. 2019) by supporting intrinsic motivation and engagement in learning (Saperstein et al. 2021).

3.5 *Current Limitations and Future Directions*

CR is increasingly recognized as an effective treatment for cognitive performance deficits in schizophrenia. The field is now considering large-scale implementation and dissemination. However, this type of scaling up may be a challenge for two reasons. First, there are a wide range of evidence-based CR interventions for schizophrenia. It is not clear which interventions are best suited for dissemination in community settings. For example, it remains unclear who should administer these interventions (i.e., level of training and education of facilitator) and the optimal parameters, including the duration (e.g., weeks, months, etc.) dosage (i.e., frequency of practice), and intensity (i.e., decision algorithms determining difficulty level) of cognitive training. Second, most CR interventions involve supplementary human guidance or psychiatric rehabilitation to generalize improvements to community functioning. These treatments are time and labor intensive and require a level of clinical stability and motivation that is not always present.

Alternative approaches are emerging to address these challenges to broader dissemination. First, technology can be used to deliver CR treatments remotely (Medalia et al. 2021). Beyond remote administration of training exercises, virtual reality (VR) interventions (e.g., mock job interviews) provide a platform for participants to practice cognitive skills in situations that closely mirror real life (Smith et al. 2015) but without the time and labor costs. Some additional advantages of VR include: easy dissemination, increased access (i.e., training at home), more frequent usage, structured practice, and automatic adaptation of difficulty based on performance and habits. Another active area of research involves the combination of pharmacological agents with CR. Pharmacological agents are being used to boost the effectiveness of CR without the use of burdensome interventions that require human guidance. For example, some currently approved and novel medications might increase alertness or motivation and thereby enhance training efficiency and performance (Harvey and Bowie 2012).

4 Transdiagnostic Considerations for Clinical Trials

One of the more complicated decisions about clinical trials for CIAS is whether to include or exclude potential participants who have disorders other than schizophrenia. In the initial FDA-NIMH-MATRICS Guidelines (Buchanan et al. 2005), the recommendation was nuanced, and a bit confusing:

> Schizophrenia and schizoaffective disorder share a similar pattern of cognitive impairments, which is distinct from patterns in major depression, bipolar disorder, and Alzheimer's dementia. However, because the current approach of the FDA to approval/labeling reflects greater diagnostic specificity of the targeted population, studies of potential cognitive-enhancers should initially include only patients with schizophrenia.

Before unpacking the recommendation, we wish to note that the first diagnostic challenge for the MATRICS Initiative was the need to show that cognitive impairment in schizophrenia was distinct from that seen in dementia. Because cognitive treatments were already approved for dementia, why was an indication needed for the same impairment, but in a different disorder? The answer was that the pattern of the impairment was quite different in the two disorders; for example, retention is nearly normal in schizophrenia but heavily impacted in dementia (Green et al. 2004; Heaton et al. 1994). After demonstrating that the existing indication and treatments for dementia would not extend to schizophrenia, the diagnostic question then moved to other psychotic disorders.

The recommendation of the consensus panel was an in-between position – that the cognitive impairments in schizophrenia are not entirely diagnostically specific (i.e., they appear to be identical to those in schizoaffective disorder), but they are partly diagnostically specific (i.e., they appear different enough from those in mood disorders and dementia). There were two factors that influenced the recommendation. First, at that point in time, the FDA's approach to labeling in psychiatry was heavily based on DSM conditions (a posture that has become more flexible over time). Second, there was a constraint by precedent. Specifically, almost all the planned clinical trials of CIAS were going to add a novel drug onto an antipsychotic, and that antipsychotic was approved only for schizophrenia. As a result, the panel recommended that recruitment be limited to a DSM diagnosis of schizophrenia. When the guidelines were updated this recommendation was not changed (Buchanan et al. 2011).

4.1 Looking Across Diagnoses

The many studies conducted since the initial recommendations in 2005 have not fully resolved the question of who to include in clinical trials of CIAS. The similarities of the cognitive impairments in schizophrenia and schizoaffective disorders remain well-supported and many studies include both disorders as a single group. Thus, there is no clear empirical reason to exclude people with a diagnosis of schizoaffective disorder from clinical trials of CIAS.

Furthermore, some investigators have made broader claims that cognitive impairment is similar across a broad range of psychiatric disorders including schizophrenia, depression, bipolar disorder, and anxiety disorders (Goodkind et al. 2015; McTeague et al. 2020). This sweeping transdiagnostic approach to cognition is consistent with the RDoC project which is designed to examine key dimensions across diagnoses (Cuthbert 2014; Insel et al. 2010). It is also consistent with the studies of personality factors that identify a common psychopathology (i.e., "p") dimension (Kotov et al. 2017).

However, a finer grain scrutiny of these studies raises the question as to whether cognitive impairment, which is indeed seen across psychiatric disorders, is exactly the same impairment and derives from the same underlying neural process. For example, work from our lab has shown that schizophrenia and bipolar disorder show different patterns of social versus non-social cognitive deficits: individuals with schizophrenia have proportionately larger deficits in social than in non-social cognition, and individuals with bipolar disorder have the opposite pattern (Lee et al. 2013). Also, the trajectories of cognitive impairment in schizophrenia and bipolar disorder differ in that those with schizophrenia start to show decline earlier in life (Kahn 2020; Mollon and Reichenberg 2018).

Even when studies report common neural abnormalities based on neuroimaging across a broad range of psychiatric disorders, a closer examination of the patterns and the specific brain regions often shows that the nature of the abnormalities differ between psychotic and nonpsychotic conditions. One example (described in (Barch 2020)) shows that the conclusions from a meta-analysis of functional neuroimaging studies of cognitive control across disorders (schizophrenia bipolar, depression, anxiety, substance use) depended on the brain region in question (McTeague et al. 2017). Whereas right insula hypoactivation appeared to be transdiagnostic, left prefrontal hypoactivation was predominantly seen in schizophrenia.

Overall, the extension of recruitment for treatment studies of cognition to anyone with a cognitive impairment, regardless of diagnosis, might be counter-productive if the neural basis of the impairments differs among subsamples. If so, the effect of a drug and its mechanism of action may benefit only a subset of participants for whom that change is relevant to their impairment. In contrast to pharmacological studies, the question about the neural basis of cognitive impairment across psychiatric disorders is not a preoccupation for cognitive remediation. It is assumed that the interventions (both restorative and compensatory) are less tied to a specific neural process compared with a drug intervention that would have a specific mechanism of action.

A middle ground between overly broad and overly narrow diagnostic requirements for treatment studies of CIAS might be to include those with schizoaffective disorder, or perhaps all those with a psychotic disorder. At any rate, it appears that ongoing treatment studies of CIAS are starting with schizophrenia alone before branching to other conditions.

4.2 *Looking Within Schizophrenia*

An inverse problem with diagnosis and CIAS is whether the diagnosis of schizophrenia is itself too broad and/or includes multiple meaningful cognition-related subgroups. The heterogeneity of the disorder, as well as the frequent reference to Bleuler's phrase of the "group of schizophrenias" (Bleuler 1950) raises the question as to whether a given drug with a specific mechanism of action will work only on a subgroup of people with schizophrenia. This problem has been handled in a couple of ways. First, clinical trials frequently try to select those with schizophrenia who have cognitive impairment in the first place for inclusion in clinical trials that are designed to enhance cognition. The logic is clear – it is difficult to improve a non-deficit. However, one can make the argument that nearly everyone with schizophrenia is cognitively reduced from where they would have been if they had not developed schizophrenia (Keefe et al. 2005). This argument is based on comparisons to expected cognitive abilities, for example, based on parental education or achievement of siblings.

An alternative way to address this problem is to parse the heterogeneity of schizophrenia by identifying subgroups that presumably share the same underlying neural pathophysiology. This approach is consistent with the NIMH RDoC project in that it focuses on a set of dimensions that are thought to underlie cognitive impairment regardless of diagnostic boundaries. While subtyping of schizophrenia has a long history based on symptoms alone (e.g., paranoid versus non-paranoid), more recent attempts have included brain-based measures such as electroencephalography (EEG) and functional magnetic resonance imaging (fMRI) to aid in the identification of subgroups. Subgroups can also be defined or validated based on their response to intervention. For example, an early sign of malleability (i.e., change from baseline after the initial 1-h dose of cognitive remediation) for two event-related potentials (mismatch negativity and P3a) identified those participants who were going to respond to the full 30-h cognitive remediation program (Hochberger et al. 2019).

A more ambitious approach is to look *both* across and within psychiatric disorders to identify "biotypes" that essentially create alternative subgroup boundaries that are different from DSM diagnoses and may have more grounding in neural processes (Clementz et al. 2016; Tamminga et al. 2017). Whether identified subtypes can inform individual differences in response to novel interventions for CIAS has yet to be determined.

5 Conclusions

Treatment development for CIAS is a complex endeavor. It involves intersecting scientific, trial implementation, regulatory, and resource dependencies. Navigating these complexities has been a major challenge for treatment developers. Since the establishment of a regulatory pathway through the MATRICS initiative in the early 2000s, we still do not have an approved drug for CIAS. However, we have learned a great deal and the field has continued to push forward on several encouraging fronts over the last 3 years.

Regarding pharmacological approaches, despite a fairly challenging early history, the field is poised for a potential breakthrough. The glyT1 inhibitor BI425809 is currently being evaluated in a set of large, global Phase III trials using state-of-the-art methods. If successful, this drug could receive FDA approval within the next 2–3 years, which would constitute a landmark achievement in schizophrenia therapeutics. Other promising glutamatergic agents are currently being evaluated for CIAS in Phase II trials, and drugs targeting a variety of novel mechanisms are also examining cognitive outcomes in early clinical development.

Regarding cognitive remediation, several types of approaches administered in an adequate dose (e.g., 3–6 months) can improve cognitive task performance. However, optimal generalization of these benefits appears to require a concomitant psychosocial intervention that bridges cognitive skills to real-world functional improvements. These approaches are time and resource intensive and require a level of stability and motivation/commitment that is often difficult for patients to sustain. Thus, a large-scale implementation is a major challenge. Current efforts focus on using technology so treatments can be delivered remotely or to enhance the ecological validity (e.g., VR) of training exercises. Combining cognitive rehabilitation with pharmacological or other interventions is another promising way to boost effectiveness.

There has also been a steady scientific push toward new ways of approaching treatment development for cognitive impairment as it relates to the diagnostic category of schizophrenia. Although the FDA currently issues indication-specific approvals, transdiagnostic approaches include both looking beyond schizophrenia to encompass other conditions, as well as looking within schizophrenia to identify more homogenous subgroups. While these alternative approaches have attracted considerable attention, they raise complex scientific questions for drug development. Furthermore, a regulatory pathway for drug development programs based on these newer paradigms does not currently exist.

We anticipate that the next several years will be an interesting period for treatment development for CIAS. It is encouraging that many different approaches to treatment development are currently being applied to the complex challenge of CIAS, as enhancing cognition remains one of the most promising approaches to improve the functional disability that has characterized this disorder for over a century.

Disclosures WPH is a full-time employee at WCG VeraSci. MFG has been a paid consultant for Biogen, Otsuka, and Teva. MFG is also an officer in a non-profit organization, MATRICS Assessment, Inc., but receives no financial compensation. LTC has no disclosures.

References

Allott K, Van-Der-El K, Bryce S, Parrish EM, McGurk SR, Hetrick S, Bowie CR, Kidd S, Hamilton M, Killackey E, Velligan D (2020) Compensatory interventions for cognitive impairments in psychosis: a systematic review and meta-analysis. Schizophr Bull 46:869–883

Balu DT, Coyle JT (2015) The NMDA receptor ‘glycine modulatory site’ in schizophrenia: D-serine, glycine, and beyond. Curr Opin Pharmacol 20:109–115

Barch DM (2020) What does it mean to be transdiagnostic and how would we know? Am J Psychiatry 177:370–372

Barlati S, Deste G, Galluzzo A, Perin AP, Valsecchi P, Turrina C, Vita A (2019) Factors associated with response and resistance to cognitive remediation in schizophrenia: a critical review. Front Pharmacol 9:1542

Best MW, Bowie CR (2017) A review of cognitive remediation approaches for schizophrenia: from top-down to bottom-up, brain training to psychotherapy. Expert Rev Neurother 17:713–723

Bioque M, Gonzalez-Rodriguez A, Garcia-Rizo C, Cobo J, Monreal JA, Usall J, Soria V, Group P, Labad J (2021) Targeting the microbiome-gut-brain axis for improving cognition in

schizophrenia and major mood disorders: a narrative review. Prog Neuro-Psychopharmacol Biol Psychiatry 105:110130
Bleuler E (1950) Dementia praecox or the group of schizophrenias. International Universities Press, New York
Bowie CR, Bell MD, Fiszdon JM, Johannesen JK, Lindenmayer JP, McGurk SR, Medalia AA, Penadés R, Saperstein AM, Twamley EW, Ueland T, Wykes T (2020) Cognitive remediation for schizophrenia: an expert working group white paper on core techniques. Schizophr Res 215: 49–53
Brannon S (2017) The difficulties in going from P2 to P3 in CNS trials: red flags from a recent CIS program. In: 13th annual scientific meeting of the Internaltional Society of CNS Clincial Trials, Washington
Buchanan RW, Davis M, Goff D, Green MF, Keefe RSE, Leon AC, Nuechterlein KH, Laughren T, Levin R, Stover E, Fenton W, Marder SR (2005) A summary of the FDA-NIMH-MATRICS workshop on clinical trial design for neurocognitive drugs for schizophrenia. Schizophr Bull 31: 5–19
Buchanan RW, Keefe RS, Umbricht D, Green MF, Laughren T, Marder SR (2011) The FDA-NIMH-MATRICS guidelines for clinical trial design of cognitive-enhancing drugs: what do we know 5 years later? Schizophr Bull 37:1209–1217
Carter CS, Barch DM, Buchanan RW, Bullmore E, Krystal JH, Cohen J, Geyer M, Green M, Nuechterlein KH, Robbins T, Silverstein S, Smith EE, Strauss M, Wykes T, Heinssen R (2008) Identifying cognitive mechanisms targeted for treatment development in schizophrenia: an overview of the first meeting of the cognitive neuroscience treatment research to improve cognition in schizophrenia initiative. Biol Psychiatry 64:4–10
Cella M, Price T, Corboy H, Onwumere J, Shergill S, Preti A (2020) Cognitive remediation for inpatients with psychosis: a systematic review and meta-analysis. Psychol Med 50:1062–1076
Chen Q, Cao T, Li N, Zeng C, Zhang S, Wu X, Zhang B, Cai H (2021) Repurposing of anti-diabetic agents as a new opportunity to alleviate cognitive impairment in neurodegenerative and neuropsychiatric disorders. Front Pharmacol 12:667874
Ciullo V, Spalletta G, Caltagirone C, Banaj N, Vecchio D, Piras F, Piras F (2021) Transcranial direct current stimulation and cognition in neuropsychiatric disorders: systematic review of the evidence and future directions. Neuroscientist 27:285–309
Clementz BA, Sweeney JA, Hamm JP, Ivleva EI, Ethridge LE, Pearlson GD, Keshavan MS, Tamminga CA (2016) Identification of distinct psychosis biotypes using brain-based biomarkers. Am J Psychiatr 173:373–384
Cotter J, Barnett JH, Granger K (2019) The use of cognitive screening in pharmacotherapy trials for cognitive impairment associated with schizophrenia. Front Psych 10:648
Cummings JL, Morstorf T, Zhong K (2014) Alzheimer's disease drug development pipeline: few candidates, frequent failures. Alzheimers Res Ther 6:1–7
Cummings J, Lee G, Ritter A, Sabbagh M, Zhong K (2020) Alzheimer's disease drug development pipeline: 2020. Alzheimers Dement (N Y) 6:e12050
Cuthbert BN (2014) The RDoC framework: facilitating transition from ICD/DSM to dimensional approaches that integrate neuroscience and psychopathology. World Psychiatry 13:28–35
Cuthbert BN, Morris SE (2021) Evolving concepts of the schizophrenia spectrum: a research domain criteria perspective. Front Psych 12:641319
Davis MC, Horan WP, Marder SR (2014) Psychopharmacology of the negative symptoms: current status and prospects for progress. Eur Neuropsychopharmacol 24:788–799
Dickerson F, Origoni A, Katsafanas E, Squire A, Newman T, Fahey J, Xiao JC, Stallings C, Goga J, Khushalani S, Yolken R (2021) Randomized controlled trial of an adjunctive sulforaphane nutraceutical in schizophrenia. Schizophr Res 231:142–144
Fleischhacker WW, Podhorna J, Groschl M, Hake S, Zhao Y, Huang S, Keefe RSE, Desch M, Brenner R, Walling DP, Mantero-Atienza E, Nakagome K, Pollentier S (2021) Efficacy and safety of the novel glycine transporter inhibitor BI 425809 once daily in patients with

schizophrenia: a double-blind, randomised, placebo-controlled phase 2 study. Lancet Psychiatry 8:191–201

Georgiades A, Davis VG, Atkins AS, Khan A, Walker TW, Loebel A, Haig G, Hilt DC, Dunayevich E, Umbricht D, Sand M, Keefe RSE (2017) Psychometric characteristics of the MATRICS consensus cognitive battery in a large pooled cohort of stable schizophrenia patients. Schizophr Res 190:172–179

Gold JM (2004) Cognitive deficits as treatment targets in schizophrenia. Schizophr Res 72:21–28

Goodkind M, Eickhoff SB, Oathes DJ, Jiang Y, Chang A, Jones-Hagata LB, Ortega BN, Zaiko YV, Roach EL, Korgaonkar MS, Grieve SM, Galatzer-Levy I, Fox PT, Etkin A (2015) Identification of a common neurobiological substrate for mental illness. JAMA Psychiat 72:305–315

Granger K, Cotter J, Baker E, Evenden J, Barnett J, Sand M (2018) Exploring participant-level trajectories of cognitive performance among patients with schizophrenia in a multi-national trial. Schizophr Bull 44:S353–S353

Green MF, Nuechterlein KH, Gold JM, Barch DM, Cohen J, Essock S, Fenton WS, Frese F, Goldberg TE, Heaton RK, Keefe RSE, Kern RS, Kraemer H, Stover E, Weinberger DR, Zalcman S, Marder SR (2004) Approaching a consensus cognitive battery for clinical trials in schizophrenia: the NIMH-MATRICS conference to select cognitive domains and test criteria. Biol Psychiatry 56:301–307

Green MF, Harris JG, Nuechterlein KH (2014) The MATRICS consensus cognitive battery: what we know 6 years later. Am J Psychiatry 171:1151–1154

Green MF, Horan WP, Lee J (2019) Nonsocial and social cognition in schizophrenia: current evidence and future directions. World Psychiatry 18:146–161

Harvey PD, Bowie CR (2012) Cognitive enhancement in schizophrenia. Pharmacological and cognitive remediation approaches. Psychiatr Clin N Am 35:683–698

Harvey PD, McGurk SR, Mahncke H, Wykes T (2018) Controversies in computerized cognitive training. Biol Psychiatr Cogn Neurosci Neuroimaging 3:907–915

Heaton R, Paulsen JS, McAdams LA, Kuck J, Zisook S, Braff D, Harris J, Jeste DV (1994) Neuropsychological deficits in schizophrenics: relationship to age, chronicity, and dementia. Arch Gen Psychiatry 51:469–476

Heinrichs RW, Zakzanis KK (1998) Neurocognitive deficit in schizophrenia: a quantitative review of the evidence. Neuropsychology 12:426–445

Hochberger WC, Joshi YB, Thomas ML, Zhang W, Bismark AW, Treichler EBH, Tarasenko M, Nungaray J, Sprock J, Cardoso L, Swerdlow N, Light GA (2019) Neurophysiologic measures of target engagement predict response to auditory-based cognitive training in treatment refractory schizophrenia. Neuropsychopharmacology 44:606–612

Hong J, Bang M (2020) Anti-inflammatory strategies for schizophrenia: a review of evidence for therapeutic applications and drug repurposing. Clin Psychopharmacol Neurosci 18:10–24

Hufford MR, Davis VG, Hilt D, Dgetluck N, Geffen Y, Loebel A, Haig G, Santarelli L, Keefe RS (2014) Circadian rhythms in cognitive functioning among patients with schizophrenia: impact on signal detection in clinical trials of potential pro-cognitive therapies. Schizophr Res 159:205–210

Insel T, Cuthbert B, Garvey M, Heinssen R, Pine DS, Quinn K, Sanislow C, Wang P (2010) Research domain criteria (RDoC): toward a new classification framework for research on mental disorders. Am J Psychiatr 167:748–751

Javitt DC (2009) Glycine transport inhibitors for the treatment of schizophrenia: symptom and disease modification. Curr Opin Drug Discov Devel 12:468–478

Joshi YB, Thomas ML, Braff DL, Green MF, Gur RC, Gur RE, Nuechterlein KH, Stone WS, Greenwood TA, Lazzeroni LC, MacDonald LR, Molina JL, Nungaray JA, Radant AD, Silverman JM, Sprock J, Sugar CA, Tsuang DW, Tsuang MT, Turetsky BI, Swerdlow NR, Light GA (2021) Anticholinergic medication burden-associated cognitive impairment in schizophrenia. Am J Psychiatry 178:838–847

Kahn RS (2020) On the origins of schizophrenia. Am J Psychiatry 177:291–297

Kambeitz-Ilankovic L, Betz LT, Dominke C, Haas SS, Subramaniam K, Fisher M, Vinogradov S, Koutsouleris N, Kambeitz J (2019) Multi-outcome meta-analysis (MOMA) of cognitive remediation in schizophrenia: revisiting the relevance of human coaching and elucidating interplay between multiple outcomes. Neurosci Biobehav Rev 107:828–845

Keefe RSE (2019) Why are there no approved treatments for cognitive impairment in schizophrenia? World Psychiatry 18:167–168

Keefe RSE (2021) Where do we cut the bell-shaped curve of CIAS? Schizophenia Res 228:633–634

Keefe RS, Harvey PD (2008) Implementation considerations for multisite clinical trials with cognitive neuroscience tasks. Schizophr Bull 34:656–663

Keefe RS, Eesley CE, Poe MP (2005) Defining a cognitive function decrement in schizophrenia. Biol Psychiatry 57:688–691

Keefe RS, Fox KH, Harvey PD, Cucchiaro J, Siu C, Loebel A (2011) Characteristics of the MATRICS consensus cognitive battery in a 29-site antipsychotic schizophrenia clinical trial. Schizophr Res 125:161–168

Keefe RS, Buchanan RW, Marder SR, Schooler NR, Dugar A, Zivkov M, Stewart M (2013) Clinical trials of potential cognitive-enhancing drugs in schizophrenia: what have we learned so far? Schizophr Bull 39:417–435

Keefe RS, Meltzer HA, Dgetluck N, Gawryl M, Koenig G, Moebius HJ, Lombardo I, Hilt DC (2015) Randomized, double-blind, placebo-controlled study of encenicline, an alpha7 nicotinic acetylcholine receptor agonist, as a treatment for cognitive impairment in schizophrenia. Neuropsychopharmacology 40:3053–3060

Keefe RS, Haig GM, Marder SR, Harvey PD, Dunayevich E, Medalia A, Davidson M, Lombardo I, Bowie CR, Buchanan RW, Bugarski-Kirola D, Carpenter WT, Csernansky JT, Dago PL, Durand DM, Frese FJ, Goff DC, Gold JM, Hooker CI, Kopelowicz A, Loebel A, McGurk SR, Opler LA, Pinkham AE, Stern RG (2016) Report on ISCTM consensus meeting on clinical assessment of response to treatment of cognitive impairment in schizophrenia. Schizophr Bull 42:19–33

Keefe RSE, Davis VG, Harvey PD, Atkins AS, Haig GM, Hagino O, Marder S, Hilt DC, Umbricht D (2017) Placebo response and practice effects in schizophrenia cognition trials. JAMA Psychiat 74:807–814

Keefe RSE, Harvey PD, Khan A, Saoud JB, Staner C, Davidson M, Luthringer R (2018) Cognitive effects of MIN-101 in patients with schizophrenia and negative symptoms: results from a randomized controlled trial. J Clin Psychiatry 79(3):17m11753

Kirkpatrick B, Fenton WS, Carpenter WT Jr, Marder SR (2006) The NIMH-MATRICS consensus statement on negative symptoms. Schizophr Bull 32:214–219

Kotov R, Krueger RF, Watson D, Achenbach TM, Althoff RR, Bagby RM, Brown TA, Carpenter WT, Caspi A, Clark LA, Eaton NR, Forbes MK, Forbush KT, Goldberg D, Hasin D, Hyman SE, Ivanova MY, Lynam DR, Markon K, Miller JD, Moffitt TE, Morey LC, Mullins-Sweatt SN, Ormel J, Patrick CJ, Regier DA, Rescorla L, Ruggero CJ, Samuel DB, Sellbom M, Simms LJ, Skodol AE, Slade T, South SC, Tackett JL, Waldman ID, Waszczuk MA, Widiger TA, Wright AGC, Zimmerman M (2017) The hierarchical taxonomy of psychopathology (HiTOP): a dimensional alternative to traditional nosologies. J Abnorm Psychol 126:454–477

Lee J, Altshuler L, Glahn DC, Miklowitz DJ, Ochsner K, Green MF (2013) Social and nonsocial cognition in bipolar disorder and schizophrenia: relative levels of impairment. Am J Psychiatr 170:334–341

Lejeune JA, Northrop A, Kurtz MM (2021) A meta-analysis of cognitive remediation for schizophrenia: efficacy and the role of participant and treatment factors. Schizophr Bull 47:997–1006

Levkovitz Y, Mendlovich S, Riwkes S, Braw Y, Levkovitch-Verbin H, Gal G, Fennig S, Treves I, Kron S (2010) A double-blind, randomized study of minocycline for the treatment of negative and cognitive symptoms in early-phase schizophrenia. J Clin Psychiatry 71:138–149

Marder SR (2006) The NIMH-MATRICS project for developing cognition-enhancing agents for schizophrenia. Dialogues Clin Neurosci 8:109–113

Marder SR, Fenton W (2004) Measurement and treatment research to improve cognition in schizophrenia: NIMH MATRICS initiative to support the development of agents for improving cognition in schizophrenia. Schizophr Res 72:5–9

Marder SR, Laughren T, Romano SJ (2017) Why are innovative drugs failing in phase III? Am J Psychiatry 174:829–831

Marx W, Skvarc DR, Mohebbi M, Walker AJ, Meehan A, Turner A, Baker A, Dodd S, Cotton SM, Scott JG, Kavanagh BE, Ashton MM, Brown E, McGrath JJ, Berk M, Dean OM (2021) The effect of adjunctive mangosteen pericarp on cognition in people with schizophrenia: secondary analysis of a randomized controlled trial. Front Psych 12:626486

McClure MM, Graff F, Triebwasser J, Perez-Rodriguez M, Rosell DR, Koenigsberg H, Hazlett EA, Siever LJ, Harvey PD, New AS (2019) Guanfacine augmentation of a combined intervention of computerized cognitive remediation therapy and social skills training for schizotypal personality disorder. Am J Psychiatry 176:307–314

McTeague LM, Huemer J, Carreon DM, Jiang Y, Eickhoff SB, Etkin A (2017) Identification of common neural circuit disruptions in cognitive control across psychiatric disorders. Am J Psychiatry 174:676–685

McTeague LM, Rosenberg BM, Lopez JW, Carreon DM, Huemer J, Jiang Y, Chick CF, Eickhoff SB, Etkin A (2020) Identification of common neural circuit disruptions in emotional processing across psychiatric disorders. Am J Psychiatry 177:411–421

Medalia A, Saperstein AM, Hansen MC, Lee S (2018) Personalised treatment for cognitive dysfunction in individuals with schizophrenia spectrum disorders. Neuropsychol Rehabil 28: 602–613

Medalia A, Saperstein AM, Stefancic A, Meyler S, Styke S, Qian M, Liu J, Cabassa LJ (2021) Feasibility and acceptability of remotely accessed cognitive remediation for schizophrenia in public health settings. Psychiatry Res 301:113956

Mollon J, Reichenberg A (2018) Cognitive development prior to onset of psychosis. Psychol Med 48:392–403

Nuechterlein KH, Green MF, Kern RS, Baade LE, Barch DM, Cohen JD, Essock S, Fenton WS, Frese FJ 3rd, Gold JM, Goldberg T, Heaton RK, Keefe RS, Kraemer H, Mesholam-Gately R, Seidman LJ, Stover E, Weinberger DR, Young AS, Zalcman S, Marder SR (2008) The MATRICS consensus cognitive battery, part 1: test selection, reliability, and validity. Am J Psychiatry 165:203–213

Prikken M, Konings MJ, Lei WU, Begemann MJH, Sommer IEC (2019) The efficacy of computerized cognitive drill and practice training for patients with a schizophrenia-spectrum disorder: a meta-analysis. Schizophr Res 204:368–374

Recio-Barbero M, Segarra R, Zabala A, Gonzalez-Fraile E, Gonzalez-Pinto A, Ballesteros J (2021) Cognitive enhancers in schizophrenia: a systematic review and meta-analysis of alpha-7 nicotinic acetylcholine receptor agonists for cognitive deficits and negative symptoms. Front Psych 12:631589

Reser MP, Slikboer R, Rossell SL (2019) A systematic review of factors that influence the efficacy of cognitive remediation therapy in schizophrenia. Aust N Z J Psychiatry 53:624–641

Saperstein AM, Kurtz MM (2013) Current trends in the empirical study of cognitive remediation for schizophrenia. Can J Psychiatr 58:311–318

Saperstein AM, Choi CJ, Jahshan C, Lynch DA, Wall M, Green MF, Medalia A (2021) Predicting response to cognitive training for schizophrenia using results from two studies with different outcomes. Schizophr Res 231:61–66

Seccomandi B, Agbedjro D, Bell M, Keefe RSE, Keshavan M, Galderisi S, Fiszdon J, Mucci A, Cavallaro R, Ojeda N, Peña J, Müller D, Roder V, Wykes T, Cella M (2021a) Exploring the role of age as a moderator of cognitive remediation for people with schizophrenia. Schizophr Res 228:29–35

Seccomandi B, Agbedjro D, Bell M, Keefe RSE, Keshavan M, Galderisi S, Fiszdon J, Mucci A, Cavallaro R, Bechi M, Ojeda N, Peña J, Wykes T, Cella M (2021b) Can IQ moderate the response to cognitive remediation in people with schizophrenia? J Psychiatr Res 133:38–45

Singer P, Dubroqua S, Yee BK (2015) Inhibition of glycine transporter 1: the yellow brick road to new schizophrenia therapy? Curr Pharm Des 21:3771–3787

Sinkeviciute I, Begemann M, Prikken M, Oranje B, Johnsen E, Lei WU, Hugdahl K, Kroken RA, Rau C, Jacobs JD, Mattaroccia S, Sommer IE (2018) Efficacy of different types of cognitive enhancers for patients with schizophrenia: a meta-analysis. NPJ Schizophr 4:22

Smith MJ, Fleming MF, Wright MA, Roberts AG, Humm LB, Olsen D, Bell MD (2015) Virtual reality job interview training and 6-month employment outcomes for individuals with schizophrenia seeking employment. Schizophr Res 166:86–91

Smucny J, Barch DM, Gold JM, Strauss ME, MacDonald AW 3rd, Boudewyn MA, Ragland JD, Silverstein SM, Carter CS (2019) Cross-diagnostic analysis of cognitive control in mental illness: insights from the CNTRACS consortium. Schizophr Res 208:377–383

Tamminga CA, Pearlson GD, Stan AD, Gibbons RD, Padmanabhan J, Keshavan M, Clementz BA (2017) Strategies for advancing disease definition using biomarkers and genetics: the bipolar and schizophrenia network for intermediate phenotypes. Biol Psychiatr Cogn Neurosci Neuroimaging 2:20–27

Thomas DW, Burns J, Audette J, Carroll A, Dow-Hygelund C, Hay M (2016) Clinical development success rates 2006–2015. Biotechnology Innovation Organization, Washington

Umbricht D, Keefe RS, Murray S, Lowe DA, Porter R, Garibaldi G, Santarelli L (2014) A randomized, placebo-controlled study investigating the nicotinic alpha7 agonist, RG3487, for cognitive deficits in schizophrenia. Neuropsychopharmacology 39:1568–1577

Van Duin D, De Winter L, Oud M, Kroon H, Veling W, Van Weeghel J (2019) The effect of rehabilitation combined with cognitive remediation on functioning in persons with severe mental illness: systematic review and meta-analysis. Psychol Med 49:1414–1425

Vita A, Barlati S, Ceraso A, Nibbio G, Ariu C, Deste G, Wykes T (2021) Effectiveness, core elements, and moderators of response of cognitive remediation for schizophrenia: a systematic review and meta-analysis of randomized clinical trials. JAMA Psychiat 78:848–858

Wykes T, Huddy V, Cellard C, McGurk SR, Czobor P (2011) A meta-analysis of cognitive remediation for schizophrenia: methodology and effect sizes. Am J Psychiatr 168:472–485

The Relationship Between Cannabis, Cognition, and Schizophrenia: It's Complicated

Hakan Kayir, Jessica Ruffolo, Patrick McCunn, and Jibran Y. Khokhar

Contents

Abstract The consequences of cannabis use, especially in the context of schizophrenia, have gained increased importance with the legalization of cannabis in North America and across the globe. Cannabis use has multifaceted impacts on cognition in schizophrenia patients and healthy subjects. Healthy subjects, particularly those

H. Kayir
Department of Biomedical Sciences, Ontario Veterinary College, University of Guelph, Guelph, ON, Canada

J. Ruffolo
Hotchkiss Brain Institute, Cumming School of Medicine, University of Calgary, Calgary, AB, Canada

P. McCunn
Department of Anatomy and Cell Biology, Schulich School of Medicine and Dentistry, University of Western Ontario, London, ON, Canada

J. Y. Khokhar (✉)
Department of Biomedical Sciences, Ontario Veterinary College, University of Guelph, Guelph, ON, Canada

Department of Anatomy and Cell Biology, Schulich School of Medicine and Dentistry, University of Western Ontario, London, ON, Canada
e-mail: jibran.khokhar@schulich.uwo.ca

Curr Topics Behav Neurosci (2023) 63: 437–462
https://doi.org/10.1007/7854_2022_396
Published Online: 2 November 2022

who initiated cannabis use at earlier ages and used high-potency cannabis for longer durations, exhibited poorer cognition mainly in working memory and attention. Cannabis use in schizophrenia has been associated with symptom exacerbation, longer and more frequent psychotic episodes, and poorer treatment outcomes. However, cannabis-using patients have better overall cognitive performance compared to patients who were not cannabis users. Interestingly, these effects were only apparent in lifetime cannabis users, but not in current (or within last 6 months) users. Moreover, higher frequency and earlier age of cannabis use initiation (i.e., before 17 years of age) were associated with better cognitive performance, although they had an earlier illness onset. Three possible hypotheses seem to come forward to explain this paradox. First, some components of cannabis may have antipsychotic or cognitive-enhancing properties. Secondly, chronic cannabis use may alter endocannabinoid signaling in the brain which could be a protective factor for developing psychosis or cognitive impairments. A third explanation could be their representation of a phenotypically distinct patient group with more intact cognitive functioning and less neurodevelopmental pathology. Multiple factors need to be considered to understand the complex relationship between cannabis, cognitive function, and schizophrenia. In short, age at initiation, duration and rate of cannabis use, abstinence duration, co-use of substances and alcohol, prescribed medications, relative cannabinoid composition and potency of cannabis, presence of genetic and environmental vulnerability factors are prominent contributors to the variability in outcomes. Animal studies support the disruptive effects of Δ9-tetrahydrocannabinol (THC) administration during adolescence on attention and memory performance. They provide insights about interaction of cannabinoid receptors with other neurotransmitter systems, such as GABA and glutamate, and other regulatory molecules, such as PSD95 and synaptophysin. Cannabidiol (CBD), on the other hand, can improve cognitive deficits seen in neurodevelopmental and chemically-induced animal models of schizophrenia. Future studies focusing on bridging the translational gaps between human and animal studies, through the use of translationally relevant methods of exposure (e.g., vaping), consistent behavioral assessments, and congruent circuit interrogations (e.g., imaging) will help to further clarify this complex picture.

Keyword Animal models · Cannabinoid(s) · Cannabis · Clinical research · Cognition · Human study · Psychosis · Schizophrenia

1 Cannabis Use in Schizophrenia Patients

The high incidence of substance and alcohol use among patients with schizophrenia presents a significant concern for psychiatry. A recent meta-analysis of 123 studies covering 165,811 subjects estimated the lifetime substance use disorder (SUD) prevalence as 41.7% in schizophrenia spectrum disorders (Hunt et al. 2018). The odds of having a co-occurring SUD are three to six times higher among patients with schizophrenia, as compared to the risk of SUD in the general population. Nicotine is the most frequently used substance among schizophrenia patients with a lifetime prevalence between 60 and 90% (Volkow 2009). The meta-analysis also showed that 26.2% of schizophrenia patients have a co-occurring cannabis use disorder, making cannabis the third most used drug right after alcohol in this patient group.

Legislative changes in the legal status of cannabis have swept across North America. The possible effects of these transitions on the general population, as well as on vulnerable populations such as adolescents and those with psychiatric disorders have become an emerging focus of research (Murray and Hall 2020). A growing number of studies have evaluated the effects of this transition on cannabis use and its health-related effects. However, since this transition is very recent, varies geographically, and the product landscape is continuously changing, many studies have produced conflicting results. The studies examining the effects of cannabis decriminalization or legalization for longer periods may provide better insight, but these studies are very rare. As an example, Portugal decriminalized cannabis together with other abused substances in 2001, and hospitalizations due to cannabis related psychosis increased almost 30-fold between 2000 and 2015 (Gonçalves-Pinho et al. 2020). During this time, rate of hospitalizations for schizophrenia and other psychotic disorders accompanied by cannabis use disorder increased from 0.87 to 10.6% (Gonçalves-Pinho et al. 2020). However, it remains unknown whether this rate is related to increased reporting or increased incidence. Schizophrenia patients with cannabis use disorder may be expected to report cannabis use history more readily in a state that has decriminalized or legalized cannabis compared to a state that has not. Similarly, when historical results are compared in a country before and after legalization, the likelihood of self-reporting of drug use would remain a confounding factor (Livne et al. 2022). Moreover, in a place where cannabis is illegal, the process of procuring cannabis may require different cognitive and social abilities. As a result, studies from different countries may report patient profiles representing distinct subgroups, which would require a more measured approach by researchers hoping to compare and reconcile between these findings.

Another important issue worth mentioning is the changing composition of cannabis. The concentration of the main psychotropic ingredient in cannabis, Δ9-tetrahydrocannabinol (THC), has been constantly increasing while the non-stimulant ingredient cannabidiol (CBD) concentration remains stable. According to the analyses of samples obtained from Drug and Enforcement Administration (DEA), THC concentrations increased from 4 to 12% during the years of 1995–2014. Because CBD content has not changed, the ratio of THC/CBD has increased from 14 to 80 during this time period (Freeman et al. 2021) and the risk of developing psychosis is doubled with the use of higher potency cannabis (>10% THC concentration) (Di Forti et al. 2019).

Although the epidemiological evidence is strong, the origins of SUD and schizophrenia co-occurrence have not been well understood. Several theories have been proposed to explain this relationship. The oft-discussed self-medication hypothesis suggests that schizophrenia patients use substance to lessen their primary symptoms or side effects of the antipsychotic treatments (Schofield et al. 2006). Tobacco smoking has been commonly proposed to be driven by self-medication in schizophrenia patients (Leonard et al. 2007). Because nicotinic receptors play an important role in several cognitive functions such as attention and memory, it usually seemed plausible for the researchers. However, not all existing literature supports this hypothesis with a variety of studies showing findings contrary to self-medication (Manzella et al. 2015).

Conversely, the diathesis-stress (two-hit) model suggests that drugs serve as an environmental risk factor contributing to the manifestation of the disease in vulnerable individuals (Maynard et al. 2001). Stimulants such as cocaine and amphetamine are widely accepted as risk factors for schizophrenia development (Bramness et al. 2012). Recently cannabis use, especially during adolescence, has also been suggested to contribute to the risk for schizophrenia. A meta-analysis including almost 67,000 subjects showed that heavy cannabis users have a fourfold increased risk for psychotic disorders compared to non-users (Marconi et al. 2016). A recent systemic review of 13 meta-analyses of longitudinal studies on cannabis use showed that 10 of them indicated a significantly increased risk of psychosis compared with non-users, while two of the remaining three pointed to an increased likelihood (Sideli et al. 2020).

The biological vulnerability hypothesis proposes that both schizophrenia and addictive substances share common biological and genetic features (Chambers et al. 2001). It differs from the self-medication and diathesis-stress hypotheses mainly by accepting both SUD and schizophrenia as primary diseases and the independent manifestations of a common neuropathology. These competing hypotheses are not necessarily mutually exclusive (Khokhar et al. 2018). Deficits in brain reward circuit function or reward deficiency syndrome have been proposed as a common source of addiction and schizophrenia symptoms. Such a deficiency could create a vulnerable state for initiation of substance use prior to onset of psychotic symptoms and lead to a diathesis-stress to induce psychosis. On the other hand, patients might self-medicate their reward deficiency through their continued use of substances (Green et al. 2007). For the primary psychotic disorder, reward deficiency could also be related with negative symptoms such as anhedonia and even cognitive deficits related with goal-directed behaviors, response inhibition, and performance monitoring (Gold et al. 2008; Strauss et al. 2014).

Although addictive drugs have initially distinct effects, they all produce some common effects on brain reward circuits. The main component of these reward circuits is mesocorticolimbic dopaminergic pathway that originates from ventral tegmental area and projects to nucleus accumbens and prefrontal cortex. The reward pathway is mostly inclined to be evaluated as a standalone system just mediating reward, but it has far more complex functions such as encoding attention, expectancy of reward and effort, disconfirmation of reward expectancy, optimal decision-making, and incentive motivation (Hauser et al. 2017; Kesby et al. 2018). Furthermore, during chronic use of the addictive drugs, other brain areas and circuits develop dysregulated adaptations that worsen over time. These adaptations leading to SUD are conceptualized as a recurring cycle and involve neuroplastic changes in the brain reward, stress, and executive function systems (Koob and Volkow 2016). CB1 receptors and their endogenous ligands anandamide and 2-arachidonoylglycerol (2-AG) are abundant in dopaminergic pathways. These endogenous cannabinoids modulate dopaminergic neurotransmission acting as a retrograde feedback system on presynaptic glutamatergic and γ-aminobutyric acid (GABA) nerve terminals (Michael A.P. Bloomfield et al. 2016).

On the other hand, malfunctioning mesocorticolimbic dopaminergic pathways is one of the most studied hypotheses in the etiology of schizophrenia. It is well known that all of the current antipsychotic drugs block striatal D2 receptors at clinical doses, and occupancy of D2 receptors is correlated with the treatment response (Nordström et al. 1993). Accordingly, increased dopaminergic neurotransmission primarily in the associative striatum (or cognitive striatum that establishes major connections with the frontal lobe) was consistently reported in these patients. Dopamine serves as a major regulator of communication between striatum and prefrontal cortex. Normal functioning of this system is needed for flexible updating of working memory, and protecting against memory interference, which are crucial components of cognitive control (Orellana and Slachevsky 2013). Noise or imbalance in these circuits could lead to a range of symptoms related to several cognitive domains, including attention, reward learning, goal-directed action and decision-making (Orellana and Slachevsky 2013; McCutcheon et al. 2019).

These two conditions, cannabis use and schizophrenia, seem to share similarities at genetic, etiologic, epidemiologic, and brain circuit levels. Although this overlap remains very complex, current studies in humans and experimental animals provide some insights into these multifaceted associations. A large-scale genome-wide association study (GWAS) found a significant correlation between lifetime cannabis use and schizophrenia. Furthermore, a Mendelian randomization approach indicated strong causal evidence for increased cannabis use in schizophrenia patients and weaker evidence for cannabis use to increased risk of schizophrenia (Pasman et al. 2018). However, another Mendelian randomization analysis used SNPs associated with ever use of cannabis and reported a significant causal link for the increased risk of schizophrenia in cannabis use (Vaucher et al. 2018). The current chapter focuses on the effects of cannabis on cognitive functions (capturing some of the Research Domain Criteria [RDoC] Cognitive Systems Domains, where possible) in healthy subjects and in patients with schizophrenia. Preclinical studies are also valuable at dissecting the causal basis of these associations, and we have summarized studies related to the effects of cannabinoids in experimental models of healthy and impaired cognitive function.

2 Cannabis and Cognition in Healthy Individuals

While cannabis use is common and widespread, the implications and consequences of this use are still unclear both during the acute and chronic stages of use. The traditional view of cannabis largely held that it produced overall cognitive decline in healthy users, in a time- and dose-dependent manner. Many studies suggest a decline in several cognitive domains, particularly in attention and memory functions in cannabis users compared to non-users (Shrivastava et al. 2011). The temporal nature of this cognitive decline is the subject of much debate. Acute effects of cannabis on cognition have been shown in many studies, but again vary greatly based on use history, route of administration, and behavioral metric tested. The body of research focused on long-term effects due to cannabis is similarly divergent and varies greatly based on experimental setup and measured outcomes.

One area where there is some agreement amongst the research literature is that the age of onset of cannabis use, which shows a relationship with the severity of cognitive decline when that decline is observed. This relationship comes as no surprise though, as cannabis use usually initiates during critical developmental periods of adolescence and could induce persistent changes to brain structure and function. At this stage it should be noted that cannabis use during adolescence increases the risk for schizophreniform disorders up to 46% in large nationwide studies (Niemi-Pynttäri et al. 2013). The effects of cannabis on healthy individuals will be discussed first in this chapter followed by patients with psychosis. Suffice to say it is essential to discuss the cannabis use literature with an eye toward contextual factors that may contribute to the relationship between cannabis use and cognition.

2.1 *Effects of Cannabis on Attention*

Impaired attention has long been considered an effect of cannabis use. Several studies have supported the notion that acute exposure to cannabinoids impairs focused, divided, or sustained attention, often in a dose-dependent manner (D'Souza et al. 2004, 2008; Hunault et al. 2009; Wesnes et al. 2010; Bedi et al. 2013; Theunissen et al. 2015). When considering all the evidence available, it appears that this impairment is mild and does not produce severe cognitive impairment or deficits (Shrivastava et al. 2011). Often the effects are subtle and become unmeasurable after a brief period of abstinence (Bosker et al. 2013). In cases where lesser impairments were observed, this has been attributed to tolerance among daily users, but may also point to differential effects amongst individual users (Ramaekers et al. 2009; Ramesh et al. 2013). However, it remains unknown if long-term heavy cannabis use can result in permanent changes in attention.

Chronic cannabis use has also been associated with deficits in attention, but again substantial variation is seen in the results, which may be attributed to methodological differences, such as inclusion criteria, tasks used to assess attention, prior use, or a myriad of other factors (Scott et al. 2018). Studies have shown regular cannabis users exhibited poor performance compared to controls across several tasks measuring attention, after both brief and longer abstinence periods (Solowij and Battisti 2008; Lisdahl and Price 2012; Dougherty et al. 2013). Conversely, other studies have shown that regular cannabis users did not differ in attentional task performance compared to controls (Fried et al. 2005; Grant et al. 2012; Becker et al. 2014). For most individuals, chronic cannabis use does not appear to lead to significant impairment in attention or attentional processing, but can result in mild, but measurable, cognitive difficulties (Accordino and Hart 2006; Lisdahl and Price 2012). Based on these findings, many individuals who regularly use cannabis would perform reasonably well on routine, everyday life tasks, but might encounter difficulties when performing complex tasks requiring focused attention or careful multi-tasking.

One particular area of focus is cannabis use in early adolescence that continues through to young adulthood. Individuals who initiate regular cannabis use early in life are more likely to display attention deficits (Ehrenreich et al. 1999; Scott et al. 2018). Among studies examining the relationship between chronic cannabis use and attention, impairments were more commonly reported among adolescents (Harvey et al. 2007; Medina et al. 2007; Hanson et al. 2010; Dougherty et al. 2013). Users abstinent for 23 days remained impaired relative to control subjects, despite improvements in sustained and divided attention with increasing abstinence; poor attentional performance was also associated with younger age of onset (Bosker et al. 2013). However, no difference or improvements between abstinent former users and control subjects on broader measures of attention were also reported (Lyons et al. 2004; Fried et al. 2005; Hooper et al. 2014; Thames et al. 2014). Whether those deficits are reversible through abstinence still remain an area of continued research.

2.2 *Effects of Cannabis on Working Memory*

Memory function has been the most consistently studied cognitive domain in relation to the effects of cannabis. The literature surrounding cannabis use and its effects on memory largely mirrors that of its effects on attention. Deficits in memory function are associated with regular cannabis use (Solowij and Battisti 2008; Scott et al. 2018) but the evidence to support or refute that association is inconsistent, due in part to widely varying methodological approaches. Many studies have shown a link between frequent cannabis use and memory deficits (Dougherty et al. 2013; Becker et al. 2014), particularly amongst those who have engaged in long-term cannabis use (Becker et al. 2018). Conversely, several studies have shown no differences in memory function amongst those who engage in frequent cannabis use and those that do not (Lisdahl and Price 2012; McKetin et al. 2016). Some studies point to abstinence as a factor in these disparate findings (Bhattacharyya and Schoeler 2013) and propose a relationship by which memory deficits due to cannabis use progressively weaken as the length of abstinence grows (Scott et al. 2018).

Working memory, in particular, is an area of focus of much literature surrounding cannabis use. Working memory refers to a form of short-term memory that allows an individual to store and manipulate information in their mind for a short period of time, and it is closely related to attention (Baddeley 1992). Impairment of working memory, much like other cognitive function, shows varied effects amongst cannabis users, but it has a relatively consistent pattern of impairment during acute cannabis administration or use. Chronic cannabis use impairs working memory in young adults, as shown in immediate recall, verbal reasoning, and working memory tasks; also, spatial working memory impairments are common in adolescent cannabis users (Hamidullah et al. 2020; Thorpe et al. 2020). Acute intoxication appears to impair working memory in a dose-dependent fashion (Hart et al. 2001). While some studies have shown that this working memory impairment persists, the impairment is generally short-term and resolves quickly following a period of abstinence. Pope and Yurgelun-Todd (1996) found no differences in working memory abilities between recently abstinent (19 h) heavy and light cannabis users compared with control subjects. In addition, no significant differences were found in working memory abilities of recently abstinent cannabis users across multiple studies (Kanayama et al. 2004; Whitlow et al. 2004; Jager et al. 2006; Fisk and Montgomery 2008).

In contrast to the acute effects, less consistency exists regarding the long-term effects of cannabis use on neurocognitive functioning. The long-term impacts of frequent cannabis use on cognition, if present, appear to be strongest in individuals who engage in heavy cannabis use early in life (Solowij and Battisti 2008; Gruber et al. 2012). As a whole, the available evidence suggests that chronic and heavy cannabis use is related to attention and working memory difficulties that might be entirely reversible, except among individuals who initiated regular use early in life and have been using cannabis for a significant part of their life but have not developed a clinically significant psychiatric or neurological disorder (Bhattacharyya and Schoeler 2013). On the other hand, if these individuals have received a psychiatric diagnosis, then they are evaluated under another group such as schizophrenia or dual diagnosis, and the effect of cannabis may interact with the risk for those disorders to produce the effects on cognition.

3 Effects of Cannabinoids on Attention and Memory in Schizophrenia Patients

Cannabis use among healthy populations has been associated with cognitive impairments, especially working memory and attention. However, among patients with schizophrenia the association is less clear. Cannabis use in schizophrenia has been associated with symptom exacerbation, longer and more frequent psychotic episodes, and poorer treatment outcomes (Grech et al. 2005; Jenkins and Khokhar 2021). While there are studies showing acute THC administration to schizophrenia patients can aggravate the disease symptoms including cognitive functions (D'Souza et al. 2005), CBD, the other psychoactive, but not psychotomimetic, component in cannabis shows antipsychotic properties (Batalla et al. 2019). On the other hand, chronic cannabis users with schizophrenia have been found to have superior cognitive functioning compared to non-users, at least in certain subgroups of patients (Jockers-Scherübl et al. 2007). Thus, while cannabis use is usually associated with cognitive impairment in healthy subjects, the association is more complex in the case of schizophrenia pathology. With relatively fewer studies in this domain, most studies have not separated attention and memory in patients with schizophrenia

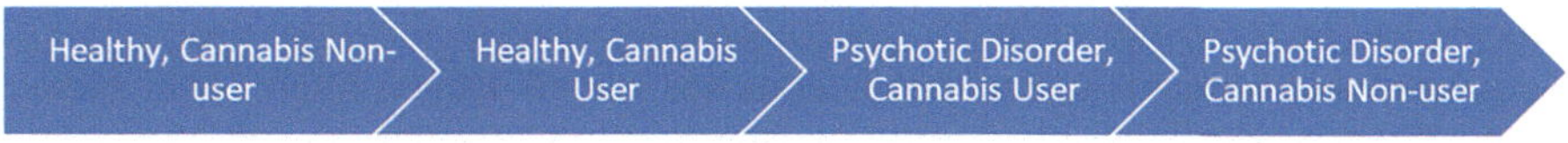

Fig. 1 Hierarchical order for cognitive functioning in different groups of subjects

as the studies in healthy subjects have; therefore, we will discuss them together in this section.

The cognitive effects of cannabinoids on schizophrenia patients are under the influence of various factors. These variables, such as the relative cannabinoid content of the cannabis (THC, CBD, etc.) of the administered or consumed drug (Jenkins et al. 2022), administration dose and route, previous cannabis usage, age of initiation, abstinence time prior to study, age, and gender are confounding factors in studies on healthy subjects already. In schizophrenia patients several others such as current antipsychotic treatment, age of onset and duration of the illness, severity of the disease, and concomitant use of other substances (mainly nicotine and alcohol) can also contribute to variability in outcomes.

A meta-analysis study comparing the effect of cannabis use on 11 different memory domains in 7,697 healthy subjects and 3,261 subjects with a psychotic disorder showed that cannabis use significantly impaired global memory in healthy cannabis users compared to non-users. Conversely, in patients with psychosis, cannabis use was associated with better performance in these tasks compared to patients who do not use cannabis (Fig. 1) (Schoeler et al. 2016). In the healthy sample, most of the memory dimensions were significantly impaired by cannabis use. The most obvious impairment was observed in prospective memory domain. The patients with cannabis use had either no impairments or performed significantly better especially in working memory, visual immediate recall, visual recognition, verbal recognition domains compared to those without cannabis use. Interestingly, in this study, healthy cannabis users showed higher levels of depressive symptoms while cannabis users in the patient sample had lower levels of depressive symptoms compared to non-user counterparts.

Another meta-analysis comparing 572 patients with schizophrenia with and without comorbid cannabis use, investigated broader cognitive functioning including attention, planning, processing speed, and various types of memory domains. Cannabis-using schizophrenia patients had better overall cognitive performance compared to patients who were not cannabis users. They had faster processing speeds, better verbal memory and working memory, better planning, and reasoning abilities. Interestingly, these effects were only apparent in lifetime cannabis users but not in current (or within last 6 months) users. Moreover, higher frequency and earlier age of cannabis use initiation (i.e., before 17 years of age) were associated with better cognitive performance although they had an earlier illness onset. However, cannabis-using patients did have more severe positive symptoms (Yucel et al. 2012). This study provided valuable insights about the cannabis use profile in patients with schizophrenia and first-episode psychosis (FEP). Similar, but less profound, effects of previous cannabis use in FEP patients were also observed; cannabis-using FEP patients had better visual memory, planning, and reasoning than non-users. Again, the subgroup of cannabis-using FEP patients that started using cannabis at an earlier age (<17 years) did better in several tests compared to later starting subgroups, and recent cannabis use was negatively association with these outcomes. Another subgroup analysis revealed that comorbid amphetamine or alcohol use did not have any effect on cognitive function (Yucel et al. 2012).

A recent study in a large group of FEP patients (948 patients and 1,313 controls from 6 countries) revealed that occasional cannabis users had 8 points higher IQ compared with their never-user counterparts in FEP patients and 3 points higher IQ in control group. On the other hand, daily cannabis users from patient and control groups had lower academic achievement scores. For social functioning, occasional and daily cannabis-using patients had better scores (i.e., less social withdrawal) compared to never-using counterparts (Ferraro et al. 2020).

Several hypotheses have been put forward to explain this paradoxical relationship. Firstly, the chemical composition of cannabis, aside from the psychotomimetic THC, may have properties that may be protective against cognitive decline in psychosis. THC and CBD are known as major psychoactive cannabinoids, and they have potentially opposing effects; while THC is psychotomimetic, CBD has proposed antipsychotic activity. Currently, there are six published studies and 13 ongoing studies (according to clinicaltrials.gov) examining the effects of CBD in psychotic disorders. In one of these published studies, CBD was administered as a monotherapy, and in the five other studies it was used as an adjunct therapy (Kirkland et al. 2022). In the monotherapy study, 800 mg daily dose of CBD had similar effects with amisulpride in improving Positive and Negative Syndrome Scale (PANSS) scores, but CBD had fewer side effects (Leweke et al. 2012). Overall, three of these six studies showed positive effects of CBD in PANSS score, however they failed to show any significant positive effects on cognitive functions. However, based on meta-analysis studies showing that recency of cannabis use had a negative impact on cognition, the long-term outcomes of these therapeutic applications would be a better approach than assessing the acute impact of CBD on cognition.

Most cannabis use studies in humans do not provide details about the composition of consumed cannabis product; a few studies have loosely defined them as high or low potency according to the used cannabis type. Sinsemilla type cannabis containing more than 10% THC is accepted as high potency while hash or resin types are thought to be low potency. These studies indicate a strong association between increased incidence of FEP and THC-rich, high-potency cannabis use (Di Forti et al. 2019). An interesting finding from a meta-analysis by Schoeler et al. (2016) was the almost two-fold increase in the memory disrupting effects of cannabis in healthy subjects in studies published after 2000 compared to the previous period. This study provided findings only for healthy subjects, with most of the studies in patients with psychosis being performed after year 2000. A possible explanation for this difference is the consistent increases in THC content in the cannabis products over time. THC and CBD concentrations in confiscated cannabis products have been monitored since 1984 (Mehmedic et al. 2010). According to an assessment from 1995 to 2014, THC content of cannabis plant material has consistently risen from 4% to 12%. On the other hand, the CBD content first increased to 0.28% until 2001 but then decreased to less than 0.15% in 2014. As a result, the ratio of THC to CBD was around 14:1 until 2001 and then increased to 80: 1 in 2014 (ElSohly et al. 2016). A more recent analysis of the same monitoring data indicated that the THC:CBD ratio had reached 103.48 in 2017. However, possibly due to widespread legalization, a decrease in THC:CBD ratio was recorded in later years with a ratio of 24.58 being observed in 2019 (ElSohly et al. 2021). Future studies in healthy and patient groups should include additional details on the potency and composition of the consumed cannabis products in order to provide a deeper understanding of the impact of cannabis composition on cognitive function in both healthy and clinical populations. Developing better, easier, and cheaper methods to describe the potency of cannabis products would be another approach. Expanding the study of the effects of THC and CBD on cognitive functions in clinical trials has also been recommended as an urgent need in this area (Rømer Thomsen et al. 2017).

Furthermore, the cannabis plant contains more than 560 compounds, 120 of which are cannabinoids, and 60 of which are unique to cannabis, with these numbers increasing with more research (ElSohly et al. 2021). We have limited information on the other cannabinoids such as Δ8-tetrahydrocannabinol, Δ9-tetrahydrocannabivarin, cannabinol, cannabidivarin, cannabigerol, and they could possibly have distinct effects on brain (Turner et al. 2017). Also, the unique complement of cannabinoids and terpenes found in the cannabis plant has been suggested to produce an "entourage effect"; however, this suggestion remains contentious. Furthermore, besides their acute or chronic effects, these compounds might also have distinct effects on brain development, making this an important area for future research.

A second possible explanation could be the modulation of endogenous cannabinoid-based neurotransmission by cannabis and their effects on the cognition. The lipid-based endogenous mediators, anandamide (AEA) and 2-arachidonoylglycerol (2-AG) are the best studied endocannabinoid molecules; 2-AG is a high efficacy agonist for both CB1 and CB2 receptors, and AEA is a low efficacy agonist at CB1 receptors and a very low efficacy agonist at CB2 receptors. There is strong evidence that endocannabinoids can bind other receptors too including the transient receptor potential cation channel subfamily V member 1 (TRPV1, capsaicin receptor) which plays a role in AEA mediating pain transmission (Di Marzo and De Petrocellis 2012). They may also regulate many distinct physiological functions such as cognition, sleep, energy metabolism, and inflammation through indirect modulation of different neurotransmitter systems such as dopamine, glutamate, and γ-aminobutyric acid (GABA) (Lu and Mackie 2021).

Cannabis has long-lasting effects on the endocannabinoid system. Increases in CB1 and CB2 receptor mRNA expression in blood cells, and increased serum concentration of 2-AG in chronic cannabis users have also been reported (Nong et al. 2002). Another study showed the persistence of cannabis-induced changes in the endocannabinoid system; even after 6 months of abstinence, increased CB2 receptor mRNA expression and increased serum AEA levels could be detected in peripheral blood samples of subjects that used cannabis more than 20 times in their lifetime (Muhl et al. 2014). The frequent (>10 times/month) cannabis users have higher AEA levels in cerebrospinal fluid (CSF) samples and lower 2-AG levels in peripheral serum samples compared to infrequent users. Despite the small sample size, the study also showed that higher levels of CSF AEA levels are associated with a lower risk of psychotic symptoms following cannabis use or psychotic symptoms observed during a drug-free state (Morgan et al. 2013). The aforementioned clinical trials investigating CBD as an antipsychotic, showed that CBD increased serum AEA levels, and this increase inversely correlated with psychotic symptoms and positively correlated with clinical improvements. A postponed and lower transition rate from initial prodromal states into psychosis was observed in the patients with higher AEA levels (Leweke et al. 2012).

A meta-analysis of studies measuring endocannabinoids in CSF and/or blood in psychosis showed that CSF and blood AEA levels are consistently high in patients compared to healthy controls. Increased CSF AEA levels were observed at any stage of psychosis (prodromal, first-episode, and multi-episode) and independent from antipsychotic treatment and cannabis usage. Moreover, AEA levels are inversely associated with symptom severity including cognitive performance. Reduced expression of synthesizing enzymes and increased expression of degrading enzymes in peripheral immune cells in more severe cases were also supported by findings from AEA measurement studies. While there are conflicting reports, the majority of these studies suggest that AEA elevation in psychosis may reflect a compensatory adaptation to the disease state (Minichino et al. 2019). Patients using cannabis may use cannabis to modulate their endogenous cannabinoid functioning to prevent the debilitating progression of the disease itself. Exploring the potential of CBD, or other drug candidates modulating endocannabinoids in the treatment of psychotic disorders is warranted, especially for improving impaired cognitive functioning which does not benefit from current therapeutics (Mielnik et al. 2021).

A third explanation for the paradoxical cognitive-enhancing effects of cannabis in schizophrenia patients could be their representation of a phenotypically distinct patient group with more intact cognitive functioning and less neurodevelopmental pathology, especially in places where cannabis may not be legalized and therefore more difficult to obtain. Cannabis use in schizophrenia patients usually starts at an early age, mainly during adolescence, and associations of increased risk exist with high-dose and high-potency cannabis use (Schoeler et al. 2016). On the other hand, abstinence duration before the cognitive tests is associated with better performance, and recency of cannabis use having the opposite effect (Rabin et al. 2013). Early and heavy cannabis use can induce psychosis or facilitate the transition to psychotic states in a group of patients that might otherwise not have experienced psychosis (Schoeler et al. 2016). Because these patients may not carry a substantial neurodevelopmental and genetic burden of schizophrenia, they are not as vulnerable as patients with genetic risk of schizophrenia to the disruptive effects of cannabis-induced psychosis. When they cease cannabis use, they may experience remission sooner, compared to those that have a tendency for psychosis.

This subgroup of schizophrenia patients was also considered to have better social skills before starting use of cannabis, because they needed to be socialized to facilitate drug-seeking behavior (Rabin et al. 2013). These patients may belong to a subgroup of schizophrenia distinct from those that experience drug-induced psychosis. According to DSM-5, the distinction between substance-induced psychosis and schizophrenia is the persistence of psychosis more than 1 month after last exposure to the substance (American Psychiatric Association 2013). A recent Swedish registry-based study revealed the 7-year follow-up results of 7,606 individuals diagnosed of substance-induced psychotic disorder between 1997 and 2015, showing that 11.3% of these patients developed schizophrenia in general and the risk increased to 18% in cannabis users (Kendler et al. 2019). Previously, a nationwide Finnish study including 18,478 individuals calculated the cumulative risk ratio for development of schizophrenia spectrum disorders as 46% for cannabis users (Niemi-Pynttäri et al. 2013). Cannabis use had the highest risk compared to other drugs in both studies, and they both showed that this transition took almost 3 years after the first substance use diagnosis (Niemi-Pynttäri et al. 2013; Kendler et al. 2019). Furthermore, the Swedish study analyzed the familial risk scores calculated from first-, second-, and third-degree relatives for nonaffective psychosis, drug abuse, and alcohol use disorder. Individuals with substance-induced psychotic disorder had higher familial risk score for drug and alcohol use disorder compared to familial risk for psychosis. On the other hand, the familial risk scores for nonaffective psychosis were higher in the patients who converted from substance-induced psychotic disorder to schizophrenia. In short, substance-induced psychosis may be more prevalent in those with low psychosis vulnerability, but high familial vulnerability to drugs and alcohol, whereas schizophrenia following substance-induced psychosis may be better described as the precipitation of the disorder by drug use in vulnerable individuals (Kendler et al. 2019). Thus, developing clinical interventions to monitor and reduce cannabis use in individuals having familial risk or known vulnerability may prove beneficial.

4 Cognition-Related Effects of Cannabinoids in Animal Models

In this section of the chapter, we will attempt to summarize multiple animal studies on the cognitive sequelae of cannabis exposure, particularly exposure to the cannabinoids THC and CBD, investigating the alterations across several cognitive RDoC-relevant domains such as sensorimotor gating, higher order functioning, learning, memory, and sociability. The potential relationship between cannabis and schizophrenia has a multifactorial etiology with a variety of environmental factors and genetic predispositions playing a role in the pathology. Thus, utilizing animal models with face, construct, and predictive validity provides an opportunity to elucidate the causal cannabis-induced cognitive consequences and relate these behavioral outcomes relevant to schizophrenia. This allows for controlled experiments without the confounds inherent in human studies including the frequency and amount of cannabis used, the composition of the cannabinoid, polydrug use, and comorbid mental illness. The most prominent differences between animal and human studies are the composition of the drugs used and route of administration. While human studies rarely evaluate the effects of parenterally administered pure THC or selective CB receptor agonists, animal studies rarely use cannabis vapor. This impacts the face validity of animal studies but increases the controllability of drug effects. Recent studies using vape systems in animals provide promising results in order to increase the validity of cannabis related models (Jenkins et al. 2022).

In human studies working memory tests usually reflect the functioning of prefrontal cortex and its intrinsic connectivity with other brain regions (Goldman-Rakic and Selemon 1997). However, working memory is often conceptualized differently in humans and animals (Dudchenko et al. 2013). In animals, standard working memory tests require learning information, usually related to visuospatial cues, about a desired outcome, and retaining it for a limited duration. They are usually assessed using delayed alternation of goals in maze-based tasks within a single session, but not typically between session (i.e., radial arm maze (RAM), Morris water maze [MWM] with alternating platform and T-maze). On the other hand, delayed non-matching-to-sample (DNMS) tasks can be performed in mazes or in operant boxes, by using objects or odors. The DNMS tasks assess the animal's ability to remember a stimulus that is no longer present after a variable delay interval (Dudchenko 2004). Thus, these tests may involve spatial memory and engage the hippocampus and may require temporary forms of consolidation in order to sustain behavioral performance in these tasks. However, working memory deficits in schizophrenia are not observed in delay dependent tasks. RDoC specifies goal maintenance, interference control, and span capacity aspects of working memory, and the animal models aiming to represent these features would better reflect the situation observed in patients. These differences should be taken into consideration for evaluating findings from rodent working memory test tasks (Dudchenko et al. 2013).

The age of exposure is another critical determinant of the effects of cannabis on cognitive functions. Accordingly, during adolescence, neuronal changes and synaptic remodeling take place to increase cognitive efficiency, and these functional and structural changes lead to maturation of brain circuits. During this period, limbic brain regions drive impulsive and risky behaviors, as prefrontocortical control is slower to develop. These changes occur together with rebalancing of excitatory/inhibitory glutamate/GABA circuitry, as well as myelination and reorganization of brain areas such as amygdala and hippocampus (Spear 2000). Thus, given the ongoing maturation at this time, adolescence is a period of elevated susceptibility to cannabinoid-induced neuronal and behavioral changes. At this stage, disruptions to the neurodevelopmental trajectories by cannabis exposure could be an important factor for triggering the psychotic disorders or cognitive deficits. It is still under debate that whether cannabis exposure is enough to induce a disruption at a sensitive neurodevelopmental period, or it uncovers latent predispositions in vulnerable populations.

4.1 Effects of THC on Cognition in Rodents

Although there is controversy among adult animals with respect to the lasting effects of THC on cognition, THC exposure during adolescence demonstrates significant cognitive impairments when animals are tested in adulthood period. For instance, adolescents that have been repeatedly exposed to THC exhibit heightened sensitivity and demonstrate greater spatial and recognition memory impairments when tested as adults (Cha et al. 2007; Rubino et al. 2009; Zamberletti et al. 2014; Hamidullah et al. 2020). More importantly, these effects continued beyond the cessation of THC treatment, thus resulting in long-lasting residual cognitive changes. Adult THC treatment did not induce long-term cognitive dysfunctions as compared to the adolescent exposure (Murphy et al. 2017). Thereby indicating the severity of the effects of cannabis is also dependent on the age that the exposure takes place.

The type of behavioral test is also an important factor that contributes to the variability in outcomes observed after cannabis or cannabinoid exposure. Although there are contradictory findings, MWM, fear conditioning, and passive avoidance for cognitive assessments seem less sensitive compared to RAM, Y-maze, novel object recognition, and active avoidance for the long-lasting effects of THC (Stark et al. 2021). Interestingly, intravenous THC self-administration during adolescence can increase the performance in delayed match-to-sample (DMTS) task during adulthood in rats (Stringfield and Torregrossa 2021). Such an increase in performance in DMTS task was also shown not only with cannabis smoke but also placebo smoke exposure, that was known to produce carbon monoxide and possibly other molecules that might interfere with neurodevelopmental stages (Hernandez et al. 2021). Besides these effects on learning and memory, adolescent THC exposure induced disruptions in pre-pulse inhibition (PPI) in adult animals, but not when administered only in adulthood (Renard et al. 2017; Abela et al. 2019).

Among studies examining the relationship between THC and attentional capacity, common assessments include the 5-choice serial reaction time task (5-CSRT). 5-CSRT requires animals to allocate their attention toward different spatial locations to achieve optimal performance. The deleterious effects of THC on attention are observed following chronic THC exposure in a 5-CSRT, where THC-exposed rats exhibit long-lasting deficits in response accuracy (Irimia et al. 2015). The attentional-set-shifting task (ASST) assesses an animal's ability to shift attentional bias between different perceptual features of complex stimuli, and it requires cognitive flexibility and sustained attention. Both acute and chronic THC exposure have shown to have no impact on outcomes of ASST (Szkudlarek et al. 2019; Weimar et al. 2020). These incompatible results may be reliant on the task's ability to recruit different neuronal pathways in relation to attentional processing.

Many different mechanisms have been proposed to explain the effect of THC on the developing brain. Primarily, CB1 receptor expression levels were reduced in the prefrontal cortex, hippocampus, periaqueductal gray and ventral midbrain, amygdala, VTA, and nucleus accumbens of adult rats treated with THC during adolescence. Interestingly, these changes were more widespread in female rats compared to males (Rubino et al. 2008; Burston et al. 2010; Renard et al. 2017). Because CB1 receptors provide retrograde feedback for GABA and glutamate neurotransmission, it is not surprising to find changes in these systems. Decreased numbers of GABAergic cells and decreased expression of GABA synthesis machinery in cortical areas were observed along with increases in NMDA and AMPA receptor subunits such as GluN2B, GluA1, and GluA2 in hippocampal post-synaptic fractions. These changes may indicate an imbalance between glutamate and GABA systems induced by adolescence THC exposure (Zamberletti et al. 2014, 2016). Among the other changes, increased dopamine levels in nucleus accumbens core (in contrast to a decrease in shell subregion), and the upregulation of dopamine transporter in striatum could have significant effects on the observed behavioral changes. Increases in dopamine D1 receptors in nucleus accumbens and D2 receptor in cortex, but decreases in hippocampus may also contribute to altered cognitive and affective states. Similar to changes in cannabinoid system, the other effects of adolescence THC exposure are appeared to be sex specific (Michael A. P. Bloomfield et al. 2016; Renard et al. 2017). Furthermore, reduced synaptic plasticity has been found in the hippocampus and cortex of rats exposed to THC. The expression levels of the synaptic plasticity markers such as synaptophysin, PSD95, β-catenin were decreased in the hippocampus and cortex of adult rats exposed to THC during adolescence, further supporting a dysregulation in hippocampus–prefrontal cortex pathway (Renard et al. 2017).

4.2 *Effects of CBD on Cognition in Rodents*

CBD may have some antipsychotic and anxiolytic properties in both rodents and humans. In rodents, CBD improves cognition and social interaction deficits in adult male rat offspring exposed to maternal immune activation (MIA), a developmental model of schizophrenia (Osborne et al. 2017). CBD reversed amphetamine- and MK-801-induced disruption of PPI, as well as PPI disruption seen in spontaneously hypertensive rats (SHR) (Stark et al. 2021), a common model of ADHD. CBD effectively ameliorated the recognition learning and memory disruptions in novel object recognition (NOR) test produced by the MIA model. Importantly, chronic CBD treatment does not cause any other behavioral or metabolic dysfunctions when evaluated either immediately after the treatments or 1 month after CBD discontinuation (Peres et al. 2018).

Gestational methylazoxymethanol acetate (MAM) treatment induces adult-onset phenotypes relevant to schizophrenia in rat offspring, including cognitive deficits and dopaminergic dysfunction. In this neurodevelopmental model of schizophrenia, CBD restored cannabinoid/GABAergic signaling deficits, and reversed the increased CB1 and dopamine D3 receptor mRNA expressions (Stark et al. 2020). CBD has also been proposed to act as a partial agonist on D2High receptors in a very similar manner to the antipsychotic aripiprazole (Seeman 2016). However, in animal studies, no direct effect of CBD on dopamine D2 receptors or dopamine levels was observed (Hasbi et al. 2020). It seems that CBD can modulate mesolimbic dopaminergic pathway activity without directly acting on D1 and D2 receptors, possibly through less studied signaling pathways such as mTOR/70-kDa ribosomal protein S6 kinase (p70S6K) (Renard et al. 2016). A recent study supports the functional role of mTOR/p70S6K pathway in the effects of CBD. Administration of CBD directly into the prefrontal cortex of rats induces cognitive dysfunction by disrupting latent inhibition and spontaneous oddity discrimination tasks. Latent inhibition represents the ability of inhibiting previously learned associations in a new situation while oddity discrimination represents recognition memory. Interestingly, CBD impairs those cognitive functions via activation of 5-HT1A receptors and reduced phosphorylation of p70S6K (Szkudlarek et al. 2021).

These studies in animal models provide valuable insights about the effects of THC and CBD for understanding the cannabinoid system in development and pathogenesis of schizophrenia. However, studies evaluating the effects of other routes of administration, such as vapor or edible forms are extremely rare. When the cannabis plant is used for vapor administration, the plant may contain different ratios of THC and CBD, which is further impacted by heat, vaporization, and inhalation, producing a unique complement of cannabinoid and non-cannabinoid components. These chemicals may have direct psychoactive effects and/or indirect effects such as altering the metabolism of active molecules. Cannabis containing edible consumption is another popular administration route in humans. Ingestion of cannabis could lead to early metabolism of THC and CBD, but may also involve the production of other active metabolites. Thus, using these alternate administration routes and substances could reflect the human condition in a better way, and it has a potential for providing further developments of cannabis use related effects in experimental models and humans.

One caveat in animal models especially for testing cognitive functions originates from conceptual differences in human and animal studies. Although the tested cognitive domains are classified under the same categories, e.g., working memory and attention, they are often tested in different ways and usually influenced by different factors across species. The nature of the animal tests may force the animals to use different cognitive strategies and brain regions while subject-related individual factors such as personality, motivation, and social factors could have an impact in human studies – although motivation can influence outcome in cognition in schizophrenia (Bismark et al. 2018). Animal studies rarely control for individual differences in sensory and motor functions, that can have important impacts on the results.

5 Future Directions

The paucity of research on the effects of cannabis on cognition in schizophrenia made it difficult to employ a RDoC framework in assessing the complex interplay between these three factors: no studies to date in patients with schizophrenia or those with cannabis use disorders have employed this approach. However, the complicated nature of these interactions underscores the need for the use of the RDoC framework to understand the potential factors and subgroup differences that give rise to the cognitive enhancements observed in cannabis-using patients with schizophrenia, especially in the context of cognitive changes related to cannabis use that might be trans-diagnostic (as has been suggested for other domains like social functioning (Karhson et al. 2016)) and in relation to dual disorders more broadly (Hakak-Zargar et al. 2022). Furthermore, this framework would also improve our ability to perform cross-species research that could inform the causal influences of cannabis exposure on cognition, both with and without the interactions with risk factors for psychopathology. Studies in preclinical models designed with the RDoC framework in mind may avoid some of the shortcomings associated with any given model of schizophrenia, and better inform the forward- and reverse-translation of findings in humans and animals on the impact of cannabis on cognition (Young et al. 2017).

6 Conclusions

Multiple factors need to be considered to understand the complex relationship between cannabis, cognitive function, and schizophrenia. Among others, age at initiation, duration of cannabis use, relative cannabinoid composition, and potency of cannabis contribute prominently to the variability in outcomes. Also, it should be noted that these factors can produce differential impacts in schizophrenia patients compared to healthy subjects. The available evidence suggests that chronic and heavy cannabis use is related to reversible attention and working memory difficulties, except in individuals who initiate the use of high-dose or high-potency cannabis during adolescence, but do not develop a clinically significant psychiatric or neurological disorder. In schizophrenia patients, recent cannabis use has been associated with symptom exacerbation, longer and more frequent psychotic episodes, and poorer treatment outcomes. However, large cohort studies show that chronic cannabis users with schizophrenia have superior cognitive functioning compared to non-users, even though they have more severe positive symptoms. Interestingly, these effects are only present in lifetime and past cannabis users, but not in current users. These patients usually have higher social functioning and have a higher familial risk for drug and alcohol use.

The constituents of the cannabis used may also contribute to variability in outcomes in patients. While CBD has potential antipsychotic properties, THC may aggravate schizophrenia symptoms including cognitive function. Moreover, other less studied components of cannabis could have possible effects on cognitive functioning in schizophrenia patients. Most cannabis use studies in humans do not provide details about the potency and contents of consumed cannabis products. Lack of a standardized method for classifying cannabis products makes interpreting these studies harder. Recently the increase in the product variety in the cannabis market creates another uncontrolled variable for clinical studies. Especially the cannabis products containing extremely high THC:CBD ratios remain a risk factor for developing psychotic disorders. Moreover, the potential for an impact of the non-THC/CBD components in the cannabis plant on schizophrenia and cognition should not be ignored.

Animal studies provide a valuable heuristic to study the causal impacts of cannabis use on cognition and schizophrenia risk. Animal models have been valuable in helping to identify the outcomes of maternal and/or adolescence cannabis exposure, evaluating the effects of different cannabinoids (either a single compound or a mixture of various constituents) given through different administration routes, and defining the brain pathways and neurotransmitter systems impacted by these exposures. However, improving the validity of these animal models is crucial to expanding our understanding of the effects of cannabis use, particularly for use of tests with translational relevance, particularly if tied to RDoC domains. Currently, there is a push toward implementing vapor administration systems into animal research to increase the face validity of the animal research. Implementing other administration routes such as edibles would also provide better modeling of human use via these routes.

Acknowledgments This work was supported by a Canadian Institute of Health Research Project Grant PJT-173442 (JYK).

References

Abela AR et al (2019) Adolescent exposure to Δ9-tetrahydrocannabinol delays acquisition of paired-associates learning in adulthood. Psychopharmacology (Berl) 236(6):1875–1886. https://doi.org/10.1007/s00213-019-5171-1

Accordino M, Hart CL (2006) Neuropsychological deficits in long-term frequent cannabis users. Neurology:1902. https://doi.org/10.1212/01.wnl.0000249081.67635.ef

American Psychiatric Association (2013) DSM 5. Am J Psychiatry. https://doi.org/10.1176/appi.books.9780890425596.744053

Baddeley A (1992) Working memory. Science 255(5044):556–559. https://doi.org/10.1126/science.1736359

Batalla A et al (2019) The potential of cannabidiol as a treatment for psychosis and addiction: who benefits most? A systematic review. Clin Med 8(7). https://doi.org/10.3390/JCM8071058

Becker MP, Collins PF, Luciana M (2014) Neurocognition in college-aged daily marijuana users. J Clin Exp Neuropsychol 36(4):379–398. https://doi.org/10.1080/13803395.2014.893996

Becker MP et al (2018) Longitudinal changes in cognition in young adult cannabis users. J Clin Exp Neuropsychol 40(6):529–543. https://doi.org/10.1080/13803395.2017.1385729

Bedi G, Cooper ZD, Haney M (2013) Subjective, cognitive and cardiovascular dose-effect profile of nabilone and dronabinol in marijuana smokers. Addict Biol 18(5):872–881. https://doi.org/10.1111/J.1369-1600.2011.00427.X

Bhattacharyya S, Schoeler T (2013) The effect of cannabis use on memory function: an update. Subst Abuse Rehabil 4:11. https://doi.org/10.2147/SAR.S25869

Bismark AW et al (2018) Relationship between effortful motivation and neurocognition in schizophrenia. Schizophr Res 193:69–76. https://doi.org/10.1016/J.SCHRES.2017.06.042

Bloomfield MAP et al (2016) The effects of δ9-tetrahydrocannabinol on the dopamine system. Nature 539(7629):369–377. https://doi.org/10.1038/nature20153

Bosker WM et al (2013) Psychomotor function in chronic daily cannabis smokers during sustained abstinence. PLoS One 8(1). https://doi.org/10.1371/JOURNAL.PONE.0053127

Bramness JG et al (2012) Amphetamine-induced psychosis – a separate diagnostic entity or primary psychosis triggered in the vulnerable? BMC Psychiatry 12:221. https://doi.org/10.1186/1471-244X-12-221

Burston JJ et al (2010) Regional enhancement of cannabinoid CB1 receptor desensitization in female adolescent rats following repeated Δ9-tetrahydrocannabinol exposure. Br J Pharmacol 161(1):103. https://doi.org/10.1111/J.1476-5381.2010.00870.X

Cha YM et al (2007) Sex differences in the effects of Δ9-tetrahydrocannabinol on spatial learning in adolescent and adult rats. Behav Pharmacol 18(5–6):563–569. https://doi.org/10.1097/FBP.0b013e3282ee7b7e

Chambers RA, Krystal JH, Self DW (2001) A neurobiological basis for substance abuse comorbidity in schizophrenia. Biol Psychiatry:71–83. https://doi.org/10.1016/S0006-3223(01)01134-9

D'Souza DC et al (2004) The psychotomimetic effects of intravenous delta-9-tetrahydrocannabinol in healthy individuals: implications for psychosis. Neuropsychopharmacology 29(8):1558–1572. https://doi.org/10.1038/SJ.NPP.1300496

D'Souza DC et al (2005) Delta-9-tetrahydrocannabinol effects in schizophrenia: implications for cognition, psychosis, and addiction. Biol Psychiatry 57(6):594–608. https://doi.org/10.1016/j.biopsych.2004.12.006

D'Souza DC et al (2008) Effects of haloperidol on the behavioral, subjective, cognitive, motor, and neuroendocrine effects of Delta-9-tetrahydrocannabinol in humans. Psychopharmacology (Berl) 198(4):587–603. https://doi.org/10.1007/S00213-007-1042-2

Di Forti M et al (2019) The contribution of cannabis use to variation in the incidence of psychotic disorder across Europe (EU-GEI): a multicentre case-control study. Lancet Psychiatry 6(5):427–436. https://doi.org/10.1016/S2215-0366(19)30048-3

Di Marzo V, De Petrocellis L (2012) Why do cannabinoid receptors have more than one endogenous ligand? Philos Trans R Soc B Biol Sci 367(1607):3216–3228. https://doi.org/10.1098/rstb.2011.0382

Dougherty DM et al (2013) Impulsivity, attention, memory, and decision-making among adolescent marijuana users. Psychopharmacology (Berl) 226(2):307–319. https://doi.org/10.1007/s00213-012-2908-5

Dudchenko PA (2004) An overview of the tasks used to test working memory in rodents. Neurosci Biobehav Rev 28(7):699–709. https://doi.org/10.1016/J.NEUBIOREV.2004.09.002

Dudchenko PA et al (2013) Animal models of working memory: a review of tasks that might be used in screening drug treatments for the memory impairments found in schizophrenia. Neurosci Biobehav Rev 37(9 Pt B):2111–2124. https://doi.org/10.1016/J.NEUBIOREV.2012.03.003

Ehrenreich H et al (1999) Specific attentional dysfunction in adults following early start of cannabis use. Psychopharmacology (Berl) 142(3):295–301. https://doi.org/10.1007/S002130050892

ElSohly MA et al (2016) Changes in cannabis potency over the last 2 decades (1995–2014): analysis of current data in the United States. Biol Psychiatry 79(7):613–619. https://doi.org/10.1016/j.biopsych.2016.01.004

ElSohly MA et al (2021) A comprehensive review of cannabis potency in the United States in the last decade. Biol Psychiatry Cogn Neurosci Neuroimaging 6(6):603–606. https://doi.org/10.1016/j.bpsc.2020.12.016

Ferraro L et al (2020) Premorbid adjustment and IQ in patients with first-episode psychosis: a multisite case-control study of their relationship with cannabis use. Schizophr Bull 46(3):517–529. https://doi.org/10.1093/schbul/sbz077

Fisk J, Montgomery C (2008) Real-world memory and executive processes in cannabis users and non-users. J Psychopharmacol 22(7):727–736. https://doi.org/10.1177/0269881107084000

Freeman TP et al (2021) Changes in delta-9-tetrahydrocannabinol (THC) and cannabidiol (CBD) concentrations in cannabis over time: systematic review and meta-analysis. Addiction 116(5):1000–1010. https://doi.org/10.1111/add.15253

Fried PA, Watkinson B, Gray R (2005) Neurocognitive consequences of marihuana – a comparison with pre-drug performance. Neurotoxicol Teratol 27(2):231–239. https://doi.org/10.1016/J.NTT.2004.11.003

Gold JM et al (2008) Reward processing in schizophrenia: a deficit in the representation of value. Schizophr Bull:835–847. https://doi.org/10.1093/schbul/sbn068

Goldman-Rakic PS, Selemon LD (1997) Functional and anatomical aspects of prefrontal pathology in schizophrenia. Schizophr Bull 23(3):437–458. https://doi.org/10.1093/schbul/23.3.437

Gonçalves-Pinho M, Bragança M, Freitas A (2020) Psychotic disorders hospitalizations associated with cannabis abuse or dependence: a nationwide big data analysis. Int J Methods Psychiatr Res 29(1):2020–2021. https://doi.org/10.1002/mpr.1813

Grant JE et al (2012) Neuropsychological deficits associated with cannabis use in young adults. Drug Alcohol Depend 121(1–2):159–162. https://doi.org/10.1016/J.DRUGALCDEP.2011.08.015

Grech A et al (2005) Cannabis use and outcome of recent onset psychosis. Eur Psychiatry 20(4): 349–353. https://doi.org/10.1016/j.eurpsy.2004.09.013

Green AI et al (2007) Schizophrenia and co-occurring substance use disorder. Am J Psychiatry 164(3):402–408. https://doi.org/10.1176/ajp.2007.164.3.402

Gruber SA et al (2012) Age of onset of marijuana use and executive function. Psychol Addict Behav 26(3):496–506. https://doi.org/10.1037/a0026269

Hakak-Zargar B et al (2022) The utility of research domain criteria in diagnosis and management of dual disorders: a mini-review. Front Psych 13. https://doi.org/10.3389/FPSYT.2022.805163

Hamidullah S et al (2020) Adolescent substance use and the brain: behavioral, cognitive and neuroimaging correlates. Front Hum Neurosci 14. https://doi.org/10.3389/fnhum.2020.00298

Hanson KL et al (2010) Longitudinal study of cognition among adolescent marijuana users over three weeks of abstinence. Addict Behav 35(11):970–976. https://doi.org/10.1016/j.addbeh.2010.06.012

Hart CL et al (2001) Effects of acute smoked marijuana on complex cognitive performance. Neuropsychopharmacology 25:757–765. https://www.nature.com/articles/1395716. Accessed 12 Nov 2021

Harvey MA et al (2007) The relationship between non-acute adolescent cannabis use and cognition. Drug Alcohol Rev 26(3):309–319. https://doi.org/10.1080/09595230701247772

Hasbi A et al (2020) Δ-tetrahydrocannabinol increases dopamine D1-D2 receptor heteromer and elicits phenotypic reprogramming in adult primate striatal neurons. iScience 23(1):100794. https://doi.org/10.1016/j.isci.2019.100794

Hauser TU, Eldar E, Dolan RJ (2017) Separate mesocortical and mesolimbic pathways encode effort and reward learning signals. Proc Natl Acad Sci U S A 114(35):E7395–E7404. https://doi.org/10.1073/pnas.1705643114

Hernandez CM et al (2021) Effects of repeated adolescent exposure to cannabis smoke on cognitive outcomes in adulthood. J Psychopharmacol 35(7):848–863. https://doi.org/10.1177/0269881120965931

Hooper SR, Woolley D, De Bellis MD (2014) Intellectual, neurocognitive, and academic achievement in abstinent adolescents with cannabis use disorder. Psychopharmacology (Berl) 231(8): 1467–1477. https://doi.org/10.1007/s00213-014-3463-z

Hunault CC et al (2009) Cognitive and psychomotor effects in males after smoking a combination of tobacco and cannabis containing up to 69 mg delta-9-tetrahydrocannabinol (THC). Psychopharmacology (Berl) 204(1):85–94. https://doi.org/10.1007/S00213-008-1440-0

Hunt GE et al (2018) Prevalence of comorbid substance use in schizophrenia spectrum disorders in community and clinical settings, 1990–2017: systematic review and meta-analysis. Drug Alcohol Depend 191:234–258. https://doi.org/10.1016/j.drugalcdep.2018.07.011

Irimia C et al (2015) Persistent effects of chronic Δ9-THC exposure on motor impulsivity in rats. Psychopharmacology (Berl) 232(16):3033–3043. https://doi.org/10.1007/s00213-015-3942-x

Jager G et al (2006) Long-term effects of frequent cannabis use on working memory and attention: an fMRI study. Psychopharmacology (Berl) 185(3):358–368. https://doi.org/10.1007/s00213-005-0298-7

Jenkins BW, Khokhar JY (2021) Cannabis use and mental illness: understanding circuit dysfunction through preclinical models. Front Psych 12. https://doi.org/10.3389/fpsyt.2021.597725

Jenkins BW et al (2022) Cannabis vapor exposure alters neural circuit oscillatory activity in a neurodevelopmental model of schizophrenia: exploring the differential impact of cannabis constituents. Schizophr Bull Open 3(1). https://doi.org/10.1093/schizbullopen/sgab052

Jockers-Scherübl MC et al (2007) Cannabis induces different cognitive changes in schizophrenic patients and in healthy controls. Prog Neuropsychopharmacol Biol Psychiatry 31(5): 1054–1063. https://doi.org/10.1016/j.pnpbp.2007.03.006

Kanayama G et al (2004) Spatial working memory in heavy cannabis users: a functional magnetic resonance imaging study. Psychopharmacology (Berl) 176(3–4):239–247. https://doi.org/10.1007/s00213-004-1885-8

Karhson DS, Hardan AY, Parker KJ (2016) Endocannabinoid signaling in social functioning: an RDoC perspective. Transl Psychiatry 6(9). https://doi.org/10.1038/TP.2016.169

Kendler KS et al (2019) Prediction of onset of substance-induced psychotic disorder and its progression to schizophrenia in a Swedish National Sample. Am J Psychiatry 176(9): 711–719. https://doi.org/10.1176/appi.ajp.2019.18101217

Kesby JP et al (2018) Dopamine, psychosis and schizophrenia: the widening gap between basic and clinical neuroscience. Transl Psychiatry 8(1):1–12. https://doi.org/10.1038/s41398-017-0071-9

Khokhar JY et al (2018) The link between schizophrenia and substance use disorder: a unifying hypothesis. Schizophr Res 194:78–85. https://doi.org/10.1016/j.schres.2017.04.016

Kirkland AE et al (2022) A scoping review of the use of cannabidiol in psychiatric disorders. Psychiatry Res 308:114347. https://doi.org/10.1016/j.psychres.2021.114347

Koob GF, Volkow ND (2016) Neurobiology of addiction: a neurocircuitry analysis. Lancet Psychiatry:760–773. https://doi.org/10.1016/S2215-0366(16)00104-8

Leonard S, Mexal S, Freedman R (2007) Smoking, genetics and schizophrenia: evidence for self medication. J Dual Diagn 3(3–4):43–59. https://doi.org/10.1300/J374v03n03_05

Leweke FM et al (2012) Cannabidiol enhances anandamide signaling and alleviates psychotic symptoms of schizophrenia. Transl Psychiatry 2(3):e94. https://doi.org/10.1038/tp.2012.15

Lisdahl KM, Price JS (2012) Increased marijuana use and gender predict poorer cognitive functioning in adolescents and emerging adults. J Int Neuropsychol Soc 18(4):678–688. https://doi.org/10.1017/S1355617712000276

Livne O et al (2022) Association of cannabis use-related predictor variables and self-reported psychotic disorders: U.S. adults, 2001-2002 and 2012-2013. Am J Psychiatry 179(1):36–45. https://doi.org/10.1176/appi.ajp.2021.21010073

Lu HC, Mackie K (2021) Review of the endocannabinoid system. Biol Psychiatry Cogn Neurosci Neuroimaging 6(6):607–615. https://doi.org/10.1016/j.bpsc.2020.07.016

Lyons MJ et al (2004) Neuropsychological consequences of regular marijuana use: a twin study. Psychol Med 34(7):1239–1250. https://doi.org/10.1017/S0033291704002260

Manzella F, Maloney SE, Taylor GT (2015) Smoking in schizophrenic patients: a critique of the self-medication hypothesis. World J Psychiatry 5(1):35. https://doi.org/10.5498/WJP.V5.I1.35

Marconi A et al (2016) Meta-analysis of the association between the level of cannabis use and risk of psychosis. Schizophr Bull 42(5):1262–1269. https://doi.org/10.1093/SCHBUL/SBW003

Maynard TM et al (2001) Neural development, cell-cell signaling, and the "Two-Hit" hypothesis of schizophrenia. Schizophr Bull 27(3):457–476. https://doi.org/10.1093/oxfordjournals.schbul.a006887

McCutcheon RA, Abi-Dargham A, Howes OD (2019) Schizophrenia, dopamine and the striatum: from biology to symptoms. Trends Neurosci 42(3):205–220. https://doi.org/10.1016/j.tins.2018.12.004

McKetin R et al (2016) A longitudinal examination of the relationship between cannabis use and cognitive function in mid-life adults. Drug Alcohol Depend 169:134–140. https://doi.org/10.1016/j.drugalcdep.2016.10.022

Medina KL et al (2007) Neuropsychological functioning in adolescent marijuana users: subtle deficits detectable after a month of abstinence. J Int Neuropsychol Soc 13(5):807. https://doi.org/10.1017/S1355617707071032

Mehmedic Z et al (2010) Potency trends of Δ9-THC and other cannabinoids in confiscated cannabis preparations from 1993 to 2008*. J Forensic Sci 55(5):1209–1217. https://doi.org/10.1111/j.1556-4029.2010.01441.x

Mielnik CA et al (2021) A novel allosteric modulator of the cannabinoid CB1 receptor ameliorates hyperdopaminergia endophenotypes in rodent models. Neuropsychopharmacology 46(2):413–422. https://doi.org/10.1038/s41386-020-00876-5

Minichino A et al (2019) Measuring disturbance of the endocannabinoid system in psychosis: a systematic review and meta-analysis. JAMA Psychiat:914–923. https://doi.org/10.1001/jamapsychiatry.2019.0970

Morgan CJA et al (2013) Cerebrospinal fluid anandamide levels, cannabis use and psychotic-like symptoms. Br J Psychiatry 202(5):381–382. https://doi.org/10.1192/bjp.bp.112.121178

Muhl D et al (2014) Increased CB2 mRNA and anandamide in human blood after cessation of cannabis abuse. Naunyn Schmiedebergs Arch Pharmacol 387(7):691–695. https://doi.org/10.1007/S00210-014-0984-2

Murphy M et al (2017) Chronic adolescent Δ 9 -tetrahydrocannabinol treatment of male mice leads to long-term cognitive and behavioral dysfunction, which are prevented by concurrent cannabidiol treatment. Cannabis Cannabinoid Res 2(1):235–246. https://doi.org/10.1089/can.2017.0034

Murray RM, Hall W (2020) Will legalization and commercialization of cannabis use increase the incidence and prevalence of psychosis? JAMA Psychiat 77(8):777. https://doi.org/10.1001/jamapsychiatry.2020.0339

Niemi-Pynttäri JA et al (2013) Substance-induced psychoses converting into schizophrenia: a register-based study of 18,478 Finnish inpatient cases. J Clin Psychiatry 74(1):20155. https://doi.org/10.4088/JCP.12m07822

Nong L et al (2002) Altered cannabinoid receptor mRNA expression in peripheral blood mononuclear cells from marijuana smokers. J Neuroimmunol 127(1–2):169–176. https://doi.org/10.1016/S0165-5728(02)00113-3

Nordström AL et al (1993) Central D2-dopamine receptor occupancy in relation to antipsychotic drug effects: a double-blind PET study of schizophrenic patients. Biol Psychiatry 33(4):227–235. https://doi.org/10.1016/0006-3223(93)90288-O

Orellana G, Slachevsky A (2013) Executive functioning in schizophrenia. Front Psych 4:35. https://doi.org/10.3389/FPSYT.2013.00035/BIBTEX

Osborne AL et al (2017) Improved social interaction, recognition and working memory with cannabidiol treatment in a prenatal infection (poly I:C) rat model. Neuropsychopharmacology 42(7):1447–1457. https://doi.org/10.1038/npp.2017.40

Pasman JA et al (2018) GWAS of lifetime cannabis use reveals new risk loci, genetic overlap with psychiatric traits, and a causal influence of schizophrenia. Nat Neurosci 21(9):1161–1170. https://doi.org/10.1038/s41593 018-0206-1

Peres FF et al (2018) Cannabidiol administered during peri-adolescence prevents behavioral abnormalities in an animal model of schizophrenia. Front Pharmacol 9(AUG). https://doi.org/10.3389/fphar.2018.00901

Pope HG, Yurgelun-Todd D (1996) The residual cognitive effects of heavy marijuana use in college students. JAMA 275(7):521–527. https://doi.org/10.1001/jama.275.7.521

Rabin RA et al (2013) Effects of cannabis use status on cognitive function, in males with schizophrenia. Psychiatry Res 206(2–3):158–165. https://doi.org/10.1016/j.psychres.2012.11.019

Ramaekers JG et al (2009) Neurocognitive performance during acute THC intoxication in heavy and occasional cannabis users. J Psychopharmacol 23(3):266–277. https://doi.org/10.1177/0269881108092393

Ramesh D, Haney M, Cooper ZD (2013) Marijuana's dose-dependent effects in daily marijuana smokers. Exp Clin Psychopharmacol 21(4):287–293. https://doi.org/10.1037/A0033661

Renard J et al (2016) Cannabidiol counteracts amphetamine-induced neuronal and behavioral sensitization of the mesolimbic dopamine pathway through a novel mTOR/p70S6 kinase signaling pathway. J Neurosci 36(18):5160–5169. https://doi.org/10.1523/JNEUROSCI.3387-15.2016

Renard J et al (2017) Adolescent THC exposure causes enduring prefrontal cortical disruption of GABAergic inhibition and dysregulation of sub-cortical dopamine function. Sci Rep 7(1). https://doi.org/10.1038/S41598-017-11645-8

Rømer Thomsen K, Callesen MB, Feldstein Ewing SW (2017) Recommendation to reconsider examining cannabis subtypes together due to opposing effects on brain, cognition and behavior. Neurosci Biobehav Rev 80:156–158. https://doi.org/10.1016/j.neubiorev.2017.05.025

Rubino T et al (2008) Chronic Δ9-tetrahydrocannabinol during adolescence provokes sex-dependent changes in the emotional profile in adult rats: behavioral and biochemical correlates. Neuropsychopharmacology 33(11):2760–2771. https://doi.org/10.1038/sj.npp.1301664

Rubino T et al (2009) Changes in hippocampal morphology and neuroplasticity induced by adolescent THC treatment are associated with cognitive impairment in adulthood. Hippocampus 19(8):763–772. https://doi.org/10.1002/hipo.20554

Schoeler T et al (2016) The effects of cannabis on memory function in users with and without a psychotic disorder: findings from a combined meta-analysis. Psychol Med 46(1):177–188. https://doi.org/10.1017/S0033291715001646

Schofield D et al (2006) Reasons for cannabis use in psychosis. Aust N Z J Psychiatry 40(6–7):570–574. https://doi.org/10.1080/J.1440-1614.2006.01840.X

Scott JC et al (2018) Association of cannabis with cognitive functioning in adolescents and young adults a systematic review and meta-analysis. JAMA Psychiat:585–595. https://doi.org/10.1001/jamapsychiatry.2018.0335

Seeman P (2016) Cannabidiol is a partial agonist at dopamine D2High receptors, predicting its antipsychotic clinical dose. Transl Psychiatry 6(10):e920. https://doi.org/10.1038/TP.2016.195

Shrivastava A, Tsuang M, Johnston M (2011) Cannabis use and cognitive dysfunction. Indian J Psychiatry 53(3):187. https://doi.org/10.4103/0019-5545.86796

Sideli L et al (2020) Cannabis use and the risk for psychosis and affective disorders. J Dual Diagn 16(1):22–42. https://doi.org/10.1080/15504263.2019.1674991

Solowij N, Battisti R (2008) The chronic effects of cannabis on memory in humans: a review. Curr Drug Abuse Rev 1(1):81–98. https://doi.org/10.2174/1874473710801010081

Spear LP (2000) The adolescent brain and age-related behavioral manifestations. Neurosci Biobehav Rev 24(4):417–463. https://doi.org/10.1016/S0149-7634(00)00014-2

Stark T et al (2020) Altered dopamine D3 receptor gene expression in MAM model of schizophrenia is reversed by peripubertal cannabidiol treatment. Biochem Pharmacol 177. https://doi.org/10.1016/j.bcp.2020.114004

Stark T, Di Martino S, Drago F, Wotjak CT et al (2021) Phytocannabinoids and schizophrenia: focus on adolescence as a critical window of enhanced vulnerability and opportunity for treatment. Pharmacol Res 174:105938. https://doi.org/10.1016/j.phrs.2021.105938

Strauss GP, Waltz JA, Gold JM (2014) A review of reward processing and motivational impairment in schizophrenia. Schizophr Bull:107–116. https://doi.org/10.1093/schbul/sbt197

Stringfield SJ, Torregrossa MM (2021) Intravenous self-administration of delta-9-THC in adolescent rats produces long-lasting alterations in behavior and receptor protein expression. Psychopharmacology (Berl) 238(1):305–319. https://doi.org/10.1007/s00213-020-05684-9

Szkudlarek HJ et al (2019) Δ-9-tetrahydrocannabinol and Cannabidiol produce dissociable effects on prefrontal cortical executive function and regulation of affective behaviors. Neuropsychopharmacology 44(4):817. https://doi.org/10.1038/S41386-018-0282-7

Szkudlarek HJ et al (2021) THC and CBD produce divergent effects on perception and panic behaviours via distinct cortical molecular pathways. Prog Neuropsychopharmacol Biol Psychiatry 104:110029. https://doi.org/10.1016/j.pnpbp.2020.110029

Thames AD, Arbid N, Sayegh P (2014) Cannabis use and neurocognitive functioning in a non-clinical sample of users. Addict Behav 39(5):994–999. https://doi.org/10.1016/J.ADDBEH.2014.01.019

Theunissen EL et al (2015) Rivastigmine but not vardenafil reverses cannabis-induced impairment of verbal memory in healthy humans. Psychopharmacology (Berl) 232(2):343–353. https://doi.org/10.1007/S00213-014-3667-2

Thorpe HHA et al (2020) Adolescent neurodevelopment and substance use: receptor expression and behavioral consequences. Pharmacol Ther. https://doi.org/10.1016/j.pharmthera.2019.107431

Turner SE et al (2017) Molecular pharmacology of phytocannabinoids. In: Progress in the chemistry of organic natural products. Springer, Cham, pp 61–101. https://doi.org/10.1007/978-3-319-45541-9_3

Vaucher J et al (2018) Cannabis use and risk of schizophrenia: a Mendelian randomization study. Mol Psychiatry 23(5):1287–1292. https://doi.org/10.1038/mp.2016.252

Volkow ND (2009) Substance use disorders in schizophrenia – clinical implications of comorbidity. Schizophr Bull:469–472. https://doi.org/10.1093/schbul/sbp016

Weimar HV et al (2020) Long-term effects of maternal cannabis vapor exposure on emotional reactivity, social behavior, and behavioral flexibility in offspring. Neuropharmacology 179: 108288. https://doi.org/10.1016/j.neuropharm.2020.108288

Wesnes KA et al (2010) Nabilone produces marked impairments to cognitive function and changes in subjective state in healthy volunteers. J Psychopharmacol 24(11):1659–1669. https://doi.org/10.1177/0269881109105900

Whitlow CT et al (2004) Long-term heavy marijuana users make costly decisions on a gambling task. Drug Alcohol Depend 76(1):107–111. https://doi.org/10.1016/j.drugalcdep.2004.04.009

Young JW et al (2017) Research domain criteria versus DSM V: how does this debate affect attempts to model corticostriatal dysfunction in animals? Neurosci Biobehav Rev 76 (Pt B):301–316. https://doi.org/10.1016/J.NEUBIOREV.2016.10.029

Yucel M et al (2012) The impact of cannabis use on cognitive functioning in patients with schizophrenia: a meta-analysis of existing findings and new data in a first-episode sample. Schizophr Bull 38(2):316–330. https://doi.org/10.1093/schbul/sbq079

Zamberletti E et al (2014) Alterations of prefrontal cortex GABAergic transmission in the complex psychotic-like phenotype induced by adolescent delta-9-tetrahydrocannabinol exposure in rats. Neurobiol Dis 63:35–47. https://doi.org/10.1016/j.nbd.2013.10.028

Zamberletti E et al (2016) Long-term hippocampal glutamate synapse and astrocyte dysfunctions underlying the altered phenotype induced by adolescent THC treatment in male rats. Pharmacol Res 111:459–470. https://doi.org/10.1016/j.phrs.2016.07.008

Sex Differences in Cognition in Schizophrenia: What We Know and What We Do Not Know

Hyun Bin Freeman and Junghee Lee

Contents

Abstract Cognitive impairment is a core feature of schizophrenia. This selective review examines whether schizophrenia patients show preserved sexual dimorphism in cognition. Existing studies using performance tasks largely show comparable sex effects between schizophrenia patients and healthy populations. This pattern appears to be similar across multiple cognitive domains and across phase of illness. Our selective review also identifies several unresolved questions about sex differences in cognition in schizophrenia. A better understanding of sex differences in cognition in schizophrenia may provide important clues to probing the relationship between cognitive impairment and pathophysiological processes of the disorder.

Keywords Nonsocial cognition · Schizophrenia · Sex differences · Social cognition

H. B. Freeman
Department of Psychology, University of Alabama at Birmingham, Birmingham, AL, USA

J. Lee (✉)
Department of Psychiatry and Behavioral Neurobiology, The University of Alabama at Birmingham, Birmingham, AL, USA

Comprehensive Neuroscience Center, The University of Alabama at Birmingham, Birmingham, AL, USA
e-mail: jungheelee@uabmc.edu

Curr Topics Behav Neurosci (2023) 63: 463–474
https://doi.org/10.1007/7854_2022_394
Published Online: 22 October 2022

1 Introduction

Schizophrenia, one of the most severe mental illnesses, affects approximately 1% of the population worldwide. Although sex differences in the incidence and expression of schizophrenia are not as pronounced as those observed in other neurodevelopmental disorders such as autism, sex differences in several key features of the illness have been well documented. For instance, a higher incidence rate was found in males than in females (e.g., 1.4 ratio) (He et al. 2020; McGrath et al. 2004), although prevalence appears to be comparable between males and females (Charlson et al. 2018; Saha et al. 2005). Compared to male patients, female patients tend to have later age of onset (Eranti et al. 2013; Zhang et al. 2012), better premorbid functioning (Allen et al. 2013; Larsen et al. 1996; Segarra et al. 2012), and better outcomes, especially during the early course of illness (Ayesa-Arriola et al. 2020; Grossman et al. 2008). A similar pattern of sex differences in symptoms and functioning is also emerging in studies with individuals who are at risk for psychosis (Rietschel et al. 2017; Walder et al. 2013). This pattern of sex differences in clinical characteristics of schizophrenia indicates that sex moderates the way the illness is manifested over the course of the illness.

In this review, we will focus on sex differences in cognitive impairments in schizophrenia – a core feature of the illness that is an important determinant of poor functional outcome and is closely related to the underlying pathophysiological processes of the disorder (Green et al. 2019). We will first examine whether sex effects in cognitive performance are similar between schizophrenia patients and healthy populations. We will then examine whether sex effects in cognition in schizophrenia are similar across phase of illness. We will finally discuss the implications of sex differences in cognition in schizophrenia by presenting unresolved questions for future studies on this topic.

Of note, sex and gender have been interchangeably used in the literature. However, during the past decade, there has been an increasing awareness that sex is distinct from gender as sex is defined as a biological trait that concerns primarily a reproductive system, whereas gender is defined as a social construct that is shaped by societal influence and/or norms on expected gender roles (American Psycholoical Association Committee on Lesbina 2011). While we acknowledge that it is important to separate the effect of biological sex and the effect of socially influenced gender, it was often difficult to determine how gender is defined (i.e., gender as distinct from sex) and measured when the term, gender, was used in schizophrenia research. Thus, we will use the term "sex" in this review unless studies specifically measured gender as defined above and examined the effect of gender on cognition.

2 Sex Differences in Cognition in Schizophrenia: Preserved Sexual Dimorphism or Not?

There is a widely held belief that neurotypical males and females perform differently on cognitive tasks, especially when tasks rely on spatial ability, verbal skills, or emotional processing. Extant studies indicate that sex difference in cognition is more nuanced than commonly believed. For instance, a small male advantage (Cohen's $d = 0.155$, 95% confidence interval [CI] = 0.087–0.223) was found in a meta-analytic review on spatial working memory (Voyer et al. 2017), whereas a small female advantage (Cohen's $d = 0.028$, 95% CI = 0.006–0.050) was found in a meta-analytic review on verbal working memory (Voyer et al. 2021). These studies also showed substantial heterogeneity in effect sizes, partly explained by specific features of the task (e.g., the types of the task, stimulus type) and age of the participants. Of note, while specific task features were significant moderators for both meta-analytic reviews, moderator analyses did not reveal larger effect sizes for certain types of the task, suggesting that task heterogeneity itself is unlikely to explain small effects of sex on working memory performance. Another meta-analytic review (Gaillard et al. 2021) found a lack of sex differences in three types of executive function tasks: performance monitoring, response inhibition, and cognitive set-shifting (Hedges' $g = -0.08$, 95% CI = −0.21–0.05; Hedges' $g = -0.01$, 95% CI = −0.15–0.13; and Hedges' $g = -0.06$, 95% CI = −0.26–0.13, respectively). This meta-analysis also found substantial heterogeneity in effect sizes, but did not formally evaluate potential moderators due to a small number of studies for each category. For emotional processing, a small female advantage was found for recognizing emotion of non-verbal stimuli (Cohen's $d = 0.186$, 95% CI = 0.155–0.217) (Thompson and Voyer 2014). Similar to nonsocial cognitive tasks, substantial heterogeneity was found, which was partly explained by the types of emotion and age of the participants. To summarize, existing evidence suggests small effects of sex on cognitive performance across multiple domains in neurotypical adults. The extent to which specific feature of the task or other factors explain the observed heterogeneity of these studies (Gaillard et al. 2021; Thompson and Voyer 2014; Voyer et al. 2017, 2021) remains to be determined.

In schizophrenia research, the existing body of work that examined sex differences in schizophrenia across multiple cognitive domains can be largely divided into two categories. The first category includes studies that examined sex differences within schizophrenia patients. While these studies provided detailed information about differences in performance between female patients and male patients, their findings were not informative in determining the extent to which sex differences in schizophrenia follow a normative pattern. Studies in the second category, on the contrary, focused on comparing sex differences in cognition of schizophrenia patients to those of control participants from the general community, thus allowing us to infer whether sex interacts with the pathophysiological processes of the disease to affect cognitive processes of patients. The focus of this review is studies in the second category.

For nonsocial cognition, the majority of studies that compared sex differences between patients and controls employed neuropsychological assessments, and produced mixed findings. For executive function, one study found a significant sex effect on executive function only in the schizophrenia patient group such that female patients performed poorer than male patients, whereas males and females in the control group performed in a similar way (Goldstein et al. 1998). Another study reported a larger sex effect of patients such that a sex effect of males performing poorer than females was larger in the patient group than control group (Seidman et al. 1997). Both studies included a small sample size (e.g., less than 40 participants in each group). Another study with a slightly larger sample (about 100 patients) reported that in both patient and control groups, males and females performed comparably (Bozikas et al. 2010).

For attention, several studies found no sex effect in either patient or control group (Han et al. 2012; Lee et al. 2020; Zhang et al. 2017). One study (Goldstein et al. 1998) reported a sex effect that was similar across both patients and controls such that females performed better than males. Another study (Mu et al. 2020) reported a significant sex effect only in the patient group such that female patients performed poorer than male patients. For working memory, several studies reported no sex effect in either patient or control group (Bozikas et al. 2010; Lee et al. 2020; Minor and Park 1999; Mu et al. 2020; Roesch-Ely et al. 2009). One study (Zhang et al. 2017) reported a differential sex effect in working memory. In this study, a sex effect was found only in the control group such that male controls performed better than female controls, whereas female patients and male patients showed comparable performance.

For spatial memory, several studies did not find any sex effect in either patient or control group (Bozikas et al. 2010; Goldstein et al. 1998; Mu et al. 2020). One study (Zhang et al. 2017) reported a sex effect only in the patient group such that male patients performed poorer than controls. Similarly, for verbal memory, several studies showed comparable performance between females and males which was presented in both patient and control groups (Bozikas et al. 2010; Goldstein et al. 1998; Lee et al. 2020; Mu et al. 2020). One study (Zhang et al. 2017) found a significant effect of sex only in the patient group, where male patients performed poorer than female patients.

Considerably fewer studies compared sex differences in schizophrenia patients and controls in social cognition, but the overall pattern of findings suggests that sex did not differentially affect performance of patients. For example, studies on emotion perception did not find sex differences in either schizophrenia patients or healthy controls (Ferrer-Quintero et al. 2021; Lee et al. 2020; Mossaheb et al. 2018). Both schizophrenia patients and healthy controls showed a lack of sex differences in other social cognitive domains, including empathy (Ferrer-Quintero et al. 2021), theory of mind (Navarra-Ventura et al. 2021; Walsh-Messinger et al. 2019), and emotion regulation (Rodriguez-Jimenez et al. 2015).

As described above, existing studies on sex differences in cognition in schizophrenia do not provide strong support for differential sex effects. Considering small sex effects found in neurotypical adults (Gaillard et al. 2021; Thompson and Voyer

2014; Voyer et al. 2017, 2021), it is not surprising that several studies did not find a sex effect in either patient or control group. When a differential sex effect was found, however, the pattern was not consistent across cognitive domains. While it is possible that schizophrenia may be associated with differential sex differences in certain cognitive domains, this differential sex effect might not be strong enough to be consistently found across studies, especially when studies included a small sample size. As most of the studies described above assessed patients with chronic schizophrenia and demographically matched controls, the next logical question is whether a similar pattern is present across phase of illness.

3 Sex Differences in Cognition in Schizophrenia Across Phase of Illness

While fewer studies examined sex differences in cognition with patients who recently experienced their first psychotic episode, a pattern of findings is similar to what was found with chronic patients. For executive function, both patients with first-episode psychosis and demographically matched controls did not show a significant sex effect (Buck et al. 2020). For verbal memory, several studies found a female advantage for both patients and controls (Albus et al. 1997; Ayesa-Arriola et al. 2014; Buck et al. 2020; Ittig et al. 2015). For visual memory, one study did not find any sex effect in either patient or control group (Buck et al. 2020), whereas another study found that males performed better than females across both patients and controls (Ayesa-Arriola et al. 2014). Similarly, for speed of processing, one study did not find any sex effect in either group (Buck et al. 2020), whereas another study found better performance of males compared to females across both patients and controls (Ittig et al. 2015).

Notably, a similar pattern of findings has also been reported in studies with individuals at risk for psychosis. For instance, a similar pattern of sex differences was found across individuals at-risk mental state (ARMS) and controls such that across both groups males performed better on reaction time measures and poorer on verbal learning and memory compared to females (Ittig et al. 2015). Another study found that across both ARMS groups and control groups, females performed better than males in speed of processing and verbal learning, but females and males showed comparable performance in working memory, problem solving, and facial affect recognition (Menghini-Muller et al. 2020). In non-help seeking youth from the Philadelphia Neurodevelopmental Cohort, psychosis spectrum youth and typically developing youth showed differential patterns of sex differences in neurocognitive development such that in the psychosis spectrum group, neurocognitive developmental lag was found across multiple domains, including memory, reasoning, and social cognition, across all age groups in males, but only in reasoning at a latter age group in females (Gur et al. 2014).

4 Outstanding Questions About Sex Differences in Cognition in Schizophrenia

As reviewed above, a large body of work examined sex differences in cognition in schizophrenia using a range of cognitive tasks. Existing evidence largely supports a normalized pattern of sex differences in cognition in schizophrenia across phases of illness. This body of work also highlights several gaps in our knowledge of sex differences in cognition in schizophrenia. We will briefly discuss a few examples of outstanding questions in this section.

One may wonder whether preserved sexual dimorphism in cognition in schizophrenia indicates that sex does not interact with the way schizophrenia affects cognition. However, existing evidence reviewed above does not provide a clear answer to this question. For example, female patients are shown to have better premorbid functioning than male patients (Segarra et al. 2012). Considering that better premorbid functioning is related to better post-onset cognitive performances in schizophrenia patients (Bucci et al. 2018; Stefanatou et al. 2018), better premorbid functioning might have protected female patients from further impairments in cognitive function. Similarly, female patients and male patients also differ in several clinical characteristics that have been shown to be related to cognitive impairments, such as negative symptoms (Maric et al. 2003). It is possible that the neurodevelopmental process of schizophrenia may differentially affect these clinical features between male patients and female patients, which in turn affects cognitive ability. Thus, a finding of preserved sexual dimorphism in cognition in schizophrenia does not necessarily suggest that biological sex does not interact with the illness process to affect cognitive performance of schizophrenia patients. It will be important to determine the extent to which cognitive performance in female and male patients is related to clinical and other illness-related features that also differ between females and males, as well as the extent to which these relationships change over the course of the illness.

While the role of cognition in functioning is well documented, few studies examined whether this relationship is similar between female patients and male patients or not. Cognitive impairment is increasingly viewed as an important treatment target for improving poor functioning of patients and as a result substantial effort has been devoted to develop and evaluate novel interventions (e.g., pharmacological treatments, neuromodulation, cognitive training). If female patients and male patients show similar relationship between cognition and functioning, one could assume that the same intervention could be effective for both male patients and female patients in a similar way. If the relationship between cognition and functioning differs quantitively between female patients and male patients, as shown in one recent study (Ferrer-Quintero et al. 2021), one could focus on identifying right "dose" for female patients and male patients when evaluating effectiveness of novel interventions. If the relationship differs qualitatively, an intervention that benefits female patients may not be effective at all in improving cognitive impairments of male patients. Thus, it will be important to systematically examine the extent to which sex moderates the relationship between cognition and community functioning in schizophrenia.

It is important to note that most of the studies reviewed above focused on performance of patients on cognitive tasks (e.g., accuracy or reaction time). While these indices can be considered the final product or outcome of processes that are necessary to perform a cognitive task, comparable levels of performance between male and female patients do not indicate that female patients and male patients utilize the same processes. For example, to perform a working memory task, one needs to encode a stimulus, maintain the representation of a stimulus on-line while inhibiting any internal or external distraction, and produce an appropriate motor response. Problems at any stage could lead to incorrect responses, but an incorrect response alone does not inform how incorrect responses occurred. In other words, comparable levels of performance between males and females across schizophrenia patients and healthy controls fail to offer any insights on the possibility that female patients and female controls use different strategies to arrive at the same response. It will be important to examine the mechanistic pathway of behavioral outputs to further understand whether a similar pattern of sex differences between schizophrenia patients and controls arise from similar underlying processes or not. Recent advances in computational psychiatry offer several models and tools to probe the underlying processes of behavioral outputs (Gold et al. 2020; Murray et al. 2017; Niv 2019; Radulescu and Niv 2019).

Further, few studies examined whether comparable sex differences in cognitive performance between schizophrenia patients and controls also involve the same neural underpinnings. It is well known that neurotypical females and males show differences in brain structures (Ge et al. 2021; Wierenga et al. 2022) and brain function (de Lacy et al. 2019; Zhao et al. 2021). Emerging evidence also demonstrates that sex differences in brain structures may differ between patients and controls. For instance, in the Philadelphia Developmental Cohort, individuals at high risk for psychosis and controls showed differential sex effects in striatal–cortical functional connectivity (Jacobs et al. 2019), but not in the thalamocortical functional connectivity (Huang et al. 2021). Individuals at high risk for psychosis also showed greater sex differences in thalamic volume than typically developing youth (Jacobs et al. 2019). When examining the volume of cerebellum, one study found that vermis volume was larger for males than females in controls, whereas the opposite pattern was found in schizophrenia patients (Womer et al. 2016). The findings of divergent sexual dimorphism of schizophrenia at a neural level raise an intriguing question as to whether a similar pattern of sex differences in cognition between schizophrenia patients and controls may arise from different neural underpinnings. It will be important to examine the effects of sex on cognition–brain relationships in schizophrenia in a systematic way.

Few studies that examined sex differences in cognition in schizophrenia considered the effect of menstrual cycle or sex hormones on cognition. Hormonal fluctuation across the menstrual cycles are shown to be related to fluctuation of clinical symptoms in female schizophrenia patients (Seeman 2012), and menstrual dysfunction is common among female schizophrenia patients (Gleeson et al. 2016).

Emerging evidence also suggests that menstrual cycles may have subtle effects on cognitive performance (Weis et al. 2011), volumes of several brain areas (Pletzer et al. 2018; Rehbein et al. 2021), and functional organization of brain regions (Pritschet et al. 2020). Thus, it is plausible that evaluating female patients at different phases of the menstrual cycle would affect cognitive performance or other assessments, which could affect the comparison of performance between females and males. It remains to be determined to which extent the menstrual cycle affects cognition and related neural substrates in females and the extent to which the effect of menstrual cycle may differ between schizophrenia patients and controls.

5 Concluding Remarks

In this perspective, we reviewed previous findings on sex differences in cognition in schizophrenia, with a focus on studies that compared sex differences in cognition between schizophrenia patients and controls. The majority of studies showed either comparable sex effects across patients or controls or did not find sex effects in either patient or control groups. Further, when differential sex effects were found, the pattern of sex differences varied across cognitive domains and across studies. Considering that sex effects in cognition in neurotypical adults were not as pronounced as commonly believed, it is possible that differential sex effects in cognition in schizophrenia may not be large enough to be consistently found across studies, especially when studies used different paradigms and included a small sample size. Thus, while existing evidence largely support the lack of differential sex effects in cognition in schizophrenia across phase of illness, it does not provide a conclusive answer to a question as to whether sex moderates the way schizophrenia is manifested over the course of illness to affect cognitive processes. A thorough investigation of unresolved questions listed above may provide important clues to answering this question and offer novel insights into probing potential mechanisms of heterogeneous etiology of the disorder.

References

Albus M, Hubmann W, Mohr F, Scherer J, Sobizack N, Franz U, Hecht S, Borrmann M, Wahlheim C (1997) Are there gender differences in neuropsychological performance in patients with first-episode schizophrenia? Schizophr Res 28:39–50

Allen DN, Strauss GP, Barchard KA, Vertinski M, Carpenter WT, Buchanan RW (2013) Differences in developmental changes in academic and social premorbid adjustment between males and females with schizophrenia. Schizophr Res 146:132–137

American Psycholoical Association Committee on Lesbina, G., Bisexual, and Transgender Concerns Office and Public and Member Communication (2011) Answers to your questions about transgender people, gender identity and gender expression

Ayesa-Arriola R, Rodriguez-Sanchez JM, Gomez-Ruiz E, Roiz-Santianez R, Reeves LL, Crespo-Facorro B (2014) No sex differences in neuropsychological performance in first episode psychosis patients. Prog Neuropsychopharmacol Biol Psychiatry 48:149–154

Ayesa-Arriola R, de la Foz VO, Setien-Suero E, Ramirez-Bonilla ML, Suarez-Pinilla P, Son JM, Vazquez-Bourgon J, Juncal-Ruiz M, Gomez-Revuelta M, Tordesillas-Gutierrez D, Crespo-Facorro B (2020) Understanding sex differences in long-term outcomes after a first episode of psychosis. NPJ Schizophr 6:33

Bozikas VP, Kosmidis MH, Peltekis A, Giannakou M, Nimatoudis I, Karavatos A, Fokas K, Garyfallos G (2010) Sex differences in neuropsychological functioning among schizophrenia patients. Aust N Z J Psychiatry 44:333–341

Bucci P, Galderisi S, Mucci A, Rossi A, Rocca P, Bertolino A, Aguglia E, Amore M, Andriola I, Bellomo A, Biondi M, Cuomo A, dell'Osso L, Favaro A, Gambi F, Giordano GM, Girardi P, Marchesi C, Monteleone P, Montemagni C, Niolu C, Oldani L, Pacitti F, Pinna F, Roncone R, Vita A, Zeppegno P, Maj M, Italian Network for Research on Psychoses (2018) Premorbid academic and social functioning in patients with schizophrenia and its associations with negative symptoms and cognition. Acta Psychiatr Scand 138:253–266

Buck G, Lavigne KM, Makowski C, Joober R, Malla A, Lepage M (2020) Sex differences in verbal memory predict functioning through negative symptoms in early psychosis. Schizophr Bull 46: 1587–1595

Charlson FJ, Ferrari AJ, Santomauro DF, Diminic S, Stockings E, Scott JG, McGrath JJ, Whiteford HA (2018) Global epidemiology and burden of schizophrenia: findings from the global burden of disease study 2016. Schizophr Bull 44:1195–1203

de Lacy N, McCauley E, Kutz JN, Calhoun VD (2019) Sex-related differences in intrinsic brain dynamism and their neurocognitive correlates. Neuroimage 202:116116

Eranti SV, MacCabe JH, Bundy H, Murray RM (2013) Gender difference in age at onset of schizophrenia: a meta-analysis. Psychol Med 43:155–167

Ferrer-Quintero M, Green MF, Horan WP, Penn DL, Kern RS, Lee J (2021) The effect of sex on social cognition and functioning in schizophrenia. NPJ Schizophr 7:57

Gaillard A, Fehring DJ, Rossell SL (2021) A systematic review and meta-analysis of behavioural sex differences in executive control. Eur J Neurosci 53:519–542

Ge R, Liu X, Long D, Frangou S, Vila-Rodriguez F (2021) Sex effects on cortical morphological networks in healthy young adults. Neuroimage 233:117945

Gleeson PC, Worsley R, Gavrilidis E, Nathoo S, Ng E, Lee S, Kulkarni J (2016) Menstrual cycle characteristics in women with persistent schizophrenia. Aust N Z J Psychiatry 50:481–487

Gold JM, Bansal S, Anticevic A, Cho YT, Repovs G, Murray JD, Hahn B, Robinson BM, Luck SJ (2020) Refining the empirical constraints on computational models of spatial working memory in schizophrenia. Biol Psychiatry Cogn Neurosci Neuroimaging 5:913–922

Goldstein JM, Seidman LJ, Goodman JM, Koren D, Lee H, Weintraub S, Tsuang MT (1998) Are there sex differences in neuropsychological functions among patients with schizophrenia? Am J Psychiatry 155:1358–1364

Green MF, Horan WP, Lee J (2019) Nonsocial and social cognition in schizophrenia: current evidence and future directions. World Psychiatry 18:146–161

Grossman LS, Harrow M, Rosen C, Faull R, Strauss GP (2008) Sex differences in schizophrenia and other psychotic disorders: a 20-year longitudinal study of psychosis and recovery. Compr Psychiatry 49:523–529

Gur RC, Calkins ME, Satterthwaite TD, Ruparel K, Bilker WB, Moore TM, Savitt AP, Hakonarson H, Gur RE (2014) Neurocognitive growth charting in psychosis spectrum youths. JAMA Psychiat 71:366–374

Han M, Huang XF, Chen DC, Xiu MH, Hui L, Liu H, Kosten TR, Zhang XY (2012) Gender differences in cognitive function of patients with chronic schizophrenia. Prog Neuropsychopharmacol Biol Psychiatry 39:358–363

He H, Liu Q, Li N, Guo L, Gao F, Bai L, Gao F, Lyu J (2020) Trends in the incidence and DALYs of schizophrenia at the global, regional and national levels: results from the global burden of disease study 2017. Epidemiol Psychiatr Sci 29:e91

Huang AS, Rogers BP, Sheffield JM, Vandekar S, Anticevic A, Woodward ND (2021) Characterizing effects of age, sex and psychosis symptoms on thalamocortical functional connectivity in youth. Neuroimage 243:118562

Ittig S, Studerus E, Papmeyer M, Uttinger M, Koranyi S, Ramyead A, Riecher-Rossler A (2015) Sex differences in cognitive functioning in at-risk mental state for psychosis, first episode psychosis and healthy control subjects. Eur Psychiatry 30:242–250

Jacobs GR, Ameis SH, Ji JL, Viviano JD, Dickie EW, Wheeler AL, Stojanovski S, Anticevic A, Voineskos AN (2019) Developmentally divergent sexual dimorphism in the cortico-striatal-thalamic-cortical psychosis risk pathway. Neuropsychopharmacology 44:1649–1658

Larsen TK, McGlashan TH, Johannessen JO, Vibe-Hansen L (1996) First-episode schizophrenia: II. Premorbid patterns by gender. Schizophr Bull 22:257–269

Lee J, Green MF, Nuechterlein KH, Swerdlow NR, Greenwood TA, Hellemann GS, Lazzeroni LC, Light GA, Radant AD, Seidman LJ, Siever LJ, Silverman JM, Sprock J, Stone WS, Sugar CA, Tsuang DW, Tsuang MT, Turetsky BI, Gur RC, Gur RE, Braff DL (2020) The effects of age and sex on cognitive impairment in schizophrenia: findings from the consortium on the genetics of schizophrenia (COGS) study. PLoS One 15:e0232855

Maric N, Krabbendam L, Vollebergh W, de Graaf R, van Os J (2003) Sex differences in symptoms of psychosis in a non-selected, general population sample. Schizophr Res 63:89–95

McGrath J, Saha S, Welham J, El Saadi O, MacCauley C, Chant D (2004) A systematic review of the incidence of schizophrenia: the distribution of rates and the influence of sex, urbanicity, migrant status and methodology. BMC Med 2:13

Menghini-Muller S, Studerus E, Ittig S, Valmaggia LR, Kempton MJ, van der Gaag M, de Haan L, Nelson B, Bressan RA, Barrantes-Vidal N, Jantac C, Nordentoft M, Ruhrmann S, Sachs G, Rutten BP, van Os J, Riecher-Rossler A, EU-GEI High Risk Study Group (2020) Sex differences in cognitive functioning of patients at-risk for psychosis and healthy controls: results from the European gene-environment interactions study. Eur Psychiatry 63:e25

Minor K, Park S (1999) Spatial working memory: absence of gender differences in schizophrenia patients and healthy control subjects. Biol Psychiatry 46:1003–1005

Mossaheb N, Kaufmann RM, Schlogelhofer M, Aninilkumparambil T, Himmelbauer C, Gold A, Zehetmayer S, Hoffmann H, Traue HC, Aschauer H (2018) The impact of sex differences on odor identification and facial affect recognition in patients with schizophrenia spectrum disorders. Front Psych 9:9

Mu L, Liang J, Wang H, Chen D, Xiu M, Zhang XY (2020) Sex differences in association between clinical correlates and cognitive impairment in patients with chronic schizophrenia. J Psychiatr Res 131:194–202

Murray JD, Jaramillo J, Wang XJ (2017) Working memory and decision-making in a frontoparietal circuit model. J Neurosci 37:12167–12186

Navarra-Ventura G, Vicent-Gil M, Serra-Blasco M, Massons C, Crosas JM, Cobo J, Jubert A, Jodar M, Fernandez-Gonzalo S, Goldberg X, Palao D, Lahera G, Vieta E, Cardoner N (2021) Group and sex differences in social cognition in bipolar disorder, schizophrenia/schizoaffective disorder and healthy people. Compr Psychiatry 109:152258

Niv Y (2019) Learning task-state representations. Nat Neurosci 22:1544–1553

Pletzer B, Harris T, Hidalgo-Lopez E (2018) Subcortical structural changes along the menstrual cycle: beyond the hippocampus. Sci Rep 8:16042

Pritschet L, Santander T, Taylor CM, Layher E, Yu S, Miller MB, Grafton ST, Jacobs EG (2020) Functional reorganization of brain networks across the human menstrual cycle. Neuroimage 220:117091

Radulescu A, Niv Y (2019) State representation in mental illness. Curr Opin Neurobiol 55:160–166

Rehbein E, Hornung J, Sundstrom Poromaa I, Derntl B (2021) Shaping of the female human brain by sex hormones: a review. Neuroendocrinology 111:183–206

Rietschel L, Lambert M, Karow A, Zink M, Muller H, Heinz A, de Millas W, Janssen B, Gaebel W, Schneider F, Naber D, Juckel G, Kruger-Ozgurdal S, Wobrock T, Wagner M, Maier W, Klosterkotter J, Bechdolf A, Group, P.S. (2017) Clinical high risk for psychosis: gender differences in symptoms and social functioning. Early Interv Psychiatry 11:306–313

Rodriguez-Jimenez R, Dompablo M, Bagney A, Santabarbara J, Aparicio AI, Torio I, Moreno-Ortega M, Lopez-Anton R, Lobo A, Kern RS, Green MF, Jimenez-Arriero MA, Santos JL, Nuechterlein KH, Palomo T (2015) The MCCB impairment profile in a Spanish sample of patients with schizophrenia: effects of diagnosis, age, and gender on cognitive functioning. Schizophr Res 169:116–120

Roesch-Ely D, Hornberger E, Weiland S, Hornstein C, Parzer P, Thomas C, Weisbrod M (2009) Do sex differences affect prefrontal cortex associated cognition in schizophrenia? Schizophr Res 107:255–261

Saha S, Chant D, Welham J, McGrath J (2005) A systematic review of the prevalence of schizophrenia. PLoS Med 2:e141

Seeman MV (2012) Menstrual exacerbation of schizophrenia symptoms. Acta Psychiatr Scand 125: 363–371

Segarra R, Ojeda N, Zabala A, Garcia J, Catalan A, Eguiluz JI, Gutierrez M (2012) Similarities in early course among men and women with a first episode of schizophrenia and schizophreniform disorder. Eur Arch Psychiatry Clin Neurosci 262:95–105

Seidman LJ, Goldstein JM, Goodman JM, Koren D, Turner WM, Faraone SV, Tsuang MT (1997) Sex differences in olfactory identification and Wisconsin card sorting performance in schizophrenia: relationship to attention and verbal ability. Biol Psychiatry 42:104–115

Stefanatou P, Karatosidi CS, Tsompanaki E, Kattoulas E, Stefanis NC, Smyrnis N (2018) Premorbid adjustment predictors of cognitive dysfunction in schizophrenia. Psychiatry Res 267:249–255

Thompson AE, Voyer D (2014) Sex differences in the ability to recognise non-verbal displays of emotion: a meta-analysis. Cognit Emot 28:1164–1195

Voyer D, Voyer SD, Saint-Aubin J (2017) Sex differences in visual-spatial working memory: a meta-analysis. Psychon Bull Rev 24:307–334

Voyer D, Saint Aubin J, Altman K, Gallant G (2021) Sex differences in verbal working memory: a systematic review and meta-analysis. Psychol Bull 147:352–398

Walder DJ, Holtzman CW, Addington J, Cadenhead K, Tsuang M, Cornblatt B, Cannon TD, McGlashan TH, Woods SW, Perkins DO, Seidman LJ, Heinssen R, Walker EF (2013) Sexual dimorphisms and prediction of conversion in the NAPLS psychosis prodrome. Schizophr Res 144:43–50

Walsh-Messinger J, Stepanek C, Wiedemann J, Goetz D, Goetz RR, Malaspina D (2019) Normal sexual dimorphism in theory of mind circuitry is reversed in schizophrenia. Soc Neurosci 14: 583–593

Weis S, Hausmann M, Stoffers B, Sturm W (2011) Dynamic changes in functional cerebral connectivity of spatial cognition during the menstrual cycle. Hum Brain Mapp 32:1544–1556

Wierenga LM, Doucet GE, Dima D, Agartz I, Aghajani M, Akudjedu TN, Albajes-Eizagirre A, Alnaes D, Alpert KI, Andreassen OA, Anticevic A, Asherson P, Banaschewski T, Bargallo N, Baumeister S, Baur-Streubel R, Bertolino A, Bonvino A, Boomsma DI, Borgwardt S, Bourque J, den Braber A, Brandeis D, Breier A, Brodaty H, Brouwer RM, Buitelaar JK, Busatto GF, Calhoun VD, Canales-Rodriguez EJ, Cannon DM, Caseras X, Castellanos FX, Chaim-Avancini TM, Ching CR, Clark VP, Conrod PJ, Conzelmann A, Crivello F, Davey CG, Dickie EW, Ehrlich S, Van't Ent D, Fisher SE, Fouche JP, Franke B, Fuentes-Claramonte P, de Geus EJ, Di Giorgio A, Glahn DC, Gotlib IH, Grabe HJ, Gruber O, Gruner P, Gur RE, Gur RC, Gurholt TP, de Haan L, Haatveit B, Harrison BJ, Hartman CA, Hatton SN, Heslenfeld DJ, van den Heuvel OA, Hickie IB, Hoekstra PJ, Hohmann S, Holmes AJ, Hoogman M, Hosten N, Howells FM, Hulshoff Pol HE, Huyser C, Jahanshad N, James AC, Jiang J, Jonsson EG, Joska JA, Kalnin AJ, Karolinska Schizophrenia Project Consortium, Klein M, Koenders L, Kolskar KK, Kramer B, Kuntsi J, Lagopoulos J, Lazaro L, Lebedeva IS, Lee PH, Lochner C, Machielsen

MW, Maingault S, Martin NG, Martinez-Zalacain I, Mataix-Cols D, Mazoyer B, McDonald BC, McDonald C, McIntosh AM, McMahon KL, McPhilemy G, van der Meer D, Menchon JM, Naaijen J, Nyberg L, Oosterlaan J, Paloyelis Y, Pauli P, Pergola G, Pomarol-Clotet E, Portella MJ, Radua J, Reif A, Richard G, Roffman JL, Rosa PG, Sacchet MD, Sachdev PS, Salvador R, Sarro S, Satterthwaite TD, Saykin AJ, Serpa MH, Sim K, Simmons A, Smoller JW, Sommer IE, Soriano-Mas C, Stein DJ, Strike LT, Szeszko PR, Temmingh HS, Thomopoulos SI, Tomyshev AS, Trollor JN, Uhlmann A, Veer IM, Veltman DJ, Voineskos A, Volzke H, Walter H, Wang L, Wang Y, Weber B, Wen W, West JD, Westlye LT, Whalley HC, Williams SC, Wittfeld K, Wolf DH, Wright MJ, Yoncheva YN, Zanetti MV, Ziegler GC, de Zubicaray GI, Thompson PM, Crone EA, Frangou S, Tamnes CK (2022) Greater male than female variability in regional brain structure across the lifespan. Hum Brain Mapp 43:470–499

Womer FY, Tang Y, Harms MP, Bai C, Chang M, Jiang X, Wei S, Wang F, Barch DM (2016) Sexual dimorphism of the cerebellar vermis in schizophrenia. Schizophr Res 176:164–170

Zhang XY, Chen DC, Xiu MH, Yang FD, Haile CN, Kosten TA, Kosten TR (2012) Gender differences in never-medicated first-episode schizophrenia and medicated chronic schizophrenia patients. J Clin Psychiatry 73:1025–1033

Zhang B, Han M, Tan S, De Yang F, Tan Y, Jiang S, Zhang X, Huang XF (2017) Gender differences measured by the MATRICS consensus cognitive battery in chronic schizophrenia patients. Sci Rep 7:11821

Zhao S, Wang G, Yan T, Xiang J, Yu X, Li H, Wang B (2021) Sex differences in anatomical Rich-Club and structural-functional coupling in the human brain network. Cereb Cortex 31:1987–1997

Rethinking Immunity and Cognition in Clinical High Risk for Psychosis

Siân Lowri Griffiths, Rachel Upthegrove, Fabiana Corsi-Zuelli, and Bill Deakin

Contents

S. L. Griffiths and R. Upthegrove
Institute for Mental Health, University of Birmingham, Birmingham, UK

F. Corsi-Zuelli
Institute for Mental Health, University of Birmingham, Birmingham, UK

Division of Psychiatry, Department of Neuroscience and Behaviour, Ribeirao Preto Medical School, University of São Paulo, São Paulo, Brazil

B. Deakin (✉)
Division of Neuroscience and Experimental Psychology, Faculty of Biology, Medicine and Health, School of Biological Sciences, University of Manchester, Manchester, UK
e-mail: bill.deakin@manchester.ac.uk

Curr Topics Behav Neurosci (2023) 63: 475–498
https://doi.org/10.1007/7854_2022_399
Published Online: 22 November 2022

Abstract It is well known that schizophrenia is associated with cognitive impairment, reduced cortical grey matter and increased circulating concentrations of inflammatory cytokines. However, the relationship between these findings is not clear. We outline the influential neuroinflammatory hypotheses that raised cytokines provoke a damaging immune response in microglia that results in reduced grey matter and associated cognitive performance. We investigated whether such an interaction might be detectable in the prodromal period as illness emerges from the Clinical High Risk for Psychosis (CHR-P). Meta-analyses suggest that compared with controls, impaired cognition and reduced grey matter are already present by the prodrome and that greater decrements are present in those who later develop symptoms. In contrast, the few cytokine studies report no abnormalities in CHR-P except that interleukin-6 (IL-6) levels were raised versus controls and to a greater extent in the future patients, in one study. We noted that cognitive impairment and less cortical grey matter are more severe in schizophrenia than in affective disorders, but that increased cytokine levels are similarly prevalent across disorders. We found no studies correlating cytokine levels with cognitive impairment in CHR-P but such correlations seem unlikely given the minimal relationship reported in a recent meta-analysis of the many cytokine-cognition studies in established illness. From this and other evidence, we conclude that neuroinflammation is not a core feature of schizophrenia nor a substrate for reduced grey matter volume or cognitive function. We draw attention instead to the emerging evidence that brain-resident immune cells and signalling molecules such as Tregs and IL-6, which are influenced by schizophrenia risk genes, regulate and are necessary for the development and function of neuron–glia interaction. We suggest that cognitive impairment in schizophrenia can be seen as a convergence of genetic and immune-neurodevelopmental dysregulation whereas raised cytokines are a consequence of impaired Tregs control of systemic inflammation.

Keywords Cognitive function · Cytokines · Genetics · Inflammation · IQ · Schizoprenia risk · Treg cells

1 Cognition and the Emergence of Psychosis from Risk

1.1 Overview

Impaired cognitive functioning is a core component of the schizophrenia spectrum and is detrimental to quality of life and social and occupational functioning. It is evident across all stages of illness (Green 1996); prior to onset of illness with origins in early development, and may progress in some around the time of illness onset and with chronicity (Khandaker et al. 2011). The profile of schizophrenia risk genes overlaps considerably with other neurodevelopmental disorder profiles; they relate to synaptic function and neurodevelopment and contribute to cognitive impairment in neurodevelopmental disorders (Kim et al. 2021; Trubetskoy et al. 2022). In this chapter we address the question of whether immune mechanisms and inflammation contribute to the evolution of cognitive impairment in schizophrenia.

The fact that psychotic symptoms do not emerge until early adulthood and usually from a clear prodromal phase, is suggestive of an active brain process underlying transition and this is one attraction of the inflammatory hypothesis. The clinical high-risk state for psychosis (CHR-P) is defined by the presence of either attenuated psychotic symptoms (APS), brief limited intermittent psychotic symptoms (BLIPS), or by genetic vulnerability and deterioration (Fusar-Poli et al. 2012; Yung et al. 2005). The presence of these syndromes predicts increased risk of transition to psychosis of around 20% at 12 months, and 30% at 3 years, which is significantly higher than the general population (Fusar-Poli et al. 2012). This predictability has inspired the prospect of preventing the development of psychosis with appropriate interventions in those with CHR-P (Fusar-Poli et al. 2020; Yung et al. 2007). However, a major difficulty is that the substantial majority who will not develop psychosis will risk unnecessary interventions and potential adverse side effects. Furthermore, there is considerable variation in the pattern of symptoms, severity and prognosis in CHR-P, which makes it difficult to target and evaluate preventative interventions. These issues have led to major efforts and longitudinal cohort studies to find categorical subtypes and dimensions of the CHR-P based on clinical features, cognitive profiling and molecular biomarkers, which will better identify risk and identify pathogenesis.

The influential neuroinflammatory hypothesis of schizophrenia proposes that mild peripheral immune activation gives rise to an inflammatory response in the brain and the neurobiological changes associated with illness onset and cognitive impairment. The origin of the immune activation is not well specified but exposure to prior infection in utero or in early life is a risk factor for psychosis that might sensitise immune responses to later stressors or infection. We discuss the meta-analytic evidence that circulating concentrations of interleukin 6 (IL-6) and other inflammatory proteins such as C-reactive protein (CRP) are increased in people with schizophrenia compared with controls and may precede illness by many years. The neuroinflammatory hypothesis has generally assumed that microglia, the brain's resident immune cells, are activated and pathogenic in schizophrenia as supported by some traditional neuropathological studies and by initial in-vivo positron emission tomography (PET) imaging studies (Corsi-Zuelli et al. 2021). Inflammatory damage might also account for evidence of oxidative stress from MRS glutathione studies (Perkins et al. 2020). There has been much interest in the possibility that cognitive impairment is a manifestation of brain dysfunction caused by inflammation in schizophrenia (Kogan et al. 2020; Khandaker et al. 2015).

In this chapter we review the literature on inflammation and neurocognition in the CHR-P population relying as far as possible on meta-analytic evidence. We will first present evidence of the cognitive profiles of CHR-P individuals and the associated risk of conversion to psychosis. Second, we will introduce the literature on immune dysfunction and the current neuroinflammation framework of pathogenesis of psychosis. We will examine evidence of the inflammatory signature within the different stages of psychosis and whether they relate to cognitive and grey matter changes. We will critically rethink the current framework.

1.2 Assessment of Cognitive Function

Over the last century many studies have reported that patients with schizophrenia perform less well than controls on tests of IQ and tests of specific mental abilities. However, there has been considerable variation in tests and techniques, which has hindered consensus and generalisable conclusions on the nature and role of cognitive impairment in the pathogenesis of schizophrenia. To address these limitations, the National Institute of Mental Health Research (NIMH) Measurement and Treatment to Improve Cognition in Schizophrenia (MATRICS) consensus developed a cognitive battery for use in clinical trials in psychosis (Green et al. 2008; Nuechterlein et al. 2008). MATRICS assesses seven cognitive domains that are consistently impaired within psychosis: Speed of Processing, Attention/Vigilance, Working Memory, Verbal Learning and Memory, Visual Learning and Memory, Reasoning and Problem Solving and Verbal Comprehension (Green et al. 2000, 2004; Nuechterlein et al. 2008) (Table 1). Although the MATRCIS tasks assess different cognitive domains, it is important to note that a single general factor, probably relating to IQ, accounts for much of the variance.

1.3 Cognitive Impairment in CHR-P

The most recent and largest systematic and meta-analytic review of cognitive impairment in CHR-P covered 78 studies up to 2020 giving a sample of 5,162 participants (Catalan et al. 2021). They reported medium to large neurocognitive impairments across the MATRICS domains and in a number of other tests with the

Table 1 MATRICS consensus cognitive test battery

Cognitive function	MATRICS subtest
Speed of processing	Symbol coding subtest (brief assessment of cognition in schizophrenia)
Speed of processing	Category fluency test, animal naming
Speed of processing	Trail making test, part A
Attention/vigilance	Continuous performance test, identical pairs version
Verbal learning	Hopkins verbal learning test – revised, immediate recall
Working memory (verbal)	Letter-number span test
Working memory (non-verbal)	Verbal learning Wechsler memory scale, third ed., spatial span subtest
Reasoning and problem solving	Mazes subtest (neuropsychological assessment battery)

largest effects on executive functions and verbal learning (Hedges $g = >0.86$) and the least on premorbid levels of intelligence. Taking a categorical approach, two studies agree in finding that 45% of CHR-P scored below normative values and 55% were within 1.5 SD of the normal range (Velthorst et al. 2019; Haining et al. 2022).

Social cognition, which is typically considered a separable domain of cognition and is defined as the mental operations underlying social interactions, is impaired in psychosis, and there is evidence of impairment in CHR-P, particularly in relation to Theory of Mind (ToM) (Thompson et al. 2012; Catalan et al. 2021; Ntouros et al. 2018). Evidence of impairments in other social cognitive domains is inconsistent, with some studies finding impairments in CHR-P compared to healthy controls, and other studies reporting no differences (Catalan et al. 2021).The inclusion of different tasks to measure the separate domains of social cognition may in part account for this observation.

1.4 Cognitive Performance in CHR-P Predicts Onset of Psychosis

Several studies have shown that more severe performance deficits in the CHR-P population are associated with greater risk of subsequent onset of psychosis, and initial impairment can approach that of FEP individuals ($\geq$1 SD below the normative mean) (Carrión et al. 2018; Fusar-Poli et al. 2012; Bora et al. 2014). Large deficits across a number of cognitive domains have been reported in those who later transition, including impairments in general intelligence, processing speed, attention, working memory, attention/vigilance, verbal fluency, visual and verbal memory and executive function (Addington et al. 2017; Fusar-Poli et al. 2012; Riecher-Rössler et al. 2009; Seidman et al. 2016). One study reported that CHR-P who transition had lower scores on social cognition, in particular, Theory of Mind (ToM) (Kim et al. 2011). There have been no statistical tests on whether cognitive domains are differentially predictive of psychosis onset.

Beyond CHR-P populations, longitudinal epidemiological studies consistently report that lower IQ is a risk factor for schizophrenia (Khandaker et al. 2011). A meta-analysis of 15 longitudinal studies of birth cohorts, army conscripts, and other cohorts, lower premorbid IQ was associated with the risk of a formal diagnosis of schizophrenia; the relationship was linear and predicted earlier age of onset (Khandaker et al. 2011). More recent analyses of the Dunedin and ALSPAC birth cohorts show an early deficit in verbal IQ by 7–8 years which remains static with a later developing lag in non-verbal IQ. The profiles are specific to future schizophrenia as they were not seen in those who developed depressive symptoms. Progressive deterioration is not obvious in these studies. The evidence is therefore strongly in favour of an early neurodevelopmental impairment that hinders future cognitive development.

1.5 CHR-P: Cognition, Grey Matter and Polygenic Risk

There is clear evidence that the CHR-P is associated with changes in brain structure (Lawrie et al. 1999) and exaggerated in those who transition (Pantelis et al. 2003). The compellingly large ENIGMA CHR-P consortium compared 1792 CHR-P individual MRI scans (253 converters) with 1,377 healthy controls. There were global reductions in grey matter (GM) thickness and surface areas, and intracranial volumes in the CHR-P vs. controls and bilateral graduated decreases across converters, non-converters and healthy controls in fusiform and paracentral gyri and other areas (Jalbrzikowski et al. 2021). A number of longitudinal studies have been carried out that might address the issue of when the GM loss occurs. In a systematic review of 36 papers from 15 longitudinal studies in CHR-P with interscan intervals of mostly <6 years, better identification of transition came from the longitudinal data than baseline alone. GM thickness and volume reduction occur in normal development from late childhood to early adulthood through pruning and myelination. This pattern was not seen in the high-risk groups in which GM thickness remained low throughout and declined further in the converters (Merritt et al. 2021; Cannon et al. 2015).

The CHR-P cognitive and imaging data so far discussed would appear to cohere in suggesting that early neurodevelopment is disturbed and gives rise to the CHR-P. Although there are no longitudinal studies to confirm whether the developmental cognitive changes are mediated by the brain changes, a recent genetic study suggests they may be related but somewhat dissociated from genetic mechanisms of schizophrenia. In brief, Corley and colleagues showed that the microglial gene component of polygenic risk scores (PGS) for schizophrenia was associated with poorer cognitive function in patients with schizophrenia and that the effect was mediated by reduced GM volume (Corley et al. 2021). This same relationship held in the general UK Biobank population. As might be expected, the neuronal and to lesser extent the astroglial component of PGS was positively related to cognition via increased GM volume. A recent analysis from the Psychiatric Genetics Consortium found that polygenic risk for IQ in the general population predicted IQ in schizophrenia but the PGS for schizophrenia did not (Richards et al. 2020). These findings suggest that intellectual impairment is partially dissociated from the genetic track to psychosis and other explanations for the clinical association are needed; abnormal immune mechanisms of development may be one.

2 The Immune System and Its Role in the Pathogenesis of Psychosis

2.1 Overview of the Immune System

The immune system engages in highly complex and coordinated processes, involving many different cell types that provide protection from harmful pathogens. The immune system can be conceptually divided into two systems: the innate immune system, and the adaptive immune system; there is considerable interaction between the two (Ermakov et al. 2022).

The innate immune system, also known as natural or native, is our first immunological line of defence. This system exists prior to infection or tissue damage and is programmed to respond rapidly to insults. It is non-specific (antigen-independent) with no immunological memory of previous responses. The components include physical and chemical barriers (epithelium and mucous membranes), inflammatory mediators (acute phase proteins such as C-reactive protein (CRP), cytokines and the complement system), phagocytes and antigen-presenting cells (neutrophils, dendritic cells, monocytes/macrophages, natural killer cells). The cells of the innate immune system process antigens and present their peptide fragments to cells of the adaptive immune system (Upthegrove et al. 2014; Ermakov et al. 2022).

The adaptive immune system, in contrast to the innate, is slower but highly specific (antigen-dependent and antigen-specific) and is characterised by memory. It provides a delayed humoral and cellular response that is directed to specific antigens learned and subsequently recognised via the immune instruction/selection mechanism. It comprises humoral immunity, the antibodies produced by type B lymphocytes, and cellular immunity, including T (thymic) lymphocytes which recognise specific antigens (Khandaker et al. 2015). T lymphocytes or T cells can express the cluster of differentiation (CD) antigen 4 ($CD4^{+}$) or CD8+ on their exterior cell surfaces. CD4+ cells can be subdivided mainly into Th1, Th2, Th17 and Tregs, which have specific functions (Upthegrove et al. 2014; Ermakov et al. 2022). Table 2 provides a breakdown of key terms.

Among the distinct subtypes of T cells, there has been a growing interest in the role of a specialised type of regulatory cells known as regulatory T cells (Tregs) in psychosis. Tregs promote tolerance against self-antigens, protect from maternal infections and autoimmune disease and control peripheral inflammation. Tregs have been identified in the healthy human brain where they regulate the interaction between microglia and astrocytes (Corsi-Zuelli et al. 2021; Corsi-Zuelli and Deakin 2021; Pasciuto et al. 2020).

2.2 *The Brain and the Periphery: The Role of Cytokines*

Cytokines orchestrate the immune response and the communication between the innate and adaptive immune systems and communicate with the CNS via the vagus nerve and the circumventricular organ that lacks a blood brain barrier (BBB) in experimental animal studies (Khandaker and Dantzer 2016). There are pro- and anti-inflammatory cytokines; some are pleiotropic on the context or cytokine milieu. Table 3 provides an overview of key cytokines and their function. The degree to which cytokines permeate the BBB physiologically in humans is not well researched and probably varies between cytokines and whether they have active transport mechanisms, and the degree to which they are bound to soluble receptors in the

Table 2 The Immune system: overview of key terms

Key term	Description
Acute phase proteins	Part of innate system secreted in response to infection, inflammation and tissue damage (e.g., CRP). Non-specific/indirect marker of inflammation
Adaptive immune system	Antigen-dependent and antigen-specific immune memory Humoral immunity: antibody secreting B lymphocytes Cellular immunity: T lymphocytes (CD4+ and CD8+) and related cytokines
Astrocytes	Pervasive glial cells that surround and provide metabolic support to neurones and synapses. End feet on blood vessels are part of the blood brain barrier (BBB), which prevents and regulates permeability to circulating molecules, cells and invading organisms
Complement Cascade	Innate immune defence of >20 interacting proteins that control infections by opsonising (marking) pathogens and facilitating phagocytosis
Cytokines	Key signalling low molecular weight proteins that coordinate and mediate the communication between innate and adaptive systems. They can be both pro- or/and anti-inflammatory depending on the cytokine milieu
Innate immune system	Immediate immune defence triggered by recognition of bacterial and viral molecular markers and tissue damage markers. Involves barriers, acute phase proteins, complement and cells that phagocytose and present antigens – neutrophils, dendritic cells, monocytes/macrophages, natural killer cells
Macrophages	Innate immunity phagocytic cells that can sometimes present antigens to adaptive immune cells
Microglia	Glial cells in brain derived from the yolk-sack (not the marrow), with equivalent function to macrophages. Microglial processes survey the brain parenchyma to remove (prune) redundant or pathological synapses crucial for brain development. Become mobile and amoeboid in response to antigens and secrete inflammatory cytokines and other messengers
Monocytes	White blood cells that respond quickly to infections as part of the innate immune response. Can become macrophages to replenish numbers
Natural killer cells	Activated as part of the immune response with a unique ability to identify and kill infected cells in the absence of antibodies
T (thymic) lymphocytes	Key cells of adaptive immunity that are programmed in the thymus and help to shape the immune response. T-cell subtypes include those that express the cluster of differentiation 4 (CD4+) or 8 (CD8+) CD4+ cells: • T helper 1 (Th1) – promote cellular immune responses against intracellular viral and bacterial infections by producing pro-inflammatory cytokines, such as INF-γ, TNF-α and by inducing macrophages and CD8+ T-cell activation • T helper 2 (Th2) – promote response against extracellular pathogens and are involved in allergic reactions. They produce anti-inflammatory cytokines, such as IL-4, IL-5, IL-3, IL-13, which stimulate B cell expansion and antibody production • T helper 17 (Th17) – produce IL-17 and related cytokines for the clearance of helminth infections and the maintenance of mucosal barriers. Powerful drivers of inflammation and autoimmunity

(continued)

Table 2 (continued)

Key term	Description
	• Regulatory T (Treg) cells – regulate and limit inflammation to promote immunological self-tolerance. Various effectors include production of anti-inflammatory and immunosuppressive cytokines (IL-10 and TGF-β) • CD8+ T cells – promote host defence against cytosolic pathogens by killing infected cells (cells infected with viruses; cancer cells) using the perforin-granzyme pathway and death ligands
B lymphocytes	Humoral part of the adaptive arm and responsible for secreting antibodies

Table 3 Overview of cytokines implicated in the pathogenesis of psychosis

Cytokine	Function	
1L-RA	Anti-inflammatory	Soluble IL-1 receptor that binds IL-1β blocking its pro-inflammatory actions. Involved in compensatory anti-inflammatory response syndrome (CARS), a global deactivation of the immune system in response to severe infection
IL-1β	Pro-inflammatory	Secreted by macrophages and induces acute phase proteins
IL-2	Mixed	Pleiotropic cytokine. Drives T-cell growth and modulates for Th cell differentiation. Important for the differentiation and survival of Tregs
IL-4	Anti-inflammatory	Produced by Th2 cells and is important to inhibit Th1 cells and IFN-γ production
IL-6	Mixed	Pleiotropic cytokine that has both pro- and anti-inflammatory properties. It induces the release of acute phase proteins, such as CRP, from the liver
IL-10	Anti-inflammatory	Produced by Th2 and Treg lymphocytes, and anti-inflammatory monocytes/macrophages. Controls inflammatory and pro-inflammatory immune cells
TNF-α	Pro-inflammatory	Sourced from macrophages and induces acute phase proteins
TGF-β	Anti-inflammatory	Immunosuppressive cytokine with key role in cell proliferation, differentiation and morphogenesis. When combined to IL-2, induces the polarisation of Tregs
IFN-γ	Pro-inflammatory	Secreted by Th 1 lymphocytes, natural killer cells and activates macrophages

IL interleukin, *IL-1RA* Interleukin-1 Receptor Antagonist, *TGF* transforming growth factor, *TNF* tumour necrosis factor, *IFN* interferon

circulation. Whether mild non-pathological increases in circulating cytokines observed in depression and psychosis would be sufficient to induce neuroinflammation is unknown. However, according to the microglial inflammation hypothesis, a non-resolving and chronic blood inflammation damages the BBB, allowing cytokines to activate microglia and initiate neuroinflammation as depicted in Fig. 1 (Khandaker et al. 2015).

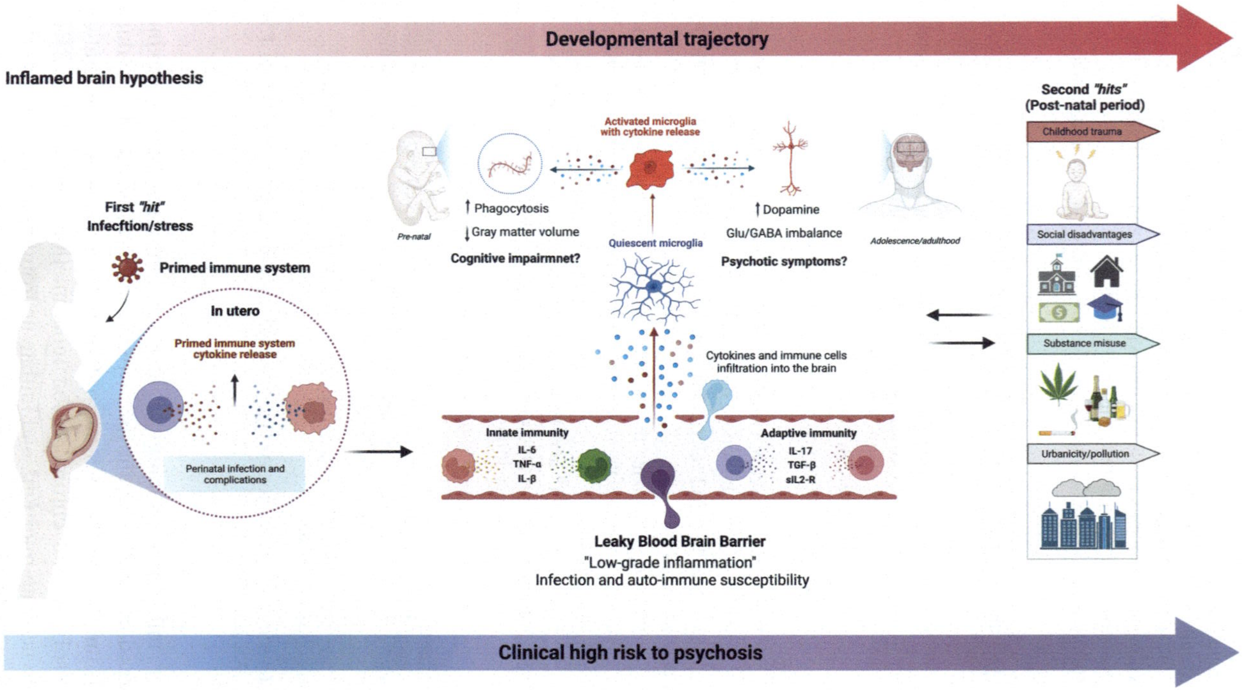

Fig. 1 The inflamed brain hypothesis of psychosis risk. Left to right. Maternal infection exposes the foetus to inflammatory cytokines which condition the developing immune system to chronic activation. Bottom: chronic systemic inflammation weakens the BBB allowing cytokines and inflammatory cells to infiltrate the brain parenchyma. Chronic inflammation may facilitate autoimmunity and mediate prevalent medical co-morbidities such as vascular disease and diabetes. Top: Infiltrated cytokines stimulate microglia to amoeboid inflamed state with phagocytosis of neuronal elements and white matter oligodendrocytes. Inflamed microglia secrete cytokines that affect neuronal function and chemokines that draw in peripheral immune cells causing further CNS disruption and inducing the CHR-P. Right: Environmental stressors and risk factors become second hits that aggravate neuroinflammation and push the CHR-P to psychosis onset

2.3 *Neuroinflammation and Psychosis: The 'Two-Hit' Vulnerability-Stress Hypothesis*

Prevalent versions of the immune hypothesis of schizophrenia propose that early exposure to elevated inflammation in gestation or in early childhood may 'prime' the brain for the development of psychotic disorders following later stressors (Giovanoli et al. 2013; Cannon et al. 2014; Föcking et al. 2016; Khandaker et al. 2015). The formative finding in a classic study was that maternal levels of CRP in 777 mothers incrementally predicted risk of later psychosis. The evidence that maternal infection may set off the inflammation is that the offspring of mothers exposed to pre-natal infections are at increased risk of psychosis. This risk is now clear for toxoplasma (OR = 1.30), HSV2 and 'infection not specified' but not as previously thought, influenza or cytomegalovirus (see meta-analysis by Davies et al. (2020)). It is likely that genetic risk, which is predominantly neurodevelopmental and synaptic (Trubetskoy et al. 2022), provides a susceptible substrate for cytokine-induced disruption together with other perinatal adversities; a family history of psychosis amplified the risk associated with maternal infection in one study (Clarke et al. 2009). The risks associated with increased CRP levels were also evident at age 15, suggesting that a persistent state of mild inflammation is part of vulnerability to second hits and the onset of illness (Metcalf et al. 2017).

According to the two-hit model, second hits such as infection, substance misuse, deprivation and physical and sexual abuse act on the primed vulnerable brain during the sensitive period of synaptic remodelling in adolescence, in part via exaggerated inflammatory responses (Fig. 1). Interestingly a meta-analysis of 25 studies in the general population reported significant effect sizes for an influence of retrospectively reported physical and sexual maltreatment on adult CRF, IL-6 and TNF-α levels (Baumeister et al. 2016). However there have only been four studies in psychosis with mixed results (Kerr et al. 2021). One careful study found that childhood abuse in first episode patients, and to a lesser extent their relatives, was associated with increased TGF-β compared to the non-abused group (Corsi-Zuelli et al. 2020). The authors concluded that stressors early in life may aggravate a hidden genetic liability to immune dysregulation that may manifest only in some subgroups of patients or their first-degree relatives.

It is now well-established that increased concentrations of circulating cytokines occur in untreated first episode psychosis, indicating a mild persistent state of systemic immune activation, with various routes by which cytokines can communicate with brain (Khandaker and Dantzer 2016). This activation has led to the current theory that cytokines penetrate the brain to activate the brains resident macrophage-like immune cells, the microglia. Inflamed microglia set off a state of brain inflammation akin to other neuroinflammatory disorders, with neurotoxic and other damaging cellular effects – the BBB becomes permeable and peripheral inflammatory cells are attracted into the brain and cause further damage (Comer et al. 2020; Monji et al. 2009; Cannon et al. 2014; Khandaker and Dantzer 2016; Goldsmith et al. 2016).

2.4 Role of Cytokines: Correlation or Causation?

Circulating cytokine levels are influenced by many environmental and internal factors and this makes it difficult to convert correlation to causality. However, recent Mendelian randomisation studies point to a causal genetic role for IL-6 underlying the risk of schizophrenia. In a birth cohort study, three functional SNPs in IL-6 and IL-6R were shown to increase the risk of schizophrenia in direct proportion to the increase in IL-6 levels predicted by the variants. The results demonstrate that the association between high IL-6 levels and schizophrenia is not due to confounding factors such as smoking but rather indicates high IL-6 levels have a causal role in schizophrenia. They found tentative effects among 20 cytokines and other inflammatory markers but only the IL-6 findings survived statistical corrections; IL-6 was also related to depression (Perry et al. 2021).

In a Mendelian randomisation study on brain structure using UK Biobank data ($n = 20{,}688$), the authors demonstrated that genes influencing IL-6 levels overlapped with those associated with GM volume of the Middle Temporal Gyrus (MTG). Furthermore, risk genes for schizophrenia as well as IL-6 pathway proteins are overexpressed in MTG compared to other brain regions according to the Allen Brain Atlas (Williams et al. 2022). Importantly, other cytokines including IL-1 and CRP did not show such effects. A study remarkable for its fMRI measures of brain connectivity in neonates showed that the measures could accurately retrospectively estimate maternal IL-6 concentrations measured during gestation, which also accounted for variance in working memory at 2 years of age (Rudolph et al. 2018). These studies suggest that the IL-6 pathway may be a key physiological player in early neurodevelopment, which, through genetic predisposition or early exposure to infection, may predispose to aberrant responses to later environmental influences.

2.5 Cytokine Profiles and Clusters in Established Psychosis

Several influential meta-analyses and systematic reviews have reported increased circulating cytokine concentrations in people with schizophrenia (Goldsmith et al. 2016; Miller et al. 2011; Zhou et al. 2021; Momtazmanesh et al. 2019; Potvin et al. 2008). A recent meta-analysis concluded that pro-inflammatory cytokines including IL-6, IL-12, IL-1β, TNF-α and TGF-β were the most consistently increased (Ermakov et al. 2022). However, meta-analyses do not all agree, and the results obviously depend on which studies have been selected. Considerable caution is required in interpreting results because a variety of factors may influence blood cytokine concentrations; three specific confounds are smoking, BMI and exposure to antipsychotics, with the latter confounded by duration of illness (Capuzzi et al. 2017). In the three most recent meta-analyses of studies in rigorously defined drug-naive patients in a first episode, IL-6, IFN-γ and IL-17 were consistently increased, TNF-α and IL-1β changes were uncertain and IL-2, IL-4, IL-8 and CRP were consistently not increased but even this summary is debateable (Upthegrove et al. 2014; Dunleavy et al. 2022; Pillinger et al. 2018). Increased cytokines have been detected in cerebro-spinal fluid (CSF) from patients with schizophrenia, bipolar disorder and major depression which were paralleled by increases in blood (Wang and Miller 2018). The elevated CSF cytokine levels suggest the brain can be exposed to increased circulating levels.

We draw attention to three further factors about cytokines. First, it is important to note that increases in cytokines are mild in comparison with values seen in inflammatory diseases, therefore, the functional significance must remain uncertain especially since unmeasured molecules such as soluble receptors for IL-6 determine how much IL-6 is seen by target membrane-bound receptors. Cytokines have important signalling functions within the CNS, and much is known about the roles of IL-6, so there is much opportunity for interaction, for instance with microglia, but little evidence of the actuality. More detailed discussion can be found in additional articles (Corsi-Zuelli et al. 2021; Goldsmith et al. 2016).

Second, cytokine increases are observed to an equal extent in major depression, bipolar disorder and autism. This finding has led to suggestions that cytokine changes reflect a transdiagnostic dimension of illness such as depression, fatigue, or anhedonia, which is common to the major mental illnesses (Goldsmith et al. 2016). Equally, the mild immune activation could reflect a shared exposure to prevalent environmental adversities. Schizophrenia is distinguished from depression by the severity of cognitive impairment, and this militates against a causal role for CNS effects of peripheral inflammation in cognitive impairment in schizophrenia.

Third, there is little evidence that immune subtypes of schizophrenia can be defined by cytokine levels alone. This premise was explored in one meta-analysis which reported that there was generally less variation in cytokine levels in patients than in controls and no evidence of bimodality (Pillinger et al. 2018). This evidence suggests mild immune activation is present to some degree in most patients. However, there is evidence that high CRP relates to cognitive decline as indicated by the difference between current and premorbid IQ, but non-specifically in psychosis and bipolar patients (Millett et al. 2021; Watson et al. 2022). Several groups, including our own, are applying machine learning and clustering techniques to cytokine profiles to define inflammatory subtypes in large datasets, externally validated by cognitive profiles and structural brain changes, with promising, but as yet, unpublished results. One study has sought such evidence although not in a CHR-P group (Fillman et al. 2016). In a whole blood cytokine gene expression analysis ignoring diagnosis, 44 patients (with illnesses averaging 11 years) and 33 controls were defined by high and low inflammation status. The immune cluster had higher expression of IL-1β, IL-8, IL-6 and IL-2 and contained 40% of the patients and 21% of the controls. There were no differences between the clusters on full-scale or premorbid IQ, or the 8 subtests. Patients scored 1 SD less than controls and this was not influenced by high vs. low inflammation except on a word- association subtest. A similar pattern was seen in grey matter in selected regions of interest. In short, there was little evidence that an immune cytokine-defined transdiagnostic subtype impacted cognitive impairment or grey matter volumes.

3 Inflammatory Profiles in the Prodrome

3.1 *Inflammatory Profiles and Onset of Psychosis*

A considerable advantage in studying immune mechanism of CHR-P is that the correlates of vulnerability are free of confounds of illness and drug treatment. The most consistent finding in a recent meta-analysis of 7 cytokine studies was that IL-6 concentrations were significantly greater in CHR-P ($n = 81$) versus 148 controls in the 5 studies in which it was measured (Park and Miller 2020). The effect size was moderate at 0.35 (SMD) without significant between-study heterogeneity. However, there was no difference in IL-6 levels between those who later became psychotic and those who did not (3 studies). In contrast IL1-B levels (2 studies) were reduced in the CHR group with a large negative effect size of 0.66 vs. controls. These differences were not influenced by age, sex or BMI in a meta-regression. Since IL-1β is seen as a driver of inflammation and other cytokines did not change, it is difficult to see the significance of the finding.

The North American Prodrome Longitudinal Study (NAPLS) recruits to a cohort of people with CHR-P aiming to discover a predictive profile of conversion based on a broad range of assessments. They measured 117 analytes in a multiplex assay to assess inflammation, oxidative stress, hormones and metabolism. They identified 15 predictors including IL-1β, IL-7, IL-8 and Matrix Metalloproteinase-8 (MMP-8) in 32 converters at 2 years, 35 controls and 40 non-converters (Perkins et al. 2015). CHR-P cohort studies such as NAPLS and PRONIA are developing multimodal risk calculators, which include inflammatory predictors, with clinically useful accuracy to guide interventions and to identify new treatment mechanisms (Kambeitz-Ilankovic et al. 2022). In summary, there is evidence for raised IL-6 in CHR, but only the NAPLS preliminary data suggest baseline increases may predict transition.

So far, we have concluded that cognitive impairment occurs in the CHR-P and predicts transition to psychosis. Similarly GM loss, which is a possible surrogate for cognitive impairment, is also reduced in CHR-P and declines in those who transition to psychosis. In this section, a limited literature suggests IL-6 is also increased in CHR-P but does not predict transition. Cognitive impairment, brain and cytokine changes appear to begin well before the CHR-P period. In the next section we discuss whether cytokines correlate with neuropsychological impairment or GM loss in the CHR transition.

3.2 *Inflammatory Profiles and Grey Matter and Cognitive Performance*

In one of the longitudinal GM studies included in the Merritt review, Cannon and colleagues found steeper rates of GM thinning in the right superior middle and orbital frontal cortical cortex in the transition group of 35 compared to 239 non-converters and 135 controls (Cannon et al. 2015). The rates of decline in 14 converters were predicted by a baseline summed index of pro-inflammatory cytokines (TNF-α, IFN-γ and IL-2) selected for their association with the inflamed microglial phenotype. The correlation in the non-converters was also significant but less marked. The results suggest an acute decline in GM thickness takes place over an average 10 months to onset possibly driven by inflammatory cytokines. It is not clear whether such a decline would initiate a corresponding decline in cognitive function – longitudinal studies are needed to establish this link. It seems unlikely that the inflammatory state of microglia would be determined by peripherally circulating cytokines. The results of further longitudinal studies from current CHR-P cohorts are eagerly awaited.

It is a popular and plausible idea that neuroinflammation as measured by cytokines would impact and correlate with cognitive impairment in people with schizophrenia and indeed with bipolar disorder and depression. However, the idea appears to be false. A remarkable meta-analysis covering 75 studies in all 3 disorders, 27 in schizophrenia, on global cognition and sub-domains, reports exceedingly small effect sizes (all <0.14) for correlations with every conceivable cytokine or other peripheral biomarker of inflammation (Morrens et al. 2022). This revelation makes it difficult to imagine there might be significant correlations between cytokine and cognition in CHR-P. This meta-analysis calls into question whether neuroinflammation causes cognitive impairment, whether peripheral cytokine levels are valid indicators of neuroinflammation and indeed whether neuroinflammation is a core process in schizophrenia. These considerations do not exclude the possibility that transdiagnostic increases in, for example, IL-6 (genetic or environmental) could evoke transdiagnostic symptoms such as anhedonia and social withdrawal via direct neuronal effects without causing neuroinflammation.

4 Rethinking Immunity and Cognition: A Paradigm Shift

The major difficulty for the inflamed brain hypothesis is the absence of a hallmark neuropathology of schizophrenia (Corsi-Zuelli and Deakin 2021). There is no gross microglial activation, astrogliosis, cellular debris, scarring or atrophy. The major practical difficulty is the absence, for obvious reasons, of direct measures of neuroinflammation in living humans. PET radioligand binding to protein markers of glial activation status is a way forward (Conen et al. 2021). Inflamed microglia express increased levels of translocator protein (TSPO). Radioligand TSPO binding studies, far from finding increases in schizophrenia, report an overall reduction across seven studies and one with cytokine data found no correlation (Meyer et al. 2020). The inference that microglia are not inflamed in schizophrenia is borne out by large-scale transcriptomic studies in post-mortem brain consortia which also report no change or reduction in microglial gene expression. The absence of microglial inflammation may explain why the anti-microglial and anti-inflammatory antibiotic,

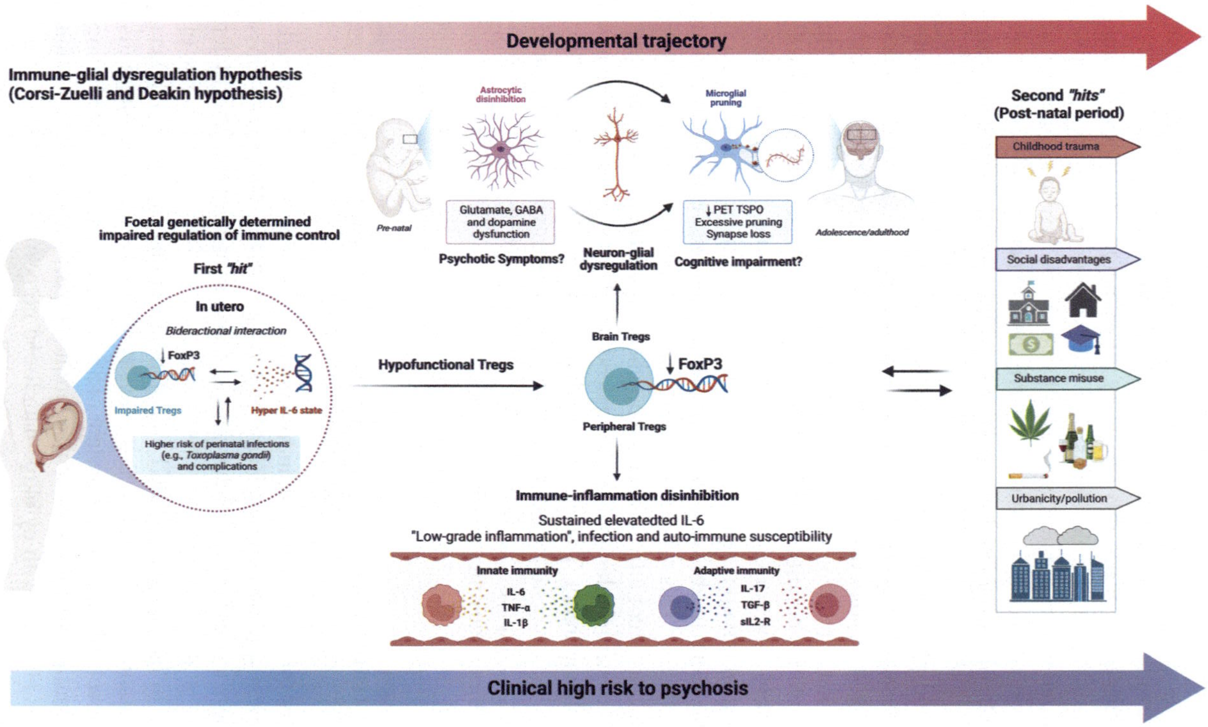

Fig. 2 Immune-glial dysregulation hypothesis (Corsi-Zuelli et al. 2021). Left to right. Hypofunctional Tregs in foetus due to schizophrenia risk genes that reduce expression of FoxP3 (key to Treg functioning) and increase IL-6 exposure, aggravated by predisposition to perinatal infection and complications. Bottom: Impaired Tregs fail to control immune responses resulting in tendency to co-morbid medical autoimmunity. Top: Tregs fail to control astrocytic development and action which drives microglia into non-inflamed developmental pruning mode that slows cognitive development. Astrocytes modify dopamine and cortical neurotransmission. Right: Environmental stressors and risk factors further destabilise Treg control of immunity and glial function. NB: The changes depicted were completely reproduced in adult rodents exposed in utero to maternal response to toxoplasma antigens. The behavioural and CNS changes were reversed by infusions of Tregs in adulthood (https://doi.org/10.1038/s41593-021-00837-1)

minocycline, had no benefit in large trials in recent onset and established schizophrenia (Deakin et al. 2018).

Reduced markers of inflammation suggest microglia are shifted to their non-inflamed synaptic pruning or housekeeping state as has been demonstrated in vitro with human stem-cell derived microglia from patients and controls (Sellgren et al. 2019). Excessive pruning would account for the loss of neuropil increasingly recognised as the mechanism of grey matter loss in schizophrenia and quite possibly the developmental neurocognitive lag in schizophrenia as discussed in previous sections (Onwordi et al. 2020; Osimo et al. 2019). Astroglial cells surround and support neurons and maintain microglia in a non-inflamed state. Transcriptomic studies suggest astroglia are overactive or more numerous and this may be driving microglia into their pruning phenotype.

It is increasingly understood that both peripheral immune responses and brain glial function are regulated by specialised regulatory T cells (Tregs), Fig. 2 (Corsi-Zuelli and Deakin 2021). Hypoactive Tregs result in systemic immune disinhibition in autoimmune disease and new restorative Treg therapies are rapidly developing. A subset of Tregs residing in healthy brain parenchyma has recently been described where they regulate astroglial–microglial interaction (Pasciuto et al. 2020). Hypoactive Tregs in schizophrenia would provide a unifying account that in schizophrenia, (1) systemic immune activation is a consequence of disinhibition and results in susceptibility to autoimmune disease including atherosclerosis and diabetes, and (2) disinhibition of glial interactions results in excessive microglial synapse elimination, loss of neuropil and cognitive impairment, the subject of this article. There are a number of therapies that directly or indirectly promote Treg function (Corsi-Zuelli and Deakin 2021) but effectiveness in cognition would likely require early preventative treatment although it is possible that synaptic regrowth and drugs which enhance plasticity could restore some function.

Acknowledgments The graphics in this chapter were created in BioRender.com.

References

Addington J, Liu L, Perkins DO, Carrion RE, Keefe RS, Woods SW (2017) The role of cognition and social functioning as predictors in the transition to psychosis for youth with attenuated psychotic symptoms. Schizophr Bull 43(1):57–63. https://doi.org/10.1093/schbul/sbw152

Baumeister D, Akhtar R, Ciufolini S, Pariante CM, Mondelli V (2016) Childhood trauma and adulthood inflammation: a meta-analysis of peripheral C-reactive protein, interleukin-6 and tumour necrosis factor-α. Mol Psychiatry 21(5):642–649. https://doi.org/10.1038/mp.2015.67

Bora E, Lin A, Wood SJ, Yung AR, McGorry PD, Pantelis C (2014) Cognitive deficits in youth with familial and clinical high risk to psychosis: a systematic review and meta-analysis. Acta Psychiatr Scand 130(1):1–15. https://doi.org/10.1111/acps.12261

Cannon M, Clarke MC, Cotter DR (2014) Priming the brain for psychosis: maternal inflammation during fetal development and the risk of later psychiatric disorder. Am J Psychiatry 171(9): 901–905. https://doi.org/10.1176/appi.ajp.2014.14060749

Cannon TD, Chung Y, He G, Sun D, Jacobson A, van Erp TG, McEwen S, Addington J, Bearden CE, Cadenhead K, Cornblatt B, Mathalon DH, McGlashan T, Perkins D, Jeffries C, Seidman LJ, Tsuang M, Walker E, Woods SW, Heinssen R (2015) Progressive reduction in cortical thickness as psychosis develops: a multisite longitudinal neuroimaging study of youth at elevated clinical risk. Biol Psychiatry 77(2):147–157. https://doi.org/10.1016/j.biopsych.2014.05.023

Capuzzi E, Bartoli F, Crocamo C, Clerici M, Carrà G (2017) Acute variations of cytokine levels after antipsychotic treatment in drug-naïve subjects with a first-episode psychosis: a meta-analysis. Neurosci Biobehav Rev 77:122–128. https://doi.org/10.1016/j.neubiorev.2017.03.003

Carrión RE, Walder DJ, Auther AM, McLaughlin D, Zyla HO, Adelsheim S, Calkins R, Carter CS, McFarland B, Melton R, Niendam T, Ragland JD, Sale TG, Taylor SF, McFarlane WR, Cornblatt BA (2018) From the psychosis prodrome to the first-episode of psychosis: no evidence of a cognitive decline. J Psychiatr Res 96:231–238. https://doi.org/10.1016/j.jpsychires.2017.10.014

Catalan A, Salazar de Pablo G, Aymerich C, Damiani S, Sordi V, Radua J, Oliver D, McGuire P, Giuliano AJ, Stone WS, Fusar-Poli P (2021) Neurocognitive functioning in individuals at clinical high risk for psychosis: a systematic review and meta-analysis. JAMA Psychiat. https://doi.org/10.1001/jamapsychiatry.2021.1290

Clarke MC, Tanskanen A, Huttunen M, Whittaker JC, Cannon M (2009) Evidence for an interaction between familial liability and prenatal exposure to infection in the causation of schizophrenia. Am J Psychiatry 166(9):1025–1030. https://doi.org/10.1176/appi.ajp.2009.08010031

Comer AL, Carrier M, Tremblay M-È, Cruz-Martín A (2020) The inflamed brain in schizophrenia: the convergence of genetic and environmental risk factors that lead to uncontrolled Neuroinflammation. Front Cell Neurosci 14. https://doi.org/10.3389/fncel.2020.00274

Conen S, Gregory CJ, Hinz R, Smallman R, Corsi-Zuelli F, Deakin B, Talbot PS (2021) Neuroinflammation as measured by positron emission tomography in patients with recent onset and established schizophrenia: implications for immune pathogenesis. Mol Psychiatry 26(9):5398–5406. https://doi.org/10.1038/s41380-020-0829-y

Corley E, Holleran L, Fahey L, Corvin A, Morris DW, Donohoe G (2021) Microglial-expressed genetic risk variants, cognitive function and brain volume in patients with schizophrenia and healthy controls. Transl Psychiatry 11(1):490. https://doi.org/10.1038/s41398-021-01616-z

Corsi-Zuelli F, Deakin B (2021) Impaired regulatory T cell control of astroglial overdrive and microglial pruning in schizophrenia. Neurosci Biobehav Rev 125:637–653. https://doi.org/10.1016/j.neubiorev.2021.03.004

Corsi-Zuelli F, Loureiro CM, Shuhama R, Fachim HA, Menezes PR, Louzada-Junior P, Mondelli V, Del-Ben CM (2020) Cytokine profile in first-episode psychosis, unaffected siblings and community-based controls: the effects of familial liability and childhood maltreatment. Psychol Med 50(7):1139–1147. https://doi.org/10.1017/s0033291719001016

Corsi-Zuelli F, Deakin B, de Lima MHF, Qureshi O, Barnes NM, Upthegrove R, Louzada-Junior P, Del-Ben CM (2021) T regulatory cells as a potential therapeutic target in psychosis? Current challenges and future perspectives. Brain Behav Immun Health 17:100330. https://doi.org/10.1016/j.bbih.2021.100330

Davies C, Segre G, Estradé A, Radua J, De Micheli A, Provenzani U, Oliver D, Salazar de Pablo G, Ramella-Cravaro V, Besozzi M, Dazzan P, Miele M, Caputo G, Spallarossa C, Crossland G, Ilyas A, Spada G, Politi P, Murray RM, McGuire P, Fusar-Poli P (2020) Prenatal and perinatal risk and protective factors for psychosis: a systematic review and meta-analysis. Lancet Psychiatry 7(5):399–410. https://doi.org/10.1016/s2215-0366(20)30057-2

Deakin B, Suckling J, Barnes TRE, Byrne K, Chaudhry IB, Dazzan P, Drake RJ, Giordano A, Husain N, Jones PB, Joyce E, Knox E, Krynicki C, Lawrie SM, Lewis S, Lisiecka-Ford DM, Nikkheslat N, Pariante CM, Smallman R, Watson A, Williams SCR, Upthegrove R, Dunn G (2018) The benefit of minocycline on negative symptoms of schizophrenia in patients with recent-onset psychosis (BeneMin): a randomised, double-blind, placebo-controlled trial. Lancet Psychiatry 5(11):885–894. https://doi.org/10.1016/S2215-0366(18)30345-6

Dunleavy C, Elsworthy RJ, Upthegrove R, Wood SJ, Aldred S (2022) Inflammation in first-episode psychosis: the contribution of inflammatory biomarkers to the emergence of negative symptoms, a systematic review and meta-analysis. Acta Psychiatr Scand. https://doi.org/10.1111/acps.13416

Ermakov EA, Melamud MM, Buneva VN, Ivanova SA (2022) Immune system abnormalities in schizophrenia: an integrative view and translational perspectives. Front Psych 13:880568. https://doi.org/10.3389/fpsyt.2022.880568

Fillman SG, Weickert TW, Lenroot RK, Catts SV, Bruggemann JM, Catts VS, Weickert CS (2016) Elevated peripheral cytokines characterize a subgroup of people with schizophrenia displaying poor verbal fluency and reduced Broca's area volume. Mol Psychiatry 21(8):1090–1098. https://doi.org/10.1038/mp.2015.90

Föcking M, Dicker P, Lopez LM, Cannon M, Schäfer MR, McGorry PD, Smesny S, Cotter DR, Amminger GP (2016) Differential expression of the inflammation marker IL12p40 in the at-risk mental state for psychosis: a predictor of transition to psychotic disorder? BMC Psychiatry 16(1):326. https://doi.org/10.1186/s12888-016-1039-7

Fusar-Poli P, Bonoldi I, Yung AR, Borgwardt S, Kempton MJ, Valmaggia L, Barale F, Caverzasi E, McGuire P (2012) Predicting psychosis: meta-analysis of transition outcomes in individuals at high clinical risk. Arch Gen Psychiatry 69(3):220–229. https://doi.org/10.1001/archgenpsychiatry.2011.1472

Fusar-Poli P, Salazar de Pablo G, Correll CU, Meyer-Lindenberg A, Millan MJ, Borgwardt S, Galderisi S, Bechdolf A, Pfennig A, Kessing LV, van Amelsvoort T, Nieman DH, Domschke K, Krebs M-O, Koutsouleris N, McGuire P, Do KQ, Arango C (2020) Prevention of psychosis: advances in detection, prognosis, and intervention. JAMA Psychiat 77(7):755–765. https://doi.org/10.1001/jamapsychiatry.2019.4779

Giovanoli S, Engler H, Engler A, Richetto J, Voget M, Willi R, Winter C, Riva MA, Mortensen PB, Feldon J, Schedlowski M, Meyer U (2013) Stress in puberty unmasks latent neuropathological consequences of prenatal immune activation in mice. Science 339(6123):1095–1099. https://doi.org/10.1126/science.1228261

Goldsmith DR, Rapaport MH, Miller BJ (2016) A meta-analysis of blood cytokine network alterations in psychiatric patients: comparisons between schizophrenia, bipolar disorder and depression. Mol Psychiatry 21(12):1696–1709. https://doi.org/10.1038/mp.2016.3

Green MF (1996) What are the functional consequences of neurocognitive deficits in schizophrenia? Am J Psychiatry

Green MF, Kern RS, Braff DL, Mintz J (2000) Neurocognitive deficits and functional outcome in schizophrenia: are we measuring the "Right Stuff"? Schizophr Bull 26(1):119–136. https://doi.org/10.1093/oxfordjournals.schbul.a033430

Green MF, Kern RS, Heaton RK (2004) Longitudinal studies of cognition and functional outcome in schizophrenia: implications for MATRICS. Schizophr Res 72(1):41–51. https://doi.org/10.1016/j.schres.2004.09.009

Green MF, Penn DL, Bentall R, Carpenter WT, Gaebel W, Gur RC, Kring AM, Park S, Silverstein SM, Heinssen R (2008) Social cognition in schizophrenia: an NIMH workshop on definitions, assessment, and research opportunities. Schizophr Bull 34(6):1211–1220. https://doi.org/10.1093/schbul/sbm145

Haining K, Gajwani R, Gross J, Gumley AI, Ince RAA, Lawrie SM, Schultze-Lutter F, Schwannauer M, Uhlhaas PJ (2022) Characterising cognitive heterogeneity in individuals at clinical high-risk for psychosis: a cluster analysis with clinical and functional outcome prediction. Eur Arch Psychiatry Clin Neurosci 272(3):437–448. https://doi.org/10.1007/s00406-021-01315-2

Jalbrzikowski M, Hayes RA, Wood SJ, Nordholm D, Zhou JH, Fusar-Poli P, Uhlhaas PJ, Takahashi T, Sugranyes G, Kwak YB, Mathalon DH, Katagiri N, Hooker CI, Smigielski L, Colibazzi T, Via E, Tang J, Koike S, Rasser PE, Michel C, Lebedeva I, Hegelstad WTV, de la Fuente-Sandoval C, Waltz JA, Mizrahi R, Corcoran CM, Resch F, Tamnes CK, Haas SS, Lemmers-Jansen ILJ, Agartz I, Allen P, Amminger GP, Andreassen OA, Atkinson K,

Bachman P, Baeza I, Baldwin H, Bartholomeusz CF, Borgwardt S, Catalano S, Chee MWL, Chen X, Cho KIK, Cooper RE, Cropley VL, Dolz M, Ebdrup BH, Fortea A, Glenthøj LB, Glenthøj BY, de Haan L, Hamilton HK, Harris MA, Haut KM, He Y, Heekeren K, Heinz A, Hubl D, Hwang WJ, Kaess M, Kasai K, Kim M, Kindler J, Klaunig MJ, Koppel A, Kristensen TD, Kwon JS, Lawrie SM, Lee J, León-Ortiz P, Lin A, Loewy RL, Ma X, McGorry P, McGuire P, Mizuno M, Møller P, Moncada-Habib T, Muñoz-Samons D, Nelson B, Nemoto T, Nordentoft M, Omelchenko MA, Oppedal K, Ouyang L, Pantelis C, Pariente JC, Raghava JM, Reyes-Madrigal F, Roach BJ, Røssberg JI, Rössler W, Salisbury DF, Sasabayashi D, Schall U, Schiffman J, Schlagenhauf F, Schmidt A, Sørensen ME, Suzuki M, Theodoridou A, Tomyshev AS, Tor J, Værnes TG, Velakoulis D, Venegoni GD, Vinogradov S, Wenneberg C, Westlye LT, Yamasue H, Yuan L, Yung AR, van Amelsvoort T, Turner JA, van Erp TGM, Thompson PM, Hernaus D (2021) Association of structural magnetic resonance imaging measures with psychosis onset in individuals at clinical high risk for developing psychosis: an ENIGMA working group mega-analysis. JAMA Psychiat 78(7):753–766. https://doi.org/10.1001/jamapsychiatry.2021.0638

Kambeitz-Ilankovic L, Koutsouleris N, Upthegrove R (2022) The potential of precision psychiatry: what is in reach? Br J Psychiatry 220(4):175–178. https://doi.org/10.1192/bjp.2022.23

Kerr DM, McDonald J, Minnis H (2021) The association of child maltreatment and systemic inflammation in adulthood: a systematic review. PLoS One 16(4):e0243685. https://doi.org/10.1371/journal.pone.0243685

Khandaker GM, Dantzer R (2016) Is there a role for immune-to-brain communication in schizophrenia? Psychopharmacology (Berl) 233(9):1559–1573. https://doi.org/10.1007/s00213-015-3975-1

Khandaker GM, Barnett JH, White IR, Jones PB (2011) A quantitative meta-analysis of population-based studies of premorbid intelligence and schizophrenia. Schizophr Res 132(2):220–227. https://doi.org/10.1016/j.schres.2011.06.017

Khandaker GM, Cousins L, Deakin J, Lennox BR, Yolken R, Jones PB (2015) Inflammation and immunity in schizophrenia: implications for pathophysiology and treatment. Lancet Psychiatry 2(3):258–270. https://doi.org/10.1016/s2215-0366(14)00122-9

Kim H, Shin N, Jang J, Kim E, Shim G, Park H, Hong K, Kwon JS (2011) Social cognition and neurocognition as predictors of conversion to psychosis in individuals at ultra-high risk. Schizophr Res 130:170–175. https://doi.org/10.1016/j.schres.2011.04.023

Kim M, Haney JR, Zhang P, Hernandez LM, Wang L-K, Perez-Cano L, Loohuis LMO, de la Torre-Ubieta L, Gandal MJ (2021) Brain gene co-expression networks link complement signaling with convergent synaptic pathology in schizophrenia. Nat Neurosci 24(6):799–809. https://doi.org/10.1038/s41593-021-00847-z

Kogan S, Ospina LH, Mittal VA, Kimhy D (2020) The impact of inflammation on neurocognition and risk for psychosis: a critical review. Eur Arch Psychiatry Clin Neurosci 270:793–802. https://doi.org/10.1007/s00406-019-01073-2

Lawrie SM, Whalley H, Kestelman JN, Abukmeil SS, Byrne M, Hodges A, Rimmington JE, Best JJ, Owens DG, Johnstone EC (1999) Magnetic resonance imaging of brain in people at high risk of developing schizophrenia. Lancet 353(9146):30–33

Merritt K, Luque Laguna P, Irfan A, David AS (2021) Longitudinal structural MRI findings in individuals at genetic and clinical high risk for psychosis: a systematic review. Front Psych 12. https://doi.org/10.3389/fpsyt.2021.620401

Metcalf SA, Jones PB, Nordstrom T, Timonen M, Mäki P, Miettunen J, Jääskeläinen E, Järvelin M-R, Stochl J, Murray GK, Veijola J, Khandaker GM (2017) Serum C-reactive protein in adolescence and risk of schizophrenia in adulthood: a prospective birth cohort study. Brain Behav Immun 59:253–259. https://doi.org/10.1016/j.bbi.2016.09.008

Meyer JH, Cervenka S, Kim M-J, Kreisl WC, Henter ID, Innis RB (2020) Neuroinflammation in psychiatric disorders: PET imaging and promising new targets. Lancet Psychiatry 7(12): 1064–1074. https://doi.org/10.1016/S2215-0366(20)30255-8

Miller BJ, Buckley P, Seabolt W, Mellor A, Kirkpatrick B (2011) Meta-analysis of cytokine alterations in schizophrenia: clinical status and antipsychotic effects. Biol Psychiatry 70(7): 663–671. https://doi.org/10.1016/j.biopsych.2011.04.013

Millett CE, Perez-Rodriguez M, Shanahan M, Larsen E, Yamamoto HS, Bukowski C, Fichorova R, Burdick KE (2021) C-reactive protein is associated with cognitive performance in a large cohort of euthymic patients with bipolar disorder. Mol Psychiatry 26(8):4096–4105. https://doi.org/10.1038/s41380-019-0591-1

Momtazmanesh S, Zare-Shahabadi A, Rezaei N (2019) Cytokine alterations in schizophrenia: an updated review. Front Psych 10. https://doi.org/10.3389/fpsyt.2019.00892

Monji A, Kato T, Kanba S (2009) Cytokines and schizophrenia: microglia hypothesis of schizophrenia. Psychiatry Clin Neurosci 63(3):257–265. https://doi.org/10.1111/j.1440-1819.2009.01945.x

Morrens M, Overloop C, Coppens V, Loots E, Van Den Noortgate M, Vandenameele S, Leboyer M, De Picker L (2022) The relationship between immune and cognitive dysfunction in mood and psychotic disorder: a systematic review and a meta-analysis. Mol Psychiatry. https://doi.org/10.1038/s41380-022-01582-y

Ntouros E, Karanikas E, Floros G, Andreou C, Tsoura A, Garyfallos G, Bozikas VP (2018) Social cognition in the course of psychosis and its correlation with biomarkers in a male cohort. Cogn Neuropsychiatry 23(2):103–115. https://doi.org/10.1080/13546805.2018.1440201

Nuechterlein KPD, Green MFPD, Kern RS, Baade LE, Barch DM, Cohen JD, Essock S, Fenton WS, Frese FJ, Gold JM, Goldberg T, Heaton RK, Keefe RSE, Kraemer H, Mesholam-Gately R, Seidman LJ, Stover E, Weinberger DR, Young AS, Zalcman S, Marder SR (2008) The MATRICS consensus cognitive battery, part 1: test selection, reliability, and validity. Am J Psychiatry 165(2):203–213. https://doi.org/10.1176/appi.ajp.2007.07010042

Onwordi EC, Halff EF, Whitehurst T, Mansur A, Cotel MC, Wells L, Creeney H, Bonsall D, Rogdaki M, Shatalina E, Reis Marques T, Rabiner EA, Gunn RN, Natesan S, Vernon AC, Howes OD (2020) Synaptic density marker SV2A is reduced in schizophrenia patients and unaffected by antipsychotics in rats. Nat Commun 11(1):246. https://doi.org/10.1038/s41467-019-14122-0

Osimo EF, Beck K, Reis Marques T, Howes OD (2019) Synaptic loss in schizophrenia: a meta-analysis and systematic review of synaptic protein and mRNA measures. Mol Psychiatry 24(4): 549–561. https://doi.org/10.1038/s41380-018-0041-5

Pantelis C, Velakoulis D, McGorry PD, Wood SJ, Suckling J, Phillips LJ, Yung AR, Bullmore ET, Brewer W, Soulsby B, Desmond P, McGuire PK (2003) Neuroanatomical abnormalities before and after onset of psychosis: a cross-sectional and longitudinal MRI comparison. Lancet 361(9354):281–288. https://doi.org/10.1016/S0140-6736(03)12323-9

Park S, Miller BJ (2020) Meta-analysis of cytokine and C-reactive protein levels in high-risk psychosis. Schizophr Res 226:5–12. https://doi.org/10.1016/j.schres.2019.03.012

Pasciuto E, Burton OT, Roca CP, Lagou V, Rajan WD, Theys T, Mancuso R, Tito RY, Kouser L, Callaerts-Vegh Z, de la Fuente AG, Prezzemolo T, Mascali LG, Brajic A, Whyte CE, Yshii L, Martinez-Muriana A, Naughton M, Young A, Moudra A, Lemaitre P, Poovathingal S, Raes J, De Strooper B, Fitzgerald DC, Dooley J, Liston A (2020) Microglia require CD4T cells to complete the fetal-to-adult transition. Cell 182(3):625–640.e624. https://doi.org/10.1016/j.cell.2020.06.026

Perkins DO, Jeffries CD, Addington J, Bearden CE, Cadenhead KS, Cannon TD, Cornblatt BA, Mathalon DH, McGlashan TH, Seidman LJ, Tsuang MT, Walker EF, Woods SW, Heinssen R (2015) Towards a psychosis risk blood diagnostic for persons experiencing high-risk symptoms: preliminary results from the NAPLS project. Schizophr Bull 41(2):419–428. https://doi.org/10.1093/schbul/sbu099

Perkins DO, Jeffries CD, Do KQ (2020) Potential roles of redox dysregulation in the development of schizophrenia. Biol Psychiatry 88(4):326–336. https://doi.org/10.1016/j.biopsych.2020.03.016

Perry BI, Upthegrove R, Kappelmann N, Jones PB, Burgess S, Khandaker GM (2021) Associations of immunological proteins/traits with schizophrenia, major depression and bipolar disorder: a bi-directional two-sample mendelian randomization study. Brain Behav Immun 97:176–185. https://doi.org/10.1016/j.bbi.2021.07.009

Pillinger T, Osimo EF, Brugger S, Mondelli V, McCutcheon RA, Howes OD (2018) A meta-analysis of immune parameters, variability, and assessment of modal distribution in psychosis and test of the immune subgroup hypothesis. Schizophr Bull 45(5):1120–1133. https://doi.org/10.1093/schbul/sby160

Potvin S, Stip E, Sepehry AA, Gendron A, Bah R, Kouassi E (2008) Inflammatory cytokine alterations in schizophrenia: a systematic quantitative review. Biol Psychiatry 63(8):801–808. https://doi.org/10.1016/j.biopsych.2007.09.024

Richards AL, Pardiñas AF, Frizzati A, Tansey KE, Lynham AJ, Holmans P, Legge SE, Savage JE, Agartz I, Andreassen OA, Blokland GAM, Corvin A, Cosgrove D, Degenhardt F, Djurovic S, Espeseth T, Ferraro L, Gayer-Anderson C, Giegling I, van Haren NE, Hartmann AM, Hubert JJ, Jönsson EG, Konte B, Lennertz L, Olde Loohuis LM, Melle I, Morgan C, Morris DW, Murray RM, Nyman H, Ophoff RA, Investigators G, van Os J, EUGEI WP2 Group, Schizophrenia Working Group of the Psychiatric Genomics Consortium, Petryshen TL, Quattrone D, Rietschel M, Rujescu D, Rutten BPF, Streit F, Strohmaier J, Sullivan PF, Sundet K, Wagner M, Escott-Price V, Owen MJ, Donohoe G, O'Donovan MC, Walters JTR (2020) The relationship between polygenic risk scores and cognition in schizophrenia. Schizophr Bull 46(2):336–344. https://doi.org/10.1093/schbul/sbz061

Riecher-Rössler A, Pflueger MO, Aston J, Borgwardt SJ, Brewer WJ, Gschwandtner U, Stieglitz R-D (2009) Efficacy of using cognitive status in predicting psychosis: a 7-year follow-up. Biol Psychiatry 66(11):1023–1030. https://doi.org/10.1016/j.biopsych.2009.07.020

Rudolph MD, Graham AM, Feczko E, Miranda-Dominguez O, Rasmussen JM, Nardos R, Entringer S, Wadhwa PD, Buss C, Fair DA (2018) Maternal IL-6 during pregnancy can be estimated from newborn brain connectivity and predicts future working memory in offspring. Nat Neurosci 21(5):765–772. https://doi.org/10.1038/s41593-018-0128-y

Seidman LJ, Shapiro DI, Stone WS, Woodberry KA, Ronzio A, Cornblatt BA, Addington J, Bearden CE, Cadenhead KS, Cannon TD, Mathalon DH, McGlashan TH, Perkins DO, Tsuang MT, Walker EF, Woods SW (2016) Association of neurocognition with transition to psychosis: baseline functioning in the second phase of the North American Prodrome Longitudinal Study. JAMA Psychiat 73(12):1239–1248. https://doi.org/10.1001/jamapsychiatry.2016.2479

Sellgren CM, Gracias J, Watmuff B, Biag JD, Thanos JM, Whittredge PB, Fu T, Worringer K, Brown HE, Wang J, Kaykas A, Karmacharya R, Goold CP, Sheridan SD, Perlis RH (2019) Increased synapse elimination by microglia in schizophrenia patient-derived models of synaptic pruning. Nat Neurosci 22(3):374–385. https://doi.org/10.1038/s41593-018-0334-7

Thompson A, Papas A, Bartholomeusz C, Allott K, Amminger GP, Nelson B, Wood S, Yung A (2012) Social cognition in clinical "at risk" for psychosis and first episode psychosis populations. Schizophr Res 141(2):204–209. https://doi.org/10.1016/j.schres.2012.08.007

Trubetskoy V, Pardiñas AF, Qi T, Panagiotaropoulou G, Awasthi S, Bigdeli TB, Bryois J, Chen C-Y, Dennison CA, Hall LS, Lam M, Watanabe K, Frei O, Ge T, Harwood JC, Koopmans F, Magnusson S, Richards AL, Sidorenko J, Wu Y, Zeng J, Grove J, Kim M, Li Z, Voloudakis G, Zhang W, Adams M, Agartz I, Atkinson EG, Agerbo E, Al Eissa M, Albus M, Alexander M, Alizadeh BZ, Alptekin K, Als TD, Amin F, Arolt V, Arrojo M, Athanasiu L, Azevedo MH, Bacanu SA, Bass NJ, Begemann M, Belliveau RA, Bene J, Benyamin B, Bergen SE, Blasi G, Bobes J, Bonassi S, Braun A, Bressan RA, Bromet EJ, Bruggeman R, Buckley PF, Buckner RL, Bybjerg-Grauholm J, Cahn W, Cairns MJ, Calkins ME, Carr VJ, Castle D, Catts SV, Chambert KD, Chan RCK, Chaumette B, Cheng W, Cheung EFC, Chong SA, Cohen D, Consoli A, Cordeiro Q, Costas J, Curtis C, Davidson M, Davis KL, de Haan L, Degenhardt F, DeLisi LE, Demontis D, Dickerson F, Dikeos D, Dinan T, Djurovic S, Duan J, Ducci G, Dudbridge F, Eriksson JG, Fañanás L, Faraone SV, Fiorentino A, Forstner A, Frank J, Freimer NB, Fromer M, Frustaci A, Gadelha A, Genovese G, Gershon ES, Giannitelli M, Giegling I, Giusti-Rodríguez P,

Godard S, Goldstein JI, González Peñas J, González-Pinto A, Gopal S, Gratten J, Green MF, Greenwood TA, Guillin O, Gülöksüz S, Gur RE, Gur RC, Gutiérrez B, Hahn E, Hakonarson H, Haroutunian V, Hartmann AM, Harvey C, Hayward C, Henskens FA, Herms S, Hoffmann P, Howrigan DP, Ikeda M, Iyegbe C, Joa I, Julià A, Kähler AK, Kam-Thong T, Kamatani Y, Karachanak-Yankova S, Kebir O, Keller MC, Kelly BJ, Khrunin A, Kim S-W, Klovins J, Kondratiev N, Konte B, Kraft J, Kubo M, Kučinskas V, Kučinskiene ZA, Kusumawardhani A, Kuzelova-Ptackova H, Landi S, Lazzeroni LC, Lee PH, Legge SE, Lehrer DS, Lencer R, Lerer B, Li M, Lieberman J, Light GA, Limborska S, Liu C-M, Lönnqvist J, Loughland CM, Lubinski J, Luykx JJ, Lynham A, Macek M, Mackinnon A, Magnusson PKE, Maher BS, Maier W, Malaspina D, Mallet J, Marder SR, Marsal S, Martin AR, Martorell L, Mattheisen M, McCarley RW, McDonald C, McGrath JJ, Medeiros H, Meier S, Melegh B, Melle I, Mesholam-Gately RI, Metspalu A, Michie PT, Milani L, Milanova V, Mitjans M, Molden E, Molina E, Molto MD, Mondelli V, Moreno C, Morley CP, Muntané G, Murphy KC, Myin-Germeys I, Nenadić I, Nestadt G, Nikitina-Zake L, Noto C, Nuechterlein KH, O'Brien NL, O'Neill FA, Oh S-Y, Olincy A, Ota VK, Pantelis C, Papadimitriou GN, Parellada M, Paunio T, Pellegrino R, Periyasamy S, Perkins DO, Pfuhlmann B, Pietiläinen O, Pimm J, Porteous D, Powell J, Quattrone D, Quested D, Radant AD, Rampino A, Rapaport MH, Rautanen A, Reichenberg A, Roe C, Roffman JL, Roth J, Rothermundt M, Rutten BPF, Saker-Delye S, Salomaa V, Sanjuan J, Santoro ML, Savitz A, Schall U, Scott RJ, Seidman LJ, Sharp SI, Shi J, Siever LJ, Sigurdsson E, Sim K, Skarabis N, Slominsky P, So H-C, Sobell JL, Söderman E, Stain HJ, Steen NE, Steixner-Kumar AA, Stögmann E, Stone WS, Straub RE, Streit F, Strengman E, Stroup TS, Subramaniam M, Sugar CA, Suvisaari J, Svrakic DM, Swerdlow NR, Szatkiewicz JP, Ta TMT, Takahashi A, Terao C, Thibaut F, Toncheva D, Tooney PA, Torretta S, Tosato S, Tura GB, Turetsky BI, Üçok A, Vaaler A, van Amelsvoort T, van Winkel R, Veijola J, Waddington J, Walter H, Waterreus A, Webb BT, Weiser M, Williams NM, Witt SH, Wormley BK, Wu JQ, Xu Z, Yolken R, Zai CC, Zhou W, Zhu F, Zimprich F, Atbaşoğlu EC, Ayub M, Benner C, Bertolino A (2022) Mapping genomic loci implicates genes and synaptic biology in schizophrenia. Nature 604(7906):502–508. https://doi.org/10.1038/s41586-022-04434-5

Upthegrove R, Manzanares-Teson N, Barnes NM (2014) Cytokine function in medication-naive first episode psychosis: a systematic review and meta-analysis. Schizophr Res 155(1):101–108. https://doi.org/10.1016/j.schres.2014.03.005

Velthorst E, Meyer EC, Giuliano AJ, Addington J, Cadenhead KS, Cannon TD, Cornblatt BA, McGlashan TH, Perkins DO, Tsuang MT (2019) Neurocognitive profiles in the prodrome to psychosis in NAPLS-1. Schizophr Res 204:311–319

Wang AK, Miller BJ (2018) Meta-analysis of cerebrospinal fluid cytokine and tryptophan catabolite alterations in psychiatric patients: comparisons between schizophrenia, bipolar disorder, and depression. Schizophr Bull 44(1):75–83. https://doi.org/10.1093/schbul/sbx035

Watson AJ, Harrison L, Preti A, Wykes T, Cella M (2022) Cognitive trajectories following onset of psychosis: a meta-analysis. Br J Psychiatry:1–8. https://doi.org/10.1192/bjp.2022.131

Williams JA, Burgess S, Suckling J, Lalousis PA, Batool F, Griffiths SL, Palmer E, Karwath A, Barsky A, Gkoutos GV, Wood S, Barnes NM, David AS, Donohoe G, Neill JC, Deakin B, Khandaker GM, Upthegrove R, Collaboration P (2022) Inflammation and brain structure in schizophrenia and other neuropsychiatric disorders: a Mendelian randomization study. JAMA Psychiat 79:498. https://doi.org/10.1001/jamapsychiatry.2022.0407

Yung AR, Pan Yuen H, Mcgorry PD, Phillips LJ, Kelly D, Dell'Olio M, Francey SM, Cosgrave EM, Killackey E (2005) Mapping the onset of psychosis: the comprehensive assessment of at-risk mental states. Aust N Z J Psychiatry 39(11–12):964–971

Yung AR, McGorry PD, Francey SM, Nelson B, Baker K, Phillips LJ, Berger G, Amminger GP (2007) PACE: a specialised service for young people at risk of psychotic disorders. Med J Aust 187(S7):S43–S46. https://doi.org/10.5694/j.1326-5377.2007.tb01336.x

Zhou X, Tian B, Han H-B (2021) Serum interleukin-6 in schizophrenia: a system review and meta-analysis. Cytokine 141:155441. https://doi.org/10.1016/j.cyto.2021.155441

The manufacturer's authorised representative in the EU is Springer Nature Customer Service Centre GmbH, Europaplatz 3, 69115 Heidelberg, Germany. If you have any concerns regarding our products, please contact ProductSafety@springernature.com

Printed and bound by CPI Group (UK) Ltd, Croydon, CR0 4YY
01/10/2026
02225851-0019